E. JAMES POTCHEN, M.D., *Consulting Editor*

Professor of Radiology
The Johns Hopkins University School of Medicine
Baltimore, Maryland; formerly Professor of Radiology
The Edward Mallinckrodt Institute of Radiology
Washington University School of Medicine
St. Louis, Missouri

Published

Forthcoming Monographs

Volume 4 in the Series
SAUNDERS
MONOGRAPHS
IN CLINICAL
RADIOLOGY

THE HAND
IN
RADIOLOGIC
DIAGNOSIS

ANDREW K. POZNANSKI, M.D.

Professor of Radiology, The University of Michigan; Co-Director of
Pediatric Radiology, C. S. Mott Children's Hospital,
The University of Michigan; Research Scientist,
Center for Human Growth and Development,
The University of Michigan, Ann Arbor, Michigan

W. B. SAUNDERS COMPANY • *Philadelphia* • *London* • *Toronto*

W. B. Saunders Company: West Washington Square
Philadelphia, Pa. 19105

12 Dyott Street
London, WC1A   1DB

833 Oxford Street
Toronto, Ontario M8Z 5T9, Canada

The Hand in Radiologic Diagnosis   ISBN 0-7216-7327-9

Print No.:   9   8   7   6   5   4   3   2

TO ELVA,
DIANA AND SUZANNE

CONTRIBUTORS

JOSEPH J. BOOKSTEIN, M.D.

Professor of Radiology, Chief of Cardiovascular Radiology,
University of Michigan Medical Center, Ann Arbor, Michigan

DEAN S. LOUIS, M.D.

Assistant Professor of Surgery—Orthopedics, Chief of Orthopedic
Hand Clinic, University of Michigan Medical Center, Ann Arbor,
Michigan; Chief of Orthopedics, Wayne County General Hospital,
Eloise, Michigan

ANDREW K. POZNANSKI, M.D.

Professor of Radiology, Co-Director of Pediatric Radiology,
C. S. Mott Children's Hospital, University of Michigan, Ann Arbor,
Michigan; Research Scientist, Center for Human Growth and
Development, University of Michigan, Ann Arbor, Michigan

TOM W. STAPLE, M.D.

Professor of Radiology, Mallinckrodt Institute of Radiology,
Washington University School of Medicine, St. Louis, Missouri

EDITOR'S FOREWORD

> If the hand be held between the discharge-tube and the [fluorescent] screen, the darker shadow of the bones is seen within the slightly dark shadow-image of the hand itself.... For brevity's sake I shall use the expression "rays" and to distinguish them from others of this name, I shall call them "x-rays."
>
> WILHELM CONRAD ROENTGEN, 1895

This historic incident was no accident, but rather presaged the hand as a model for radiographic studies of bones and soft tissue. Early studies devoted much of their attention to the diagnosis of infectious diseases and trauma. These studies were followed by the recognition that the hand x-rays provided important diagnostic information on systemic disease processes ranging from abnormal body growth to metabolic diseases of bone. More recently, there has been renewed emphasis on the use of the hand x-ray to classify genetic abnormalities. The remarkable recent growth of medical genetics as a discipline is largely related to a combination of a better understanding of molecular genetics and a greater precision in clinical classification. The ability to discern more subtle differences between people has been nowhere more apparent than in the improved classification made possible by recognizing many of these abnormalities on the hand x-ray.

Some years ago I was taken by an excellent review article written by Dr. McAfee and Dr. Donner entitled The Differential Diagnosis of Radiographic Changes of the Hand, in which is stated, "Like the funduscope examination of the eyes, the bones of the hand frequently serve as 'mirrors' of systemic disease." The recognition of this precept has led to the wider application of the hand x-ray in the diagnosis of disease. However, their admonition "that routine radiographs of the hand deserve a wider role in the diagnosis of systemic disease" still holds true. This monograph was therefore invoked in an effort to enhance an appreciation for the use of the hand x-ray in the management of patients with infectious, metabolic, occupational and congenital diseases. It is envisioned that a more comprehensive understanding of the subtle differences seen in hand x-rays may lead to a renewed interest in this important diagnostic modality, based on a sound appreciation of the current state of the art.

We are indeed fortunate that Dr. Poznanski has accepted this challenge and has produced a scholarly monograph in a lucid and erudite style that clearly portrays the radiology of the hand and all its implications. Dr. Poznanski, a native of Poland and a graduate of McGill University, studied radiology at the Henry Ford Hospital. For the past six years, he has been on the faculty of the University of Michigan Medical Center and is currently the Co-

Director of Pediatric Radiology at the C. F. Mott Children's Hospital. Although his interests have ranged widely through the technical and clinical aspects of pediatric radiology, he personally has been involved in clarifying our understanding of the skeletal manifestations of congenital disease. While many radiologists have come to appreciate his work on the thumb and carpals in congenital malformation syndromes, most are unaware of his contribution to the field of physical anthropology, best exemplified in a paper entitled Disharmonic Maturation of the Hand in Congenital Malformation Syndromes.

As the recognized authority on the hand x-ray, Dr. Poznanski has complemented his publication of some 80 research articles with an extensive interest in teaching radiology. His contribution not only to the development of new knowledge but to its dissemination is amply documented in this monograph. Dr. Poznanski's characteristic aura of excellence has resulted in a work that is a fitting sequel to the previous monographs in this series.

E. James Potchen, M.D.

PREFACE

For centuries the hand has been known as a mirror of disease. Similarly, the hand radiograph reflects a wide range of disease states. Although the hand responds to various disorders as does the remainder of the skeleton, many of the hand manifestations are unique, particularly in the congenital malformation syndromes. The goal in writing this book was to gather data about the various diseases as they affect the hand, so that the information would be readily available for reference.

After the discovery of the roentgen ray, the hand was the first portion of the body to be studied radiologically in a systematic fashion. This was partly because the hand is an accessible portion of the skeleton and has relatively little overlying soft tissue. Today the hand is still a diagnostically useful region. Because of the hand's thinness, films can be obtained without screens, allowing excellent visualization of fine trabecular structure. The hand is also remote enough from the body to be radiographed freely without significant bone marrow or gonadal dose.

There are four main sections of this book. The first (Chapters 1 through 5) deals with the normal hand, its development, skeletal maturation and measurement, and various special radiologic techniques.

The second section (Chapters 6 through 10) describes the normal variants and congenital anomalies of the hand. Although many of the congenital anomalies alone have no clinical significance, when they are associated with other congenital anomalies they may be diagnostic of certain congenital malformation syndromes. The aim of this section is to help the reader differentiate between the normal and the abnormal, and to determine whether a certain radiologic finding is isolated or whether it is related to a malformation syndrome. To attain this goal, tables are presented, listing other findings that are associated with the variants or anomalies discussed in the text. By referring to these tables, the physician should be able to identify the conditions in which a certain finding may occur.

The third section (Chapters 11 through 13) deals with congenital malformation syndromes. Chapter 13 is an alphabetical listing of a number of syndromes which have some roentgen manifestations in the hand. Each discussion includes a brief clinical description as well as a brief summary of other radiologic findings that may be helpful in diagnosis. The references have been kept to a minimum and should be used to obtain further information about these conditions.

The fourth section (Chapters 14 through 21) deals with the hand manifestations of acquired disorders. Sometimes the distinction between the acquired and the congenital is not clear. For example, several of the hematologic disorders are due to a congenital defect, as is the case for sickle cell anemia. They have nevertheless been included in the section on acquired disorders because the radiologic manifestations are mainly secondary to the hematologic disorder.

A large portion of this book is devoted to the study of normal variants and congenital disorders of the hand, in particular the child's hand. This partially reflects my own personal bias as a pediatric radiologist, and also the facts that more variations are possible in the child's hand and that the spectrum of abnormalities on the basis of congenital disorders is probably wider than that due to acquired conditions. Normal variations are also much more common in the pediatric patient. Differentiation between the various congenital malformation syndromes is often possible by means of the radiograph of the child's hand, whereas when maturation has taken place, such identification may be impossible.

ANDREW K. POZNANSKI, M.D.

ACKNOWLEDGMENTS

Many individuals have been of considerable help to me in the preparation of this book, and their efforts are deeply appreciated.

Four chapters were prepared for me by three friends and colleagues. They deal with subjects in which they have much expertise, and their efforts are greatly appreciated. Dr. Joseph Bookstein, Professor of Radiology at the University of Michigan, wrote the section on angiography of the hand. Dr. Dean Louis, Assistant Professor of Surgery at the University of Michigan, prepared the section on trauma to the hand. Dr. Tom Staple, Professor of Radiology at Washington University in St. Louis, Missouri, wrote the chapter on the arthritides.

Dr. John Holt, Professor of Radiology at the University of Michigan, has helped and encouraged me in the preparation of this book. He has had a great interest in the hand; in fact, in 1944 at the joint meeting of the American Roentgen Ray Society and Radiological Society of North America, he presented an exhibit entitled "The Bones of Hands as an Index of Local and Systemic Disease." Dr. Holt has over many years collected many excellent radiographs which he made freely available to me. He also made many helpful comments as the text was being written.

Dr. Stanley M. Garn, a Fellow of the Center of Human Growth and Development and Professor of Nutrition in the School of Public Health at the University of Michigan, has been a source of stimulation and information. Over the past five years we have collaborated in numerous research projects dealing with the hand. He has freely supplied me with radiographs showing normal variants, as well as much normative data which he has derived. Some of his published, and previously unpublished, data are included in this book. He also assisted greatly by critically reviewing the chapters on measurement and maturation.

A number of other physicians have been extremely helpful in reviewing the manuscript. Dr. Lawrence Kuhns, a new colleague in the Division of Pediatric Radiology, carefully read most of the chapters and made many useful comments. He also provided some translations from the German literature. A number of pediatricians lent their expertise in reviewing the chapters in their special areas of interest. Dr. Roy Schmickel reviewed the chapters on the chromosomal abnormalities and on the malformation syndromes; Dr. Joseph Baublis, the chapter on infectious disease; Dr. George Bacon, the discussion of endocrine disease; and Dr. Al Burdi, from the Anatomy Department of the University of Michigan, reviewed the section on embryology.

Dr. Aaron Stern, Dr. John Gall and Dr. Roy Schmickel, as well as many of the other staff and residents in pediatrics, radiology and orthopedics at the University of Michigan have been very helpful in finding me interesting and unusual cases.

Most of the illustrations used in this book came from the files of the University of Michigan, but a significant number of cases were from my alma mater, the Henry Ford Hospital in Detroit. Drs. William Reynolds and Max Clark from the Henry Ford Hospital, and Dr. William McAlister from Washington University, St. Louis, Missouri, were particularly cooperative in sending me many interesting films which added significantly to the scope of this book. Many other individuals have been kind enough to send me tabular and illustrative material. They include Drs. L. Ackerman, F. P. Agha, R. J. Allen, D. P. Babbitt, J. W. Barber, G. Baylin, M. H. Becker, W. E. Berdon, D. E. Boblitt, S. P. Bohrer, S. H. Boswell, J. W. Bowerman, C. Bream, W. R. Breg, H. H. Brueckner, A. Burdi, C. J. Campbell, M. P. Capp, J. Carr, W. P. Cockshott, D. P. Corbett, W. A. Crabbe, G. Currarino, M. K. Dalinka, J. E. Desautels, H. Dick, J. P. Dorst, D. Elzinga, C. D. Enna, W. Eyler, G. Fine, R. J. Fosmoe, B. Frame, K. Gefferth, A. Giedion, B. Gompels, R. J. Gorlin, J. L. Gwinn, R. Hall, R. C. Hildreth, E. Hooper, C. S. Houston, E. S. Huckins, B. S. Jones, R. C. Juberg, I. Krieger, K. Krufky, J. P. Kuhn, T. R. Lawrie, F. A. Lee, D. S. Louis, R. I. Macpherson, S. Markel, P. Maroteaux, W. Martel, V. McKusick, H. E. Meema, D. C. Moses, M. E. Mottram, R. J. Neviaser, M. B. Ozonoff, B. L. Pear, J. A. Pitcock, H. J. Pollock, R. V. Pozderac, R. Rapp, S. Reuter, W. Riggs, A. S. Romer, H. D. Rosenbaum, R. R. Schreiber, G. Shackelford, L. Shapiro, R. S. Sherman, F. N. Silverman, T. W. Staple, G. I. Sugarman, Y. Sugiura, D. Swindler, L. E. Swischuk, S. P. S. Teotia, M. Ting, D. Tinkle, J. M. Tishler, W. Walker, A. Weinstein, R. Weiss, W. J. Weston, A. A. White, III, D. Wilner, R. Carroll, R. D'Alonzo, and W. Glat.

The original research in this book was done mainly in conjunction with Dr. Stanley M. Garn and has been supported in part by two grants: (1) the James Picker Foundation on recommendation of the Committee on Radiology, National Academy of Sciences–National Research Council (Grant RG 72-10), and (2) National Institute of Child Health and Human Development (Grant HDO7134).

Mrs. Helen Harper was responsible for many of the bone length measurements and the pattern profile plots. She also assisted me in preparation of material for photography and library research. Her careful efforts are appreciated.

Dr. James Potchen, the Consulting Editor of the Saunders Monographs in Clinical Radiology, stimulated me to write this book. My thanks also go to Mr. Jack Hanley, Medical Editor of the W. B. Saunders Company, for his support during this work, and to Ms. Pamela Herr for her copy editorial work. Miss Marie Ayres and Mrs. Judy Davids typed and retyped the manuscript many times with great care. The Photography Department at the University of Michigan, under the direction of Mr. Edgar Sherman, was most helpful in producing the majority of the prints for this book.

A. K. P.

CONTENTS

Part I

THE NORMAL HAND AND TECHNIQUES OF ITS EVALUATION

Chapter 1

HISTORY, RADIOGRAPHIC ANATOMY, EMBRYOLOGY AND COMPARATIVE ANATOMY

The hand is one of the features that distinguish man from other animals. Man is the only animal which effectively uses the hand. As stated by Alpenfels,[1] "Man alone has a hand. He uses it as a tool, as a symbol, and as a weapon. A whole literature of legend, folklore, superstition and myth has been built around the human hand. As an organ of performance, it serves as eyes for the blind; the mute talk with it; and it has become a symbol of salutation, supplication and condemnation. The hand has played a part in the creative life of every known society and has come to be symbolic or representative of the whole person in art, in drama, and in dance." The right-handedness of most men has been given varying significance in different societies. For example, in some cultures the right hand is used for cooking and eating, while the left is used for bathing,

elimination and activities associated with sex.[1] The right and left hands have become symbolic of good and evil. The hand has been used to express feeling in various forms of art, ranging from the primitive to the present.[1, 5] Durer (1471–1528) devoted much of his life to the study of the hand, as evidenced in his paintings, and Rodin (1840–1917) used the expressiveness of the hand in many of his sculptures.

The derivation of the word "hand" has been used for many words of action,[1] including manipulate, mandate and dexterous (having two right hands). The term "right" or "true" arises from right-handedness, as does the French word *droit*, meaning right or law. Similarly, the word "left" symbolizes "evil" and the Latin term *sinister*, meaning left, also has negative meanings.

The hand has been used for counting.

3

Units of measurement, including the inch, were derived from the hand. In the past, various tools were constructed using measurements in terms of numbers of hands.[1] The hand has been used for identification; fingerprints have been used for identification since ancient times. In China fingerprints were used to sign paintings,[1] while a present-day security system uses the hand configuration as a means of identification.* The hand has also had much symbolic and metaphysical significance. The art of palmistry or chiromancy was practiced in ancient times, but it was a physician named Hartlieb[4] who wrote one of the notable books on the subject in 1448. The hand is used as a mode of expression, particularly in certain national groups, although most individuals use their hands when talking. A formalized hand language has been developed for the deaf, and the tactile sensation of the hand has been used by the blind in interpreting braille.

REFERENCES

1. Alpenfels, E. J.: The Anthropology and Social Significance of the Human Hand. *Artif. Limbs*, 2:4–21, 1955.
2. Goff, C. W.: Comparative Anthropology of Man's Hand. *Clin. Orthop.*, 13:9–23, 1959.
3. Krogman, W. M.: The Anthropology of the Hand. *Ciba Symposium*, 4:1294–1306, 1942.
4. Mierzecki, H.: Symbolism and Pathognomy of the Hand. *Ciba Symposium*, 4:1319–1322, 1942.
5. Reininger, W.: The Hand in Art. *Ciba Symposium*, 4:1323–1327, 1942.
6. Vesely, D. G.: Sculpture of the Hand. A Dramatization of Anatomy. *Clin. Orthop.*, 89:94–102, 1972.

RADIOLOGY OF THE HAND

Historical Facets

On November 15, 1895, the first radiograph of a human being was produced, and was that of a hand. An early hand radiograph obtained on December 22, 1895, is illustrated in Figure 1–1. In 1896 over a thousand articles appeared in the world literature on the use of radiography;[1] most

---

*Identimation, Northvale, New Jersey 07647.

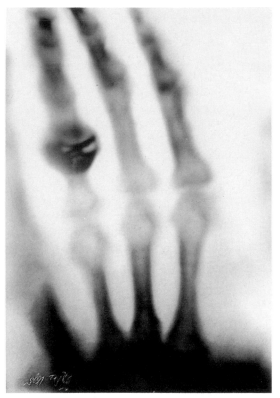

Figure 1–1. This is one of the first radiographs of a portion of the human body. December 22, 1895. (Courtesy Deutsches Museum, Munich.)

of these dealt with the hand. Partially because of the relatively low output of the x-ray machines in those days, the hand was the only part of the body thin enough to be easily radiographed.

Grigg[1] lists some of the firsts in radiology of the hand. These include the following: In January 1896 Jastrowitz published a description of a radiograph of a glass splinter within the hand. Also in January 1896 Haschek and Lindenthal outlined the arteries of a severed hand of a cadaver by injecting radiopaque material, thus producing the first angiogram. The use of a radiograph for aiding in the extraction of a bullet from the hand was reported in January of 1896 by Mosetig-Moorhof. In February 1896 Zenger described destruction of phalanges, probably from osteomyelitis. Wertheim-Salomonson, in February 1896, described a spina ventosa, hypertrophic pulmonary osteoarthropathy, and gave the first description of the appearance of a hand of a young child. He described the cartilage as being translucent to x-rays and predicted that this could be useful in determining the degree of ossification and in diagnosing rickets. Rowland, also in February 1896, described ankylosis of the distal interphalangeal joint, which was subsequently operated on. In April 1896 Hoppe-Seyler demonstrated the calcification of arteriosclerosis. Smith, in 1896,[2] published a radiograph of the hand of a Down's syndrome child and described shortening of the fifth metacarpal. Thus we can see that the hand served as a model for the early experiments in radiography of man.

REFERENCES

1. Grigg, E. R. N.: *In* Bruwer, Andre J. (Ed.): *Classic Descriptions in Roentgenology.* Charles C Thomas, Publisher, Springfield, Illinois, 1964, Vol. 1, pp. 47–70.
2. Smith, T. T.: Peculiarity in Shape of Hand in Idiots of Mongol Type. *Pediatrics*, 2:315–320, 1896.

Normal Radiographic Anatomy of the Hand

The hand usually contains 8 carpal bones, 5 metacarpals and 5 proximal, 4 middle and 5 distal phalanges (Fig. 1–2). The

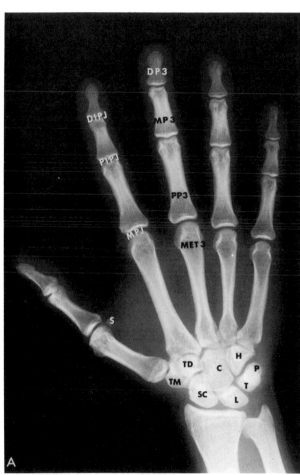
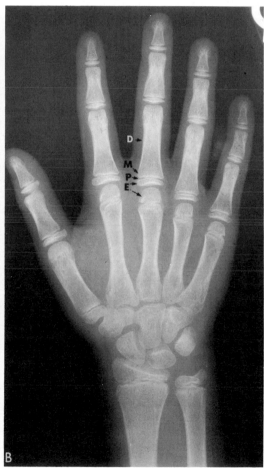

Figure 1–2. *A,* Normal adult. PA of the hand. The carpal bones are the trapezium (TM), trapezoid (TD), capitate (C), hamate (H), scaphoid (SC), lunate (L), triquetrum (T) and pisiform (P). The metacarpals (MET), proximal phalanges (PP), middle phalanges (MP), distal phalanges (DP), metacarpophalangeal joint (MPJ), proximal interphalangeal joint (PIPJ) and distal interphalangeal joint (DIPJ) are numbered according to the ray involved, starting with the thumb as number 1. The sesamoid (S) over the head of the first metacarpal is usually present.

B, Child. Posteroanterior view of the hand. The diaphysis (D), metaphysis (M), physis or epiphyseal plate (P) and epiphysis (E) can be seen.

thumb has only 2 phalanges. In many ways the metacarpal of the thumb behaves like a proximal phalanx. Its epiphysis during childhood (Fig. 1–2B) is located on its proximal end, as in the phalanges and different from the other metacarpals, where epiphyses are distal in position. The nomenclature used for the carpals in this book will be that of the Birmingham revision (1933) of the Basel *Nomina Anatomica*. The terms commonly used in the surgical literature are listed in parentheses. The carpals in the distal row, from radial to ulnar side, are the trapezium (greater multangular), trapezoid (lesser multangular), capitate and hamate. In the proximal row are the scaphoid (navicular), lunate, triquetrum and pisiform.

Positioning in Radiography of the Hand

Many positions of the hand for radiography have been used and are well illustrated in textbooks on technique, including those by Clark,[1] Merrill[2] and Meschan.[3] A radiograph of the hand in the PA projection is illustrated in Figure 1–2A. In the child (Fig. 1–2B) the appearance of the hand depends on age, and this will be described in greater detail in the section on skeletal maturation.

As in radiography of any portion of the body, multiple projections are necessary to delineate anatomic form, since the hand is a three-dimensional structure. Although radiographs at right-angle projections are valuable when possible, they are not always useful since in the lateral view many of the structures of the hand are superimposed. Thus, the oblique view is often utilized. Generally speaking, when a certain portion of the hand needs to be examined, specific views can be obtained. For example, in a finger injury when only the finger is to be radiographed, AP, lateral and oblique views are easy to obtain (Fig. 1–3). In some situations multiple views are needed, particularly after injury or contracture when the hand cannot be straightened or when radiographs of the clenched bandaged hand must be obtained. Radiographs are obtained with various relationships of the hand to the film, so that in each view a different row of pha-

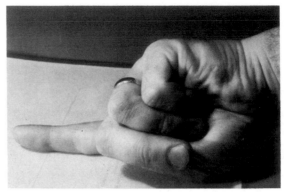

Figure 1–3. If there is question of abnormality in only one of the fingers, a lateral view of the isolated finger is easy to obtain.

langes is parallel to the film and is thus less distorted (Fig. 1–4). An additional view of the hand is sometimes useful in evaluation of early erosion in rheumatoid arthritis. It is obtained by radiographing the hand palm up with a slight degree of obliquity (Fig. 1–5).

Oblique views of the wrist are necessary, particularly in evaluation of possible carpal fractures. Various projections are used, depending on which portion of the wrist is questioned. The scaphoid is particularly important and can be well demonstrated by an oblique view of the wrist (Fig. 1–7B). The fifth finger lies on the table and the thumb is elevated so that the wrist is at about a 45° angle to the film (Fig. 1–6). This view also demonstrates the joint between the trapezium and first metacarpal. A modification of this view includes some ulnar deviation. Another scaphoid view of value is obtained with the hand flat on the film, the palm outstretched and the thumb spread away from the index finger. In the words of Meschan: "The axis of the central ray bisects the angle between the thumb and the index finger at an angle of 45° from the horizontal. The central ray is directed over the region of the scaphoid. A markedly distorted but good view of the midsection of the scaphoid is thus obtained."[3]

The lateral view of the wrist is important, particularly for evaluation of wrist dislocation. The relationship of the lunate to the capitate and of the lunate to the radius must be clearly seen (Fig. 1–8).

Another useful view of the wrist is the carpal tunnel view.[4] This can be obtained

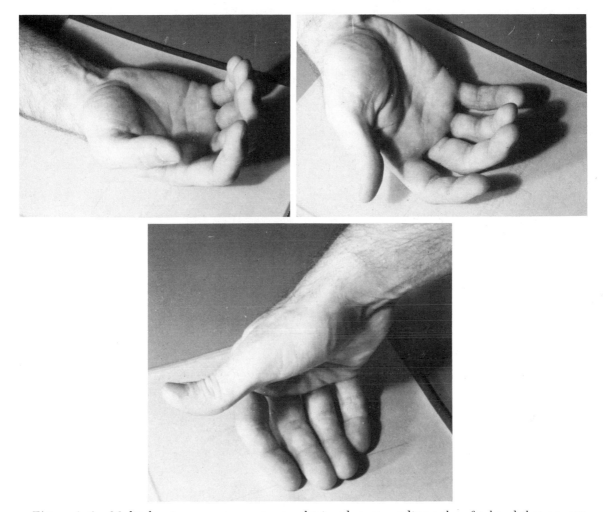

Figure 1–4. Multiple views are necessary to obtain adequate radiographs of a hand that cannot be straightened. The hand is positioned so that various portions of the digits are parallel to the table.

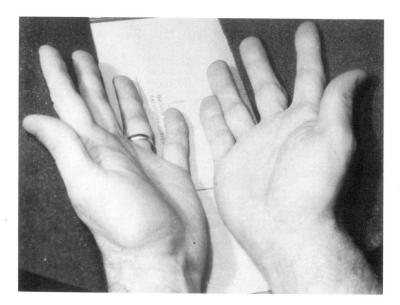

Figure 1–5. Special oblique views are useful for detecting small erosions of the metacarpal heads in rheumatoid arthritis. The hands are supported on foam blocks.

Figure 1–6. Oblique view of the scaphoid is used for study of scaphoid fractures.

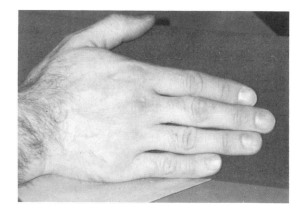

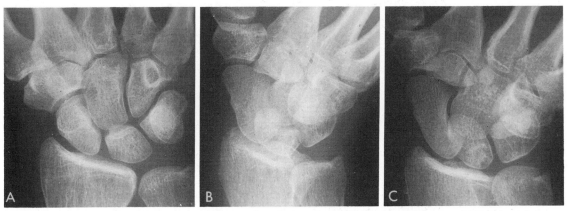

Figure 1–7. Views of the wrist. Radiographs obtained in (A) PA, (B) oblique and (C) PA with beam angulation.

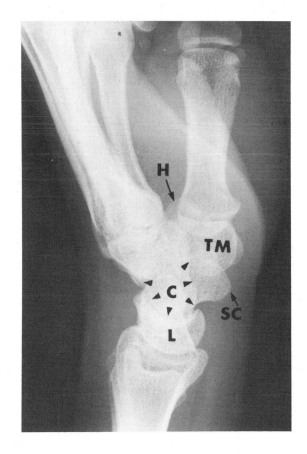

Figure 1–8. Lateral radiograph of the wrist. Note the relationship between the capitate (C) and the lunate (L). The scaphoid (SC) and the trapezium (TM) can also be visualized in this view. The hook of the hamate (H) may be seen between the first and other metacarpals.

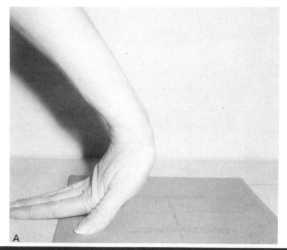

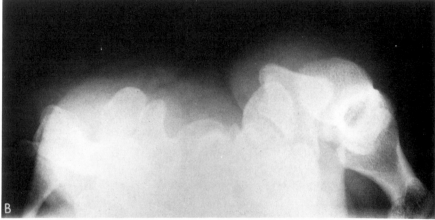

Figure 1–9. Carpal tunnel view. *A*, The hand is bent backwards on itself.
   B, Corresponding radiograph clearly shows the carpal tunnel. Abnormalities of the hook of the hamate as well as projections into the tunnel by other structures can be visualized in this view.

in two ways: either by leaning on the film with palm down, as shown in Figure 1–9, or by putting the hand on the film palm down and maximally extending the hand. In this projection the hook of the hamate is well seen. Fractures of the hamate as well as other structures projecting into the canal can be demonstrated in this fashion.

REFERENCES

1. Clark, K. C.: *Positioning in Radiography*, 8th Ed. Intercontinental Medical Book Corp., New York, 1967.
2. Merrill, V.: *Atlas of Roentgenographic Positions*, 3rd Ed. The C. V. Mosby Co., St. Louis, 1967, Vol. 1.
3. Meschan, I.: *An Atlas of Normal Radiographic Anatomy*, 2nd Ed. W. B. Saunders Company, Philadelphia, 1959.
4. Wilson, J. N.: Profiles of the Carpal Canal. *J. Bone Joint Surg.*, 36A:127–132, 1954.

Immobilization of the Hand

Since most hand radiographs are obtained with relatively long exposures (about 0.1 second at 500 milliamperes), when non-screen techniques are used some means of support for the hand are necessary to prevent motion. This is useful even for co-operative patients, since many of the positions are not stable. Support can be given in various ways, such as with simple foam blocks or wedges. In the oblique view a foam step block is useful (Fig. 1–10). Sandbags over the forearm also help to steady the hand.

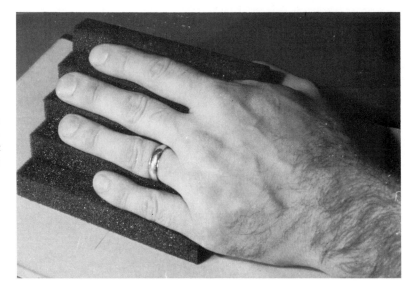

Figure 1–10. Step foam block used to assist immobilization of the hand of an adult for oblique views of the fingers.

In radiographing small infants and children, more effective modes of immobilization are necessary. A satisfactory method is to press a 1/16th-inch-thick sheet of acetate against the hand, using some weights on either side of the sheet, as shown in Figure 1–11. The forearm is also immobilized with sandbags. In young children this usually suffices. However, in the very young infant it may be somewhat more effective to have the hand lie palm up with the same mode of immobilization. In this case films are best done with the infant immobilized on the "brat board." Even then the thumb may be difficult to keep straight, since the infant will tend to flex it.

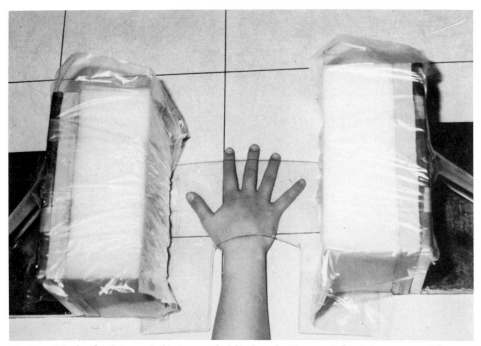

Figure 1–11. Method of immobilizing a child's hand. Sheet of flexible acetate film compressed by weights on either side flattens the hand.

Radiation Protection

When the hand is radiographed, it is most important that the central beam is directed so as not to irradiate the gonadal region. This can be done by having the patient sit at an angle to the x-ray tube. In young infants the examination is done with the child either prone or supine with the hands well away from the body. If, in some situations, the patient must sit so that his gonadal region is near the direct beam, a lead apron must be provided.

Technical Factors in Hand Radiography

The kilovoltage should be kept in the low 40s so that good contrast is obtained. The milliamperage used should be as high as possible so that the time of exposure will be as short as possible, particularly if the patient is uncooperative or has a significant tremor. Another means to shorten exposures is to decrease the film tube distance. Reduction from the usual 40 inches to 23 inches allows a threefold decrease in time. This change does not significantly affect the penumbra blur, since the hand lies directly on the film and is relatively thin.

The film used should in most cases be exposed without screens, since there is significant image blurring when screens are used (Fig. 1–12) and since the extra radiation dose to the patient is of little significance in this region of the body. Ultradetail screens offer significant improvement over conventional or high-speed screens, but still give results inferior to those from nonscreen techniques. For convenience, conventional screen film may be used without screen, either in paper-wrapped form or in a cardboard holder. This has the advantage of being automatically processable (radiographic nonscreen film cannot be processed in medical automatic processors at the present time). The dose required with conventional film is significantly larger (about four times) than that needed with radiographic nonscreen film, and the contrast is somewhat poorer.

A significant improvement in film quality may be obtained by using industrial films or Kodak RP mammographic film, which can be processed through conventional medical automatic processors. These films have an exceedingly fine grain. The use of the mammographic film still further increases patient dosage—five times the dosage with conventional film—but this may be warranted in certain situations because of the improved visualization of detail. The fine-grain films are particularly useful in detecting small flecks of calcification or fine trabecular detail (Fig. 1–13). Meema[1] has shown that by using industrial film it is easier to make the diagnosis of the finer changes, such as the increased permeative bone loss of thyrotoxicosis or the early erosions of hyperparathyroidism.

REFERENCE

1. Meema, H. E., Rabinovich, S., Meema, S., Lloyd, G. J., and Oreopoulos, D. G.: Improved Radiological Diagnosis of Azotemic Osteodystrophy. *Radiology*, 102:1–10, 1972.

Magnification Radiology

The magnification obtained by the geometry of positioning (i.e., placing the hand at a distance from the film) produces a larger image, but when nonscreen technique is used the result is usually of poorer quality than that obtained by the conventional technique. This is due to the fact that with the smallest focal spots presently available (0.3 mm.), the penumbra blurring from magnification is greater than the blurring from the grain of the film (Fig. 1–14). With screen technique, of course, magnification does allow for significant improvement. An additional problem with magnification radiography of the hand bones is that most fine-focus tubes should not be operated in this low kilovoltage range because of space-charge problems.

Radiologic Evaluation of Hand Motion

The dynamics of movement of the hand were evaluated from the early days of radiology. Bryce[4] in 1896 published a paper on evaluation of wrist motion in the living hand. Johnston[7,8] did careful anatomic studies in 1907. X-ray stereoscopy of the wrist was used by Von Bonin[10] in 1929 and by Wright[11] in 1935, while Arkless[1]

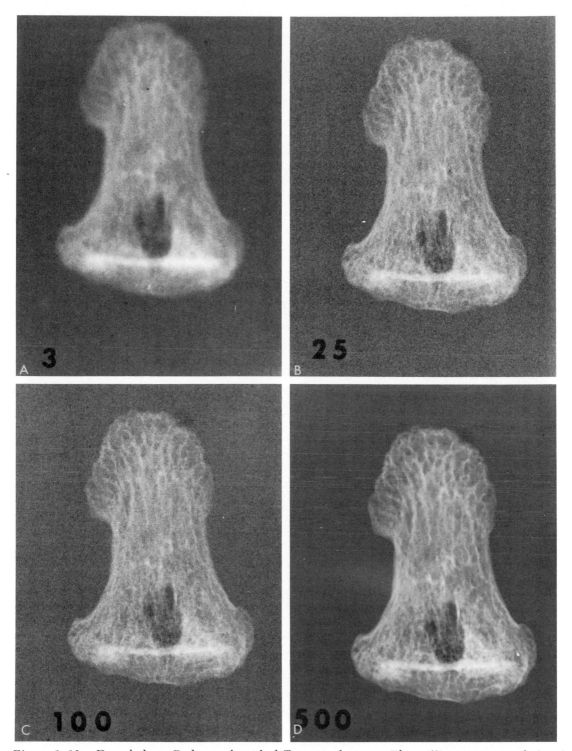

Figure 1–12. Dry phalanx. Radiograph with different techniques. The milliampere seconds (mas) required are listed at the bottom left-hand corner of the film.

A, RPL film with high-speed screen.

B, Radiographic nonscreen film.

C, RPS film without screen.

D, Kodak mammographic film, RPM.

Note the marked improvement in film detail with the mammographic film, and the rather poor rendition of detail with the use of screens.

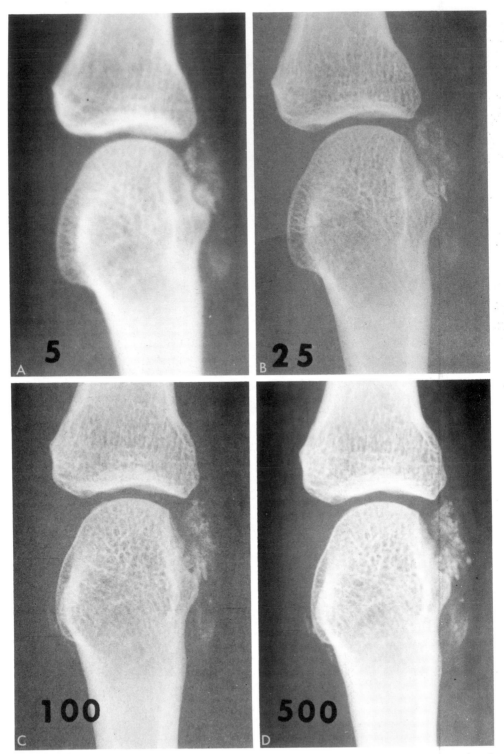

Figure 1–13. Patient with scleroderma and soft tissue calcifications. The techniques are the same as those used in Figure 1–12. Only the large calcifications can be seen with the use of screens. A greater number of calcifications are evident with the conventional nonscreen film (*B*) or with screen film used without screens (*C*), while with the use of the mammographic film (*D*) fine detail is easily perceived.

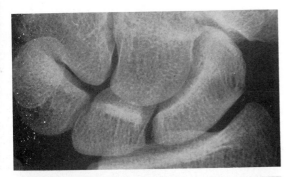

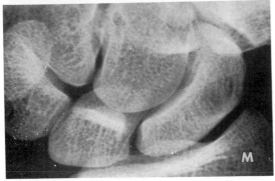

Figure 1–14. Magnification with nonscreen exposures. Two times geometric magnification using 0.3 mm. focal spot. Both the magnified film (M) and the nonmagnified film are reproduced the same size for ease of comparison. Note that there is a slight loss in detail on the magnified film.

in 1967 used cineradiography for evaluation of relative motion. Cineradiography allows more complete evaluation of motion than do still pictures at various positions, but it is not easily adaptable for publication. The study of wrist motion has found little clinical application. Arkless[1] has attempted to relate the motion of the various bones to the various methods of immobilization of fractures. In another paper[2] he shows some alterations in motion in rheumatoid arthritis. We have used cineradiography in the evaluation of the wrist in arthrogryposis as an aid in determining therapy.

Ulnar and Radial Motion of the Wrist

This is a complex motion involving several relative motions. The proximal cup of the wrist, composed of the scaphoid, lunate and triquetrum, is most flexible. The distal carpals move more as a unit with the metacarpals and there is little or no motion between the distal carpals.

In moving the hand from ulnar to radial deviation (Fig. 1–15), motion occurs between the radius and the proximal cup and between the proximal cup and the distal carpals. The relative degree of motion at these two centers varies between individuals. There is also motion between the proximal carpals themselves. In ulnar deviation the scaphoid is seen in full profile (Fig. 1–15A), while on radial deviation it rolls partially into the palm and is overlaid by the trapezium (Fig. 1–15C). Also, in ulnar deviation the lunate and triquetrum come closer to each other, the hamate overlapping the lunate, and there is palmar deviation of the lunate, which is best seen in the lateral view (Fig. 1–16).

There is no articulation between the triquetrum and the ulna, which are separated by a meniscus. The pisiform moves with the wrist in ulnar deviation, coming close to the ulna. In radial deviation there is widening of the lunate-triquetral joint.

Flexion and Extension of the Wrist

In flexion and extension of the wrist, motion occurs between the proximal and distal carpals and at the radiocarpal joint (Fig. 1–17). No motion occurs at the carpometacarpal joints except in the thumb. The relative amount of motion at the radiocarpal and intercarpal joints varies in different individuals. According to Boyes,[3] slightly more than half of the total motion takes place between lunate and radius, although this is not necessarily true in all persons. Arkless[2] states that more dorsiflexion occurs in the capitate-lunate area and more palmar flexion at the lunate-radial joint.

Motion of the Thumb

The motion of opposition is complex. Most of the motion occurs at the first metacarpotrapezium joint (Fig. 1–18). The metacarpophalangeal joint is more like the interphalangeal joints of the other fingers, allowing mainly flexion and extension. The head of the first metacarpal resembles more the heads of the proximal phalanges of the other digits than it does the meta-

(Text continued on page 21)

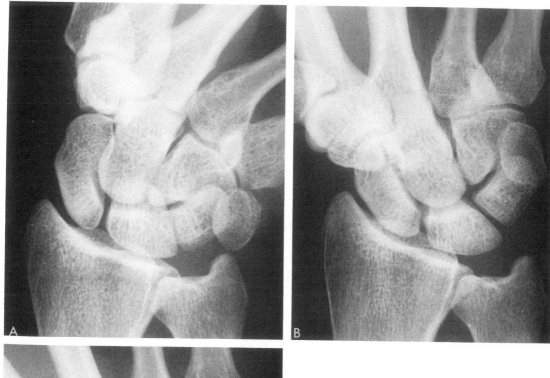

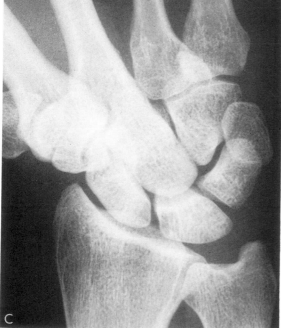

Figure 1–15. Normal adult female hand in (A) ulnar and (C) radial deviation, and in (B) midposition. Note the relative movement of the proximal row of carpals as compared to the radius, and of the distal carpals as compared to the proximal row. Note also that with rotation of the lunate in ulnar deviation it overlies a portion of the hamate. The scaphoid is better visualized in the ulnar deviation view.

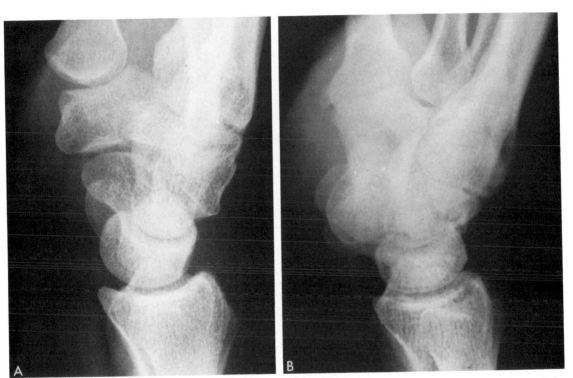

Figure 1–16. Lateral view in (A) ulnar deviation and (B) radial deviation. Note the tipping of the lunate in a palmar direction during ulnar deviation.

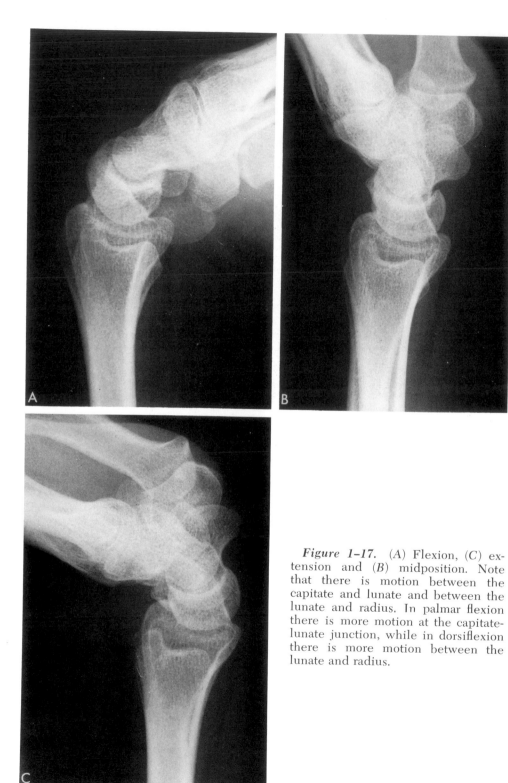

Figure 1–17. (*A*) Flexion, (*C*) extension and (*B*) midposition. Note that there is motion between the capitate and lunate and between the lunate and radius. In palmar flexion there is more motion at the capitate-lunate junction, while in dorsiflexion there is more motion between the lunate and radius.

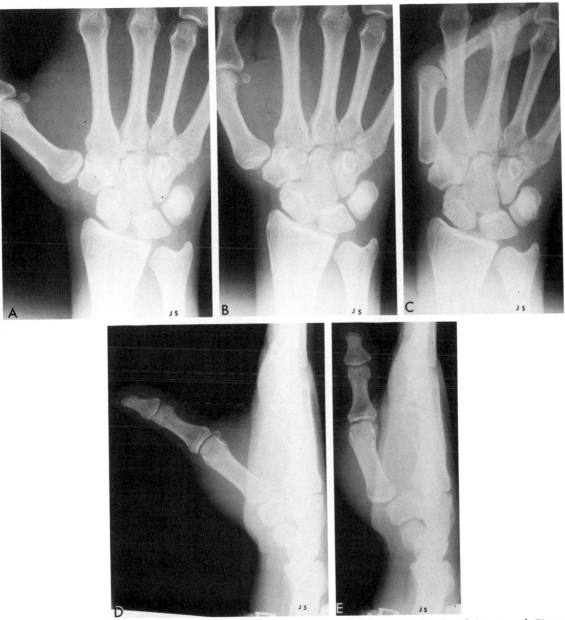

Figure 1–18. Thumb motion. Movement occurs both in the plane of the hand (*A, B* and *C*) and perpendicular to it (*D* and *E*). Note that there is relatively little carpal motion associated with the thumb motion.

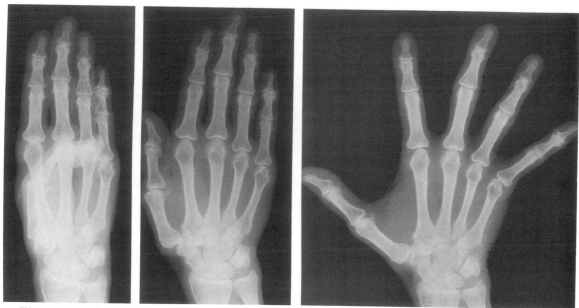

Figure 1–19. Motion of the metacarpophalangeal joints. Considerable lateral motion can occur, particularly at the metacarpophalangeal joint of the fifth finger.

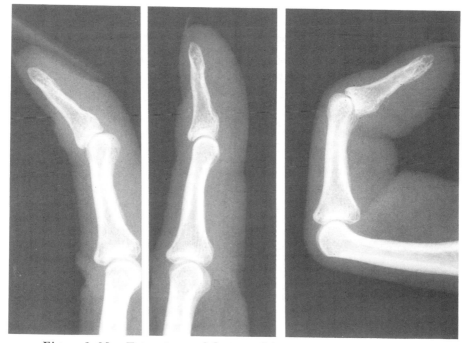

Figure 1–20. Extension and flexion of the interphalangeal joints.

carpal heads. The lateral sides and dorsum of the head of the first metacarpal are not covered with cartilage like the other metacarpal heads. The radiologic evaluation of motion of the thumb is not well documented, since the motion is complex, occurring both in the plane of the remainder of the hand and at right angles to it, so that two angles in space must be considered.[5] There is remarkably little motion of the carpals with extensive motion of the thumb (Fig. 1–18).

Other Motions of the Hand

There is some lateral deviation that occurs at the metacarpophalangeal joint (Fig. 1–19). More complex motion is evident in grasping or opposition. The metacarpal heads can be in one plane or they can form a gentle arch. The various complex motions are well described in Boyes's text,[3] but the radiologic changes associated with these motions are not well documented in the literature. Both flexion and lateral motion are possible in the metacarpophalangeal joints.

The interphalangeal joints are sliding joints (Fig. 1–20). The proximal joints flex 70 to 90°; the middle, 105 to 115°; and the distal, 45 to 90°.[3] Some lateral motion of the finger joint is possible when the hand is in extension. In flexion, this lateral motion is lost.

REFERENCES

1. Arkless, R.: Cineradiography in Normal and Abnormal Wrists. *Am. J. Roentgenol.*, 96:837–844, 1966.
2. Arkless, R.: Rheumatoid Wrists: Cineradiography. *Radiology*, 88:543–549, 1967.
3. Boyes, J. H.: *Bunnell's Surgery of the Hand*, 5th Ed. J. B. Lippincott Co., Philadelphia, 1970.
4. Bryce, T. H.: On Certain Points in the Anatomy and Mechanism of the Wrist-Joint Reviewed in the Light of a Series of Röntgen Ray Photographs of the Living Hand. *J. Anat. & Physiol.*, 31:59–79, 1896.
5. Duparc, J., and de la Caffiniere, J.–Y.: A Propos des Mouvements du Premier Métacarpien. *Presse Méd.*, 78:833–834, 1970.
6. Harris, H., and Joseph, J.: Variation in Extension of the Metacarpo-Phalangeal and Interphalangeal Joints of the Thumb. *J. Bone Joint Surg.*, 31B:547–559, 1949.
7. Johnston, H. M.: Varying Positions of the Carpal Bones in the Different Movements at the Wrist. Part I. *J. Anat. & Physiol.*, 41:109–122, 1907.
8. Johnston, H. M.: Varying Positions of the Carpal Bones in the Different Movements at the Wrist. Part II. *J. Anat. & Physiol.*, 41:280–292, 1907.
9. Kaplan, E. G.: The Participation of the Metacarpophalangeal Joint of the Thumb in the Act of Opposition. *Bull. Hosp. Joint. Dis.*, 27:39–45, 1966.
10. Von Bonin, G.: A Note on the Kinematics of the Wrist Joint. *J. Anat.*, 63:259–262, 1929.
11. Wright, R. D.: A Detailed Study of Movement of the Wrist Joint. *J. Anat.*, 70:137–143, 1935.

EMBRYOLOGY OF THE HAND

The first formation of the limb buds takes place at about four weeks postfertilization.[2, 4] The upper limb buds are formed very slightly earlier than the lower. Subsequently, each limb bud increases in length and the proximal portion develops before the distal. The finger rays become evident at about the fifth week (Fig. 1–21A). Although the skeletal elements first develop as mesodermal condensations, they are soon replaced by cartilage in a specific order (Fig. 1–21B).[4] The carpals can be noted as condensed mesenchyme at five weeks; a few days later the carpals chondrify. The metacarpals begin to chondrify at the same time as the carpals (five weeks). During the sixth week a cartilaginous os centrale is found in most fetuses. It eventually fuses with the cartilaginous scaphoid (Fig. 1–22). Similarly, a chondrifying nodule corresponding to the os triangulare is sometimes seen in the carpus of the fetus. These two ossicles are sometimes seen in adults in association with a variety of congenital malformations. The sesamoids also appear very early in development; usually they begin to chondrify at about seven weeks and their distribution is similar to that of the adult.[4] Some joint cavities begin to be formed at about nine weeks. Thus, according to O'Rahilly, the anomalies in which the number of skeletal elements is increased arise very early in intrauterine life. For example, polydactyly and ulnar dimelia must have had their beginnings before six weeks of development, either as mesodermal or chondral deficiencies. A decrease in the number of skeletal elements can, however, occur after this period, since it may be the result of postnatal changes from either destruction or failure in further development. O'Rahilly states that the cases of hypodactyly and radial hemimelia occur very early in the embryonic phase. Similarly, experience with thalidomide embryopathy has shown that different malformations can occur depending on the time of ingestion of the teratogen. When the teratogen is ingested at 50 days there is a triphalangeal thumb, while if ingestion occurs earlier there may be hypoplasia or absence of the thumb.

According to Boyes,[1] phocomelia and hemimelia occur at three weeks, polydactyly and lobster claw at three weeks, brachydactyly and syndactyly at six weeks, and brachyphalangism and symphalangism at seven weeks.

According to O'Rahilly, the earliest ossi-

fication in the hand of the fetus is in the tips of the distal phalanges, which occurs as early as seven weeks (Fig. 1–21B).[2, 4] Bone collars form in the metacarpals and proximal phalanges at 9 to 10 weeks, in the middle phalanges at 10 to 12 weeks and in the distal phalanges at 8 to 10 weeks. These are seen at the ends of the bones before the appearance of periosteal buds. Vascular invasions occur at 10 to 11 weeks in the metacarpals, at 11 to 13 weeks in the proximal phalanges, at 13 to 15 weeks in the middle phalanges and at 11 to 15 weeks in the distal phalanges. These vascular invasions herald the approach of the ossification centers. The center for the middle phalanx of the little finger may be delayed until full term. Ossification of the carpus and of the epiphyses occurs after birth and is discussed in the section on skeletal maturation (p. 50).

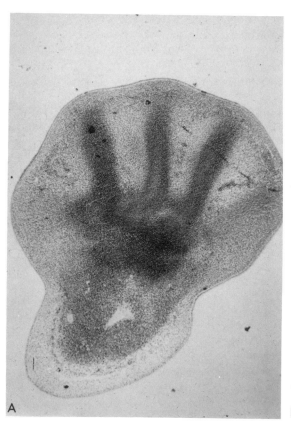

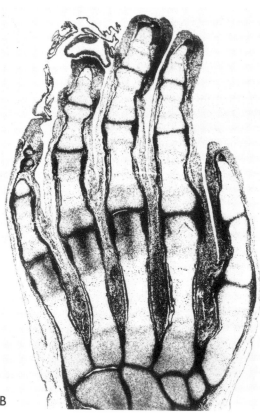

A   B

Figure 1–21.   A, Hand of a 14.5 cm. (crown-rump length) six week old embryo. Mesenchymal condensations (blastema) of the finger rays' common carpal center.
  B, Hand of a 28 mm. fetus (about eight weeks). Note the early collars of ossification in the metacarpals and phalanges. (Courtesy Dr. Alphonse Burdi, Ann Arbor, Michigan.)

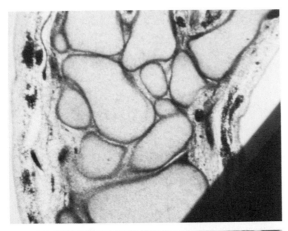

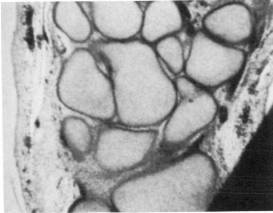

Figure 1-22. Wrist in 29 mm. embryo. The two sections are somewhat oblique to the plane of the wrist at different levels. There is partial fusion of the small os centrale to the scaphoid. (Courtesy Dr Alphonse Burdi, Ann Arbor, Michigan.)

REFERENCES

1. Boyes, J. H.: *Bunnell's Surgery of the Hand,* 5th Ed. J. B. Lippincott Co., Philadelphia, 1970.
2. Gray, D. J., Gardner, E., and O'Rahilly, R.: The Prenatal Development of the Skeleton and Joints of the Human Hand. *Am. J. Anat.,* 101: 169–223, 1957.
3. Lewis, O. J.: The Development of the Human Wrist Joint During the Fetal Period. *Anat. Rec.,* 166:499–516, 1970.
4. O'Rahilly, R., Gardner, E., and Gray, D. J.: The Skeletal Development of the Hand. *Clin. Orthop.,* 13:42–51, 1959.

COMPARATIVE ANATOMY OF THE HAND

The primitive manus (or hand) has five fingers and a carpus composed of three rows (Fig. 1–23). The proximal row consists of three bones, the ulnare, the intermedium and the radiale, which correspond in man to the triquetrum, the lunate and the scaphoid, respectively. The middle row in the very primitive animals consists of four bones, but most modern reptiles and mammals have only one or two os centrales (Fig. 1–24).[4] In man no remnants of this central row are usually present except during embryo development. As previously mentioned, an os centrale is occasionally present as an anomaly, particularly in association with certain congenital malformation syndromes, including the Holt-Oram syndrome and the hand-foot-uterus syndrome. The distal row in the primitive animals usually contains five bones, one for each digit. In most animals there is loss of the fifth, which may be used with the fourth to form the hamate. The other three form the trapezium, trapezoid and capitate in man. In some syndromes, particularly the oto-palato-digital syndrome and the Ellis-van Creveld syndrome, there may be five bones remaining in the distal row.

The wrist joint of the living hominoids differs from that of other primates by the presence of a semilunar meniscus which separates the ulna from the triquetrum and pisiform.[3] This adaptation permits pronation and supination and is essential for free brachiation and the use of tools. This meniscus may become an ossicle in the gibbon, the so-called os Daubentonii, which may be the same as the os triangulare seen in the developing fetus and occasionally in adult man.

The primate hand retains more of the pattern of the primitive manus than do other mammals's hands which have evolved for specialized functions, such as running, flying, swimming and so forth. In the primitive amphibians there are two to three digits per toe. In most primitive reptiles the phalangeal formula (the number of phalanges in each digit) is 2,3,4,5,3, while in the primitive mammals and man it is 2,3,3,3,3. A marked increase in the number of phalanges is evident in sea-dwelling mammals, such as seals and dolphins. The greatest number was in a sea-dwelling prehistoric reptile, the ichthyosaurus, which had as many as 26 phalanges to one digit. Other adaptations have also grossly changed the manus. In the mole (Fig. 1–26A), there

(Text continued on page 28)

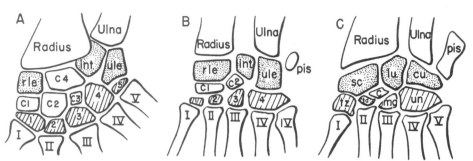

Figure 1-23. Homologies between the carpus of a (*A*) primitive tetrapod, (*B*) primitive reptile and (*C*) mammal. Proximal row elements stippled; central row and pisiform unshaded; distal row hatched. (Courtesy Romer, A. S.: *The Vertebrate Body,* 4th Ed. W. B. Saunders Company, Philadelphia, 1970.)

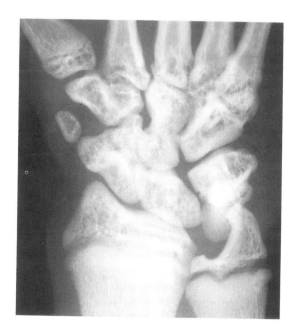

Figure 1-24. Wrist of *Macaca nemestrina* (pigtailed monkey). There are two additional ossicles in the middle row. (Courtesy Dr. Daris Swindler. Reproduced from Poznanski, A. K., and Holt, J. F.: *Am. J. Roentgenol.,* 112:443–459, 1971.)

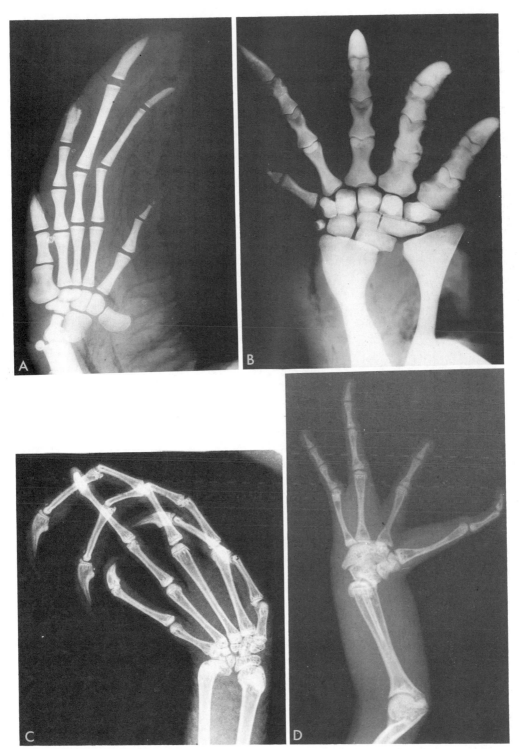

Figure 1–25. Adaptation of the manus in some reptiles. *A*, Sea turtle. The digits are not separate but form a paddle. *B*, Land turtle. *C*, Lizard. The distal phalanges are modified into better defined claws. (Courtesy Dr. D. Tinkle, Ann Arbor, Michigan.) *D*, Frog.

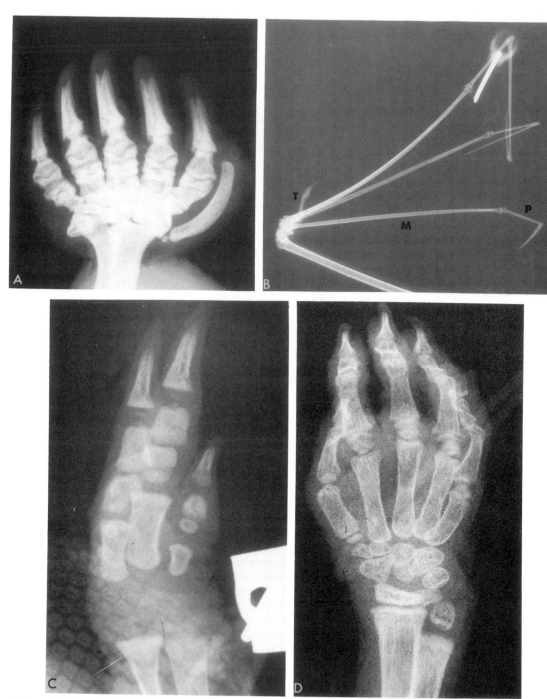

Figure 1–26. Adaptation of the manus in some mammals. *A*, Mole. There is an extraradial projection on the hand, which is a modification of a sesamoid. The hand is adapted for digging through the ground. *B*, Bat. Metacarpal (M) and phalanges (P) are slender with a web between them. The thumb (T) is small and used for grasping. *C*, Armadillo (infant). Adapted for digging with a three-claw hand. *D*, Opossum. Well-developed thumb.

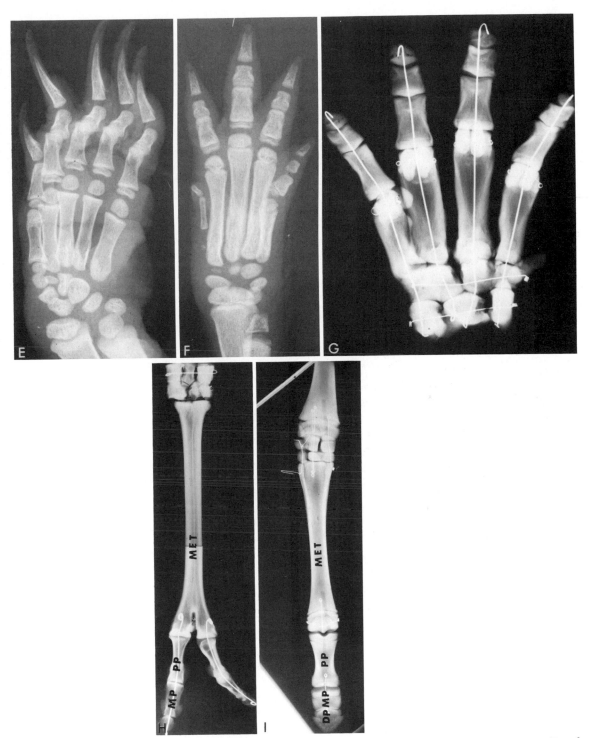

Figure 1–26. Continued. E, Coatimundi. Sharp claws and well-defined digits. F, Hyrax (South African rabbit). Hoof-like modification of the digits. G, Hippopotamus. Articulated skeleton. Four digits are evident. H, Camel. Articulated skeleton. Further modification with a single metacarpal (MET) and two sets of phalanges each with a proximal phalanx (PP), middle phalanx (MP) and distal phalanx. I, Horse (colt). Articulated skeleton. Epiphyses are still visible. There is a single digit remaining with one metacarpal (MET) and one set of phalanges (PP). The distal phalanx (DP) is incorporated into the hoof. Also shown is the middle phalanx (MP). (Animals and skeletal material courtesy Dr. E. Hooper, Ann Arbor, Michigan.)

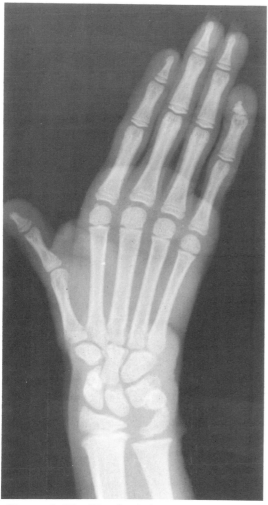

Figure 1-27. Hand of rhesus monkey. The thumb is relatively short. There is an os centrale.

has been much adaptation for digging through the ground. In the rabbit and many of the rodents the manus is modified so that these animals walk on their metacarpals. The ungulates walk on the tips of their fingers, which are usually decreased in number. In some, such as the pig, only the third and fourth are functional, the second and fifth being vestigial. In the horse the digits are reduced to one (Fig. 1–26*I*).

In birds the manus helps to form a skeleton for the wings. Most birds retain some remnant of three fingers. In bats a different modification has taken place. Four digits are elongated and a web extends between them and the body. A short thumb is present but is not incorporated in the wing and serves for grasping (Fig. 1–26*B*).

The thumb in man is biphalangeal in most cases. It is longer in man than in most other primates (Fig. 1–27).[1] The opposition of the thumb is greater in those primates that have become accustomed to terrestrial rather than to arboreal life.

REFERENCES

1. Ashley-Montagu, F. M.: On the Primate Thumb. *Amer. J. Phys. Anthropol.*, 15:291–314, 1931.
2. Kent, G. C., Jr.: *Comparative Anatomy of the Vertebrates.* The C. V. Mosby Co., St. Louis, 1965.
3. Lewis, O. J.: The Hominoid Wrist Joint. *Am. J. Phys. Anthropol.*, 30:251–268, 1969.
4. Romer, A. S.: *The Vertebrate Body*, 4th Ed. W. B. Saunders Company, Philadelphia, 1970.

Chapter 2

RADIOLOGIC ANTHROPOMETRY OF THE HAND

When you cannot measure it, when you cannot express it in numbers, you have scarcely in your thoughts advanced to the stage of science whatever the matter may be.

WILLIAM THOMPSON, LORD KELVIN[1]

LENGTHS OF THE METACARPALS AND PHALANGES
  Relative Bone Lenths
    Metacarpophalangeal Ratios
    Pattern Profile Analysis
SIZE OF CARPAL BONES
RELATIVE SLENDERNESS OF BONE

MEASUREMENT OF CORTICAL BONE
OTHER METHODS TO EVALUATE BONE
MINERALIZATION
SOFT TISSUE MEASUREMENTS
SESAMOID INDEX
CARPAL ANGLE

Measurement is becoming more useful in radiologic diagnosis as newer approaches and improved normative data are accumulated. Measurements are often necessary in the evaluation of the hand, particularly in the congenital disorders, since it is often impossible to evaluate subjectively all the 27 bones of the hand and wrist. Variations may occur in the length or width of bones, their relative slenderness, the amount of mineral within the bone or the relative size and position of the various bones. These measurements are always different in males and females and differ with different ages and populations. To be clinically meaningful the normative data to which an individual is to be compared must be based on a population that is comparable, since many of these measurements are affected by race or by nutritional or economic background of the individual.

Some of the measurements that are clinically useful and for which normative data

have been accumulated will be discussed in this chapter. Skeletal maturation, which is a form of measurement, will be discussed in Chapter 3.

REFERENCE

1. Strauss, M. B.: *Familiar Medical Quotations*. Little, Brown and Company, Boston, 1968, p. 482.

LENGTHS OF THE METACARPALS AND PHALANGES

There are many clinical entities characterized by alterations in the length of the metacarpals and phalanges. The hand is enlarged in various forms of gigantism and is reduced in size to a varying degree in many conditions associated with dwarfism. The osseous elongation or reduction in the remainder of the skeleton may not

29

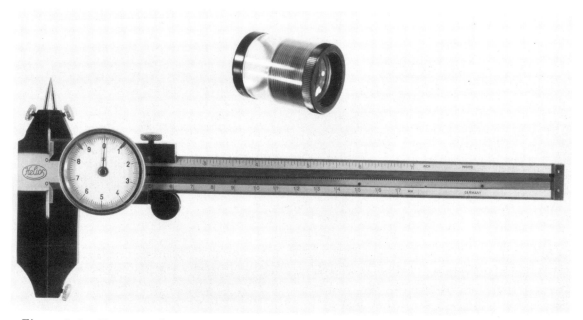

Figure 2–1. Direct reading caliper and comparator. The direct reading caliper can be used for both length and width measurements. The comparator may be useful in cortical width measurements as well.

be proportional to that of the various bones of the hand. For instance, a single segment only may be mainly involved, as in the relatively common condition of shortening of the middle phalanx of the fifth finger (brachymesophalangism 5). Alternately, entire rows as in brachydactyly A_1, or rays as in Franconi's anemia, may be reduced in size. Some method of measuring length is necessary, since subjective evaluation, particularly in children of various ages, is usually unsatisfactory.

The length of the tubular bones of the hand in skeletal material was published by Pfitzner in 1893[6] and by Lewenz and Whiteley in 1902.[5] Data at various ages and sexes derived from radiologic material were published by Garn et al.[3] and by Gefferth.[4] The Garn data were based on a population of white American children of Northern European ancestry living in Ohio. They were of above average economic status and were all healthy volunteer participants in the Fels longitudinal study.

The measurements are best made using a direct reading caliper (Fig. 2–1). The maximum length of each bone is measured along its longitudinal axis, with the exception of the third metacarpal, in which the hook is excluded since it is often variable and may be difficult to visualize (Fig. 2–2). The Garn et al. data give the length, including the epiphysis, of each of the 19 bones at one year intervals for adults and for children from age two. The standard deviation of variation is also given. Tables are available for measurements, both for males and females (Table 2–1). Unpublished data for lengths without epiphyses are also available.[2]

The Gefferth data[4] are similar but more detailed in the neonatal period. They are based on Hungarian children and may not be completely applicable to children in the United States. The portion of his data dealing with infancy is reproduced in Table 2–2. The measurements at one year of age in the Gefferth data are larger than those supplied by the Garn data without epiphysis,[2] since Gefferth's measurements include or exclude the epiphyses depending on whether they are present. With this approach, values of length in the period when the epiphyses are beginning to ossify (Chapter 3) are extremely dependent on the degree of maturation.

In normal individuals the length of the hand bones is dependent on many variables, including sex, race and familial genetic background. It is also related somewhat to body size (the correlation coefficient $r = 0.60$).[2] The hand bones are small in most congenital or acquired conditions associated with dwarfism, and large in those associated with gigantism. In some situations the hands are disproportionately small, as in the Prader-Willi syndrome (Chapter 12), while in others, such as cerebral gigantism, they are disproportionately large (Chapter 12).

(*Text continued on page 35*)

Figure 2–2. Measurements used in the Garn data. The maximum length of each bone is used, with the exception of the third metacarpal, in which the small process at the base is excluded.

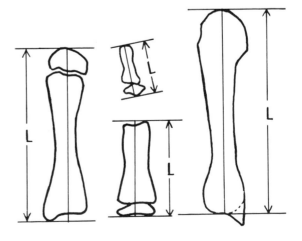

TABLE 2–1A. Standards for Metacarpal and Phalangeal Lengths and Variability (Age 2 to 10)*

BONES		2 MEAN	2 S.D.	3 MEAN	3 S.D.	4 MEAN	4 S.D.	5 MEAN	5 S.D.	6 MEAN	6 S.D.	7 MEAN	7 S.D.	8 MEAN	8 S.D.	9 MEAN	9 S.D.	10 MEAN	10 S.D.
Males																			
Distal	5	8.8	..	8.4	0.6	9.0	0.7	9.9	0.6	10.7	0.6	11.4	0.8	12.2	0.9	12.6	1.0	13.5	0.9
	4	9.2	0.7	8.9	0.8	10.5	0.8	11.5	0.8	12.3	0.9	13.1	1.0	13.9	1.0	14.4	1.0	15.3	1.2
	3	8.7	0.9	9.5	0.8	10.2	0.8	11.1	0.8	11.8	0.9	12.7	1.0	13.4	1.0	14.0	1.0	14.8	1.1
	2	8.2	0.5	8.8	1.1	9.1	1.0	10.1	0.9	10.8	0.9	11.6	1.0	12.4	1.0	13.0	1.0	13.7	1.1
	1	11.1	0.6	12.3	0.8	13.2	1.0	14.4	0.9	15.4	0.9	16.5	1.1	17.4	1.1	17.9	1.2	19.0	1.2
Middle	5	8.8	0.9	9.8	0.8	10.6	1.0	11.2	1.0	12.0	1.0	12.7	1.1	13.5	1.1	14.3	1.2	15.0	1.2
	4	13.5	0.9	14.5	1.1	15.8	0.9	16.7	1.0	17.7	1.1	18.7	1.1	19.8	1.3	20.9	1.3	21.6	1.4
	3	14.1	0.8	15.1	1.1	16.5	1.0	17.6	1.0	18.7	1.0	19.8	1.2	20.9	1.3	22.0	1.3	22.9	1.4
	2	11.2	0.7	12.3	0.9	13.5	1.0	14.4	1.0	15.3	1.0	16.1	1.1	17.1	1.1	18.1	1.2	18.8	1.2
Proximal	5	16.1	0.7	17.8	0.9	19.2	1.1	20.6	1.0	21.8	1.2	23.0	1.3	24.2	1.3	25.2	1.5	26.4	1.5
	4	20.5	0.9	22.8	1.0	24.7	1.2	26.4	1.2	27.9	1.3	29.5	1.4	31.0	1.6	32.3	1.9	33.9	1.9
	3	21.8	1.0	24.2	1.1	26.3	1.4	28.1	1.4	29.8	1.6	31.5	1.6	33.2	1.8	34.7	2.2	36.1	1.9
	2	19.5	1.0	21.9	1.1	23.7	1.3	25.4	1.2	26.8	1.5	28.3	1.3	29.7	1.8	31.4	1.9	32.5	1.9
	1	15.2	..	15.9	1.1	17.2	1.1	18.3	1.2	19.6	1.2	20.8	1.3	21.8	1.5	23.1	1.5	24.2	1.4
Metacarpal	5	23.9	1.0	26.3	1.5	28.9	1.9	32.1	2.2	34.6	2.2	36.7	2.1	38.8	2.5	40.6	2.5	42.7	2.9
	4	25.5	1.3	28.9	1.5	31.7	2.1	35.0	2.5	37.9	2.7	40.1	2.7	42.2	3.1	44.1	2.8	46.5	3.5
	3	28.6	1.3	32.3	1.8	35.6	2.3	39.3	2.8	42.6	2.8	45.3	2.8	47.6	3.5	49.8	3.0	52.3	3.7
	2	30.6	1.5	34.5	1.7	37.9	2.3	41.6	2.7	44.9	2.9	47.7	2.8	50.2	3.4	52.6	3.0	55.0	3.9
	1	19.6	1.3	22.0	1.2	24.1	1.2	26.7	1.6	29.0	1.7	30.9	1.8	32.7	2.1	34.4	2.1	36.3	2.3
Females																			
Distal	5	7.8	0.6	8.4	0.6	9.1	0.7	9.9	0.7	10.6	0.8	11.4	0.9	12.1	1.0	12.7	1.1	13.5	1.2
	4	9.1	0.7	9.9	0.7	10.6	0.8	11.5	0.8	12.4	0.9	13.2	1.1	14.0	1.1	14.4	1.2	15.5	1.4
	3	8.8	0.7	9.9	0.8	10.2	0.7	11.1	0.7	12.2	1.3	12.7	1.1	13.5	1.1	14.1	1.1	15.0	1.4
	2	8.0	0.7	8.6	0.7	9.4	0.7	10.1	0.8	10.9	0.9	11.7	1.0	12.3	1.1	13.1	1.1	13.8	1.4
	1	11.3	0.8	12.5	1.1	13.2	0.8	14.4	1.0	15.4	1.1	16.3	1.3	17.3	1.3	17.8	1.4	19.0	1.6
Middle	5	9.0	0.6	9.8	0.8	10.5	0.9	11.2	1.0	12.2	1.1	12.9	1.3	13.6	1.4	14.2	1.4	15.2	1.6
	4	13.5	0.9	14.9	1.0	15.8	1.1	16.9	1.1	18.1	1.3	19.1	1.4	20.1	1.4	20.9	1.5	22.2	1.6
	3	14.2	0.9	15.6	1.0	16.6	1.1	17.9	1.2	19.2	1.3	20.3	1.4	21.4	1.4	22.1	1.5	23.6	1.7
	2	11.6	0.9	12.8	1.0	13.6	1.1	14.8	1.1	16.0	1.2	16.8	1.2	17.8	1.4	18.1	1.5	19.6	1.7
Proximal	5	16.3	1.0	17.9	1.1	19.1	1.1	20.6	1.1	22.0	1.2	23.1	1.4	24.4	1.6	25.2	1.6	27.1	2.0
	4	20.7	1.1	22.9	1.1	24.6	1.3	26.3	1.3	28.2	1.7	29.7	1.7	31.2	2.0	32.4	2.0	34.5	2.4
	3	22.2	1.2	24.5	1.3	26.4	1.4	28.3	1.4	30.4	1.8	32.1	2.0	33.7	2.2	35.0	2.2	37.3	2.6
	2	20.1	1.2	22.3	1.3	24.0	1.8	25.8	1.8	27.7	1.7	29.2	1.9	30.7	2.0	31.5	2.4	34.0	2.4
	1	14.9	1.5	16.3	1.1	17.2	1.8	18.8	2.0	20.2	1.3	21.4	1.5	22.7	1.6	23.5	2.0	25.5	2.1
Metacarpal	5	23.7	1.5	26.0	1.9	29.4	1.8	32.6	2.0	35.1	2.1	37.2	2.4	39.4	2.1	40.8	2.5	43.8	2.8
	4	26.0	1.9	29.6	2.1	32.2	2.0	35.6	2.5	38.4	2.7	40.5	2.8	43.1	3.0	44.3	2.8	47.5	3.5
	3	29.4	2.1	33.4	2.9	36.3	2.3	40.3	2.7	43.3	3.1	45.8	3.1	48.7	3.2	49.9	3.2	53.6	3.8
	2	31.3	1.9	35.2	2.7	38.2	2.3	42.2	2.7	45.6	3.2	48.1	3.3	51.2	3.3	52.6	3.3	56.6	4.1
	1	19.9	1.6	22.7	1.6	24.8	1.7	27.3	1.8	29.6	1.9	31.5	2.0	33.5	2.1	34.8	2.4	37.4	2.6

*For each sex N ≅ 150 at age 4, 124 at age 9, 78 in adulthood, and 30–85 at intermediate ages. All values are in mm. (From Garn, S. M., et al.: *Radiology*, 105:376–377, 1972.)

TABLE 2–1B. Standards for Metacarpal and Phalangeal Lengths and Variability (Age 11 to Adult)*

BONES		11		12		13		14		15		16		17		18		ADULTS	
		MEAN	S.D.	MEAN	S.D.	MEAN	S.D.	MEAN	S.D.	MEAN	S.D.	MEAN	S.D.	MEAN	S.D.	MEAN	S.D.	MEAN	S.D.
Males																			
Distal	5	14.2	0.9	15.0	0.9	15.8	0.9	16.8	0.9	17.6	1.0	17.9	1.0	18.1	1.0	18.1	1.2	18.7	1.3
	4	16.1	1.2	17.0	1.3	17.3	1.4	18.8	1.4	19.6	1.4	20.0	1.3	20.3	1.3	20.0	1.3	20.5	1.2
	3	15.6	1.2	16.4	1.2	17.1	1.3	18.2	1.3	19.0	1.3	19.3	1.4	19.5	1.3	19.4	1.3	20.1	1.2
	2	14.3	1.1	15.0	1.3	15.7	1.4	16.7	1.3	17.5	1.2	17.8	1.4	18.2	1.4	18.1	1.5	18.8	1.4
	1	19.7	1.1	20.6	1.3	21.7	1.4	22.8	1.3	24.1	1.3	24.5	1.4	24.9	1.4	24.8	1.5	25.2	1.4
Middle	5	15.7	1.4	16.5	1.5	17.5	1.5	18.9	1.6	19.9	1.6	20.5	1.4	20.6	1.4	21.0	1.4	21.6	1.6
	4	22.6	1.5	23.6	1.5	24.8	1.7	26.5	1.7	27.7	1.5	28.4	1.5	28.7	1.6	29.1	1.5	29.6	1.6
	3	24.0	1.4	24.9	1.4	26.3	1.7	28.0	1.6	29.2	1.5	30.0	1.6	30.2	1.4	30.6	1.8	31.1	1.8
	2	19.8	1.8	20.4	1.4	21.6	1.6	23.2	1.6	24.3	1.5	25.0	1.5	25.3	1.8	25.6	1.7	26.1	1.6
Proximal	5	27.6	1.7	28.9	2.0	30.5	2.4	32.9	2.4	34.7	2.0	35.6	1.8	36.1	2.2	35.9	2.0	36.3	2.0
	4	35.3	2.0	37.0	2.4	38.8	2.9	41.6	2.8	43.7	2.6	44.9	2.3	45.4	2.3	45.2	2.5	45.5	2.3
	3	37.8	2.3	39.5	2.6	41.5	2.9	44.4	2.8	46.6	2.5	47.8	2.4	48.3	2.3	48.2	2.7	48.5	2.6
	2	33.9	2.1	35.5	2.4	37.2	2.6	39.8	2.6	41.8	2.8	42.8	2.5	43.3	2.6	43.4	2.4	43.7	2.2
	1	25.4	1.6	26.7	2.0	28.5	2.0	30.9	2.2	32.9	1.8	33.8	1.5	34.6	2.6	34.7	1.8	35.0	1.9
Metacarpal	5	44.6	2.8	47.1	3.2	49.1	4.0	52.2	3.9	55.4	3.6	57.1	2.8	57.9	2.5	57.5	2.9	58.0	3.0
	4	48.4	3.1	51.0	3.7	53.1	4.6	56.4	4.5	59.5	4.1	61.5	3.7	62.6	3.1	61.7	3.7	62.1	3.5
	3	54.6	3.5	57.3	4.0	59.5	5.1	63.1	4.9	66.7	4.1	68.7	4.1	69.7	3.1	69.0	3.7	69.0	3.8
	2	57.3	3.5	60.6	3.9	63.3	5.1	67.1	4.8	70.6	4.3	73.2	3.8	74.2	2.9	73.9	3.5	73.7	3.8
	1	38.2	2.4	40.2	2.7	42.5	3.0	45.1	2.8	47.6	2.6	48.8	2.3	49.5	2.1	49.4	2.7	49.6	2.9
Females																			
Distal	5	14.2	1.3	15.0	1.3	15.4	1.3	15.6	1.3	15.9	1.4	15.9	1.4	16.2	1.3	16.0	1.2	16.2	1.2
	4	16.2	1.4	17.1	1.4	17.6	1.4	17.9	1.3	18.0	1.4	18.0	1.3	18.1	1.4	17.9	1.3	18.0	1.3
	3	15.8	1.3	16.6	1.4	17.1	1.4	17.3	1.3	17.6	1.5	17.5	1.4	17.6	1.4	17.4	1.3	17.7	1.3
	2	14.4	1.3	15.2	1.5	15.7	1.5	15.8	1.5	16.1	1.6	16.0	1.7	16.3	1.5	16.2	1.6	16.6	1.6
	1	20.0	1.7	20.9	1.7	21.4	1.7	21.7	1.6	22.0	1.7	22.0	1.7	22.1	1.8	22.0	1.7	22.1	1.7
Middle	5	16.2	1.7	17.2	1.8	17.9	1.8	18.1	1.6	18.4	1.7	18.5	1.7	18.5	1.9	18.6	1.7	18.7	1.7
	4	23.4	1.8	24.7	1.9	25.7	1.9	25.9	1.8	26.3	1.8	26.4	1.8	26.5	1.8	26.3	1.8	26.4	1.7
	3	24.9	1.9	26.2	2.0	27.2	2.0	27.5	1.7	28.1	1.8	28.0	1.9	28.0	1.9	27.8	1.8	27.9	1.6
	2	20.6	1.8	21.8	1.9	22.7	1.8	23.0	1.8	23.5	1.8	23.3	1.9	23.4	1.9	23.1	1.6	23.2	1.6
Proximal	5	28.7	2.1	30.5	2.2	31.9	2.2	32.3	2.1	32.9	2.2	32.8	2.3	32.8	2.3	32.5	2.0	32.5	1.9
	4	36.5	2.5	38.8	2.6	40.3	2.5	40.9	2.3	41.5	2.5	41.6	2.6	41.7	2.6	41.1	2.2	40.8	2.4
	3	39.5	2.5	41.7	2.8	43.5	2.6	44.1	2.4	44.6	2.6	44.8	2.7	44.8	2.5	44.2	2.4	44.0	2.3
	2	35.9	2.6	38.0	2.6	39.5	2.6	39.9	2.4	40.6	2.6	40.6	2.6	40.7	2.6	39.9	2.3	40.0	2.3
	1	27.2	2.3	29.2	2.4	30.6	2.4	31.1	1.9	31.8	2.0	31.7	2.1	31.9	2.0	31.3	1.9	31.4	2.0
Metacarpal	5	46.3	2.9	48.7	2.9	51.8	2.8	52.1	2.8	52.6	3.0	52.8	3.0	53.0	2.7	52.0	2.7	51.9	3.6
	4	50.2	2.9	52.8	3.7	55.1	3.6	56.2	3.6	56.9	3.6	57.2	3.9	57.2	3.5	56.1	2.9	56.0	3.5
	3	56.5	4.0	59.5	4.2	62.1	4.0	63.4	4.0	63.9	3.9	64.3	4.3	64.5	4.1	63.2	3.4	62.6	4.0
	2	59.9	4.3	63.2	4.4	66.2	4.2	67.0	3.9	68.1	4.2	68.6	4.3	68.9	4.1	67.5	3.4	66.9	4.3
	1	39.7	3.0	42.0	3.0	43.8	2.7	44.4	2.5	45.3	2.4	45.0	2.8	45.0	2.6	44.6	2.2	44.2	2.6

*For each sex N ≅ 150 at age 4, 124 at age 9, 78 in adulthood, and 30–85 at intermediate ages. All values are in mm. (From Garn, S. M., et al.: *Radiology,* 105:376–377, 1972.)

TABLE 2–2A. Lengths of the Hand Bones—Males*
(MEASUREMENTS IN MILLIMETERS INCLUDE THE EPIPHYSES WHEN THEY WERE PRESENT.)

MALES		NEWBORN		2 WK.–2½ MO.		OVER 2½ MO.–4½ MO.		OVER 4½ MO.–7 MO.		ABOVE 7 MO.–11 MO.		ABOVE 11 MO.–15 MO.	
		L	S.D.	L	S.D.	L	S.D.	L	S.D.	L	S.D.	L	S.D.
DISTAL	5	4.5	0.5	4.8	0.6	5.0	0.4	5.3	0.9	5.8	0.7	6.3	0.6
	4	5.5	0.5	5.4	0.6	6.0	0.6	6.3	0.5	6.7	0.4	7.3	0.7
	3	5.6	0.5	5.3	0.9	5.9	0.7	6.3	0.8	6.5	0.6	7.1	0.9
	2	5.1	0.5	4.7	0.4	5.0	0.5	5.5	0.7	5.8	0.5	6.4	0.7
	1	5.9	0.5	6.5	0.5	6.8	0.6	7.3	0.4	7.7	0.7	8.9	0.9
MID	5	5.5	0.5	5.9	0.7	6.1	0.4	6.8	1.0	7.5	1.0	7.7	1.0
	4	7.5	0.5	8.6	1.1	8.7	0.9	9.9	0.8	10.3	0.8	11.4	1.0
	3	7.9	0.5	8.5	1.1	9.2	0.7	10.2	0.9	11.1	1.0	11.6	1.1
	2	6.5	0.6	6.9	0.7	7.2	0.6	8.1	0.8	8.5	0.7	9.3	1.1
PROXIMAL	5	8.5	0.6	9.5	1.0	10.0	1.0	11.0	1.3	12.1	1.0	13.1	1.1
	4	10.8	0.5	12.1	1.3	12.9	1.3	14.0	1.0	15.5	1.0	16.9	1.4
	3	11.7	0.6	12.8	1.2	13.5	1.0	14.9	0.9	16.0	1.2	18.0	1.3
	2	10.3	0.5	11.7	1.4	12.0	0.8	13.7	1.1	14.7	1.0	16.1	1.4
	1	7.3	0.6	8.3	0.9	8.9	0.7	9.7	1.0	10.7	0.7	11.6	1.0
METACARP.	5	11.2	0.6	12.7	0.9	13.2	1.2	14.3	1.2	15.8	1.2	17.1	1.1
	4	12.7	0.6	14.1	1.0	14.8	1.4	15.9	1.2	17.7	1.1	19.2	1.1
	3	14.2	0.8	15.8	1.5	16.5	1.0	18.3	2.3	19.7	1.6	21.3	1.2
	2	14.5	0.5	16.4	1.4	17.0	1.4	19.0	1.5	20.3	1.6	22.4	1.4
	1	9.4	0.8	10.6	1.4	11.9	0.9	12.3	1.8	13.5	1.2	14.6	1.4

*From Gefferth: *Acta Paediat. Acad. Sci. Hung.*, 13:117–124, 1972.

TABLE 2–2B. Lengths of the Hand Bones—Females*
(MEASUREMENTS IN MILLIMETERS INCLUDE THE EPIPHYSES WHEN THEY WERE PRESENT.)

FEMALES		NEWBORN		2 WK.–2½ MO.		OVER 2½ MO.–4½ MO.		OVER 4½ MO.–7 MO.		ABOVE 7 MO.–11 MO.		ABOVE 11 MO.–15 MO.	
		L	S.D.	L	S.D.	L	S.D.	L	S.D.	L	S.D.	L	S.D.
DISTAL	5	4.6	0.6	4.6	0.6	4.9	0.4	5.4	0.8	5.7	0.6	5.9	0.6
	4	5.2	0.5	5.6	0.9	5.9	0.7	6.2	0.9	6.9	0.4	7.6	0.6
	3	5.3	0.6	5.4	0.7	5.8	0.7	6.3	0.7	6.5	0.7	7.5	0.8
	2	4.8	0.7	5.0	0.4	5.2	0.8	5.7	0.6	5.8	0.9	6.4	0.8
	1	6.0	0.4	6.4	0.6	6.8	0.7	7.5	0.6	8.4	0.6	9.4	1.0
MID	5	5.6	0.5	5.5	0.5	6.2	0.6	6.6	0.7	7.5	0.8	7.9	1.1
	4	7.3	0.9	8.0	0.9	8.8	1.7	9.8	1.0	10.8	0.7	11.9	1.4
	3	7.5	0.8	8.1	1.9	9.2	0.7	9.9	0.8	11.3	1.0	12.3	1.4
	2	6.4	0.6	6.8	1.0	7.5	1.0	8.2	0.8	8.6	0.8	9.9	0.6
PROXIMAL	5	8.5	0.8	9.0	0.9	10.3	0.6	11.2	1.0	12.5	1.0	13.3	1.8
	4	10.8	0.7	11.8	0.8	12.8	1.0	14.2	1.1	16.1	1.8	18.1	1.8
	3	11.3	0.8	12.3	1.3	13.6	2.4	15.2	1.3	16.8	1.2	19.2	1.3
	2	10.4	0.6	11.1	1.1	12.5	0.8	13.5	1.0	15.0	1.4	17.3	1.6
	1	7.5	0.6	8.0	1.0	9.0	0.9	9.6	1.6	11.1	1.2	12.3	1.0
METACARP.	5	11.7	1.0	12.2	1.3	13.7	1.0	15.2	1.3	16.7	1.7	18.3	2.1
	4	12.8	1.1	13.3	1.2	14.9	1.0	16.9	1.2	18.7	1.7	20.2	1.4
	3	14.3	0.9	15.3	1.3	17.3	1.5	19.2	1.4	20.6	1.6	22.9	2.8
	2	14.8	1.3	15.6	1.0	17.8	1.9	19.5	1.6	21.7	1.9	24.5	3.0
	1	9.5	0.5	10.5	0.7	11.4	1.0	12.6	1.0	14.0	1.4	15.6	1.1

*From Gefferth: *Acta Paediat. Acad. Sci. Hung.*, 13:117–124, 1972.

REFERENCES

1. Archibald, R. M., Finby, N., and De Vito, F.: Endocrine Significance of Short Metacarpals. *J. Clin. Endocrinol.*, 19:1312–1322, 1959.
2. Garn, S. M.: Personal communication.
3. Garn, S. M., Hertzog, K., Poznanski, A. K., and Nagy, J. M.: Metacarpophalangeal Length in the Evaluation of Skeletal Malformations. *Radiology*, 105:375–381, 1972.
4. Gefferth, K.: Metrische Auswertung der kurzen Röhrenknochen der Hand von der Geburt bis zum Ende der Pubertät: Längenmasse. *Acta Paediat. Acad. Sci. Hung.*, 13:117–124, 1972.
5. Lewenz, M. A., and Whiteley, M. A.: Data for the Problem of Evolution in Man. A Second Study of the Variability and Correlation of the Hand. *Biometrika*, 1:345–360, 1902.
6. Pfitzner, W.: Beiträge zur Kenntniss des menschlichen Extremitätenskelets. V.: Anthropologische Beziehungen der Hand und Fussmaasse. *Morphologische Arbeiten*, 2:93–205, 1893.

Relative Bone Lengths

Metacarpophalangeal Ratios

In many situations it is not the actual reduction or increase in length of the hand bones that is important, but rather the length of one bone in relation to the other hand bones. In the past, various authors have attempted to establish simple techniques of comparing one bone length to another, developing several useful radiologic signs. Archibald et al.[1] described the "metacarpal sign" as a mode of evaluating relative shortening of the fourth metacarpal in Turner's syndrome (Fig. 2–3). In a normal individual a line drawn tangential to the fifth and fourth metacarpals does not intersect the third. If the fourth is short, then this line will intersect the third. There are many problems involved in using the metacarpal sign. For example, if the fifth metacarpal is also shortened, or more shortened than the fourth, the metacarpal sign can be negative even though the fourth is short. Also, the metacarpal sign may be positive in a significant percentage of normal individuals.[2] Kosowicz[5] also attempted to quantitate one bone against another by comparing the length of the fourth metacarpal to the sum of the lengths of the proximal and distal phalanges. Similarly, in attempting to determine relative

(Text continued on page 41)

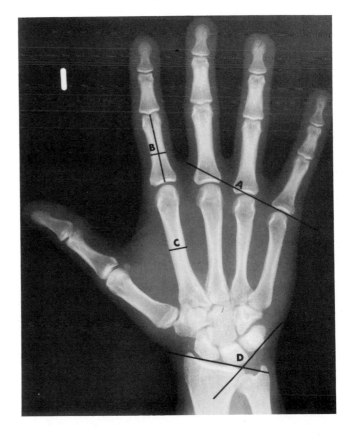

Figure 2–3. Site of some hand measurements.

(A) Metacarpal sign. A line is drawn tangential to the heads of the fourth and fifth metacarpals. It normally does not intersect the third.

(B) Measurements employed by Parish for determining the slenderness index use the minimum width and the minimum length, in contradistinction to the measurements used by Garn (Figs. 2–2 and 2–3C).

(C) Measurement site for determination of cortical thickness as measured by Garn. The measurement is obtained at the midpoint of the maximum length of the second metacarpal. The total diameter of the bone at this level equals T, the medullary cavity diameter equals M and the cortical thickness (C) equals T − M.

(D) Carpal angle. This is the angle between the line tangential to the scaphoid and lunate, and the line tangential to the lunate and triquetrum.

TABLE 2–3. Ratio Standards for Phalanges and Metacarpals with the More Distal Bone as the Numerator*

BONE RATIO, DISTAL TO PROXIMAL	MALES (AGE)								FEMALES (AGE)							
	1†		4		9		Adult†		1†		4		9		Adult†	
	Mean	S.D.	Mean	S.D.	Mean	S.D.	Mean	S.D.	Mean	S.D.	Mean	S.D.	Mean	S.D.	Mean	S.D.
Distal 5/distal 4	0.83	.04	0.85	.04	0.88	.04	0.91	.04	0.81	.06	0.86	.04	0.88	.04	0.90	.04
/distal 3	0.87	.06	0.88	.05	0.90	.04	0.93	.04	0.83	.06	0.89	.04	0.90	.04	0.92	.04
/distal 2	0.98	.08	0.99	.06	0.97	.04	1.00	.06	0.96	.11	0.98	.04	0.97	.05	0.98	.04
/distal 1	0.66	.05	0.58	.04	0.70	.03	0.74	.04	0.65	.06	0.69	.03	0.71	.04	0.73	.04
/middle 5	0.81	.09	0.86	.08	0.88	.07	0.87	.06	0.79	.09	0.88	.08	0.89	.08	0.87	.07
/middle 4	0.52	.04	0.57	.03	0.60	.03	0.63	.03	0.50	.05	0.58	.03	0.61	.04	0.61	.04
/middle 3	0.51	.05	0.55	.03	0.57	.03	0.60	.03	0.49	.05	0.55	.03	0.57	.04	0.58	.04
/middle 2	0.65	.06	0.67	.04	0.70	.04	0.72	.04	0.62	.06	0.67	.04	0.70	.05	0.70	.04
/proximal 5	0.44	.04	0.47	.03	0.50	.03	0.52	.03	0.43	.04	0.48	.03	0.50	.03	0.50	.03
/proximal 4	0.34	.03	0.37	.02	0.39	.02	0.41	.03	0.33	.03	0.37	.02	0.39	.03	0.40	.03
/proximal 3	0.33	.03	0.34	.02	0.36	.03	0.39	.02	0.31	.03	0.35	.02	0.36	.03	0.37	.02
/proximal 2	0.37	.03	0.38	.02	0.40	.02	0.43	.02	0.35	.03	0.38	.02	0.40	.04	0.40	.02
/proximal 1	0.50	.04	0.53	.03	0.55	.03	0.54	.03	0.48	.04	0.53	.04	0.54	.04	0.52	.03
/metacarpal 5	0.31	.03	0.31	.02	0.31	.02	0.32	.02	0.30	.03	0.31	.02	0.31	.02	0.31	.03
/metacarpal 4	0.28	.02	0.29	.02	0.29	.02	0.30	.02	0.27	.03	0.28	.02	0.29	.02	0.29	.03
/metacarpal 3	0.25	.02	0.25	.02	0.25	.02	0.27	.02	0.24	.02	0.25	.02	0.25	.02	0.26	.02
/metacarpal 2	0.23	.02	0.24	.02	0.24	.02	0.26	.02	0.23	.02	0.24	.02	0.24	.02	0.24	.02
/metacarpal 1	0.38	.03	0.37	.02	0.37	.02	0.38	.02	0.36	.04	0.37	.03	0.36	.03	0.37	.02
Distal 4/distal 3	1.04	.05	1.04	.03	1.03	.03	1.02	.04	1.03	.05	1.03	.03	1.02	.03	1.02	.03
/distal 2	1.18	.08	1.17	.06	1.11	.05	1.10	.06	1.20	.11	1.13	.05	1.10	.05	1.09	.06
/distal 1	0.80	.06	0.80	.04	0.80	.04	0.82	.03	0.80	.07	0.80	.03	0.81	.03	0.81	.03
/middle 5	0.97	.11	1.01	.10	1.01	.09	0.95	.07	0.97	.12	1.02	.09	1.02	.09	0.96	.08
/middle 4	0.63	.04	0.67	.04	0.69	.04	0.69	.03	0.63	.05	0.67	.04	0.69	.04	0.68	.04
/middle 3	0.61	.05	0.64	.04	0.65	.03	0.66	.03	0.60	.04	0.64	.04	0.65	.04	0.64	.04
/middle 2	0.78	.06	0.78	.05	0.80	.05	0.79	.04	0.77	.07	0.78	.05	0.79	.05	0.77	.04
/proximal 5	0.53	.04	0.55	.03	0.57	.03	0.57	.03	0.53	.04	0.55	.03	0.57	.03	0.55	.03
/proximal 4	0.41	.03	0.43	.03	0.45	.02	0.45	.03	0.41	.03	0.43	.02	0.44	.02	0.44	.02
/proximal 3	0.39	.03	0.40	.02	0.42	.03	0.42	.02	0.39	.03	0.40	.02	0.41	.03	0.41	.02

TABLE 2–3. Continued   Ratio Standards for Phalanges and Metacarpals with the More Distal Bone as the Numerator*

BONE RATIO, DISTAL TO PROXIMAL	MALES (AGE)								FEMALES (AGE)							
	1†		4		9		Adult†		1†		4		9		Adult†	
	Mean	S.D.	Mean	S.D.	Mean	S.D.	Mean	S.D.	Mean	S.D.	Mean	S.D.	Mean	S.D.	Mean	S.D.
/proximal 2	0.44	.03	0.44	.03	0.46	.03	0.47	.02	0.44	.04	0.44	.03	0.46	.04	0.45	.02
/proximal 1	0.60	.05	0.62	.04	0.62	.04	0.59	.03	0.60	.05	0.61	.04	0.61	.04	0.57	.03
/metacarpal 5	0.37	.03	0.37	.03	0.35	.02	0.36	.02	0.36	.03	0.36	.02	0.35	.02	0.35	.03
/metacarpal 4	0.34	.03	0.33	.02	0.33	.02	0.33	.02	0.33	.03	0.33	.02	0.33	.02	0.32	.02
/metacarpal 3	0.30	.03	0.30	.02	0.29	.02	0.30	.02	0.30	.03	0.29	.02	0.29	.02	0.29	.02
/metacarpal 2	0.28	.02	0.28	.02	0.27	.02	0.28	.02	0.28	.03	0.28	.02	0.27	.02	0.27	.02
/metacarpal 1	0.46	.04	0.44	.03	0.42	.02	0.42	.02	0.45	.04	0.43	.03	0.41	.02	0.41	.02
Distal 3/distal 2	1.13	.07	1.13	.06	1.08	.04	1.07	.05	1.16	.09	1.10	.04	1.08	.04	1.07	.05
/distal 1	0.77	.05	0.77	.04	0.78	.03	0.80	.04	0.78	.06	0.78	.03	0.79	.03	0.80	.03
/middle 5	0.93	.11	0.98	.10	0.98	.08	0.93	.07	0.94	.11	0.98	.09	0.99	.08	0.95	.08
/middle 4	0.61	.04	0.64	.04	0.67	.04	0.68	.04	0.61	.04	0.65	.04	0.67	.04	0.67	.04
/middle 3	0.59	.05	0.62	.04	0.64	.03	0.65	.04	0.59	.04	0.62	.03	0.64	.03	0.63	.04
/middle 2	0.75	.06	0.76	.05	0.78	.05	0.77	.04	0.75	.06	0.75	.04	0.78	.05	0.76	.04
/proximal 5	0.51	.04	0.53	.03	0.56	.03	0.56	.04	0.51	.04	0.54	.03	0.56	.03	0.54	.03
/proximal 4	0.40	.03	0.41	.03	0.43	.03	0.44	.03	0.40	.03	0.42	.02	0.43	.02	0.43	.03
/proximal 3	0.38	.03	0.39	.02	0.40	.03	0.41	.03	0.37	.03	0.39	.02	0.40	.03	0.40	.02
/proximal 2	0.43	.03	0.43	.03	0.45	.02	0.46	.03	0.42	.04	0.43	.03	0.45	.03	0.44	.03
/proximal 1	0.58	.04	0.60	.04	0.61	.04	0.58	.03	0.58	.05	0.60	.04	0.60	.04	0.56	.03
/metacarpal 5	0.35	.03	0.35	.03	0.34	.02	0.35	.03	0.35	.03	0.35	.02	0.35	.02	0.34	.03
/metacarpal 4	0.33	.03	0.32	.03	0.32	.02	0.33	.02	0.32	.03	0.32	.02	0.32	.02	0.31	.02
/metacarpal 3	0.29	.02	0.29	.02	0.28	.02	0.29	.02	0.29	.03	0.28	.02	0.28	.02	0.28	.02
/metacarpal 2	0.27	.02	0.27	.02	0.27	.02	0.27	.02	0.27	.02	0.27	.02	0.27	.02	0.26	.02
/metacarpal 1	0.44	.04	0.42	.03	0.41	.02	0.41	.03	0.43	.04	0.41	.03	0.41	.03	0.40	.02
Distal 2/distal 1	0.68	.05	0.69	.04	0.72	.03	0.75	.04	0.68	.05	0.71	.04	0.73	.03	0.75	.04
/middle 5	0.82	.11	0.87	.09	0.91	.08	0.87	.07	0.83	.11	0.90	.09	0.92	.08	0.89	.08
/middle 4	0.54	.04	0.58	.04	0.62	.04	0.63	.04	0.53	.04	0.59	.04	0.63	.04	0.63	.04
/middle 3	0.52	.04	0.55	.04	0.59	.03	0.60	.04	0.51	.04	0.56	.04	0.59	.04	0.59	.04
/middle 2	0.66	.05	0.67	.04	0.72	.04	0.72	.05	0.65	.06	0.69	.04	0.72	.05	0.71	.05
/proximal 5	0.45	.04	0.47	.04	0.52	.03	0.52	.04	0.45	.04	0.49	.03	0.52	.04	0.51	.04
/proximal 4	0.35	.03	0.37	.03	0.40	.03	0.41	.03	0.35	.03	0.38	.02	0.40	.03	0.41	.03
/proximal 3	0.33	.03	0.35	.03	0.37	.03	0.39	.03	0.33	.03	0.35	.02	0.37	.03	0.38	.03
/proximal 2	0.38	.03	0.38	.03	0.41	.02	0.43	.03	0.37	.04	0.39	.03	0.42	.04	0.41	.03
/proximal 1	0.51	.05	0.53	.04	0.56	.04	0.54	.04	0.51	.05	0.54	.04	0.56	.04	0.53	.04
/metacarpal 5	0.31	.03	0.32	.03	0.32	.02	0.32	.02	0.31	.03	0.32	.02	0.32	.02	0.32	.03
/metacarpal 4	0.29	.03	0.29	.02	0.29	.02	0.30	.02	0.28	.03	0.29	.02	0.30	.02	0.30	.02
/metacarpal 3	0.26	.02	0.26	.02	0.26	.02	0.27	.02	0.25	.03	0.26	.02	0.26	.02	0.27	.02
/metacarpal 2	0.24	.02	0.24	.02	0.25	.02	0.26	.02	0.24	.02	0.25	.02	0.25	.02	0.25	.02
/metacarpal 1	0.39	.03	0.38	.03	0.38	.02	0.38	.03	0.38	.04	0.38	.04	0.38	.03	0.38	.03

TABLE 2–3. Continued   Ratio Standards for Phalanges and Metacarpals with the More Distal Bone as the Numerator*

BONE RATIO, DISTAL TO PROXIMAL	MALES (AGE)								FEMALES (AGE)							
	1†		4		9		Adult†		1†		4		9		Adult†	
	Mean	S.D.	Mean	S.D.	Mean	S.D.	Mean	S.D.	Mean	S.D.	Mean	S.D.	Mean	S.D.	Mean	S.D.
Distal 1/middle 5	1.22	.13	1.27	.12	1.26	.10	1.17	.08	1.22	.13	1.27	.10	1.26	.10	1.19	.11
/middle 4	0.79	.05	0.84	.05	0.86	.04	0.85	.05	0.79	.05	0.83	.04	0.86	.04	0.84	.06
/middle 3	0.77	.06	0.80	.04	0.81	.04	0.81	.04	0.76	.06	0.80	.04	0.81	.04	0.79	.05
/middle 2	0.98	.08	0.98	.06	0.99	.05	0.97	.05	0.97	.09	0.97	.05	0.99	.05	0.95	.06
/proximal 5	0.67	.04	0.69	.04	0.71	.04	0.70	.04	0.66	.04	0.69	.03	0.71	.04	0.68	.04
/proximal 4	0.52	.03	0.54	.03	0.56	.03	0.55	.04	0.51	.03	0.54	.02	0.55	.03	0.54	.03
/proximal 3	0.49	.03	0.50	.03	0.52	.03	0.52	.03	0.48	.03	0.50	.02	0.51	.03	0.50	.03
/proximal 2	0.56	.03	0.56	.03	0.57	.03	0.58	.03	0.55	.03	0.55	.03	0.57	.04	0.56	.03
/proximal 1	0.75	.04	0.77	.04	0.78	.04	0.72	.04	0.75	.05	0.77	.04	0.76	.05	0.71	.04
/metacarpal 5	0.46	.03	0.46	.03	0.44	.02	0.44	.04	0.46	.03	0.45	.03	0.44	.03	0.43	.04
/metacarpal 4	0.42	.03	0.42	.03	0.41	.02	0.41	.03	0.41	.03	0.41	.02	0.40	.02	0.40	.02
/metacarpal 3	0.38	.02	0.37	.02	0.36	.02	0.37	.02	0.37	.03	0.36	.02	0.36	.02	0.35	.02
/metacarpal 2	0.35	.02	0.35	.02	0.34	.02	0.34	.02	0.35	.02	0.35	.02	0.34	.02	0.33	.02
/metacarpal 1	0.58	.03	0.55	.03	0.52	.03	0.51	.03	0.56	.04	0.53	.03	0.51	.03	0.50	.03
Middle 5/middle 4	0.66	.06	0.67	.05	0.69	.04	0.73	.03	0.65	.06	0.66	.04	0.68	.04	0.71	.03
/middle 3	0.64	.07	0.64	.05	0.65	.04	0.69	.04	0.63	.06	0.63	.04	0.65	.04	0.67	.04
/middle 2	0.81	.08	0.78	.06	0.79	.05	0.83	.05	0.80	.08	0.77	.05	0.79	.05	0.80	.05
/proximal 5	0.55	.05	0.55	.04	0.57	.03	0.60	.03	0.55	.05	0.55	.04	0.56	.04	0.58	.03
/proximal 4	0.43	.04	0.43	.04	0.44	.03	0.48	.03	0.42	.04	0.43	.03	0.44	.03	0.46	.03
/proximal 3	0.41	.04	0.40	.04	0.41	.03	0.45	.03	0.40	.04	0.40	.03	0.41	.03	0.43	.03
/proximal 2	0.46	.05	0.45	.04	0.46	.03	0.49	.03	0.45	.04	0.44	.03	0.45	.04	0.47	.03
/proximal 1	0.62	.06	0.61	.05	0.62	.04	0.62	.04	0.62	.05	0.61	.04	0.61	.04	0.60	.04
/metacarpal 5	0.38	.04	0.37	.03	0.35	.03	0.37	.02	0.38	.04	0.36	.03	0.35	.03	0.36	.03
/metacarpal 4	0.35	.04	0.33	.03	0.33	.03	0.35	.02	0.34	.04	0.33	.03	0.32	.03	0.33	.02
/metacarpal 3	0.32	.03	0.30	.03	0.29	.02	0.31	.02	0.31	.03	0.29	.03	0.29	.02	0.30	.02
/metacarpal 2	0.29	.03	0.28	.03	0.27	.02	0.29	.02	0.29	.03	0.27	.02	0.27	.02	0.28	.02
/metacarpal 1	0.48	.05	0.44	.04	0.42	.03	0.44	.03	0.46	.05	0.42	.03	0.41	.03	0.42	.03
Middle 4/middle 3	0.97	.05	0.96	.03	0.95	.03	0.95	.03	0.97	.03	0.95	.03	0.95	.03	0.95	.03
/middle 2	1.24	.07	1.17	.05	1.15	.04	1.14	.04	1.23	.07	1.16	.05	1.15	.05	1.14	.04
/proximal 5	0.84	.04	0.82	.03	0.83	.03	0.82	.03	0.84	.04	0.83	.04	0.83	.04	0.82	.03
/proximal 4	0.66	.03	0.64	.03	0.65	.03	0.65	.03	0.65	.03	0.64	.02	0.64	.02	0.65	.02
/proximal 3	0.62	.03	0.60	.02	0.60	.03	0.61	.02	0.62	.03	0.60	.03	0.60	.03	0.60	.02
/proximal 2	0.70	.04	0.67	.03	0.67	.03	0.68	.03	0.69	.04	0.66	.03	0.67	.04	0.66	.02
/proximal 1	0.95	.06	0.92	.04	0.90	.04	0.85	.04	0.95	.05	0.92	.05	0.89	.04	0.84	.03
/metacarpal 5	0.59	.04	0.55	.03	0.51	.03	0.51	.02	0.58	.04	0.54	.03	0.51	.03	0.51	.04
/metacarpal 4	0.54	.04	0.50	.03	0.47	.03	0.48	.02	0.53	.04	0.49	.03	0.47	.03	0.47	.02
/metacarpal 3	0.48	.03	0.45	.03	0.42	.02	0.43	.02	0.47	.03	0.44	.03	0.42	.02	0.42	.02
/metacarpal 2	0.45	.03	0.42	.02	0.40	.02	0.40	.02	0.44	.03	0.42	.02	0.40	.02	0.40	.02
/metacarpal 1	0.73	.05	0.66	.04	0.61	.03	0.60	.03	0.71	.05	0.64	.04	0.60	.03	0.60	.02

TABLE 2-3 Continued. Ratio Standards for Phalanges and Metacarpals with the More Distal Bone as the Numerator*

BONE RATIO, DISTAL TO PROXIMAL	MALES (AGE)								FEMALES (AGE)							
	1†		4		5		Adult†		1†		4		9		Adult†	
	Mean	S.D.	Mean	S.D.	Mean	S.D.	Mean	S.D.	Mean	S.D.	Mean	S.D.	Mean	S.D.	Mean	S.D.
Middle 3/middle 2	1.29	.10	1.22	.04	1.22	.04	1.19	.04	1.27	.05	1.22	.04	1.22	.04	1.20	.03
/proximal 5	0.88	.07	0.86	.04	0.88	.04	0.86	.04	0.88	.06	0.87	.04	0.88	.04	0.86	.04
/proximal 4	0.68	.05	0.67	.03	0.68	.03	0.69	.03	0.67	.04	0.68	.03	0.68	.03	0.68	.03
/proximal 3	0.65	.05	0.63	.03	0.64	.03	0.64	.02	0.64	.04	0.63	.03	0.63	.03	0.64	.02
/proximal 2	0.73	.06	0.69	.03	0.70	.03	0.71	.03	0.72	.04	0.69	.03	0.70	.05	0.70	.02
/proximal 1	0.98	.09	0.96	.04	0.95	.04	0.89	.04	0.99	.07	0.97	.05	0.94	.05	0.89	.03
/metacarpal 5	0.61	.05	0.57	.04	0.54	.03	0.54	.03	0.60	.05	0.56	.03	0.54	.03	0.54	.04
/metacarpal 4	0.56	.05	0.52	.03	0.50	.03	0.50	.03	0.55	.05	0.52	.03	0.50	.03	0.50	.02
/metacarpal 3	0.50	.04	0.46	.03	0.44	.02	0.45	.03	0.49	.04	0.46	.03	0.44	.03	0.45	.02
/metacarpal 2	0.46	.04	0.44	.03	0.42	.02	0.42	.03	0.46	.04	0.44	.02	0.42	.02	0.42	.03
/metacarpal 1	0.75	.07	0.69	.04	0.64	.03	0.63	.03	0.74	.06	0.67	.04	0.63	.03	0.63	.03
Middle 2/proximal 5	0.68	.05	0.70	.04	0.72	.04	0.72	.04	0.69	.05	0.71	.04	0.72	.04	0.72	.03
/proximal 4	0.53	.04	0.55	.03	0.56	.03	0.57	.03	0.53	.04	0.55	.03	0.56	.03	0.57	.02
/proximal 3	0.50	.03	0.51	.03	0.52	.03	0.54	.02	0.50	.04	0.52	.03	0.52	.03	0.53	.02
/proximal 2	0.57	.03	0.57	.03	0.58	.03	0.60	.02	0.57	.04	0.57	.03	0.58	.04	0.58	.02
/proximal 1	0.77	.05	0.79	.03	0.78	.03	0.75	.03	0.78	.06	0.79	.04	0.77	.04	0.74	.03
/metacarpal 5	0.47	.04	0.47	.04	0.45	.03	0.45	.03	0.48	.04	0.46	.03	0.44	.03	0.45	.03
/metacarpal 4	0.43	.04	0.43	.03	0.41	.03	0.42	.03	0.43	.04	0.42	.03	0.41	.03	0.42	.02
/metacarpal 3	0.39	.03	0.38	.03	0.36	.02	0.38	.02	0.39	.04	0.38	.02	0.36	.02	0.37	.02
/metacarpal 2	0.36	.03	0.36	.02	0.34	.02	0.36	.02	0.36	.03	0.36	.02	0.34	.02	0.35	.02
/metacarpal 1	0.59	.04	0.56	.03	0.53	.03	0.53	.03	0.58	.05	0.55	.03	0.52	.03	0.53	.03
Proximal 5/proximal 4	0.78	.02	0.78	.02	0.78	.02	0.80	.02	0.77	.02	0.78	.02	0.78	.02	0.80	.02
/proximal 3	0.74	.03	0.73	.02	0.73	.03	0.75	.02	0.73	.03	0.72	.02	0.72	.03	0.74	.02
/proximal 2	0.83	.03	0.81	.03	0.80	.03	0.83	.03	0.83	.04	0.80	.03	0.80	.05	0.81	.02
/proximal 1	1.12	.05	1.12	.05	1.09	.05	1.03	.05	1.13	.06	1.11	.06	1.08	.06	1.04	.04
/metacarpal 5	0.69	.03	0.67	.03	0.62	.02	0.63	.02	0.69	.03	0.65	.03	0.62	.02	0.63	.04
/metacarpal 4	0.63	.03	0.61	.03	0.57	.03	0.59	.02	0.63	.04	0.59	.03	0.57	.02	0.58	.02
/metacarpal 3	0.57	.03	0.54	.03	0.51	.02	0.53	.02	0.56	.03	0.53	.02	0.51	.02	0.52	.03
/metacarpal 2	0.53	.03	0.51	.02	0.48	.02	0.49	.02	0.53	.03	0.50	.02	0.48	.02	0.49	.03
/metacarpal 1	0.86	.05	0.80	.04	0.73	.03	0.73	.04	0.84	.05	0.77	.04	0.73	.03	0.74	.03
Proximal 4/proximal 3	0.95	.02	0.94	.02	0.93	.03	0.94	.02	0.95	.02	0.93	.03	0.93	.03	0.93	.02
/proximal 2	1.07	.04	1.04	.03	1.03	.03	1.04	.03	1.07	.04	1.03	.04	1.03	.06	1.02	.02
/proximal 1	1.45	.07	1.44	.07	1.40	.07	1.30	.06	1.47	.08	1.43	.07	1.39	.08	1.30	.04
/metacarpal 5	0.89	.04	0.86	.04	0.80	.03	0.79	.03	0.90	.04	0.84	.04	0.80	.03	0.79	.05
/metacarpal 4	0.82	.04	0.78	.04	0.73	.03	0.73	.03	0.81	.04	0.76	.04	0.73	.04	0.73	.03
/metacarpal 3	0.73	.03	0.69	.03	0.65	.02	0.66	.03	0.73	.03	0.68	.03	0.65	.03	0.65	.03
/metacarpal 2	0.68	.03	0.65	.03	0.62	.03	0.62	.02	0.68	.03	0.64	.03	0.62	.02	0.61	.03
/metacarpal 1	1.11	.06	1.02	.05	0.94	.04	0.92	.04	1.09	.06	0.99	.05	0.93	.04	0.93	.03

TABLE 2–3 Continued.   Ratio Standards for Phalanges and Metacarpals with the More Distal Bone as the Numerator*

BONE RATIO, DISTAL TO PROXIMAL	MALES (AGE)								FEMALES (AGE)							
	1†		4		9		Adult†		1†		4		9		Adult†	
	Mean	S.D.	Mean	S.D.	Mean	S.D.	Mean	S.D.	Mean	S.D.	Mean	S.D.	Mean	S.D.	Mean	S.D.
Proximal 3/proximal 2	1.12	.04	1.11	.03	1.11	.04	1.11	.02	1.13	.03	1.10	.04	1.11	.07	1.10	.02
/proximal 1	1.52	.08	1.54	.07	1.50	.08	1.39	.06	1.55	.09	1.54	.08	1.50	.09	1.40	.04
/metacarpal 5	0.94	.05	0.91	.05	0.85	.04	0.84	.03	0.95	.04	0.90	.04	0.86	.04	0.85	.06
/metacarpal 4	0.86	.04	0.83	.04	0.79	.04	0.78	.03	0.86	.04	0.82	.04	0.79	.04	0.78	.03
/metacarpal 3	0.77	.04	0.74	.03	0.70	.03	0.71	.03	0.77	.03	0.73	.03	0.70	.03	0.70	.03
/metacarpal 2	0.71	.03	0.70	.03	0.66	.03	0.66	.03	0.72	.03	0.69	.03	0.67	.03	0.66	.04
/metacarpal 1	1.17	.06	1.09	.05	1.01	.05	0.98	.04	1.15	.07	1.07	.05	1.01	.05	1.00	.03
Proximal 2/proximal 1	1.35	.06	1.39	.05	1.36	.05	1.25	.04	1.37	.07	1.39	.09	1.35	.08	1.28	.04
/metacarpal 5	0.83	.05	0.83	.05	0.77	.03	0.76	.03	0.84	.04	0.82	.05	0.77	.04	0.78	.05
/metacarpal 4	0.76	.04	0.75	.04	0.71	.03	0.71	.03	0.76	.04	0.74	.05	0.71	.04	0.71	.03
/metacarpal 3	0.69	.04	0.67	.03	0.63	.03	0.64	.03	0.68	.04	0.66	.04	0.63	.04	0.64	.03
/metacarpal 2	0.64	.03	0.63	.03	0.60	.02	0.60	.02	0.64	.03	0.63	.04	0.60	.03	0.60	.03
/metacarpal 1	1.04	.06	0.99	.04	0.91	.04	0.89	.04	1.02	.06	0.97	.06	0.91	.06	0.91	.03
Proximal 1/metacarpal 5	0.62	.03	0.60	.04	0.57	.03	0.61	.03	0.61	.04	0.59	.03	0.58	.03	0.61	.04
/metacarpal 4	0.57	.03	0.54	.03	0.53	.03	0.57	.03	0.56	.04	0.54	.03	0.53	.03	0.56	.03
/metacarpal 3	0.51	.03	0.48	.03	0.47	.03	0.51	.03	0.50	.03	0.48	.03	0.47	.03	0.50	.03
/metacarpal 2	0.47	.02	0.45	.02	0.44	.02	0.48	.02	0.47	.03	0.45	.02	0.45	.02	0.47	.03
/metacarpal 1	0.77	.04	0.71	.03	0.67	.03	0.71	.03	0.75	.04	0.70	.04	0.67	.03	0.71	.03
Metacarpal 5/metacarpal 4	0.92	.03	0.91	.03	0.92	.02	0.93	.02	0.91	.04	0.91	.02	0.92	.02	0.92	.04
/metacarpal 3	0.82	.03	0.81	.03	0.82	.02	0.84	.02	0.81	.03	0.81	.02	0.82	.02	0.83	.04
/metacarpal 2	0.76	.03	0.76	.03	0.77	.02	0.79	.02	0.76	.02	0.77	.03	0.77	.03	0.78	.05
/metacarpal 1	1.25	.05	1.20	.05	1.18	.05	1.17	.04	1.22	.07	1.19	.06	1.17	.05	1.17	.07
Metacarpal 4/metacarpal 3	0.90	.02	0.89	.02	0.89	.02	0.90	.02	0.90	.02	0.89	.02	0.89	.02	0.90	.02
/metacarpal 2	0.83	.02	0.83	.02	0.84	.02	0.84	.02	0.84	.04	0.84	.03	0.84	.03	0.84	.03
/metacarpal 1	1.36	.06	1.31	.05	1.28	.05	1.25	.05	1.35	.07	1.30	.07	1.27	.06	1.27	.05
Metacarpal 3/metacarpal 2	0.93	.03	0.94	.02	0.95	.02	0.94	.02	0.94	.03	0.95	.02	0.95	.02	0.94	.02
/metacarpal 1	1.52	.07	1.48	.06	1.45	.06	1.39	.05	1.50	.08	1.47	.07	1.44	.07	1.42	.07
Metacarpal 2/metacarpal 1	1.64	.06	1.57	.06	1.53	.05	1.49	.05	1.60	.09	1.54	.07	1.52	.06	1.52	.07

*From Garn, Poznanski, Hertzog, Nagy and Miller, in press.
†Lengths measured without epiphysis at age 2, with epiphyses at later ages, as the maximum length along the shaft, excluding only the hook at the base of the third metacarpal.

shortening of the fifth middle phalanx of Down's syndrome children, Hall[4] established a middle phalanx quotient, which was the ratio of the length of the middle phalanx to the sum of the lengths of all three phalanges of the fifth finger. A simple and more accurate approach in comparing one bone to another is to use bone length ratios.

Garn et al. published the ratios[3] for all of the hand bones for males and females, as well as the standard deviation (Table 2–3). These data were derived from the same basic data as the length measurements. They were obtained by taking the mean and the standard deviation of the various ratios for each individual in each age group. Only representative ages are tabulated, since the ratios change very little with age. The values in infancy are for measurements without epiphyses, while the others are for measurements with epiphyses.

Ratios can be useful if just two bones need be compared. Also, the most discriminatory ratio for a condition can be evaluated. In Down's syndrome the most discriminatory ratio is metacarpal 5 to metacarpal 3. Ratios have been used successfully to quantify the changes of length of the various segments of the thumb.[6] In the Holt-Oram thumb, the metacarpal to distal phalanx ratio is the most discriminatory. Abnormal ratios were seen in the Cornelia de Lange syndrome, diastrophic dwarfism, myositis ossificans progressiva and the oto-palato-digital syndrome, as well as in many other conditions. These are discussed in Chapter 13.

REFERENCES

1. Archibald, R. M., Finby, N., and De Vito, F.: Endocrine Significance of Short Metacarpals. J. Clin. Endocrinol., 19:1312–1322, 1959.
2. Bloom, R. A.: The Metacarpal Sign. Brit. J. Radiol., 43:133–135, 1970.
3. Garn, S. M., Poznanski, A. K., Hertzog, K., Nagy, J. M., and Miller, R. L.: Metacarpophalangeal Ratios in the Evaluation of Skeletal Malformations, in press.
4. Hall, B.: Mongolism in Newborns—A Clinical and Cytogenic Study. Chapter VII. Measurements of the Lengths of the Finger Phalanges in Newborn and Adult Mongoloids and in Controls. Acta Pediat. Supplement 154, pp. 65–73, 1964.
5. Kosowicz, J.: The Roentgen Appearance of the Hand and Wrist in Gonadal Dysgenesis. Am. J. Roentgenol., 93:354–361, 1965.
6. Poznanski, A. K., Garn, S. M., and Holt, J. F.: The Thumb in the Congenital Malformation Syndromes. Radiology, 100:115–129, 1971.

Relative Bone Length— Pattern Profile Analysis

Although the bone length ratios suffice when only two or three bones must be compared, another approach is needed when it is necessary to compare a larger number of hand bones. A convenient approach to this problem is that of pattern profile analysis.[2]

By using graphic technique of pattern profile presentation, it is possible to visualize dimensional alterations of all rows and rays for an individual patient or for a group. By this means, one patient may be compared to another regardless of age and sex, and a group of patients may be pooled for comparison.

Pattern profiles are derived from measurements of the hand bones as described previously in the section on bone length. Depending on age, the measurement may include or exclude the epiphyses. In most cases, when the epiphyses are present it is better to include them since the measurements are usually more accurate. The first step in data analysis is to express each bone length in standard deviation units (Z scores) relative to the mean for age and sex, using Table 2–1 or 2–2. Thus, if a bone is 3 standard deviations smaller than normal it has a Z score equal to −3. If it is 2 standard deviations above normal the Z score equals +2. The second step is graphic representation. The Z score is plotted on the ordinate and the location in the hand is on the abscissa. Since the plots are Z scores, not lengths, patients of different ages and sexes can be represented together and compared (Fig. 2–4). The plots can then be compared visually. Statistical comparison is difficult, but some measure of comparison can be obtained by using the product moment correlation (the Pearsonian r). In most of the congenital malformation syndromes the correlations are in the 0.7 to 0.9 range. Generally speaking, a pattern that has much variation within it is less affected by measurement error than one which is almost flat (Fig. 2–5).

Similarity in pattern, both visually and

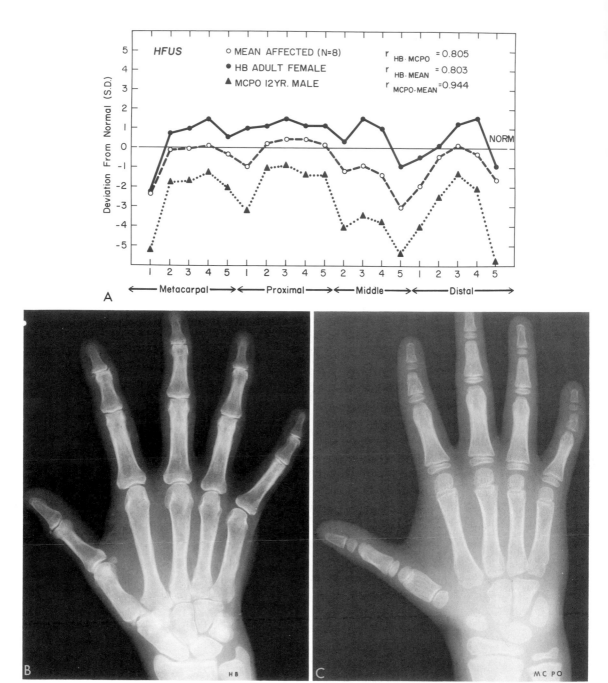

Figure 2–4. (A) Metacarpophalangeal profile pattern and (B and C) radiographs in the hand-foot-uterus syndrome. Plots of two representative members of the family and mean of the eight affected individuals. Note the relative shortening of the first metacarpal, first proximal phalanx, second middle phalanx, fifth middle phalanx and fifth distal phalanx. Although some of these findings are also evident on the radiographs, the profiles provide information far beyond the capabilities of the most experienced radiographic observer. Also, since the profiles are plotted against appropriate standards for age and sex, they allow comparison between dissimilar individuals, such as an adult female (HB = solid line) and a boy (MCPO = dotted line). (From Poznanski, A. K., et al.: *Radiology*, 104:1–11, 1972.)

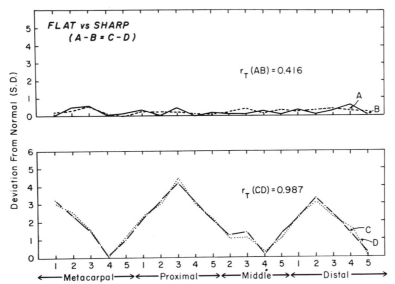

Figure 2-5. Simulation of the effects of random measuring errors on pattern similarity in two synthetic hand patterns, one of which is relatively patternless (A), while the other is highly patterned (C). The same increments were added to each bone length in A and in C, resulting in two patterns, B and D. The small increment caused a more significant dissimilarity in the flat pattern (A to B), while there was very little change when C was changed to D. The effect on similarity is evident both by inspection of the pattern and by statistical comparison (From Poznanski, A. K., et al.: *Radiology*, 104:1–11, 1972.)

statistically, refers to the ups and downs of the pattern, *not* to the height of the pattern above the mean line, since the height is simply a representation of the size of the hand bones.

In most normal and abnormal individuals there is little side-to-side asymmetry, so that either hand can be used for the measurements. There are family similarities in normal and abnormal individuals. These are highest in identical twins ($r = 0.79$)[2] and less in dizygotic twins ($r = 0.38$).

In the congenital malformation syndromes with strong patterning, such as the Holt-Oram,[1] oto-palato-digital[3] or tricho-rhino-phalangeal,[4] similarity between affected members of different families is significantly greater than between unaffected members of the same family. Pattern profiles are little affected by age and maturation[2] in both normal and abnormal individuals (Fig. 2–6).

Similarity can be seen on pattern profile plots that are not evident on simple visual

Figure 2-6. Girl with typical features of the Holt-Oram syndrome at age 10 and age 15. Note the remarkable lack of change in pattern during this time. (From Poznanski, A. K., et al.: *Birth Defects, Original Article Series*, 8:125–131, 1972.)

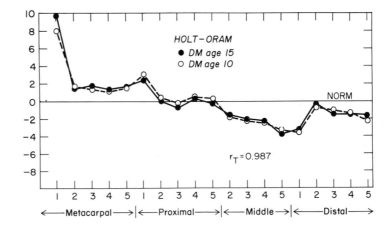

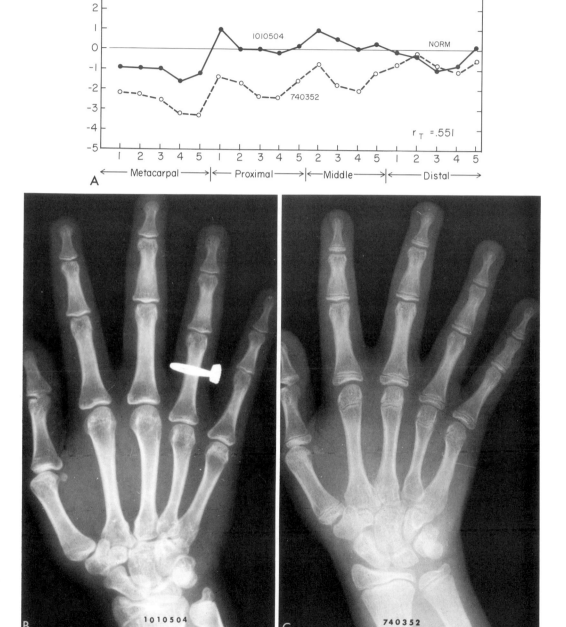

Figure 2–7. (A) Pattern profiles and (B and C) radiographs in two XO individuals (Turner's syndrome). Pattern profiles show the similarities of the hands in this syndrome, which simple visualization of the radiographs does not afford. The shortening of the fourth metacarpals is readily apparent, but the relatively long proximal phalanx of the thumbs and the middle phalanx in the second finger are not easily perceived on the radiographs. (From Poznanski, A. K., et al.: *Radiology,* 104:1–11, 1972.)

inspection of the roentgenogram. This is illustrated in two patients with Turner's syndrome (Fig. 2–7).

The use of the pattern profile can be helpful in diagnosis and in determining whether an individual is or is not affected. Characteristic patterns are seen in a number of conditions and will be described with the various syndromes (Chapters 11 and 13) in which such patterns have been determined.

REFERENCES

1. Poznanski, A. K., Garn, S. M., Gall, J. C., Jr., and Stern, A. M.: Objective Evaluation of the Hand in the Holt-Oram Syndrome. *Birth Defects, Original Article Series*, Part XV, 8:125–131, 1972.
2. Poznanski, A. K., Garn, S. M., Nagy, J. M., and Gall, J. C., Jr.: Metacarpophalangeal Pattern Profiles in the Evaluation of Skeletal Malformation. *Radiology*, 104:1–11, 1972.
3. Poznanski, A. K., Macpherson, R. I., Gorlin, R. J., Garn, S. M., Nagy, J. M., Gall, J. C., Jr., Stern, A. M., and Dijkman, D. J.: The Hand in the Oto-Palato-Digital Syndrome. *Ann. Radiol.*, 16: 203–209, 1973.
4. Poznanski, A. K., Schmickel, R. D., and Harper, H. A. S.: The Hand in the Tricho-Rhino Phalangeal Syndrome. *Birth Defects, Original Article Series*, in press.

SIZE OF CARPAL BONES

Carpal bone size variations could conceivably also be useful in diagnosis. Measurements for these bones are given by Schmid and Moll[2] but are not separated according to sex. Garn[1] has sex-specific measurements for the carpals in a large population.

One of the problems of carpal measurements is that the dimensions of these bones are very dependent on the relative position in the wrist and are also affected by radiographic position.[3]

Garn found that individuals with long slender hands have carpals that are relatively long, while individuals with short wide hands have relatively wide carpals.

REFERENCES

1. Garn, S. M.: Personal communication.
2. Schmid, F., and Moll, H.: *Atlas Der Normalen*

Und Pathologischen Handskeletenwicklund, Springer Verlag, Berlin, 1960.
3. Schulte-Brinkmann, W., and Konrad, R. M.: Zur MeBtechnik der Hand- und FuBwurzelknochen bei Kindern. *Forschr. Roentgenstr.*, 99:544–550, 1963.

RELATIVE SLENDERNESS OF BONE

Determination of relative slenderness of bone has been of value in the diagnosis of Marfan's syndrome but may have significance in other disorders as well.

Sinclair et al.[4] described a metacarpal index to be used as a measure of relative slenderness of bone. The metacarpal index was defined as the average of the ratios of the length divided by the midpoint widths of the second, third, fourth and fifth metacarpals. In a normal population of 100 individuals of unstated age, the index was less than 7.9 in all cases.[4] It was 7.5 to 7.9 in 41 per cent, 7.0 to 7.4 in 39 per cent and 6.5 to 6.9 in 16 per cent. On the other hand, in Marfan's syndrome it was above 8.4 in all 20 cases. It was 9.0 or above in 13 cases.

Joseph and Meadow[1] published values for the metacarpal index for children during the first two years. These are significantly lower than those of adults (Table 2–4). Parish[3] described the slenderness of all of the metacarpals and proximal phalanges in adults. The values were slightly different for the right and left hands. Table 2–5 lists the values for the left hand. Parish used minimum lengths rather than the maximum lengths that Garn used. Also, Parish used the minimum width of the bone rather

TABLE 2–4. Metacarpal Index During the First Two Years of Age*

Age (months)	MALES		FEMALES	
	Mean	*S.D.*	*Mean*	*S.D.*
6	5.23	0.46	5.60	0.37
12	5.30	0.41	5.75	0.41
18	5.28	0.40	5.82	0.45
24	5.40	0.43	5.84	0.43

*From Joseph and Meadow: *Arch. Dis. Child.*, 44:515–516, 1969. (Published by the *Brit. Med. J.*)

TABLE 2–5.   Relative Slenderness*†
(Left Hand)

		MALE		FEMALE	
		Mean	*S.D.*	*Mean*	*S.D.*
MET.	1	4.24	0.36	4.71	0.42
	2	7.41	0.59	8.13	0.60
	3	7.25	0.55	7.87	0.53
	4	7.99	0.60	9.05	0.80
	5	6.42	0.59	7.25	0.67
METACARPAL INDEX		7.02	0.49	7.78	0.49
PROX.	1	3.40	0.30	3.72	0.34
	2	3.80	0.22	4.20	0.25
	3	4.10	0.29	4.59	0.31
	4	4.18	0.27	4.71	0.35
	5	3.95	0.23	4.39	0.38

°From Parish: *Brit. J. Radiol.*, 39:52–62, 1966.
†Measurements are the minimal length of the bone divided by the thinnest diameter.

than measuring it at the midpoint as was done by Sinclair (Fig. 2–3).

Kosowicz[2] also published data on the relative slenderness of bone and found it to be increased in Turner's syndrome, particularly in the middle and proximal phalanges. His "normals" were based on 100 patients of various ages and were determined by dividing the length by the minimum width. The ratio for middle phalanges was 3.5 (S.D. = 0.3) and for proximal phalanges, 4.6 (S.D. = 0.4). The latter is somewhat higher than Parish's mean value and is probably due to using maximum rather than minimum length.

Kosowicz[2] also measured the ratio of the tuft width as compared to the shaft width of the distal phalanges, which was 1.3 (S.D. = 0.17). It was increased in a significant percentage of patients with gonadal dysgenesis.

REFERENCES

1. Joseph, M. C., and Meadow, S. R.: The Metacarpal Index of Infants. *Arch. Dis. Child.*, 44:515–516, 1969.
2. Kosowicz, J.: The Roentgen Appearance of the Hand and Wrist in Gonadal Dysgenesis. *Am. J. Roentgenol.*, 94:354–361, 1965.
3. Parish, J. G.: Radiographic Measurements of the Skeletal Structure of the Normal Hand. *Brit. J. Radiol.*, 39:52–62, 1966.
4. Sinclair, R. J. G., Kitchin, A. H., and Turner, R. W. D.: The Marfan Syndrome. *Quart. J. Med.*, 53:19–46, 1960.

MEASUREMENT OF CORTICAL BONE

The use of the thickness of the cortical layer of the second metacarpal as a measure of mineralization was suggested by various workers, including Virtama and Mähönen,[10] Barnett and Nordin[2] and Garn.[4] Various bones in the hand could be measured, but most authors use the second metacarpal. The measurements used by Garn[4, 6] are the outside diameter of the second metacarpal at its midpoint (T) and the diameter of the medullary space at the same level (M).[7] C is the cortical thickness. It is defined as $T - M$. T is diminished if there is lack of bone formation, and M is increased if there is increased bone resorption. It can be calculated from simple geometry that the cortical area (CA) = 0.785 $(T^2 - M^2)$ and that the percentage of cortical area (PCA) $= \dfrac{T^2 - M^2}{T^2}$. Values for T, M, C, CA and PCA, as well as their standard deviation, are given in Table 2–6. These data are based on the Fels group of Ohio whites. The values are similar to those published by Virtama and Helelä,[9] except that the Finnish children are about one year behind those in the United States in cortical mineralization. Additional values of cortex at various ages have been published by Bonnard[3] and by Gryfe et al.[7] The measurements are best made using a direct reading caliper or by using a comparator. The use of a ruler is less accurate and may be the reason some authors[1] have low replicability with this method.

The use of the second metacarpal correlates well with other methods of bone measurement.[4, 10] Its main advantage is that it is a simple and readily available technique. However, it cannot be used if a local disorder of bone, such as an old fracture, involves the second metacarpal.

The total diameter, T, does not terminate its growth after adolescence but increases slowly into old age. M, a measure of endosteal resorption, follows a different course. There is a juvenile phase of resorption, which is followed by a phase of apposition and then by a third phase of resorption lasting through old age. The loss is greater in the female than in the male. The relative changes in the bone with age and nutrition and different populations are well de-

TABLE 2–6. Standards for Metacarpal Width, Cortical Thickness, Cortical Area, and PCA

AGE (YR.)	TOTAL WIDTH (T) Mean	TOTAL WIDTH (T) S.D.	MEDULLARY WIDTH (M) Mean	MEDULLARY WIDTH (M) S.D.	CORTICAL WIDTH (C) Mean	CORTICAL WIDTH (C) S.D.	CORTICAL AREA (CA) Mean	CORTICAL AREA (CA) S.D.	PER CENT CORTICAL AREA (PCA) Mean	PER CENT CORTICAL AREA (PCA) S.D.
					Males					
1	4.50	0.34	3.04	0.45	1.46	0.30	8.63	1.65	54.22	9.40
2	5.11	0.44	3.24	0.62	1.85	0.39	12.09	2.35	59.28	10.85
4	5.53	0.49	3.04	0.62	2.48	0.37	16.65	2.54	69.49	8.47
6	6.05	0.53	3.06	0.66	2.98	0.44	21.26	3.51	73.94	8.53
8	6.57	0.54	3.13	0.66	3.43	0.45	26.08	3.90	76.88	7.29
10	7.16	0.59	3.28	0.66	3.88	0.49	31.81	4.97	78.72	6.52
12	7.73	0.65	3.43	0.72	4.29	0.60	37.66	6.37	79.87	6.67
14	8.52	0.77	3.63	0.72	4.89	0.68	46.83	8.52	81.45	5.85
16	9.11	0.72	3.81	0.75	5.29	0.51	53.82	7.53	82.29	5.14
18	9.31	0.68	3.56	0.90	5.75	0.66	57.94	7.55	84.91	6.04
30	9.36	0.68	3.41	0.81	5.94	0.43	59.59	6.62	86.49	4.67
40	9.35	0.50	3.72	0.83	5.63	0.60	57.59	5.29	83.77	5.97
50	9.65	0.88	3.84	0.93	5.81	0.63	61.54	9.64	83.85	5.67
60	9.69	0.62	4.44	0.84	5.24	0.62	58.03	6.82	78.67	6.43
70	9.38	0.58	4.61	1.05	4.76	0.73	52.99	5.28	76.25	6.23
80	9.07	0.51	4.23	0.62	4.89	0.56	50.10	5.30	76.00	5.23
					Females					
1	4.35	0.36	2.87	0.38	1.47	0.31	8.40	1.94	56.04	8.36
2	4.91	0.47	3.12	0.53	1.79	0.36	11.29	2.41	59.32	9.36
4	5.37	0.49	3.04	0.49	2.32	0.35	15.39	2.79	67.68	7.12
6	5.76	0.53	3.01	0.51	2.76	0.43	18.98	3.41	72.41	6.28
8	6.26	0.58	3.05	0.58	3.20	0.41	23.51	4.01	76.04	6.25
10	6.80	0.63	3.26	0.64	3.53	0.48	28.01	4.95	76.70	6.71
12	7.40	0.68	3.25	0.74	4.14	0.57	34.72	6.09	80.22	6.70
14	7.77	0.62	2.94	0.68	4.83	0.57	40.64	6.20	85.25	5.53
16	7.79	0.61	2.71	0.71	5.08	0.60	41.91	6.15	87.43	5.33
18	7.90	0.64	2.71	0.72	5.18	0.68	43.22	6.94	87.63	5.03
30	7.94	0.55	2.61	0.80	5.33	0.69	43.96	5.85	88.49	5.82
40	8.08	0.65	2.59	0.89	5.45	0.81	45.79	7.06	88.85	6.13
50	7.79	0.66	2.27	0.71	5.52	0.75	43.67	7.13	90.89	4.98
60	8.12	0.43	3.26	0.88	4.85	0.68	43.02	4.03	83.20	7.59
70	8.34	0.70	4.38	0.88	3.99	0.63	38.65	4.15	70.93	7.00
80	8.29	0.61	5.00	0.64	3.30	0.51	34.47	4.15	63.38	6.70

*From Garn, S. M., et al.: *Radiology,* 100:509–518, 1971.

scribed in Garn's text[4] and subsequent papers.

Although most of the adult type of bone loss occurs at the endosteal surface with increase in size of the medullary space (M), other situations may exist in childhood.[6] Some examples are listed in Table 21–1, which shows that loss or gain may occur at either surface. Thus, a single parameter of cortical bone loss cannot be used satisfactorily. Instead, several must be calculated. In clinical practice, C and PCA, T and M are probably the most significant. PCA offers one great advantage in that it is relatively independent of the size of the individual. It is, however, markedly influenced by various degrees of medullary stenosis which may occur in otherwise normal individuals.

The various cortical measurements may also be only slightly affected by conditions that more significantly affect cancellous rather than cortical bone. There may also be a permeative type of cortical bone loss which may be apparent on observation[8] but which affects the cortical measurement only slightly. This phenomenon is seen in thyrotoxicosis and with rapid bone loss such as occurs in some cases of immobilization or disuse, particularly in the initial phases. In these cases, other methods of evaluation must be used.

REFERENCES

1. Adams, P., Davies, G. T., and Sweetname, P. M.: Observer Error and Measurements of the Metacarpal. *Brit. J. Radiol.,* 42:192–197, 1969.

2. Barnett, E., and Nordin, B. E. C.: The Radiological Diagnosis of Osteoporosis: A New Approach. *Clin. Radiol.*, 11:166–174, 1960.
3. Bonnard, G. D.: Cortical Thickness and diaphysial diameter of the metacarpal bones from the age of three months to eleven years. *Helv. Paediat. Acta*, 23:445–462, 1968.
4. Garn, S. M.: *The Earlier Gain and the Later Loss of Cortical Bone in Nutritional Perspective.* Charles C Thomas, Publisher, Springfield, Illinois, 1970.
5. Garn, S. M., Miller, R. L., and Larson, K. E.: Metacarpal Lengths, Cortical Diameters and Areas From the 10-State Nutrition Survey. Personal publication, 1973.
6. Garn, S. M., Poznanski, A. K., and Nagy, J. M.: Bone Measurement in the Differential Diagnosis of Osteopenia and Osteoporosis. *Radiology*, 100:509–518, 1971.
7. Gryfe, C. I., Exton-Smith, A. N., Payne, P. R., and Wheeler, E. F.: Pattern of Development of Bone in Childhood and Adolescence. *Lancet*, 1:523–526, 1971.
8. Meema, H. E., and Schatz, D. L.: Simple Radiologic Demonstration of Cortical Bone Loss in Thyrotoxicosis. *Radiology*, 97:9–15, 1970.
9. Virtama, P., and Helelä, T.: Radiographic Measurements of Cortical Bone. Variations in a Normal Population Between 1 and 90 Years of Age. *Acta Radiol.*, Supplement 293, 1969.
10. Virtama, P., and Mähönen, H.: Thickness of the Cortical Layer as an Estimate of Mineral Content of Human Finger Bones. *Brit. J. Radiol.*, 33:60–62, 1960.

OTHER METHODS TO EVALUATE MINERALIZATION

Many methods of bone density measurements have been employed and the literature is extensive. Review of the various methods is given in detail in the Proceedings of a Conference of Progress in Methods of Bone Measurement.[5] The method of Colbert[2, 3] has been used in bone density measurements of the phalanges and metacarpals but requires a computer for its calculation. The Cameron method[3, 7] of direct photon absorptiometry has been adapted to the hand, but most work with this method has been in the region of the forearm. An additional approach to bone mass is a technique based on Compton scattering.[4]

REFERENCES

1. Balz, G.: Röntgenologisches Verfahren zur quantitativen Beurteilung des Mineralgehaltes an der Grundphalanx des Daumens. *Fortschr. Roentgenstr.*, 113:581–589, 1970.
2. Colbert, C., and Garrett, C.: Photodensitometry of Bone Roentgenograms with an On-Line Computer. *Clin. Orthop.*, 65:39–45, 1969.
3. Colbert, C., Mazess, R. B., and Schmidt, P. B.: Bone Mineral Determination in Vitro by Radiographic Photodensitometry and Direct Photon Absorptiometry. *Invest. Radiol.*, 5: 336–340, 1970.
4. Kennet, T. J., Garnett, E. S., and Webber, C. E.: An In Vivo Measurement of Absolute Bone Density. *J. Canad. Ass. Radiol.*, 23:168–170, 1972.
5. *Progress in Methods of Bone Mineral Measurement.* National Institute of Arthritis and Metabolic Diseases Conference, Bethesda, Maryland, February 15–17, 1968. U.S. Department of Health, Education and Welfare, Washington, D.C.
6. Schuster, W., Reiss, H., and Kramer, K.: The Objective Assessment of Disorders of Bone Mineralization in Congenital and Acquired Skeletal Diseases in Childhood. *Ann. Radiol.*, 13:255–265, 1970.
7. Sorenson, J. A., and Cameron, J. R.: A Reliable In Vivo Measurement of Bone-Mineral Content. *J. Bone Joint Surg.*, 49A:481–497, 1967.

SOFT TISSUE MEASUREMENTS

The evaluation of the thickness of soft tissue is of some help in the evaluation of acromegaly and possibly other disorders. Lin and Lee[1] described a soft tissue index of the second proximal phalanx. They defined this as the ratio of the middle of the phalanx at its midportion to the width of the soft tissues at the same level. Both measurements were made at right angles to the long axis of the phalanx. The index in normals was 0.45 with one S.D. = 0.05. In acromegalics the mean index was 0.40., one S.D. = 0.03.

REFERENCE

1. Lin, S. –R., and Lee, K. F.: Relative Value of Some Radiographic Measurements of the Hand in the Diagnosis of Acromegaly. *Invest. Radiol.*, 6:426–431, 1971.

SESAMOID INDEX

The measurement and size of the adductor sesamoid of the thumb have been determined because of its increase in size in acromegaly. This is further discussed in Chapter 19. The sesamoid index is defined as the product of its length times its width.[1, 2] The studies by Lin and Lee and by Kleinberg et al. used two different diameters for

TABLE 2-7.   Carpal Angle in 928 Well Individuals from the 10 State Nutrition Survey

AGE	WHITE MALE		WHITE FEMALE		BLACK MALE		BLACK FEMALE	
	Mean	S.D.	Mean	S.D.	Mean	S.D.	Mean	S.D.
4–6	123.1	5.6	127.1	6.3	130.6	6.1	131.3	7.1
6–8	127.0	11.5	130.0	10.0	131.0	8.9	133.7	8.6
8–10	133.0	7.7	124.5	7.6	139.6	7.7	138.9	8.1
10–12	132.7	7.1	135.8	8.2	138.5	11.1	138.6	8.3
12–14	131.6	8.1	129.4	8.5	141.7	8.5	141.2	9.2
14–above	133.8	9.8	129.6	8.7	141.7	9.5	138.6	8.7

obtaining this product. Normal values are 25.1 in males and 20.3 in females (one S.D. = 6.0) in the Lin and Lee[2] series and 20 in Kleinberg et al.,[1] with a range of 12 to 29. In acromegalics the range was 30 to 63.

REFERENCES

1. Kleinberg, D. L., Young, I. S., and Kupperman, H. S.: The Sesamoid Index. An Aid in the Diagnosis of Acromegaly. *Ann. Intern. Med.*, 64: 1075–1078, 1966.
2. Lin, S. –R., and Lee, K. F.: Relative Value of Some Radiographic Measurements of the Hand in the Diagnosis of Acromegaly. *Invest. Radiol.*, 6:426–431, 1971.

CARPAL ANGLE

Kosowicz[1] defined the carpal angle as the angle between two lines, one tangential to the scaphoid and lunate and the other tangential to the lunate and triquetrum (Fig. 2–3). The mean carpal angle, according to Kosowicz, is 131.5, with one S.D. = 7.2. We have measured carpal angles in a normal population from the 10 State Nutrition Survey.[1] The mean values in whites was 130.9°. The 5th to 95th percentile range was 115.0° to 146.5°. This corresponds well with Kosowicz's values. The carpal angle, however, in blacks was significantly different and was equal to 138.5°, with a 5th to 95th percentile range of 123.5 to 153.5. The carpal angle increases somewhat with age (Table 2–7).

One of the problems with the use of an angle as a parameter is that it is very dependent on the shape, structure and configuration of the carpal bones. It is also significantly affected by carpal position. In 10 controls studied, the mean carpal angle was 132.7° in neutral position, 109.7° in radial deviation and 139.4° in ulnar deviation.

REFERENCES

1. Harper, H. A. S., Poznanski, A. K., and Garn, S. M.: The Carpal Angle Effects of Age, Race and Sex, in press.
2. Kosowicz, J.: The Roentgen Appearance of the Hand and Wrist in Gonadal Dysgenesis. *Am. J. Roentgenol.*, 93:354–361, 1965.

SKELETAL MATURATION

The concept of skeletal maturation refers to the degree of development of calcification in bone. Its aspects include the presence of initial ossification centers, various modeling characteristics and epiphyseal closure. The skeletal maturation or bone age is a different entity from the size of bone. Although some relationship exists between maturation and size, each can vary independently of the other. An example of this occurs in treatment with growth hormone, where there may be a significant increase in size without a change in maturation (Fig. 3–1). Skeletal maturation (particularly epiphyseal closure) is more closely related to sexual maturity than to stature.

The hand is probably the most commonly used portion of the skeleton for evaluation of maturation. Although not completely representative of the maturation of the entire skeleton, it is satisfactory enough in most clinical situations. The use of the hand has great advantages. Well-positioned radiographs are easy to obtain. Using the hand alone gives the smallest integral radiation dosage to the patient and there is no significant bone marrow or gonadal radiation. The hand is also valuable because the greatest amount of normative data is available for it, more than for any other portion of the body. The hand, however, is of very

little value in the first year of life, particularly in retarded children, so that during early infancy other sites have to be used. In our clinical practice at the C. S. Mott Children's Hospital, we use the knee and foot at these ages.

APPLICATIONS OF EVALUATION OF MATURATION

By studying the osseous development of the hand, one can distinguish prior to puberty which children will mature early and which will be delayed. Menarche in girls, for example, occurs soon after fusion of the distal phalangeal epiphyses of the hand. When boys of the same age near puberty are arranged in order of increasing sexual maturation, their skeletal maturation will fall in approximately the same order.[17]

Skeletal maturation has many applications for the clinician. It gives some idea of how far the child has developed. In the investigation of various endocrine disorders the bone age may be of value in diagnosis and therapy. Similarly, certain patterns of dysharmonic maturation may be diagnostically useful. Bone age determinations are useful in the evaluation of the very large or the dwarfed child. The orthopedic

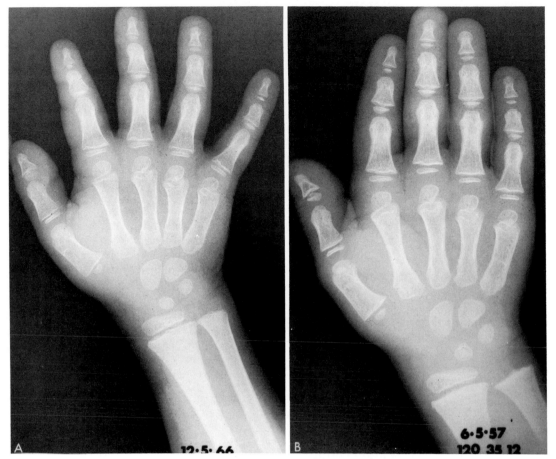

Figure 3–1. Effect of growth hormone. *(A)* Before and *(B)* six months after treatment with growth hormone. Note the marked increase in size with relatively little change in maturation.

surgeon uses skeletal maturation in the hand as a guide to when to close an epiphysis in cases of limb length discrepancy. Although it would seem more logical to use the maturation of the knee to determine relative closure, most of the available data are based on the hand.[2]

Skeletal maturation is also useful in the determination of ultimate height. Bayley and Pinneau[4] developed tables for predicting adult height from skeletal age using the Greulich and Pyle bone age standards (actually, they predicted height at 18 years). The main source of error in the evaluation of ultimate height is in the determination of the bone age and the fact that the various portions of the body may not be equally mature. Roche and French[28] have shown differences of up to 1.2 years between knee and hand maturation. These data can be applied to whites but accuracy in evaluation of blacks and of other races is less since the bone standards were derived from radiographs of white children.

The relative degree of depression or elevation of skeletal maturation, as compared to stature, will determine the eventual height of an individual. In conditions when both the maturation and stature are equally depressed, the individual will end up "normal" in height. If the skeletal maturation is advanced as compared to height the individual will end up small. If maturation is retarded as compared to stature the individual will ultimately be taller than normal. An illustration of the relationship between maturation and stature is that in some parts of the world where there is malnutrition and the height of the children is more severely depressed than skeletal maturation, the result is a relatively short adult population.

METHODS OF EVALUATING MATURATION

Pryor in 1907[23] in a study of the hand and wrist in living children did the first significant radiologic study of maturation. He discovered that maturation is usually symmetric, that the female is more advanced than the male and that variations in ossification pattern of bone are heritable traits. Rotch in 1909[30] used the term "anatomic index" to describe the present concept of skeletal maturation or bone age. These early approaches were crude, and many refinements and methods have since been developed. Many were of little value because of their approach, because they were based on antiquated standards or because they did not differentiate between the sexes. Many other individuals have contributed to the development of the concepts of skeletal maturation, but space does not permit detailed discussion.

The most used methods of evaluation of skeletal maturation in the United States which involve particularly the hand include those found in the Greulich and Pyle atlas, the Garn approach of onsets of ossification and the Tanner-Whitehouse-Healy method.

The Greulich-Pyle Atlas[17]

This is probably the most commonly used method of skeletal maturation evaluation in this country. It is certainly the most convenient to use in radiologic practice.

Todd in 1937 published an atlas on skeletal maturation which was developed into the present form by Greulich and Pyle,[17] and into the abbreviated form by Pyle, Waterhouse and Greulich.[25] The population sample used was that of white Cleveland children of families of somewhat above average economic and educational status. All of the involved children were thought to be free of major disease and were studied longitudinally. The atlas is a collection of radiographs of hands of children at various ages for both sexes. The standards were picked as the most representative for that age group. The authors also have described a number of "maturity indicators," which they define as "those features of individual bones which because they tend to recur regularly and in a definite and irreversible order mark their progress toward maturity." These maturity indicators are listed with line drawings following the standards and are described in the text adjoining each picture. The maturity indicators are different for various bones and refer mainly to alterations in shape of the bone rather than to alterations in the size. The first of these indicators is the onset of ossification of a center. Other indicators include the relationships of the epiphysis to the metaphysis, the presence of certain indentations, the capping of the epiphysis and epiphyseal fusion. The size alone is not considered to be a maturational factor.

Although the authors had a large-sized sample from which to choose, the bones in each standard still do not fit exactly in the median for the age of that bone, so that some interbone variation exists even in the most "classic" hand.

The simplest approach to evaluating bone age, which takes only a few minutes, is to look through the standards and find a radiograph which compares in maturation with the film in question. If this can be found, a crude estimation of maturation can be made. If there is considerable interbone variation in ossification, the concept of bone age becomes less meaningful. There are various approaches to this problem. Greulich and Pyle recommend that "bone age" should be found for each of the hand bones and an average value taken to obtain the bone age of the hand. This approach allows for less interobserver error and is valuable in accurate assessment. It is, however, quite time-consuming and in everyday radiologic practice somewhat impractical. If the hand does not fit well into the standard patterns, greater emphasis should be given to the phalangeal centers. Roche et al.[27,29] and Johnston and Jahina[19] have shown it may be simpler to omit the carpals entirely when using the Greulich and Pyle standards, thus simplifying the number of measurements and not significantly affecting the bone age.

The main problem with the atlas method is that it requires considerable subjective evaluation. Thus, particularly with inexperienced observers, such as new residents, the interobserver and intraobserver error can be quite high. Training significantly improves the replicability of the Greulich and Pyle readings. Also, since the standards are based on a white middle class population, the tables are of limited validity when applied to other racial groups.[7]

Atlases are also available for evaluation of the foot[18] and knee,[24] and these are used best for the younger age group, in whom relatively little change occurs in the ossification of the hand and wrist.

Range of Normal Variation

Comparison with the mean when taken in terms of chronologic age is meaningless unless it is considered in terms of standard deviation or percentiles. Tables of values of standard deviation of variation are given in the Greulich and Pyle atlas as determined from the Brush Foundation study. The standard deviation of variation varies somewhat with sex and considerably with age. The values in males, for example, range from about two months at one year of age, to nine months at six years of age to 11 months at 15 years of age. The female values are similar. Generally speaking, one can consider a range of two standard deviations above normal to two standard deviations below normal as constituting the normal range. Obviously some normal children will be outside this range.

The Garn Approach to Skeletal Maturation

Another method of evaluating bone maturation that is simple and useful in clinical practice is the Garn approach, which simply uses the onset of ossification. Garn has published tables of onset of ossification of both hands (Table 3–1)[14] (as well as of other

TABLE 3–1. Age-at-Appearance Percentiles for Postnatal Ossification Centers of the Hand (in years)*

| | PERCENTILES | | | | | |
| | Boys | | | Girls | | |
OSSIFICATION CENTER	5th	50th	95th	5th	50th	95th
Capitate	–	0.25	0.60	–	0.15	0.56
Hamate	0.03	0.31	0.82	–	0.18	0.59
Radius	0.53	1.10	2.30	0.38	0.82	1.70
3rd proximal phalanx	0.77	1.37	2.15	0.41	0.85	1.61
2nd proximal phalanx	0.78	1.41	2.17	0.40	0.87	1.64
4th proximal phalanx	0.80	1.40	2.40	0.41	0.90	1.66
1st distal phalanx	0.75	1.51	2.70	0.42	0.99	1.73
2nd metacarpal	0.93	1.61	2.82	0.64	1.09	1.69
3rd metacarpal	0.95	1.79	3.01	0.65	1.13	1.94
5th proximal phalanx	1.00	1.85	2.82	0.65	1.19	2.07
3rd middle phalanx	1.01	1.97	3.31	0.63	1.28	2.36
4th metacarpal	1.09	2.03	3.60	0.75	1.29	2.17
4th middle phalanx	1.00	2.05	3.24	0.63	1.24	2.43
5th metacarpal	1.27	2.17	3.82	0.86	1.37	2.35
2nd middle phalanx	1.30	2.19	3.31	0.67	1.36	2.54
3rd distal phalanx	1.31	2.41	3.72	0.72	1.46	2.69
Triquetrum	0.49	2.43	5.47	0.29	1.70	3.73
4th distal phalanx	1.37	2.44	3.73	0.73	1.52	2.82
1st metacarpal	1.45	2.59	4.32	0.92	1.60	2.67
1st proximal phalanx	1.84	3.00	4.57	0.93	1.71	2.84
2nd distal phalanx	1.80	3.17	4.97	1.06	2.50	3.29
5th distal phalanx	2.06	3.29	4.98	1.01	1.96	3.45
5th middle phalanx	1.94	3.40	5.84	0.88	1.97	3.54
Lunate	1.53	4.07	6.77	1.08	2.62	5.65
Scaphoid	3.59	5.63	7.81	2.35	4.12	5.99
Trapezium	3.53	5.87	8.97	1.94	4.08	6.36
Trapezoid	3.12	6.22	8.50	2.38	4.17	6.01
Ulna	5.25	7.10	9.07	3.29	5.37	7.63
Adductor sesamoid of thumb	11.03	12.76	14.62	8.67	10.72	12.68

*Modified from Garn et al.: *Med. Radiogr. Photogr.*, 43:45–66, 1967. (Published by Radiography Markets Division, Eastman Kodak Company.)

areas), including the 5th and 95th percentile values. The main advantage of the Garn approach is that it is the most objective, evaluating simply the presence or the absence of an ossification center. However, even this can sometimes be associated with some uncertainty, particularly if the ossification center is very small and has to be distinguished from artifact. The greatest disadvantage of the method is that the ages at which it can be used are somewhat limited, since it can be used only when ossification centers appear. Also, since the newly ossifying centers may occur in various parts of the body at various ages, radiographs other than those of the hand may be necessary. Another problem is that some of the centers, particularly the carpals, have little predictive value, and if, at the time the patient is examined, these are the centers which are ossifying, the range of normality can be quite large. This method is, however, a useful adjunct to the Greulich and Pyle atlas.

The Tanner-Whitehouse-Healy Method[34]

This is a scoring method which has been developed for the hand and wrist. This approach is based on a British population and is not entirely valid when compared without correction to a United States population. When children's hands are evaluated using the Tanner-Whitehouse-Healy standard, the maturation is greater than when using the Greulich and Pyle atlas.[26] At times this difference may be over one year. In the Tanner-Whitehouse-Healy system most bones are evaluated in terms of eight maturity stages. Tanner excluded the second and fourth fingers so that the average would be weighed equally by the carpals and the tubular bones. An arbitrary weighing system is also included.

One of the theoretical problems with this method is that the carpals, which are the most variable bones, are given relatively more value with this method than in the Greulich and Pyle method (in the Tanner-Whitehouse-Healy method they are weighed equally with the tubular bones). For the practicing radiologist the Tanner-Whitehouse-Healy method is also much more time consuming than simple radio-

graphic comparison, though the difference becomes not as great if each bone is evaluated separately by the Greulich and Pyle method. In comparing the Tanner-Whitehouse-Healy method to that of the Greulich and Pyle atlas, Acheson et al.[1] found that the random errors were smaller with the Tanner-Whitehouse-Healy method, but interobserver errors (systematic errors) were smaller with the Greulich and Pyle method. The Tanner-Whitehouse-Healy method is a useful research approach to bone age study if the variation between the British and the United States populations is taken into account.

Other Methods of Evaluation

A commonly used method of maturation evaluation was that of counting the number of ossification centers present. This was probably one of the poorest approaches to skeletal maturation. Garn and Rohmann[10] have shown that the number of centers at any given age correlates only moderately with the number of centers at another age ($r = 0.40$ over a four-year period). Similarly, the counts do not prove adequately representative of the remainder of the skeleton. Schmid and Moll[31] have developed standards for a German population, but the standards do not take into account sex differences. They do give the size of the carpals at various ages.

Eklöf and Ringertz[6] also devised a method of evaluating maturation based on bone length and width. This is more a measure of size than of maturation and thus measures a different entity. Sugiura[33] has published standards for both sexes for Japanese children, which should be useful.

OPERATIONAL MEANING OF MATURITY CRITERIA[9]

One of the important factors in the evaluation of maturation is that males and females are both qualitatively and quantitatively different in maturation. Thus, separate standards are unquestionably necessary, especially for some bones in which the sexual dimorphism may be great. Because of the large differences in maturation of various bones and the fact that no individual fits perfectly into a set pattern, very small changes in maturation observed by different observers, such as one-quarter year, have little meaning. The lunate, for example, has a median appearance of 4.07 years in males and 2.62 years in girls, indicating 27 per cent of maturity in boys and 19 per cent in girls.[9] Similarly, the scaphoid, trapezium and trapezoid have a very high sexual dimorphism. Differences in percentage of ossification for various centers are also evident at various ages.

Various phenomena in ossification also have little relation to each other. For example, ossification onsets and epiphyseal fusions may be unrelated.[9] It may be that a single concept of a skeletal maturity is too broad for all the uses that we presently put it to. Skeletal maturity is thus probably more than one phenomenon.

DYSHARMONIC MATURATION[21]

Unusual sequences of maturation have been termed dysharmonic.[21] This term includes right to left asymmetry, differences in degree of ossification between the carpals and the phalanges and delay or advancement of specific centers. Dysharmonic maturation may occur in normal populations, and since there are racial differences in sequence, dysharmonic maturation occurs when an individual is evaluated using a set of standards based on a different population. Dysharmonic maturation may also be the result of various disease states, and in some disorders the pattern may be characteristic (Table 3–2).

SYMMETRY OF MATURATION

Variations in maturation between the right and left hand may occur in normal populations, but the differences are only minimal.[17] The carpals, which are the most variable bones, as expected, have the greatest degree of asymmetry.[3] In a series of malnourished children, Dreizen et al.[5] found more than six months' asymmetry in only 1.5 per cent of cases. The variation in maturation between the bones of a hand was greater than the difference between the two hands in 98 per cent of cases. Asymmetry in maturation can be due to

TABLE 3–2. Causes of Dysharmonic Maturation in the Hand

A. ASYMMETRY FROM SIDE TO SIDE
    (1) Idiopathic hemihypertrophy
    (2) Silver's syndrome
    (3) Neurofibromatosis
    (4) Unilateral advancement from hyperemia
    (5) Unilateral retardation from paralysis, i.e., polio
    (6) Unilateral retardation from decreased blood supply

B. ISOLATED DYSHARMONY OF ONE OR MORE CENTERS
    (1) Advanced maturation from hyperemia
        (a) Infection
        (b) Healing fracture
        (c) Rheumatoid arthritis
    (2) Delay in maturation owing to damage of the epiphysis
        (a) Infection
        (b) Trauma, including radiation
        (c) Multiple exostoses
        (d) Tumor
        (e) Rheumatoid arthritis
    (3) Congenital
        (a) Scaphoid delay or absence in radial hypoplasia or thumb hypoplasia syndromes, including Fanconi's anemia, Juberg-Hayward syndrome
        (b) Late scaphoid in cerebral gigantism
        (c) Capitate delay in epiphyseal dysplasia
        (d) Lunate delay in homocystinuria, Seckel's syndrome
        (e) Other carpal bone delays in Morquio's, spondyloepiphyseal and spondylometaphyseal dysplasia, Hurler's syndrome, etc.
        (f) Phalangeal delay or absence in Apert's syndrome, symphalangism
        (g) Phalangeal or metacarpal advancement in some of the brachydactyly syndromes, Turner's syndrome, pseudohypoparathyroidism

C. DISPROPORTION BETWEEN CARPALS AND PHALANGES
    (1) Racial and familial variations
    (2) Trisomy 18—carpals behind phalanges
    (3) Cerebral gigantism—carpals behind phalanges
    (4) Seckel's syndrome
    (5) Beckwith-Wiedemann syndrome—carpals ahead of phalanges

a number of conditions, including increased vascularity to an extremity, such as may be caused by hemangioma, arteriovenous malformation or rheumatoid arthritis (Fig. 3–2). Hemihypertrophy (Fig. 3–3), either idiopathic or related to Silver's syndrome, is also associated in most cases with advanced maturation on the larger side. Hypoplasia of an extremity due to a decrease in vascular supply or paralysis (Fig. 3–4)

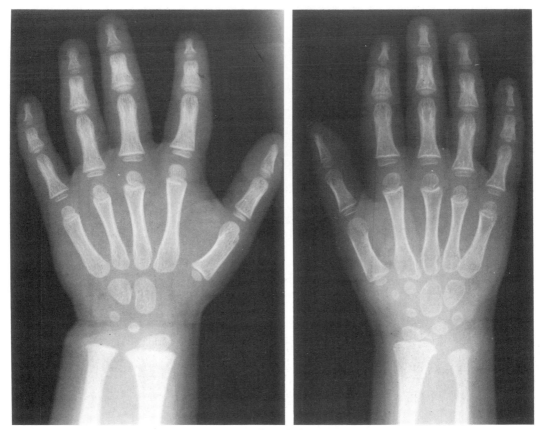

Figure 3–2. Advanced maturation associated with hyperemia. This 28 month old female had a rheumatoid arthritis-like picture on the right with marked advancement of the right ossification centers. There was associated hypoplasia of the distal radius and ulna, most likely on the basis of disuse. (From Poznanski, A. K., et al.: *Am. J. Phys. Anthropol.*, 35:417–432, 1971.)

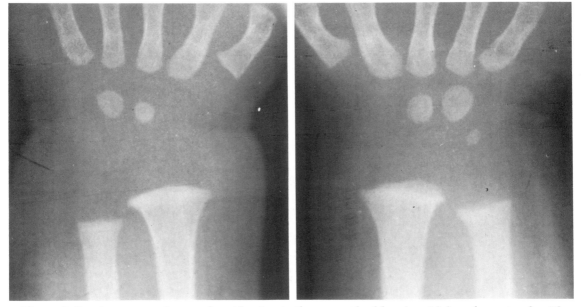

Figure 3–3. Asymmetry in carpal ossification in three month old male with hemihypertrophy. The hamate and capitate are more advanced on the right and the triquetrum is present only on the right side. (From Poznanski, A. K., et al.: *Am. J. Phys. Anthropol.*, 35:417–432, 1971.)

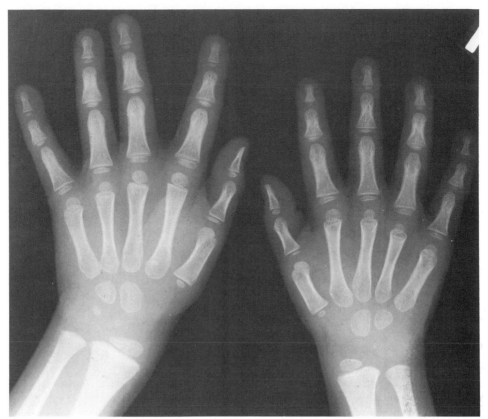

Figure 3-4. Delayed maturation due to spastic hemiplegia of unknown cause in a five year, seven month old boy. There is a definite difference in size and maturation between the two sides, the left being significantly more advanced. (From Poznanski, A. K., et al.: *Am. J. Phys. Anthropol.,* 35:417–432, 1971.)

may be associated with retardation of maturation on that side. This complication may be seen following ligation of blood vessels after brachial catheterization (Table 3–2).

SEQUENCE VARIATIONS

Considerable variation in ossification order exists in normal populations. The type of ossification sequence may vary with different populations and between the sexes. In the Stuart et al.[32] study, the triquetrum was the 16th bone to ossify in the male and the 23rd bone in the female. In Garn and Rohmann's[11] sequence the difference was not as great. Recent studies by Garn et al.[15] have shown that the lunate ossifies after the triquetrum in 93.2 per cent of white males and 100 per cent of normal white females. A late lunate is some-

what more common in blacks (Fig. 3–5).[8] The sequence of trapezium-trapezoid occurs in 41.8 per cent of males and 55.5 per cent of females. The incidence of the various ossification sequences is listed in Table 3–3 and is based on a large population.

Sequence variation is also genetically determined. Garn, Rohmann and Davis[13] found a correlation between children and their parents (0.3). The correlation was higher between siblings (0.4 to 0.6) and even higher between monozygotic twins (0.9). Osseous retardation may increase the number of abnormal sequences apparently present[12] if a longitudinal study is not used, since the sampling process tends to separate out sequences so that they are seen rather than missed.

Different sequences in maturation can also be seen in comparing children who are

TABLE 3-3. Frequency of Dichotomous Ossification Sequences in Children of European Ancestry

CENTER PRESENT	Sex	Capitate %	Capitate No.[1]	Hamate %	Hamate No.	Distal radius %	Distal radius No.	Triquetral %	Triquetral No.	Lunate %	Lunate No.	Scaphoid %	Scaphoid No.	Trapezium %	Trapezium No.	Trapezoid %	Trapezoid No.	Distal ulna %	Distal ulna No.
Capitate	M			96.0	75	97.6	42	100.0	224	100.0	403	100.0	789	100.0	823	100.0	800	100.0	1048
	F			94.9	79	100.0	23	100.0	93	100.0	208	100.0	380	100.0	371	100.0	383	100.0	614
Hamate	M	4.0	75			94.8	39	100.0	219	100.0	398	100.0	784	100.0	818	100.0	795	100.0	1043
	F	5.1	79			100.0	24	100.0	94	100.0	209	100.0	381	100.0	372	100.0	384	100.0	615
Distal radius	M	2.4	42	5.2	39			97.9	192	99.7	365	100.0	749	100.0	783	100.0	760	100.0	1008
	F	0.0	23	0.0	24			98.6	72	100.0	185	100.0	357	100.0	348	100.0	360	100.0	591
Triquetral	M	0.0	224	0.0	219	2.1	192			93.2	207*	99.8	567	99.6	603	99.8	578	100.0	824
	F	0.0	93	0.0	94	1.4	72			100.0	115	100.0	287	100.0	278	100.0	290	100.0	521
Lunate	M	0.0	403	0.0	398	0.3	365	6.8	207*			99.0	394	99.3	426*	98.3	411*	99.3	653
	F	0.0	208	0.0	209	0.0	185	0.0	115			97.7	180	95.0	181	94.0	199	98.8	416
Scaphoid	M	0.0	789	0.0	784	0.0	749	0.2	567	1.0	394			60.9	156*	53.7	149	90.8	317*
	F	0.0	380	0.0	381	0.0	357	0.0	287	2.3	180			46.2	119	51.4	103	97.5	246
Trapezium	M	0.0	823	0.0	818	0.0	783	0.4	603	0.7	426*	39.1	156*			41.8	161*	85.2	319*
	F	0.0	371	0.0	372	0.0	348	0.0	278	5.0	181	53.8	119			55.5	108	93.9	277
Trapezoid	M	0.0	800	0.0	795	0.0	760	0.2	578	1.7	411*	46.3	149	58.2	161*			90.7	304*
	F	0.0	383	0.0	384	0.0	360	0.0	290	6.0	199	48.6	103	44.5	108			97.5	243
Distal ulna	M	0.0	1048	0.0	1043	0.0	1008	0.0	824	0.7	653	9.2	317*	14.8	319*	9.3	304*		
	F	0.0	614	0.0	615	0.0	591	0.0	521	1.2	416	2.5	246	6.1	277	2.5	243		

[1] No. refers to the number of individuals exhibiting sequences involving the pair of centers in question, % refers to percentage of that number exhibiting the sequence shown, asterisks (*) designate sex differences significant at p = 0.05 or better, all data from the present study except capitate-hamate sequences taken from Garn and Rohmann (1960) for completeness. (From Garn, S. M., et al.: *Am. J. Phys. Anthropol.*, 37:111–115, 1972.)

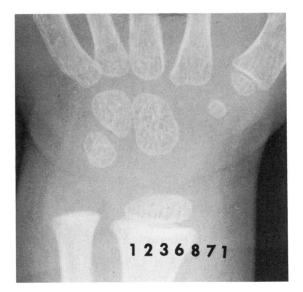

Figure 3–5. Late lunate bone in a three year old mentally retarded black girl. The late lunate is somewhat more common in blacks than in whites.

retarded in maturation to those who are advanced. Very distinct patterns were found by Poznanski et al.,[21] who compared children in the 5th percentile in the number of centers present (retarded) to those who were above the 95th percentile (advanced) (Table 3–4).

LOCAL FACTORS AFFECTING THE MATURATION OF ONLY A FEW BONES

A large number of conditions can cause some effect on the maturation of a specific ossification center. Advanced maturation

TABLE 3–4. Incidence of Sequence Variations in Advanced and Retarded Males*

		5TH PERCENTILE (retarded)		95TH PERCENTILE (advanced)	
	N	% of total in 5th percentile	N	% of total in 95th percentile	χ^2
Total males	151		96		
Total "abnormal"† sequence		59.0	47	49.0	1.06
Some relative delay of onset of					
triquetrum	43	28.5	11	11.5	7.79
lunate	4	2.6	2	2.1	0.03
scaphoid	13	8.6	8	8.3	0.02
trapezium	18	11.9	6	6.2	1.38
trapezoid	5	3.3	1	1.0	0.45
Some carpal relatively advanced to a phalangeal or metacarpal epiphysis	5	3.3	18	18.7	13.56
Triquetrum relatively advanced	2	1.3	6	6.2	3.03
Lunate relatively advanced	3	2.0	12	12.5	9.13

*This is based on children in the 10 State Nutrition Survey. (Reprinted from Poznanski et al.: *Am. J. Phys. Anthropol.*, 35:417–432, 1971.)
†Sequence used as "normal" was that described by Garn, Rohmann and Silverman, 1967.

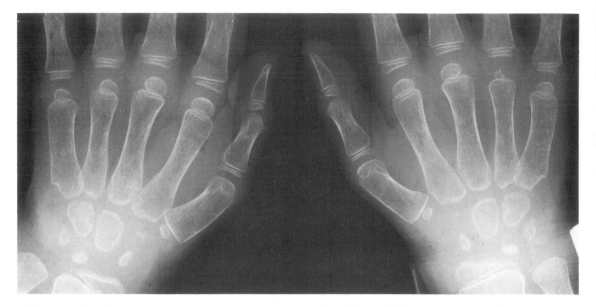

Figure 3–6. Local factors causing maturational delay. This child with rheumatoid arthritis was 5.2 years old. There is marked delay in ossification of the epiphysis of the right fourth metacarpal. Some of the carpals are also delayed. (From Poznanski, A. K., et al.: *Am. J. Phys. Anthropol.*, 35: 417–432, 1971.)

can occur from hyperemia of any cause and is not uncommon in rheumatoid arthritis, infection or healing fracture. Similarly, infection can delay the onset of maturation owing to damage of the epiphysis. Similar damage can occur from trauma, radiation therapy and adjacent tumors including multiple exostoses.

A number of congenital conditions are associated with delay or absence of a specific carpal center. Some of these are listed in Table 3–2. For example, the scaphoid is delayed or absent in any condition associated with absence of the thumb or hypoplasia of the radius. Thus, it can be seen in Franconi's anemia. Also, in hypoplasia of the thumb one of the epiphyses in the hypoplastic phalanx can be missing. Local advancement of skeletal maturation in the head of the fourth metacarpal in Turner's syndrome is responsible for the early fusion of this epiphysis and the resultant shortening of this bone. Early fusion is also seen in some of the brachydactyly syndromes. Damage to an epiphysis can cause either delayed maturation (Fig. 3–6) or advanced maturation.

Disproportion between the maturation of the carpals and phalanges can be seen in many conditions with extremes of maturation (Figs. 3–7 and 3–8). In most cases the maturation of the carpals is behind that of the phalanges, whether one had retarded maturation, as in trisomy 18, or advanced maturation, as in cerebral gigantism.

ADVANCED SKELETAL MATURATION

There are a number of conditions with advanced skeletal maturation, most of which are associated with sexual precocity. The causes of advanced maturation are listed in Table 3–5. In many of these conditions the degree of sexual maturation advance is parallel to the skeletal maturation. An exception to this is advanced maturation due to endocrine-secreting tumors, where the soft tissue changes appear to occur more rapidly than the alteration in maturation (Fig. 3–9). Obese children are generally more advanced maturationally than thin individuals. The maturational advancement in cerebral gigantism and lipodystrophy seems to be fairly parallel to the height age and bone age in these conditions, and is probably an acceleration of

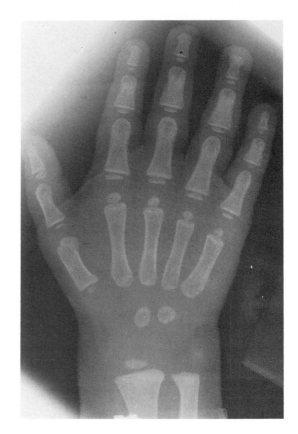

Figure 3-7. Relative advancement of phalanges over carpals. This is a 14 month old child with the salt-losing form of adrenogenital syndrome. The marked advancement is manifested mainly in the phalanges, which had a maturation of about 30 months. Metacarpals are intermediate in maturation (22 months), while the carpals are least advanced, showing maturation between 12 and 15 months. (From Poznanski, A. K., et al.: *Am. J. Phys. Anthropol.*, 35:417–432, 1971.)

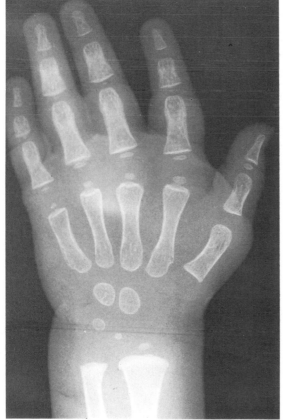

Figure 3-8. Advanced carpal over phalangeal maturation in 11.5 month old female who developed premature thelarche at two years of age. Four carpals are present while the distal phalangeal epiphyses have not yet ossified. A less significant difference was present at two years of age. The pattern of relative carpal advancement is more common in normally advanced children than in the malformation syndromes. (From Poznanski, A. K., et al.: *Am. J. Phys. Anthropol.*, 35:417–432, 1971.)

TABLE 3–5. Causes of Advanced Skeletal Maturation

A. ASSOCIATED WITH SEXUAL PRECOCITY°
  (1) True sexual precocity
    (a) Idiopathic—constitutional
    (b) Pineal gland tumors
    (c) Hypothalamic malformations—
      hamartoma, etc.
    (d) McCune-Albright syndrome—fibrous
      dysplasia
    (e) Other cerebral lesions—including other
      tumors
  (2) Gonadotropin-producing tumors
    (a) Hepatomas
    (b) Ovarian chorioepithelioma
  (3) Precocious pseudopuberty
    (a) Ovarian tumors—estrogen- or
      gonadotrophic-producing

    (b) Testicular tumors
    (c) Adrenal tumors
    (d) Drug induced
  (4) Incomplete sexual precocity
    (a) Premature thelarche
    (b) Premature adrenarche

B. OTHER CONDITIONS
  (1) Hyperthyroidism
  (2) Cerebral gigantism
  (3) Certain congenital malformation syndromes
    (a) Acrodysostosis
    (b) Beckwith-Wiedemann syndrome
    (c) Cockayne's syndrome
    (d) Marshall's syndrome
  (4) Obesity
  (5) Idiopathic

°Modified from Van Der Werff Ten Bosch: *In* Gardner, L. L. (Ed.): *Endocrine and Genetic Diseases.* W. B. Saunders Company, Philadelphia, 1969.

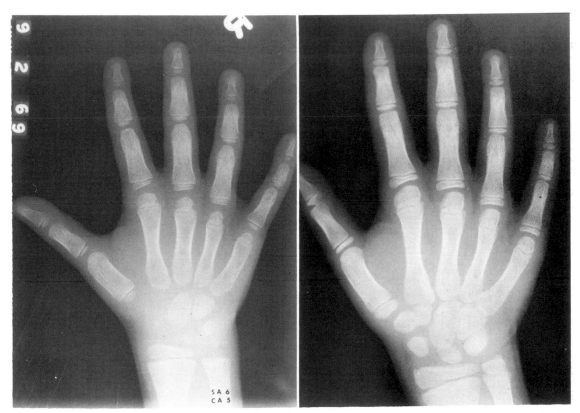

Figure 3–9. Advancement of maturation from an optic nerve glioma. This boy initially had a diencephalic syndrome from an optic nerve glioma and developed secondary sex characteristics. From age five to age seven his bone age shows a tremendous increase, changing from 6 to 12 years. The bone changes were not as advanced as the associated sexual maturation. (SA = skeletal age; CA = chronologic age.)

the entire maturation growth process rather than a specific effect on maturation alone.

CONDITIONS ASSOCIATED WITH RETARDATION OF MATURATION

A large number of conditions are associated with some skeletal maturational retardation (Table 3–6). The most dramatic retardation is probably seen in hypothyroidism, where the retardation can be five or more standard deviations away from normal. In fact, when retardation is of this degree the possibility of hypothyroidism has to be considered, whether it is on the basis of primary hypothyroidism or hypothyroidism secondary to panhypopituitarism. In true gigantism there is a paradoxical difference between maturation and growth. Despite the massive increase in size, the skeletal maturation remains the same. Growth hormone seems to have relatively little effect on maturation. When a child with hypopituitarism is treated with large doses of growth hormone, a remarkable increase in size may occur without significant increase in maturation (Fig. 3–1). Maturation is also retarded in most of the chromosomal disorders. In Down's syndrome it is slightly depressed. This is further discussed in Chapter 11. Maturation is markedly depressed in trisomy 18, in which the carpals are particularly affected.

Malnutrition is frequently associated with some bone retardation, but the maturation is not depressed as much as the growth of the individual. As a result the individuals end up as short adults, since their epiphyses fused relatively early as compared to their total growth. This explains the relatively short stature of the population in malnourished areas. Much of the secular increase in size which has been evident in the United States has been due to improved nutrition.

Many chronic illnesses tend to retard maturation. When the disease is of short duration, much of this retardation can be made up when the child recovers.[22] Congenital heart disease, particularly of the cyanotic type, is often associated with skeletal retardation.[35] Children suffering from maternal deprivation usually have a markedly retarded osseous maturation.[20] Although this may be partially associated

TABLE 3–6. Generalized Causes of Maturational Retardation

A. ENDOCRINE
 (1) Thyroid—hypothyroidism
 (2) Adrenal—Addison's disease, Cushing's disease
 (3) Gonadal—hypogonadism
 (4) Pituitary—panhypopituitarism
  —gigantism
  —craniopharyngioma

B. CHROMOSOMAL DISORDERS
 (1) Mongolism
 (2) Trisomy 18
 (3) XO
 (4) XXXXY
 (5) Most other chromosomal disorders

C. OTHER CONDITIONS
 (1) Malnutrition
 (2) Chronic illness, particularly congenital heart disease
 (3) Maternal deprivation
 (4) Bone dysplasia
 (5) Miscellaneous other malformation syndromes
 (6) Disorders of mineralization—rickets
 (7) Legg-Perthes disease
 (8) Idiopathic

with the lack of nutrition, other factors, including associated hypopituitarism, may be implicated. A large number of congenital malformation syndromes and bone dysplasias are usually associated with retarded bone age. In various rachitic conditions the lack of mineralization of the epiphyses and the relative widening of the epiphyseal plates give the appearance of marked skeletal retardation, which rapidly improves when the patient is treated.

REFERENCES

1. Acheson, R. M., Vicinus, J. H., and Fowler, G. B.: Studies in the Reliability of Assessing Skeletal Maturity from X-Rays. *Hum. Biol.*, 38:204–218, 1966. (Part III. Greulich-Pyle Atlas and Tanner-Whitehouse Method Contrasted.)
2. Anderson, M., Green, W. T., and Messner, M. B.: Growth and Predictions of Growth in the Lower Extremities. *J. Bone Joint Surg.*, 45A: 1–14, 1963.
3. Baer, M. J., and Durkatz, J.: Bilateral Asymmetry in Skeletal Maturation of the Hand and Wrist: A Roentgenographic Analysis. *Am. J. Phys. Anthropol.*, 15:181–196, 1957.
4. Bayley, N., and Pinneau, S. R.: Tables for Predicting Adult Height from Skeletal Age: Revised for Use with the Greulich-Pyle Hand Standards. *J. Pediat.*, 40:423–441, 1952.

5. Dreizen, S., Snodgrasse, R. M., Webb-Peploe, H., Parker, G. S., and Spies, T. D.: Bilateral Symmetry of Skeletal Maturation in the Human Hand and Wrist. *A.M.A. J. Dis. Child.,* 93:122–127, 1957.

6. Eklöf, O., and Ringertz, H.: A Method for Assessment of Skeletal Maturity. *Ann. Radiol.,* 10:330–336, 1967.

7. Garn, S. M.: The Applicability of North American Growth Standards in Developing Countries. *Canad. Med. Assoc. J.,* 93:914–919, 1965.

8. Garn, S. M.: Blacks Sequence Table. Personal communication, 1971.

9. Garn, S. M., Poznanski, A. K., and Nagy, J. M.: The Operational Meaning of Maturity Criteria. *Am. J. Phys. Anthropol.,* 35:319–326, 1971.

10. Garn, S. M., and Rohmann, C. G.: The Number of Hand-Wrist Centers. *Am. J. Phys. Anthropol.,* 18:293–299, 1960.

11. Garn, S. M., and Rohmann, C. G.: Variability in the Order of Ossification of the Bony Centers of the Hand and Wrist. *Am. J. Phys. Anthropol.,* 18:219–230, 1960.

12. Garn, S. M., Rohmann, C. G., and Blumenthal, T.: Ossification Sequence Polymorphism and Sexual Dimorphism in Skeletal Development. *Am. J. Phys. Anthropol.,* 24:101–115, 1966.

13. Garn, S. M., Rohmann, C. G., and Davis, A. A.: Genetics of Hand-Wrist Ossification. *Am. J. Phys. Anthropol.,* 21:33–40, 1963.

14. Garn, S. M., Rohmann, C. G., and Silverman, F. N.: Radiographic Standards for Postnatal Ossification and Tooth Calcification. *Med. Radiogr. Photogr.,* 43:45–66, 1967.

15. Garn, S. M., Sandusky, S. T., Miller, R. L., and Nagy, J. M.: Developmental Implications of Dichotomous Ossification Sequences in the Wrist Region. *Am. J. Phys. Anthropol.,* 37:111–115, 1972.

16. Garn, S. M., Silverman, F. N., and Rohmann, C. G.: A rational Approach to the Assessment of Skeletal Maturation. *Ann. Radiol.,* 7:297–307, 1964.

17. Greulich, W. W., and Pyle, S. I.: *Radiographic Atlas of Skeletal Development of the Hand and Wrist,* 2nd Ed. Stanford University Press, Stanford, California, 1959.

18. Hoerr, N. L., Pyle, S. I., and Francis, C. C.: *Radiographic Atlas of Skeletal Development of the Foot and Ankle.* Charles C Thomas, Publisher, Springfield, Illinois, 1962.

19. Johnston, F. E., and Jahina, S. B.: The Contribution of the Carpal Bones to the Assessment of Skeletal Age. *Am. J. Phys. Anthropol.,* 23:349–354, 1965.

20. Powell, G. F., Brasel, J. A., and Blizzard, R. M.: Emotional Deprivation and Growth Retardation Simulating Idiopathic Hypopituitarism. I. Clinical Evaluation of the Syndrome. *N. Engl. J. Med.,* 276:1271–1278, 1967.

21. Poznanski, A. K., Garn, S. M., Kuhns, L. R., and Sandusky, S. T.: Dysharmonic Maturation of the Hand in the Congenital Malformation Syndromes. *Am. J. Phys. Anthropol.,* 35:417–432, 1971.

22. Prader, A., Tanner, J. M., and von Harnack, G. A.: Catch-up Growth Following Illness or Starvation. An Example of Developmental Canalization in Man. *J. Pediat.,* 62:646–659, 1963.

23. Pryor, J. W.: The Hereditary Nature of Variation in the Ossification of Bones. *Anat. Rec.,* 1:84–88, 1907.

24. Pyle, S. I., and Hoerr, N. L.: *A Radiographic Standard of Reference for the Growing Knee.* Charles C Thomas, Publisher, Springfield, Illinois, 1969.

25. Pyle, S. I., Waterhouse, A. M., and Greulich, W. W.: *A Radiographic Standard of Reference for the Growing Hand and Wrist.* The Press of Case-Western Reserve University, Cleveland, Ohio, 1971.

26. Roche, A. F., Davila, G. H., and Eyman, S. L.: A Comparison Between Greulich-Pyle and Tanner-Whitehouse Assessments of Skeletal Maturity. *Radiology,* 98:273–280, 1971.

27. Roche, A. F., Davila, G. H., Pasternack, B. A., and Walton, M. J.: Some Factors Influencing the Replicability of Assessments of Skeletal Maturity (Greulich-Pyle). *Am. J. Roentgenol.,* 109:299–306, June 1970.

28. Roche, A. F., and French, N.Y.: Differences in Skeletal Maturity Levels Between the Knee and Hand. *Am. J. Roentgenol.,* 109:307–312, 1970.

29. Roche, A. F., and Johnson, J. M.: A Comparison Between Methods of Calculating Skeletal Age (Greulich-Pyle). *Am. J. Phys. Anthropol.,* 30:221–230, 1969.

30. Rotch, T. M.: A Study of the Development of the Bones in Childhood by the Roentgen Method, with the View of Establishing a Developmental Index for the Grading of and the Protection of Early Life. *Trans. Assoc. Am. Physicians,* 24:603–630, 1909.

31. Schmid, F., and Moll, H.: *Atlas Der Nonmalen und Pathologischen Handskeletenwicklung,* Springer Verlag, Berlin, 1960.

32. Stuart, H. C., Pyle, S. I., Cornoni, J., and Reed, R. B.: Onsets, Completions and Spans of Ossification in the 29 Bone-Growth Centers of the Hand and Wrist. *Pediatrics,* 29:237–249, 1962.

33. Sugiura, Y., and Nakazawa, O.: *Roentgen Diagnosis of Skeletal Development.* Chugai-Igaku Company, Tokyo, Japan.

34. Tanner, J. M., Whitehouse, R. H., and Healy, J. B.: *Standards for Skeletal Age.* 1962 International Children's Centre, Paris, France.

35. White, R. I., Jr., Jordan, C. E., Fischer, K. C., Dorst, J. P., Nagy, J. M., Garn, S. M., and Neill, C. A.: Delayed Skeletal Growth and Maturation in Adolescent Congenital Heart Disease. *Invest. Radiol.,* 6:326–332, 1971.

ARTERIOGRAPHY

by Joseph J. Bookstein, M.D.

It was in 1896, shortly after the discovery of the roentgen ray, that Haschek and Lindenthal[6] injected metallic salts into the arteries of an amputated specimen and produced the first arteriogram of the hand. Despite this precocious inauguration, however, angiography of the hand has received only limited clinical application. Recently, with the development of better contrast agents and simpler methods for intra-arterial injection, digital arteriography has been used more frequently. Its primary indication has been in the evaluation of digital ischemia. Interesting observations have been recorded in several collagen diseases, such as scleroderma and rheumatoid arthritis. To a lesser degree, digital arteriography is also useful in evaluating nonocclusive disease of the arteries, such as arteriovenous fistulas and aneurysms.

TECHNIQUE OF DIGITAL ARTERIOGRAPHY

The simplest and safest technique for performing digital arteriography is by direct puncture of the brachial artery just above the antecubital fossa, where the artery is palpable medial to the distal tendon of the biceps. In this region the artery pursues a relatively straight course and is partially fixed by the lacertus fibrosus.

By extending and variously supinating the forearm, the artery may be placed in its most palpable position. Rotation so that the thumb is superior usually is optimal. Local infiltration is performed using minimal volumes of anesthetics so as not to obscure the brachial pulse. Care must be exercised to avoid puncturing the artery during anesthesia, because of the strong tendency of the brachial artery to go into spasm. A skin nick is made, usually with an 18 gauge needle, and the artery is then punctured with a 19 or 20 gauge cannula-stylet combination. The cannula is aimed distally, and passed through both walls of the artery. The stylet is removed and the cannula gently withdrawn until blood spurts from the hub. A flexible guide wire is then advanced into the artery about 1 inch beyond the end of the cannula and the cannula is advanced over the guide wire for 1 cm. If advanced too far, the cannula is likely to enter one of the branches of the brachial artery. After successful placement, the cannula is attached to a flexible connector and the system is flushed with heparinized saline. The hand is taped in an extended position over a Schonander changer. Generally the grid is removed. By placing the hand diagonally on a 14 inch by 14 inch changer, the entire hand and most of the forearm can be filmed.

We routinely inject 15 mg. of tolazoline, diluted with 10 ml. of saline, into the cannula over a period of 30 seconds, and inject contrast medium after another 30 second delay. The tolazoline markedly accelerates blood flow and dilates the smaller and medium-sized arteries, greatly enhancing arterial visualization. It also eliminates spasm, so that any stenoses demonstrated can be ascribed to organic disease. Ten ml. of Conray* (60 per cent methylglucamine iothalamate) are injected in 1½ seconds, and films are obtained at the rate of one per second for 10 seconds. Often the serial examination is supplemented by a second injection, where a single exposure is made with the hand resting on a cardboard cassette, a technique that provides excellent resolution (see Figs. 4–4, 4–6, 4–10 and 4–14).

An alternate method for delivering contrast medium utilizes a retrograde femoral approach. By using a catheter with a gentle distal S curvature, often in combination with a C-shaped guide, a catheter can be easily passed from the arch into the distal brachial artery. Because of the slight added risk, we reserve this approach for cases where direct puncture of the brachial artery cannot be accomplished.

Other techniques for digital arteriography have been described, including a direct operative approach, puncture of the axillary artery or puncture of the subclavian artery. I believe these techniques are largely obsolete.

NORMAL ANATOMY AND THE NORMAL ARTERIOGRAM

The hand is supplied by the radial and ulnar arteries, which arise from the brachial artery shortly below the elbow. At times the brachial artery bifurcates considerably above the elbow and either the radial or ulnar artery may not be visualized by a single puncture at the level of the antecubital fossa. In about 10 per cent of cases, a persistent median artery contributes importantly to the blood supply of the hand.

The arterial anatomy varies considerably (Fig. 4–1). Typically, there are two volar

---

*Registered trademark; available from Mallinckrodt Pharmaceuticals, St. Louis, Missouri.

arches, a superficial and a deep, usually formed by terminal branches of the radial and ulnar arteries. The superficial arch is larger, and generally gives rise to three common volar digital arteries, which in turn bifurcate into proper digital arteries of the second, third, fourth and fifth digits. The deep volar arch gives rise to a radialis indicis volaris (proper digital artery to the radial aspect of the second digit), which may arise in common with or separately from the princeps pollicis artery supplying the thumb. Arcuate branches pass around the phalanges to connect the proper digital arteries. This pattern was present in about 35 per cent of 650 dissections in the series of Coleman and Anson.[3]

Variations from this basic pattern are indicated in Figure 4–1B through J. A persistent median artery was present in 9.9 per cent of the series by Coleman and Anson (Figs. 4–1D,E,I,J).[3] An arch formed entirely from the ulnar artery was present in 37 per cent (Fig. 4–1C). Twenty-one per cent demonstrated an incomplete arch, i.e., there were no important anastomoses between the two major arches of the hand, and the ulnar artery did not extend radially to supply the thumb. These arterial variations help explain the variability of symptoms after occlusion of the same artery in different patients.

A dorsal carpal rete is present, formed from the radial and interosseous arteries and perforator branches. The dorsal rete gives origin to dorsal metacarpal arteries, which then bifurcate into dorsal digital arteries. These dorsal arteries are small and usually invisible on clinical angiography.

A normal arteriogram is shown in Figure 4–2. The film represents a single exposure obtained on a cardboard cassette 4 seconds after the onset of injection. Contrast material normally appears at the wrist about 1 second after the onset of injection and reaches the tips of the digits by 4 seconds. The superficial volar arch is complete. A deep arch is not present. The dorsal carpal rete is barely visible (arrow).

The arteries are usually smooth and tapering, but not uncommonly digital stenoses or occlusions and collateral flow can be seen in elderly, otherwise normal patients. In a series of 94 cases studied with postmortem arteriography, Laws et al.[9]

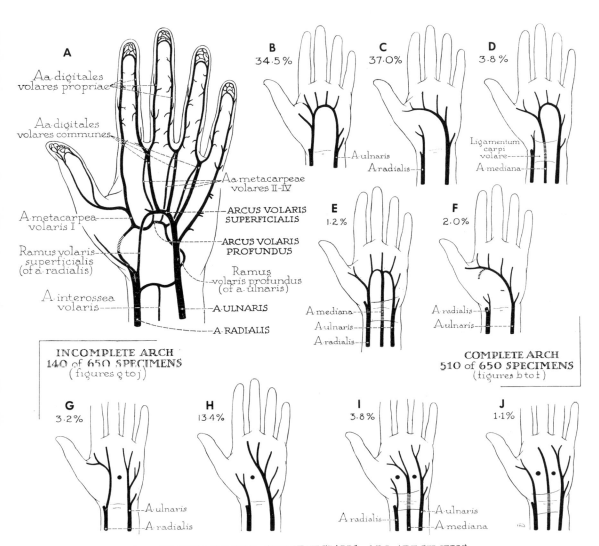

A

Aa. digitales
volares propriae

Aa. digitales
volares communes

Aa. metacarpeae
volares II–IV

A. metacarpea
volaris I

ARCUS VOLARIS
SUPERFICIALIS

Ramus volaris
superficialis
(of a. radialis)

ARCUS VOLARIS
PROFUNDUS

Ramus
volaris profundus
(of a. ulnaris)

A. interossea
volaris

A. ULNARIS

A. RADIALIS

B 34.5%

C 37.0%

A. ulnaris

A. radialis

D 3.8%

Ligamentum
carpi
volare

A. mediana

E 1.2%

A. mediana

A. ulnaris

A. radialis

F 2.0%

A. radialis

A. ulnaris

INCOMPLETE ARCH
140 of 650 SPECIMENS
(figures g to j)

COMPLETE ARCH
510 of 650 SPECIMENS
(figures b to f)

G 3.2%

A. ulnaris

A. radialis

H 13.4%

I 3.8%

A. radialis

A. ulnaris

A. mediana

J 1.1%

ARCUS VOLARIS SUPERFICIALIS, 650 SPECIMENS

Figure 4–1. Diagrammatic representations of the digital arterial supply. In *A*, the typical distribution is indicated. Parts *B* through *J* indicate common variants. (From Coleman and Anson: *Surg. Gynecol, Obstet.*, 113:409–424, 1961.)

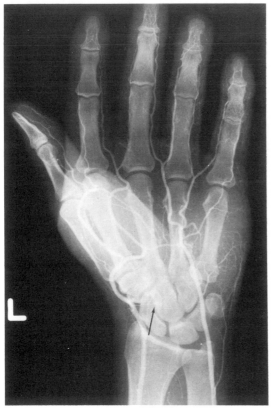

Figure 4–2. Normal digital arteriogram. Cardboard technique. There is a complete superficial palmar arch. A deep palmar arch is not present. The dorsal carpal rete is faintly demonstrated (*arrow*). Radial and ulnar proper digital arteries are present in each digit.

found occlusive lesions in 31, all but one of whom were over the age of 50. These occlusive lesions were often associated with atherosclerosis of the aorta or coronary arteries, and were presumably due to atherosclcrosis in the majority of cases.

As already mentioned, the brachial artery not infrequently bifurcates considerably above the elbow, so that nonvisualization of a radial or ulnar artery may be due to injection distal to the bifurcation and, in the absence of other signs of obstruction, should not be ascribed to occlusion.

PATHOLOGIC CONDITIONS

Digital Ischemia

By far the most common indication for digital arteriography is in the evaluation of digital ischemia. Table 4–1 presents our classification of causes of digital occlusive disease.

Arteriography may play a crucial role in differentiating organic from functional disease, in localizing the site of organic obstruction, in elucidating the cause of obstruction and in planning and evaluating therapy.

Scleroderma

At our institution, digital arteriography has been commonly employed in the investigation of patients with scleroderma. The arteriograms were part of a broad investigational work-up of these patients, which has been reported in detail elsewhere.[5]

Histologic examination of digital arteries from patients with scleroderma has revealed severe and consistent abnormalities.[11] The major abnormality is intimal thickening of the arterioles. This may appear as acute panarteritis, intimal proliferation with varying degrees of stenosis or arteriosclerotic lesions. Abnormalities are unique in degree and extent, and have even been observed in the vasa vasorum.

Angiography in scleroderma reflects the

TABLE 4–1. Causes of Digital Ischemia

A. ORGANIC
  (1) Collagen disease
      (a) Scleroderma°
      (b) Rheumatoid arthritis°
      (c) Polyarteritis°
      (d) Dermatomyositis°
      (e) Lupus erythematosus
  (2) Trauma
      (a) Hypothenar hammer syndrome°
      (b) Electrical burn°
      (c) Frostbite°
      (d) Hemodialysis shunts°
      (e) Other
  (3) Arterial disease
      (a) Arteriosclerosis°
      (b) Embolism°
      (c) Thromboangiitis obliterans°
      (d) Neurovascular compression syndrome
  (4) Intravascular Coagulopathies
      (a) Polycythemia vera
      (b) Leukemia
      (c) Thrombotic thrombocytopenic purpura
      (d) Others

B. FUNCTIONAL

°Discussed in text.

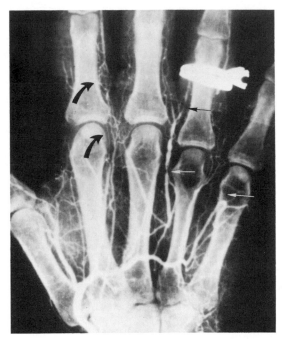

Figure 4-3. Scleroderma. Screen technique. Multiple stenoses are seen in common and proper digital arteries (*straight arrows*). The ulnar artery is occluded and does not contribute appreciably to the superficial palmar arch. Some collateral circulation is seen bridging obstructed arteries (*curved arrows*).

flow, and contrast medium often did not reach the fingertips for 10 seconds or more after injection.

In five patients, repeat arteriograms were performed after treatment with Potaba* (potassium aminobenzoate). Despite objective improvement of skin lesions in four of these patients, arterial lesions remained stable in two and progressed in three.

In summary, results in our cases have indicated that (1) almost all patients with scleroderma have organic occlusive disease of the arteries of the wrist, hand or fingers; (2) arteriography need not be performed in most patients with scleroderma, but can be helpful in diagnosing or excluding scleroderma in equivocal cases, especially when signs or symptoms of digital ischemia are present; and (3) arteriography was more reliable than plethysmography in evaluating the presence of occlusive digital arterial disease.

---

*Registered trademark; available from Glenwood Laboratories, Inc., Tenafly, New Jersey.

severe changes noted histologically. In our review of arteriograms in 31 patients,[5] severe stenoses or occlusions were present in 29 (Figs. 4-3 and 4-4). Most of these patients had multiple areas of stenosis. The ulnar arteries were involved in 11 of 31, but the radial artery was involved in only one case. The common digitals were often not involved, while the proper digital arteries were involved in 90 per cent of cases (Fig. 4-4), most commonly in the mid or distal portions. The third and fourth digits were involved in 80 to 90 per cent of patients, the second in 75 per cent, the thumb in 50 per cent and the fifth digit in 20 per cent. Collateral circulation around sites of obstruction was frequent (Fig. 4-4). In addition to discrete stenoses and occlusions, generalized narrowing of common and proper digital arteries was often observed, a feature which may simply reflect the markedly reduced blood flow to the hand. Serial films have demonstrated marked slowing of linear velocity of blood

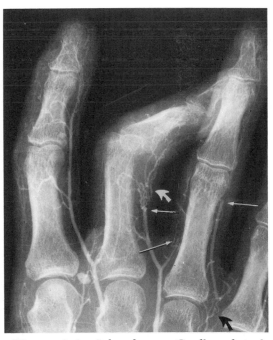

Figure 4-4. Scleroderma. Cardboard technique. Note discrete occlusions of proper digital arteries (*straight arrows*) with bridging collateral arteries (*curved arrows*).

Rheumatoid Arthritis

Histologic examination of the digital arteries of patients with rheumatoid arthritis has frequently demonstrated intimal thickening with little or no cellular reaction, and some central thrombosis with partial recanalization.[8, 13] In their series of arteriographic examinations of patients with rheumatoid arthritis, Laws et al.[8] demonstrated areas of arterial stenosis in 26 of 38 cases. Each of the four fingers was involved with equal frequency, although there was a tendency for more frequent involvement in digits showing arthritic changes. Collateral circulation occurred often, and apparently was responsible for maintaining adequate circulation to the fingertips, as opposed to the severe distal ischemic changes frequently present in patients with scleroderma. Hyperemic areas were present in 22 of 37 patients, particularly near bony erosions or in regions of synovial proliferation in joints or tendon sheaths.

In most patients with rheumatoid arthritis, arteriography is not indicated and we have accordingly performed arteriography in very few. An example is shown in Figure 4–5, in which two isolated proper digital occlusions are present. The original film demonstrated some hypervascularity over the carpal joints.

Other Collagen Diseases

In three patients with polyarteritis, Laws et al.[8] demonstrated abrupt occlusions with well-developed collateral circulation. They felt the arteriographic pattern was somewhat characteristic. In our single arteriographic examination in a patient with polyarteritis, characteristic aneurysms of digital arteries were present with associated occlusive disease (Fig. 4–6). In addition, innumerable aneurysms were seen on intestinal arteriography, although few were evident on renal arteriography.

In one patient with dermatomyositis, Laws et al.[8] observed occlusions of the digital arteries. We have studied one patient with dermatomyositis who had a normal arteriogram, and one patient with mixed scleroderma and dermatomyositis who had occlusions of the proper digital arteries. Of two patients with a diagnosis of Raynaud's disease, and one each with vasospastic disease and diffuse morphea, none had arteriographic abnormalities.

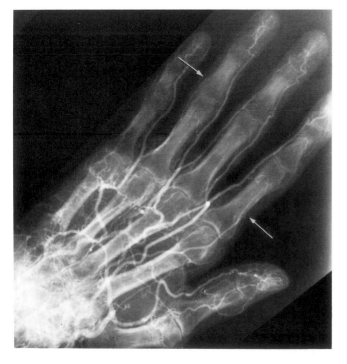

Figure 4–5. Rheumatoid arthritis. Magnification technique with high speed screen–film combination. Note that the technical quality is inferior to the cardboard technique shown in Figures 4–4 and 4–6. Isolated discrete occlusions are noted (*arrows*). There was mild hypervascularity present on later films over the wrist joints, but no hypervascularity is evident in the fingers despite low-grade activity.

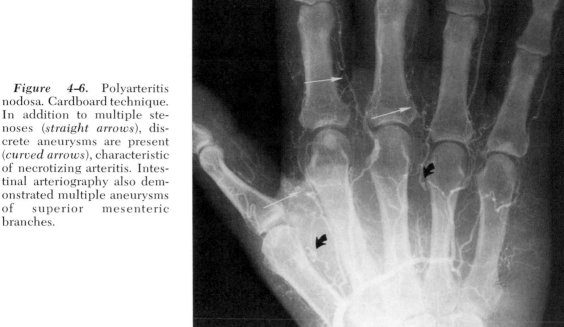

Figure 4-6. Polyarteritis nodosa. Cardboard technique. In addition to multiple stenoses (*straight arrows*), discrete aneurysms are present (*curved arrows*), characteristic of necrotizing arteritis. Intestinal arteriography also demonstrated multiple aneurysms of superior mesenteric branches.

The Hypothenar Hammer Syndrome

Single or repeated trauma to the hypothenar region can damage the ulnar artery and produce thrombosis, spasm or aneurysm. The most susceptible area is immediately beyond the volar carpal ligament, where the artery passes over the hook of the hamate bone and is protected by relatively little overlying tissue. Post-traumatic ischemia of this type has been labeled the hypothenar hammer syndrome by Conn et al.[4]

The first known case was described in 1772, and it followed repeated trauma from the butt of a coachman's whip against the palm of the hand. The syndrome is most frequent in men who use the hand repeatedly as a hammer for pushing, pounding or twisting, as in some types of factory work. The condition has also been described in karate experts, and in those constantly using a cane or crutch. Because of the variability of the arterial supply to the fingers and the associated collateral circulation (Fig. 4–1), any finger may show signs of ischemia in hypothenar hammer syndrome.

Arteriography will demonstrate narrowing, occlusion or aneurysm of the ulnar artery, usually in the vicinity of the hook of the hamate bone (Fig. 4–7). Most symptomatic patients will also show one or more occluded digital arteries and one or more incomplete palmar arches or inadequate digital or volar metacarpal arteries.[2] Arteriography plays a crucial role in diagnosis of this condition, in differentiating it from other causes of digital ischemia and in planning therapy.

Therapy may consist of endarterectomy or excision of the thrombosed arterial segment.[7] Indirect therapy, using stellate ganglion block, often supplemented by adrenergic blocking agents[4] or sympathectomy, is advocated by some.

Electrical Burns

The hands and arms are frequently injured in patients suffering electrical burns. Injury may be extremely severe, with virtual electrocoagulation of all tissues within the limb. Evaluation of potential viability may be impossible clinically, and arteriography may be helpful. Where the limb is not salvageable, multiple discrete arterial obstructions and total absence of flow to various segments may be seen (Fig. 4–8).

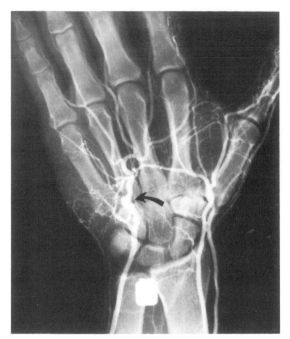

Figure 4–7. Hypothenar hammer syndrome. Right digital arteriography of a 28 year old factory worker who pounded car moldings into place with his right hand, and who complained of numbness and coldness of the second, third and fourth digits. Note multiple areas of irregularity and dilatation of the ulnar artery adjacent to the hook of the hamate bone (*arrow*). Multiple occlusions of distal proper digital arteries were also present, and could have been secondary to embolism from thrombosis within the abnormal portion of the ulnar artery. Note that the ulnar distribution of the second, third and fourth digits corresponds nicely with the symptomatic fingers.

Arterial spasm and thrombosis may also be evident.

Frostbite

The importance of vascular injury in the pathogenesis of frostbite has been recognized for some time.[12] Experimental studies have demonstrated that within minutes after thaw, capillaries and venules become occluded with thrombi. Several hours after thaw most blood flows through precapillary shunts. We have performed arteriography in one patient with old frostbite injury of the hands and demonstrated marked slowing of blood flow and apparent occlusions of multiple proper digital arteries (Fig. 4–9).

Hemodialysis Shunts

Patients may have signs and symptoms of digital ischemia after performance of shunt for hemodialysis. Usually the ischemia can be directly ascribed to occlusion of one or more major arteries supplying the hand, as well as to incomplete development of palmar arches and collateral routes.

Other Types of Trauma

Other types of injury may produce arterial spasm or thrombosis and secondary

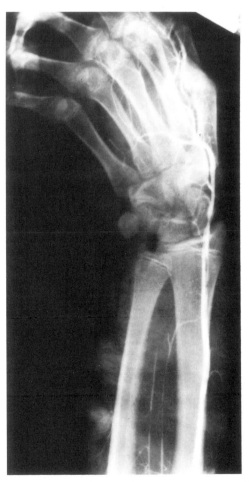

Figure 4–8. Electrical burn. Arteriography two days after burn, and after fasciotomy, demonstrates complete occlusion of the ulnar artery and multiple occluded digital arteries. Thrombosis is seen within the distal radial artery. The hand was infected. The lack of demonstrable arterial supply indicated the futility of conservative therapy, and midforearm amputation was performed.

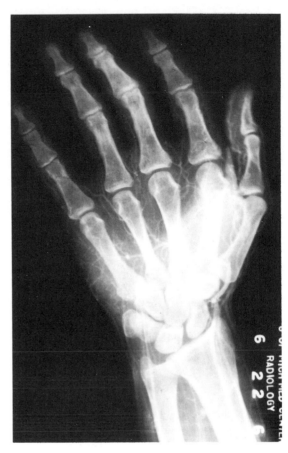

Figure 4–9. Frostbite had occurred two and a half years previously. The patient had complained of pain and numbness of the fingers since that time, especially after exposure to cold. The arteriogram demonstrates narrowing and occlusion of proper digital arteries of the second through fifth digits.

digital ischemia. Fractures of the upper extremity may be associated with arterial compression, and severe ischemic injury (Volkmann's contracture) may supervene. Bullet and knife wounds not infrequently produce arterial injury with secondary disruption, spasm or thrombosis. In these conditions it is particularly important to reduce spasm with tolazoline during arteriography so that organic changes can be clearly evaluated.

Arteriosclerosis

Occlusive lesions of the digital arteries, probably largely atherosclerotic in origin, were frequently found in the digital arteries of older patients in the arteriographic-histologic studies by Laws et al.[9] We also have frequently noted occlusions of digital arteries in otherwise normal patients. However, collateral circulation generally is abundant, and these lesions are ordinarily not associated with symptoms.

Clinically significant atherosclerotic disease involving the upper extremity is most frequent in the subclavian artery at its origin. However, description of these changes is beyond the scope of this chapter.

Embolism

Occasionally thrombotic emboli may lodge in arteries of the upper extremities. Usually this is the result of thrombosis superimposed on atherosclerosis in the proximal subclavian artery. In Figure 4–10, an arteriogram is demonstrated in a patient who developed sudden signs of ischemia of the hand. The arteriogram demonstrates evidence of organizing emboli, and an intimal web was apparent on the original film. This patient also had an impaired axillary pulse and a bruit was present low in the neck, suggesting that thromboembolism was superimposed on atherosclerotic disease of the proximal subclavian artery. Embolism to the upper extremity may also

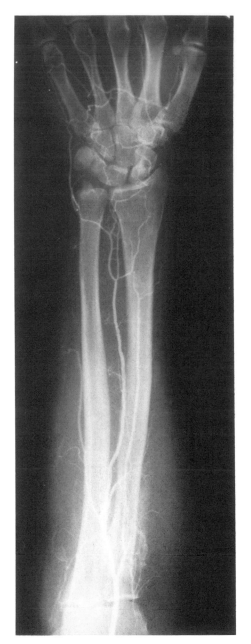

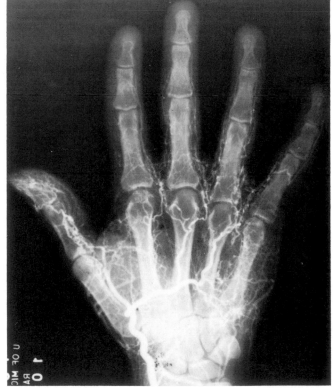

Figure 4–10. Arterial embolism. There was sudden onset of pain and pallor in the left hand several days prior to radiographic examination. The left axillary pulse was reduced and a bruit was heard over the left supraclavicular region. Arteriography demonstrates occlusion of the distal radial and ulnar arteries, with the majority of the blood supply to the hand flowing through the interosseous artery. On the original films, a web was visible in the interosseous artery, an appearance characteristic of an organized embolus. Arterial obstructions are thought to be secondary to thrombotic emboli which originate from atherosclerotic disease at the origin of the left subclavian artery.

Figure 4–11. Buerger's disease (thromboangiitis obliterans). A 45 year old male developed aching of the feet six months earlier, and cyanosis and pain of the tip of the right index finger four months earlier. Arteriography demonstrates occlusions of many proper digital arteries with extensive collateral circulation near the metacarpophalangeal joints. The size and number of collateral vessels are greater than are usually seen in scleroderma, and suggested the possibility of Buerger's disease. Later films showed abundant distal vessels.

be secondary to intracardiac clot or tumor, or bacterial endocarditis.

Thromboangiitis Obliterans

The upper extremity is involved in perhaps 50 per cent of patients with thromboangiitis obliterans.[10] In the single patient we have examined with upper extremity involvement, a rather characteristic appearance was seen (Fig. 4–11). Occlusions involved relatively larger arteries of the hand, and collateral arteries were larger, more tortuous and more abundant than we have observed in other conditions. These arteriographic features are analogous to those so well described in thromboangiitis obliterans of the lower extremities.

Nonischemic Conditions

Occasionally conditions other than digital ischemia serve as indications for digital arteriography.

Occupational Acroosteolysis

In 1967 the syndrome of occupational acroosteolysis was described by Wilson et al.[16] The syndrome is characterized primarily by resorption of portions of distal phalangeal tufts, some digital tenderness and a Raynaud-like phenomenon, and was seen in 31 of 3000 workers involved in the manufacture of polyvinylchloride. We have performed arteriography in one patient. Mild and nonspecific hypervascularity was evident adjacent to areas of bony resorption (Fig. 4–12), and the princeps pollicis was distally occluded. I am not aware of other descriptions of arteriography in this condition.

Tumors

In patients with soft tissue tumors of the hand, arteriography may clarify the nature and extent of the lesion. Figure 4–13 demonstrates the arteriogram of a patient with an arteriovenous malformation of the hand. In Figure 4–14, a close-up view of

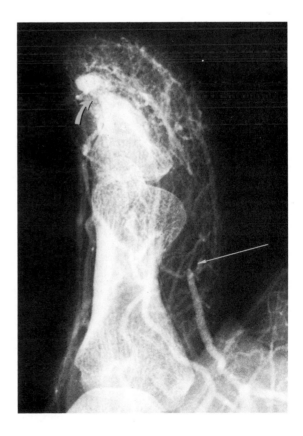

Figure 4–12. Occupational acroosteolysis. A 28 year old male with a history of two and a half years of exposure to polyvinylchloride complained of tingling and pallor of the hands on exposure to cold for two and a half years. Intermittent swelling of the hands developed after cold exposure two years previously, but permanent hand swelling was now present. X-rays of the hands had demonstrated transverse defects of the tufts of the first through fourth digits on the left, and of the third through fifth digits on the right.

Arteriography, cardboard technique, demonstrates an occlusion of the princeps pollicis (*straight arrow*). In the region of the underlying osteolytic defect (*curved arrow*) there is mild hypervascularity. In other areas, including digits which were symptomatic, no arterial occlusions were seen, and it is possible that the occlusion here is coincidental. However, there was hypervascularity adjacent to all areas of bone resorption.

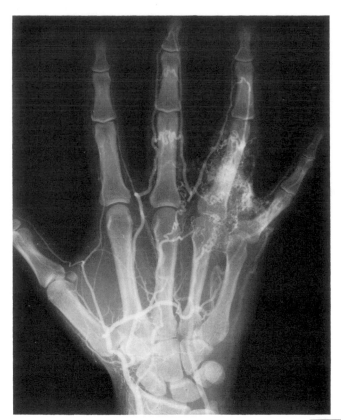

Figure 4–13. Arteriovenous malformation of the hand. Several arteries had been surgically ligated. Note numerous tortuous vessels and early venous opacification.

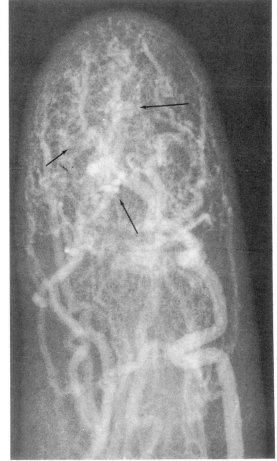

Figure 4–14. Pacinian neurofibromatosis. This 66 year old woman had exquisite pain at the tip of the second finger for one year. Arteriography demonstrated some enlarged and tortuous vessels (*arrows*). At operation, multiple pacinian neurofibromas were removed, and the symptoms completely disappeared.

the arteriogram in a patient with pacinian neurofibromatosis of the tip of the second digit is shown. In this case, the tumor was not discretely outlined on angiography, and only slight distortion of vessels and hypervascularity indicated the presence of a pathologic lesion.

Aneurysms

Traumatic and mycotic aneurysms of digital arteries have been described.[14] We have not had the opportunity to study such patients.

REFERENCES

1. Butsch, J. L., and Janes, J. J.: Injuries of the Superficial Palmar Arch. *J. Trauma*, 3:505–516, 1963.
2. Calenoff, L.: Angiography of the Hand: Guidelines for Interpretation. *Radiology*, 102:331–335, 1972.
3. Coleman, S. S., and Anson, B. J.: Arterial Patterns in the Hand Based Upon a Study of 650 Specimens. *Surg. Gynecol., Obstet.*, 113:409–424, 1961.
4. Conn, J., Bergan, J. J., and Bell, J. L.: Hypothenar Hammer Syndrome: Post-traumatic Digital Ischoemia. *Surgery*, 68:1122–1128, 1970.
5. Dabich, L., Bookstein, J., Zweifler, A., and Zarafonetis, C.: Digital Arteries in Patients with Scleroderma: Arteriographic and Plethysmographic Studies. *Arch. Int. Med.*, 130:708–714, 1972.
6. Haschek, E., and Lindenthal, O.: A Contribution to the Practical Use of the Photography According to Roentgen. *Wien. Klin. Wochneschr.*, 9:63, 1896.
7. Kleinert, H. E., and Volantes, G. J.: Thrombosis of the Palmar Arterial Arch and its Tributaries: Etiology and Newer Concepts in Treatment. *J. Trauma*, 5:447–455, 1965.
8. Laws, J. W., Lillie, J. G., and Scott, J. T.: Arteriographic Appearances in Rheumatoid Arthritis and other Disorders. *Brit. J. Radiol.*, 36:477–493, 1963.
9. Laws, J. W., Sallab, R. A., and Scott, J. T.: An Arteriographic and Histological Study of Digital Arteries. *Brit. J. Radiol.*, 40:740–747, 1967.
10. McPherson, J. R., Juergens, J. L., and Gifford, R. W.: Thromboangiitis Obliterans and Arteriosclerosis Obliterans. *Ann. Int. Med.*, 59:288–296, 1963.
11. Norton, W. L.: Vascular Disease in Progressive Systemic Sclerosis. *Ann. Int. Med.*, 73:317–324, 1970.
12. Quintanella, R., Krusen, F. H., and Esser, H. E.: Studies on Frostbite with Special Reference to Treatment and the Effect on Minute Blood Vessels. *Am. J. Physiol.*, 149:149–161, 1947.
13. Scott, J. T., Sallab, R. A., and Laws, J. W.: The Digital Artery Design in Rheumatoid Arthritis — Further Observations. *Brit. J. Radiol.*, 40:748–754, 1967.
14. Sutton, D.: Arteriography of the Upper Extremities; *In* Abrams, H. L. (Ed.): *Angiography.* Little, Brown and Company, Boston, 1971.
15. Wegelius, U.: Angiography of the Hand. Clinical and Postmortem Investigations. *Acta Radiol.*, Supplement 315, Stockholm, 1972.
16. Wilson, R., McCormick, W., Tattum, C., and Creech, J.: Occupational Acroosteolysis. *J.A.M.A.*, 201:577–581, 1967.

Chapter 5

OTHER SPECIAL PROCEDURES

TOMOGRAPHY
XERORADIOGRAPHY
ELECTRON RADIOGRAPHY
ARTHROGRAPHY AND THE STUDY OF THE
  DIGITAL SHEATHS
  Arthrography of the Wrist
  Arthrography of Other Joints in the Hand
  Injection of Digital Sheaths of the Hand

RADIODERMATOGRAPHY
THERMOGRAPHY
RADIOISOTOPE SCANNING
  Synovial Membrane Scanning
BONE SCANNING

Besides the various radiographic procedures discussed in Chapter 1 and the angiographic methods described in Chapter 4, there are a number of other techniques of imaging which may be applied to the hand. These include methods which use x-rays, as well as detection of patterns of heat (thermography) and distribution of injected radioisotopes.

The x-ray procedures include tomograms and the use of other modes of detection of x-rays, such as xeroradiography or electron radiography. Fluoroscopic evaluation of the hand has been considered in Chapter 1. Contrast media can be used to outline the joint cavities (arthrography), tendon sheaths or dermal ridges and creases (radio-dermatography).

TOMOGRAPHY

Tomography is useful in obliterating overlapping shadows that interfere with visualization of the area in question (Fig. 5–1). Tomography is not very often used for the phalanges, since they can usually be isolated by simpler radiographic techniques. There is, however, a definite place for tomography in the evaluation of the wrist and of the metacarpals, particularly around their base. It is particularly difficult to visualize normal anatomy of the metacarpals or carpals in the lateral view. By means of tomography, the localization of a lesion in these areas can be shown more clearly than by conventional filming. Tomography can be useful in the demonstration of fine fracture lines, particularly in the scaphoid, or for localization of calcifications, or in the definition of a nidus of an osteoid osteoma. It is also useful in detecting fractures of the lunate in Kienböck's disease.

The optimal tomographic technique for the hand uses thin cuts, which are produced using the complex motions such as large circles and, preferably, hypocycloids or spirals. These motions also avoid linear ghosts which may be disturbing in linear motion tomograms. To avoid this problem if only linear tomography is available, care must be taken that the direction of tube travel is not parallel to any important linear shadows that need to be defined. Geometric magnification together with tomography may improve detail of screen exposures.

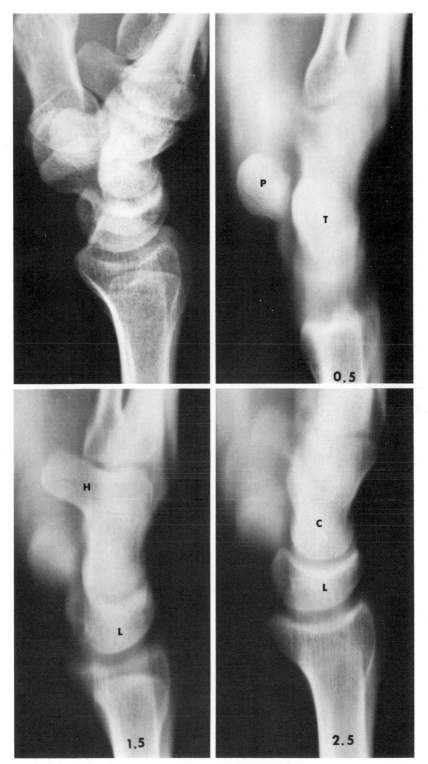

Figure 5–1. Lateral radiogram and linear tomograms of the wrist of a normal young adult male. The number on each tomogram refers to the height above table as measured from the ulnar side. Although the capitate (C), lunate (L) and scaphoid (S) are well seen on the plain view, the bone island in the scaphoid and the small radiolucencies in the lunate are seen much better on the tomograms. The hamate (H), trapezium (TM), trapezoid (TD), triquetrum (TQ) and pisiform (P) are also seen much more clearly on the tomogram.

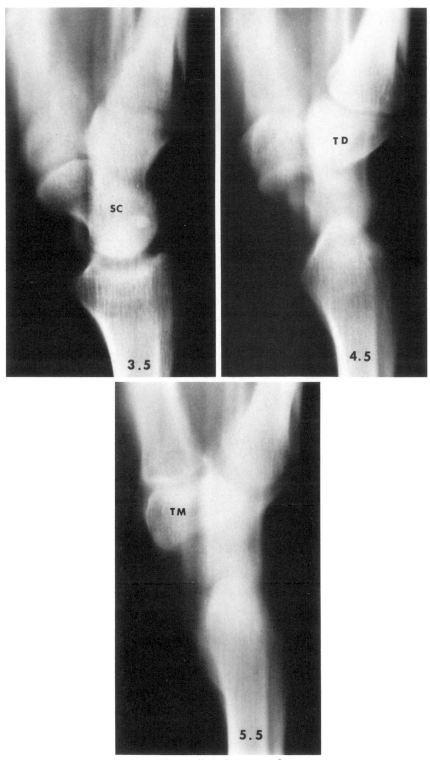

Figure 5–1 Continued.

REFERENCES

1. Gentaz, R., Lespargot, J., Levame, J.-H., and Poli, J.-P.: La Maladie de Kienböck. Approche Tomographique. Analyse de 5 Cas. *Nouv. Presse Med.*, 1:1207–1210, 1972.
2. Martin, P. L., Dunhamel, J., and Broussin, J.: Tomographie du Carpe en Incidence de Profil et Tomographie Agrandie. *J. Radiol. Electrol. Med. Nucl.*, 34:182–185, 1953.
3. Norman, A.: The Value of Tomography in the Diagnosis of Skeletal Disorders. *Radiol. Clin. North Am.*, 8:251–258, 1970.

XERORADIOGRAPHY

Xeroradiography is a technique of recording x-ray images by means of alterations in charge on semiconductors. X-radiation causes local alteration in the charge on a selenium plate. A charged powder distributes itself, depending on the intensity of the charge on the selenium plate producing an image. The powder image can be transferred to a sheet of paper or plastic, producing a permanent image that can then be viewed. One of the main advantages of xeroradiography is that there is edge enhancement (Fig. 5–2). Thus, adjacent areas with slight differences in density can be better visualized. This is particularly useful in the evaluation of foreign bodies in the hand, where the radiopacity of the foreign body differs only slightly from that of tissue. Wood, for example, is often difficult to localize with plain radiographs but is often seen much better on the xeroradiograph (Fig. 5–3). A clinical example of this is shown in Chapter 17, page 481. Another advantage of a xeroradiogram is that it shows both the dark and light portions of the film with equal advantage and makes bright lighting unnecessary. This is of less importance in the hand than in the breast, where xeroradiography has been used to a much greater extent. Another advantage of xeroradiography is its relatively large latitude, and the fact that high kilovoltage can be used while maintaining an adequate

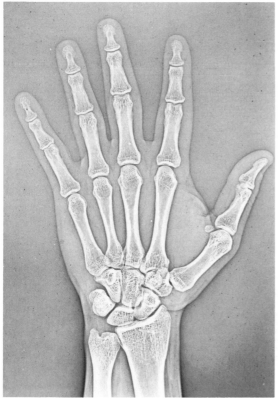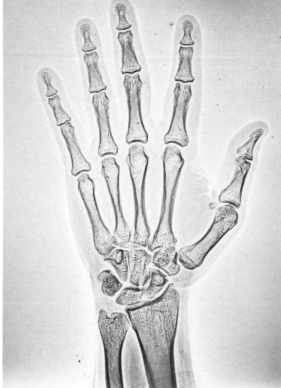

Figure 5–2. Xeroradiogram. Normal hand in negative and positive modes. Note the good visualization of soft tissue detail as well as bone trabecular structure.

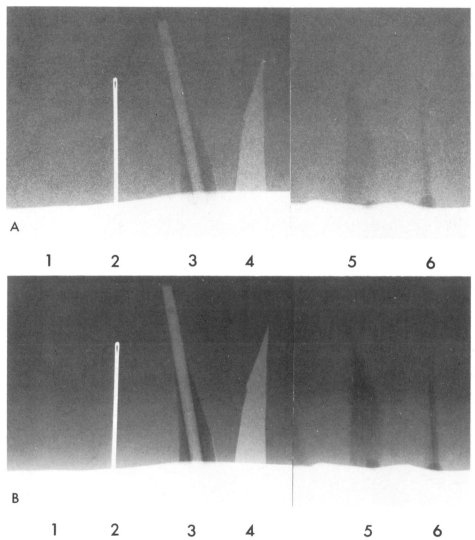

Figure 5–3. Radiographs and photographs of various objects immersed in 28 mm. of water: (*1*) a pine needle, (*2*) a metal needle, (*3*) a pencil, (*4*) a piece of glass, (*5*) a piece of wood, (*6*) a piece of wood.

A, Radiograph obtained using RPR film without screens. B, Radiograph obtained using Kodak mammography film. C, RPL film and Par Speed screens. D, Xeroradiogram, negative mode. E, Xeroradiogram, positive mode. Note that most of the objects are better seen on the Xeroradiograph.

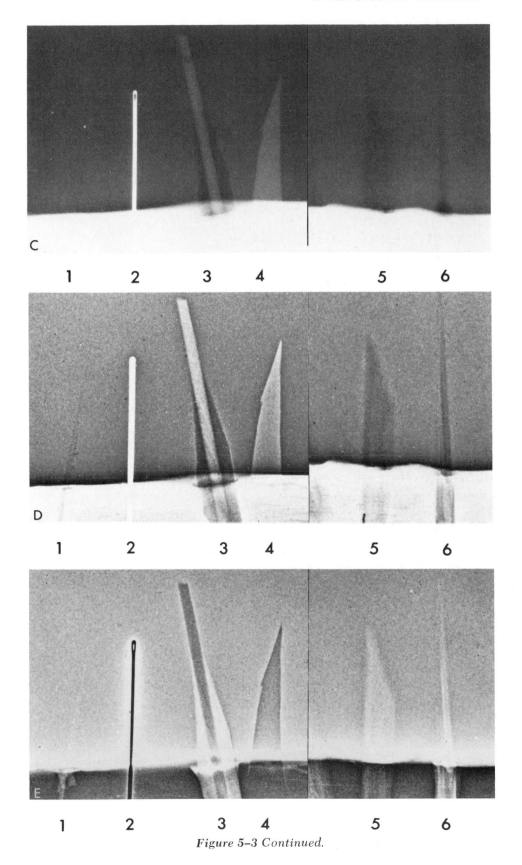

Figure 5–3 Continued.

image. Optimal hand xeroradiographs can be obtained with a kilovoltage of 120 KVP.

The xeroradiograph can be produced in either positive or negative mode, depending on the area of interest. In some situations one mode appears to be better than the other.

REFERENCES

1. Woesner, M. E., and Sanders, I.: Xeroradiography: A Significant Modality in the Detection of Nonmetallic Foreign Bodies in Soft Tissues. Am. J. Roentgenol., 115:636–640, 1972.
2. Wolfe, J. N.: Xerography of the Breast. Radiology, 91:231–240, 1968.
3. Wolfe, J. N.: Xeroradiography of the Bones, Joints, and Soft Tissues. Radiology, 93:583–587, 1969.

ELECTRON RADIOGRAPHY

Electron radiography is a newly described method in which an image is formed of a charged distribution on a dielectric plate. This is converted to a visible image by exposure to a toner in a development chamber, and finally the image is fixed. The resultant image somewhat resembles that seen in xeroradiography with enhanced edge effect.

REFERENCE

1. Stanton, L., Brady, L. W., Day, J. L., Lightfoot, D. A., and Tobin, R.: Electron-Radiographic Imaging. Scientific Exhibit. Meeting, Radiologic Society of North America, Chicago, 1972.

ARTHROGRAPHY AND THE STUDY OF THE DIGITAL SHEATHS

Arthrography of the Wrist

Contrast examination of the wrist has been done in normal individuals, as well as in patients with rheumatoid arthritis and in patients with ganglia. The indications according to Wirth[9] are for evaluation of injury to fibrocartilage, tears of the capsule, localization of symptomatic calcifications and bone fragments within the joint space, joint ganglia and osteochondritis dissecans.

The contrast medium is injected in the dorsal aspect of the wrist between the radius and the scaphoid and lunate. Wirth injects the contrast medium along the radial aspect of the extensor indicis proprius, which is easily palpable when the index finger is extended. About 2 ml. of contrast medium can be injected, preferably under fluoroscopic control.

In the normal wrist the synovial margins are smooth with two small pouches, one on the radial volar side and the other on the ulnar side near the ulnar styloid process (Fig. 5–4). In 16 per cent of cases studied by Harrison et al.,[3] there was communication between the radiocarpal and radioulnar joint. Other series reviewed by these authors showed a different incidence of this phenomenon, which may be related to the age of the patient. Communication between the radiocarpal and midcarpal joint was seen in 13 per cent of cases. In none of the 100 wrists studied was there evidence of communication between the wrist joint and the flexor or the extensor tendon sheaths.

In rheumatoid arthritis[3] there is increased irregularity of the synovial margin with a corrugated pattern. Radiocarpal and midcarpal communications, as well as radiocarpal and radiolunar communications, occur in about 70 per cent of patients. Radiocarpal and extensive tendon communications also occur in 20 per cent of cases.

Wrist ganglia can be filled by injection of the wrist joint. Andren and Eiken[1] found that 23 of 27 patients with volar wrist ganglia had a communication between the joint and the ganglion (see Fig. 20–23). In a group of 32 dorsal ganglia, 14 communicated with the wrist joint. Interestingly enough, when the contrast medium is injected into the ganglion, contrast enters the joint only very rarely, suggesting that a valve-like mechanism must be present.

Arthrography of Other Joints in the Hand

The metacarpophalangeal and interphalangeal joints can be also injected (Fig. 5–5). Weston[7] in cadavers used a 26 gauge needle to inject these joints and demonstrated their distribution. This has as yet little clinical application. These joints can

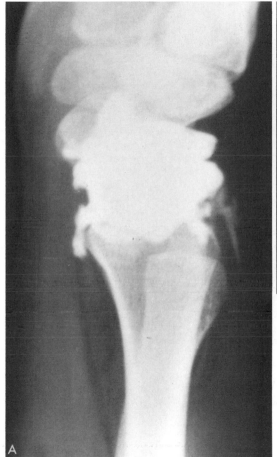

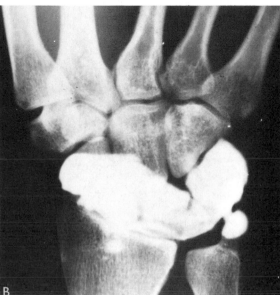

Figure 5–4. Normal arthrogram of the wrist. The contrast medium outlines the joint cavity. Two small pouches, one on the radial side and one on the ulnar side, are normal anatomic findings. (Courtesy Dr. William Reynolds, Henry Ford Hospital, Detroit, Michigan.)

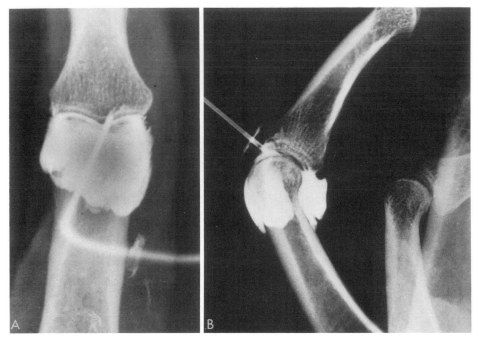

Figure 5-5. Arthrogram of the proximal interphalangeal joint of the finger. The joint space is filled and illustrates the extent of the joint. *A*, AP view. *B*, lateral view. (From Weston, W. S.: *Australas. Radiol.*, 13:211, 1969. Film courtesy Dr. W. J. Weston, New Zealand.)

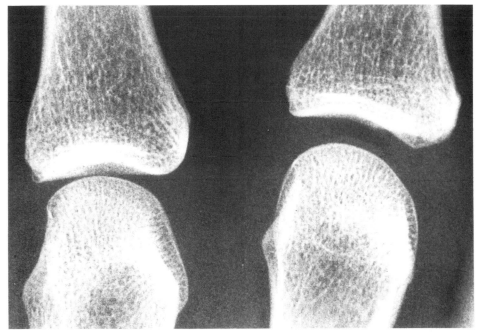

Figure 5-6. "Vacuum" arthrogram of the metacarpophalangeal joint. Traction was applied to the finger, resulting in separation at the joint space and production of vapor within the joint. The thickness of the articular cartilage can be visualized, particularly over the metacarpal head. This vacuum phenomenon is associated with cracking of the knuckles.

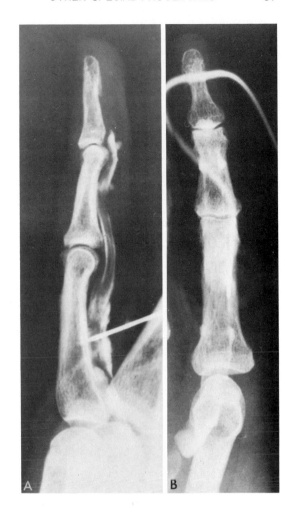

Figure 5-7. This illustrates the common sheath of the flexor digitorum sublimis and flexor digitorum profundus. In the PA view (*B*) there is accumulation of contrast above the reflection of the digital sheath at the level of the neck of the metacarpal. (From Weston, W. J.: *Australas. Radiol.*, 13:360, 1969. Films courtesy Dr. W. J. Weston, New Zealand.)

also be demonstrated by vapor produced with traction (Fig. 5-6).

Injection of Digital Sheaths of the Hand

The digital sheaths can also be demonstrated with contrast medium. Weston[8] carried out these studies postmortem (Fig. 5-7), while Semple[5] performed the examination in live individuals. By means of this study the flexor tendons can be clearly visualized, and this technique may have some value in the treatment of rheumatoid arthritis or conceivably in the evaluation of tendon injury. Brewerton[2] found that the patient with synovitis is easier to inject than the normal. He described the appearance of tenosynovitis in rheumatoid arthritis.

REFERENCES

1. Andren, L., and Eiken, O.: Arthrographic Studies of Wrist Ganglions. *J. Bone Joint Surg.*, 53A: 299–302, 1971.
2. Brewerton, D. A.: Radiographic Studies of Tendons in the Rheumatoid Hand. *Brit. J. Radiol.*, 42: 487–492, 1969.
3. Harrison, M. O., Freiberger, R. H., and Ranawat, C. S.: Arthrography of the Rheumatoid Wrist Joint. *Am. J. Roentgenol.*, 112:480–486, 1971.
4. Ranawat, C. S., Harrison, M. O., and Jordan, L. R.: Arthrography of the Wrist Joint. *Clin. Orthop.*, 83:6–12, 1972.
5. Semple, J. C.: Instrumental and Technical Notes. Radiographic Appearance of Normal Flexor Tendon Sheaths in the Hand. *Brit. J. Radiol.*, 43:271–273, 1970.
6. Weston, W. J.: The Soft-Tissue Changes of Rheumatoid Arthritis at the Wrist. *Australas. Radiol.*, 12:384–392, 1968.
7. Weston, W. J.: The Normal Arthrograms of the Metacarpo-Phalangeal, Metatarso-Phalangeal and Inter-Phalangeal Joints. *Australas. Radiol.*, 13:211–218, 1969.

8. Weston, W. J.: The Digital Sheaths of the Hand. *Australas. Radiol.*, 13:360–364, 1969.
9. Wirth, W.: *In:* Schinz, H. R., et al. (Eds.): *Roentgen Diagnosis.* 2nd American Ed. Grune & Stratton, Inc., New York, 1968, Vol. 1, pp. 359–361.

RADIODERMATOGRAPHY

Radiodermatography is a technique of radiographic demonstration of dermal ridges and creases. Any highly opaque metallic powder can be used. Although compounds of lead have been used in the past, a nontoxic metal is preferred. Tantalum powder appears to be the most practical material for this purpose. A small amount of hand cream is massaged onto the hands to make them slightly sticky, and a moderate amount of tantalum is sprinkled and rubbed lightly into the hand until the creases and spaces between the dermal ridges are filled with tantalum. They are clearly visible on inspection. Care must be taken that the dorsum of the hand is not coated. The hand is then placed palm down on the film, without smudging the tantalum. A PA film is obtained, using mammographic film or a good nonscreen film (Figs. 5–8, 5–9 and 5–10).

By means of this technique the dermatoglyphic patterns are easily visualized and the relationship of the creases to the hand bones can be clearly demonstrated. One of the shortcomings of this method is that the dermal patterns of the thumb are not

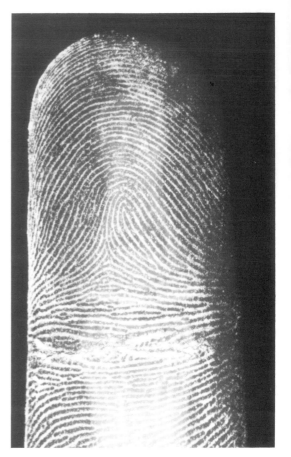

Figure 5–8. Radiodermatography. Distal portion of finger. The dermal ridges are clearly seen. The underlying phalanx is seen beneath. Both shadows were seen better simultaneously on the original radiograph.

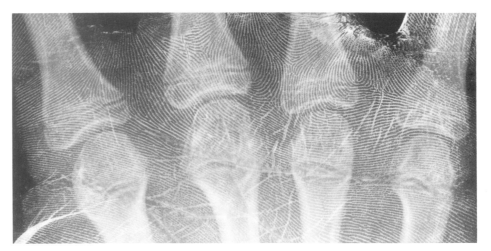

Figure 5–9. Radiodermatoglyphics of metacarpophalangeal region. Note the good visualization of the dermal ridges and the creases, as well as the osseous skeleton.

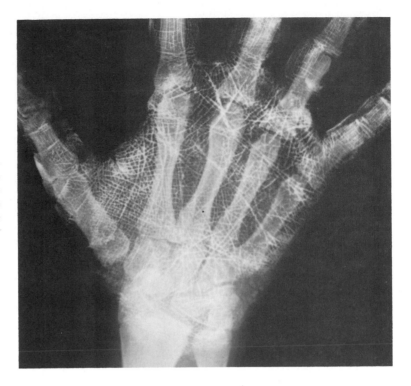

Figure 5–10. Radiodermatography of the palm of the hand of a Down's syndrome child. Note the simian crease and the unusual ridges on the palm of the hand.

demonstrated in the conventional PA view, and a separate view must be used. In newborn infants this technique is usually not successful because of the shallowness of the dermal ridges, although the creases can still be seen. This technique may also have some teaching value in relating surface landmarks to skeletal anatomy.

REFERENCES

1. Garn, S. M., Poznanski, A. K., and Gall, J. C., Jr.: Applications of Radiodermatography to Human and Primate Studies. *Am. J. Phys. Anthropol.*, 33:109–114, 1970.
2. Poznanski, A. K., Gall, J. C., Jr., and Garn, S. M.: Radiodermatography. Simultaneous Demonstration of Dermatoglyphics and Osseous Structures of the Hand. *Invest. Radiol.*, 4:340–342, 1969.

THERMOGRAPHY

Thermography is a method of graphically demonstrating the pattern of heat emission of a body. The variations in skin temperature are shown in terms of gradations of blackness or whiteness of a film or variations in color (Fig. 5–11). The main advantage of the method of thermography is that it does not require any injection material or irradiation of the patient, but actually measures the heat radiation emitted by the patient.

Although thermography has been used mainly in evaluation of the breast, it has some definite potential in the evaluation of the hand. An area of localized warmth or localized coolness in the hand can be detected by thermography (Fig. 5–12). Thermography will therefore reflect the state of the circulation in the hand. For example, in Raynaud's disease (Fig. 5–13), the circulation to the fingertips is diminished and these areas will appear cooler. If a ganglionic block is performed, thermography can be obtained for objective evaluation of the effect on the circulation. Various other causes of decreased peripheral vascularity can also be detected by this method; for example, Gershon-Cohen et al.[5] have demonstrated smoking decreases circulation.

Inflammatory changes in tissue can be detected by this means—for example, joint involvement in the arthritides, such as rheumatoid, or tendonitis in Quervain's disease. Also, osteomyelitis, sprains, frac-

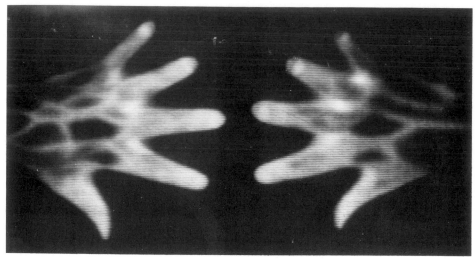

Figure 5–11. Normal hand thermogram. Note that the region of the fingertips is warmer than the remainder of the hand, but the change in warmth is gradual. Vascular structures along the dorsum of the hand are visualized as white streaks. (Courtesy Dr. W. Reynolds, Henry Ford Hospital, Detroit, Michigan.)

tures, clubbing (Fig. 5–14) and all other conditions associated with increased warmth can be demonstrated on the thermogram.

Thermography may be useful in differentiating between second and third degree burns, since in the latter the skin is cold because of decreased local vascularity, while in the former it is warm because of irritation and inflammation. Lawson, in

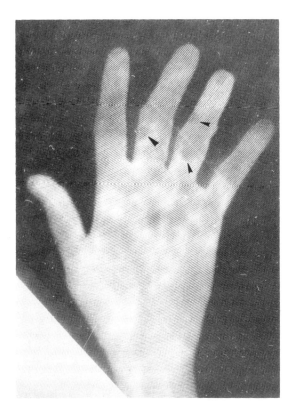

Figure 5–12. Thermogram of erythema multiforme. Nodules (*arrows*) in the fingers appear as cold areas surrounded by a region of erythema.

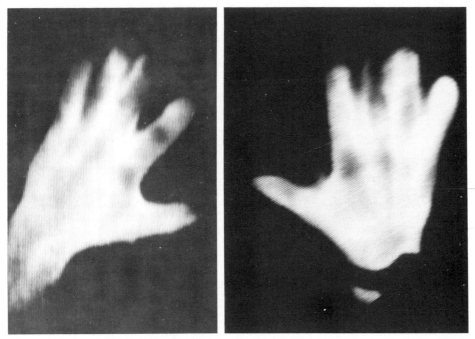

Figure 5-13. Thermogram in Raynaud's disease. Both hands of an individual with Raynaud's disease. There is evidence that the third finger bilaterally appears relatively cold as compared to the others. The black shadow along the patient's wrist region on the right is a wrist watch. (Courtesy Dr. W. Reynolds, Henry Ford Hospital, Detroit, Michigan.)

Figure 5-14. Thermogram in a patient with clubbing secondary to a pulmonary cavitary lesion. Films above and below are at two different sensitivity settings. Note that the fingertips are considerably hotter than the remainder of the hand. This is a manifestation of the increased warmth associated with the clubbing. Vascular structures along the dorsum of the hand are clearly visualized. (Courtesy Dr. W. Reynolds, Henry Ford Hospital, Detroit, Michigan.)

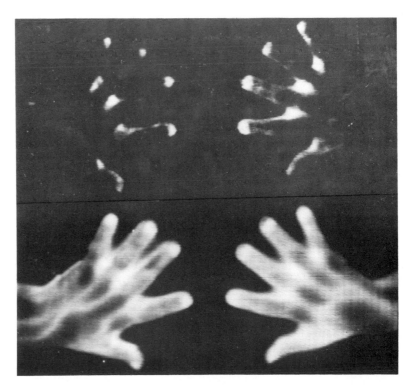

his early studies of thermography, also showed the use of this modality in the evaluation of damage from frostbite.

REFERENCES

1. Barnes, R. B.: Thermography of the Human Body. *Science*, 140:870–877, 1963.
2. Boas, N. F.: Thermography in Rheumatoid Arthritis. *Ann. N.Y. Acad. Sci.*, 121:223–234, 1964.
3. Connell, J. F., Jr., Morgan, E., and Rousselot, L. M.: Thermography in Trauma. *Ann. N.Y. Acad. Sci.*, 121:171–176, 1964.
4. Cosh, J. A., and Ring, E. F. J.: Techniques of Heat Detection Used in the Assessment of Rheumatic Diseases. *J. Radiol. Electrol. Med. Nucl.*, 48:84–89, 1967.
5. Gershon-Cohen, J., Borden, A. G. B., and Hermel, M. B.: Thermography of Extremities after Smoking; *Brit. J. Radiol.*, 42:189–191, 1969.
6. Koob, E.: Infra-Red Thermography in Hand Surgery. *Hand*, 4:65–67, 1972.
7. Lawson, R. N., Wlodek, G. D., and Webster, D. R.: Thermographic Assessment of Burns and Frostbite. *Can. Med. Assoc. J.*, 84:1129–1131, 1961.
8. Weill, F., Bonneville, J. F., Prevotat, N., Ricatte, J. P., Japy, C., and Francois, J.: Sémiologie Thermographique des Ischémies Chroniques des Membres. Corrélations Angiographiques. Le Signe de L'Hyperthermie Paradoxale. *Presse Med.*, 77:629–632, 1969.
9. Winsor, T., and Bendezu, J.: Thermography and the Peripheral Circulation. *Ann. N.Y. Acad. Sci.*, 121:135–156, 1964.

RADIOISOTOPE SCANNING

Radioisotopes can be used for imaging synovial tissues or bone. Synovial scanning probably has more clinical potential in the hand than does bone scanning, since the primary value of bone scanning is in the evaluation of metastatic disease, which occurs very rarely in the hand bones.

Synovial Membrane Scanning

Certain radiopharmaceuticals appear to localize in the inflamed synovium. Thus, scans of the extremities may be useful in detecting early synovitis. Intravenous ^{99m}Tc pertechnetate has been used for this purpose in a dose of 5 to 15 millicuries.

In the presence of synovitis, after some delay the level of radioactivity in the synovial membrane becomes higher than that in the blood. It has been shown experimentally that the localization of the radioactive material is predominantly in the synovium and not in the surrounding tissue or joint effusion.

In the normal individual the activity in the hand is uniform (Fig. 5–15). However, any type of inflammatory process will show up as a region of increased activity (Figs. 5–16 and 5–17), including rheumatoid arthritis, psoriatic arthritis, gout,

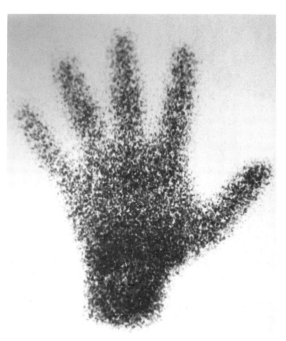

Figure 5–15. Normal synovial scan using ^{99m}Tc pertechnetate. There is relatively uniform distribution of the isotope throughout the hand. (Courtesy Dr. R. V. Pozderac, Veterans Administration Hospital, Ann Arbor, Michigan.)

Figure 5–16. Left (A) right (B) joint scan and corresponding radiographs of patient with Reiter's arthritis. The bony changes are only slight except in the left first metacarpophalangeal joint. This region appears very active on the scan. The marked increase in activity in the region of the right wrist and right third finger is associated with relatively little radiographic manifestation except for slight soft tissue swelling of that finger. The right thumb also appears to have increased activity, indicating joint involvement. (Scans courtesy Dr. R. V. Pozderac, and films courtesy Dr. R. Rapp, both of the Veterans Administration Hospital, Ann Arbor, Michigan.)

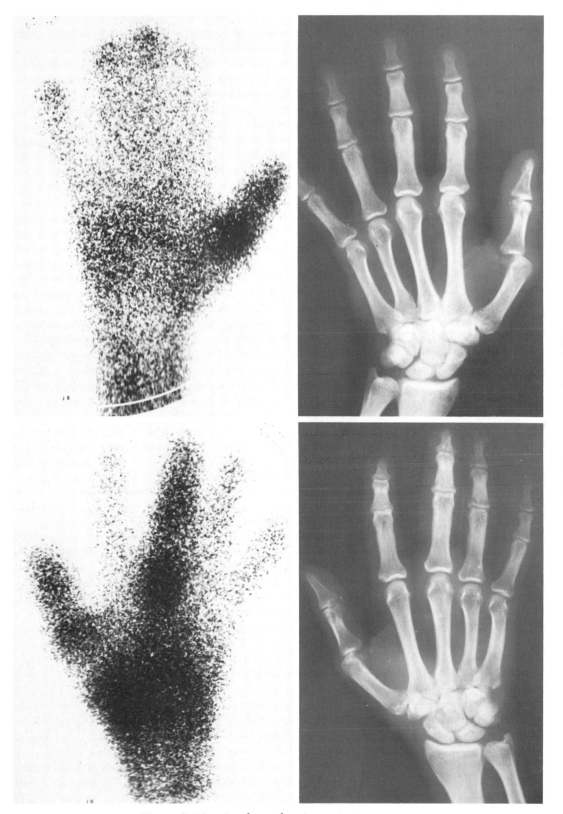

Figure 5-16. *See legend on opposite page.*

Reiter's arthritis, infectious arthritis, tendonitis and bursitis. The joint scans become positive prior to the onset of radiographic signs and sometimes even prior to the onset of clinical signs and symptoms. The scan remains positive after the clinical symptoms have subsided and eventually becomes less active even though radiographic signs of damage from the arthritis may persist.

The scan may be of value in the patient with joint pain but with negative or borderline laboratory or roentgen findings. If in these cases the scan is negative, the pain is probably not due to joint disease. If the scan is positive, this is good evidence that the patient has synovitis which will eventually be confirmed. By being able to detect subclinical synovitis, the scan may be useful in determining if a certain arthritis is indeed monarticular or whether various joints are involved. It could also be potentially used as a mode of evaluating therapy.

Synovial membrane scanning is somewhat parallel to thermography in its ability to detect early inflammation. However, according to Maxfield et al., the scanning method is more sensitive in detecting early joint changes.

One possible source of error in synovial scanning in children is that there appears to be increased activity in the carpals and in the metacarpal heads, which has been interpreted as due to activity at the site of rapidly growing cartilage.

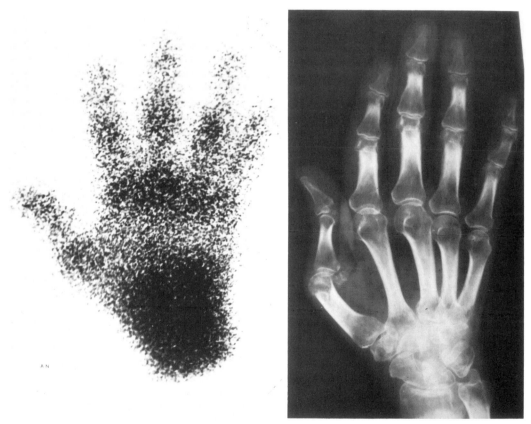

Figure 5–17. Joint scan and radiograph. Rheumatoid arthritis. Note the increased activity in the region of the wrist, the metacarpophalangeal joints and the interphalangeal joints. This is paralleled by the bony demineralization in these areas on the radiograph. (Scan courtesy Dr. R. V. Pozderac, and film courtesy Dr. R. Rapp, both of the Veterans Administration Hospital, Ann Arbor, Michigan.)

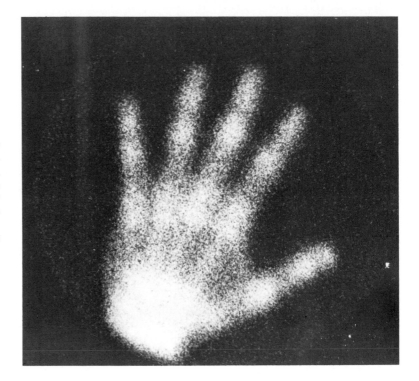

Figure 5–18. Normal bone scan using ^{99m}Tc polyphosphate. There is increased activity in the bones of the hand and there is further localization at the joint surface. (Scan courtesy Dr. D. Moses, Ann Arbor, Michigan.)

REFERENCES

1. Aprill, C. N., Schuler, S. E., and Weiss, T. E.: Peripheral Joint Imaging: Variation in Normal Children. *J. Nucl. Med.*, 13:367–372, 1972.
2. Maxfield, W. S., Weiss, T. E., and Shuler, S. E.: Synovial Membrane Scanning in Arthritic Disease. *Semin. Nucl. Med.*, 2:50–70, 1972.

BONE SCANNING

The isotope presently used for bone scanning is ^{99m}Tc polyphosphate, which is picked up by bone scanning of the bones of the hand (Fig. 5–18). It has little clinical application at this time in the evaluation of the hand.

Part II

NORMAL VARIANTS AND ANOMALIES OF THE HAND

Chapter 6

NORMAL VARIANTS AND MINOR ANOMALIES OF THE HAND

VASCULAR GROOVES
BONE-IN-BONE APPEARANCE
GROWTH LINES
LUCENT BANDS IN THE METAPHYSIS
SCLEROTIC FOCI IN BONE
EPIPHYSEAL VARIATIONS
   Dense or Ivory Epiphyses
   Pseudoepiphyses

    Multiple Epiphyseal Centers
    Cone-Shaped Epiphyses
SESAMOID BONE VARIATIONS
VARIATION IN SHAPE OF THE PHALANGES
    AND METACARPALS

    There is a wide range of variation in the shape of the hand bones. The hand may reflect the sex or the occupation of the individual. Thick, dense bones with prominent muscle attachments are seen in the male who does heavy manual labor, while slender, delicate bones may be seen in older females.

    Most of the variants that will be discussed are not clinically significant, but it is im-

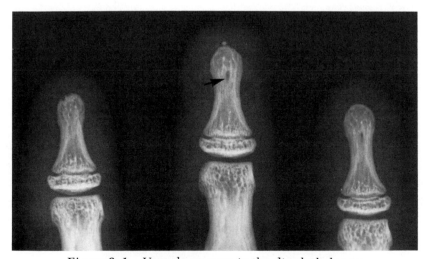

Figure 6–1. Vascular groove in the distal phalanges.

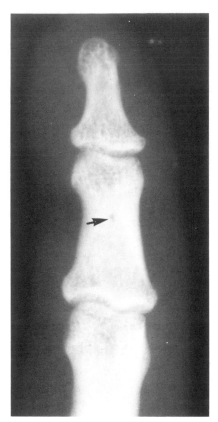

Figure 6-2. Vascular groove in the middle phalanx.

portant to be able to recognize these normal variants in order to distinguish them from pathologic changes. Some variants, however, border on the pathologic and may indeed be diagnostic of malformation syndromes. The best example of this is in the cone-shaped epiphyses. Normal variants of the wrist are discussed in Chapter 8.

VASCULAR GROOVES

A number of vascular grooves or openings may be evident in the phalanges and metacarpals of the hand. The location of these has been outlined by Ravelli[2] and by Cocchi[1] (Figs. 6-1 to 6-5).

In the distal (Fig. 6-1) and middle phalanges (Fig. 6-2) they appear as small round radiolucencies which may be con-

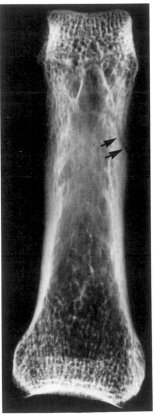

Figure 6-4. Vascular groove in a dried proximal phalanx.

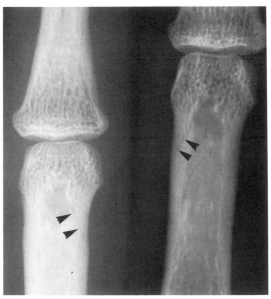

Figure 6-3. Vascular grooves in the proximal phalanges.

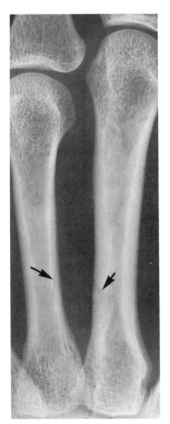

Figure 6–5. Vascular grooves in the meta-carpals.

BONE-IN-BONE APPEARANCE

The appearance of an outline of one bone within another is less common in the hand bones than in the long bones and in the spine and pelvis. Although there are many causes for this finding, including phosphorus poisoning and osteopetrosis, many times the cause is unknown and may simply reflect a growth phenomenon due to severe illness (Fig. 6–6).

GROWTH LINES

These are caused by conditions similar to those producing the bone-in-bone appearance but they may also be seen in some otherwise normal children. They are commonly seen in children who have multiple courses of chemotherapy for cancer or leukemia (Fig. 6–7), but they are much less common in the hands than in other bones of the body.

fused with cystic lesions of bone. They are much more commonly seen in the middle than in the distal phalanges and may be evident at all ages. They are probably more pronounced in various hematologic disorders.

In the proximal phalanges (Figs. 6–3 and 6–4) and metacarpals (Fig. 6–5) the vascular grooves are linear in configuration, traversing the bony cortex. Because of their linear appearance they can be easily confused with fractures.

REFERENCES

1. Cocchi, U.: Vergleichend-anatomische Studie zur Frage der Skelettreifung. *Fortschr. Geb. Roentgenstr. Nuklearmed.,* 72:32–47, 1949.
2. Ravelli, A.: Gefäßkanäle in den Fingergliedern. *Radiol. Clinica,* 22:465–469, 1953.

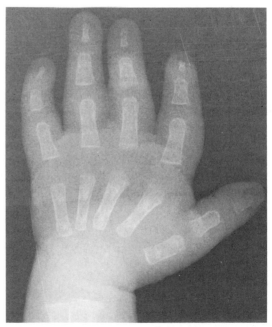

Figure 6–6. Bone-in-bone appearance in the metacarpals. This child had some serious illnesses. The central area of sclerosis surrounded by the lucency is the result of changes in the growth rate.

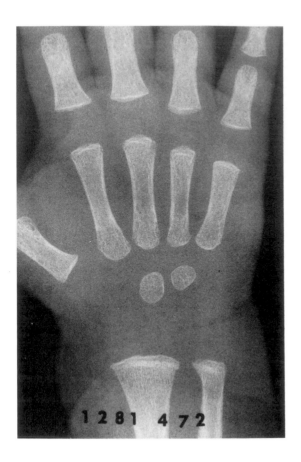

Figure 6–7. Dense "growth" line in a child treated for neuroblastoma. Distinct lines are seen in the distal ends of the metacarpals, radius and ulna.

Figure 6–8. Lucent metaphyseal bands. This child had some intrauterine growth retardation. There were lucent bands throughout the skeleton as well as in the metacarpals.

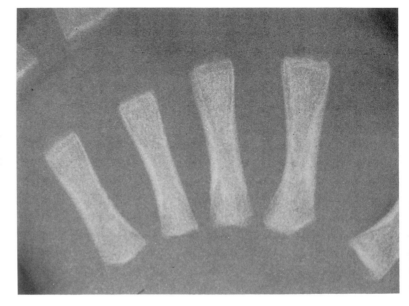

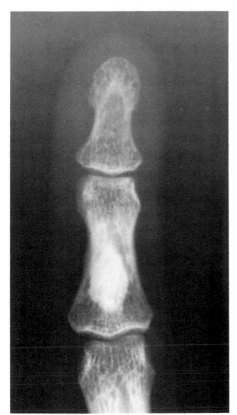

Figure 6–9. Area of bone sclerosis of unknown origin in the middle phalanx. No other areas of bone sclerosis were seen in the hand.

REFERENCES

1. Garn, S. M., Silverman, F. N., Hertzog, K. P., and Rohmann, C. G.: Lines and Bands of Increased Density. Their Implication to Growth and Development. *Med. Radiogr. Photogr.*, 44:58–89, 1968.
2. Park, E. A.: The Imprinting of Nutritional Disturbances on the Growing Bone. *Pediatrics*, Supplement 154, pp. 815–862, 1964.

LUCENT BANDS IN THE METAPHYSIS

In the newborn infant, lucent bands may be seen in the metaphysis of any bone. They are often the result of some intrauterine insult, particularly intrauterine infections. Although more commonly seen in the femur, they may occasionally affect the hand, particularly in the region of the metacarpals (Fig. 6–8).

SCLEROTIC FOCI IN BONE

Foci of increased density may occur in any of the hand bones (Figs. 6–9 to 6–11). They represent regions of compact bone within the spongiosa and are usually of no clinical significance. They vary in size and shape. Sometimes they are adjacent to the cortex. Occasionally, multiple bone densities are seen throughout the hand bones in osteopoikilosis (Fig. 6–12). Small dense sesamoid bones overlying the finger bones can sometimes be confused with these areas of increased bone density (Fig. 6–13). Oblique films or lateral films will differentiate them.

EPIPHYSEAL VARIATIONS

A number of variants occur in the epiphyses, including dense epiphysis, pseudo-

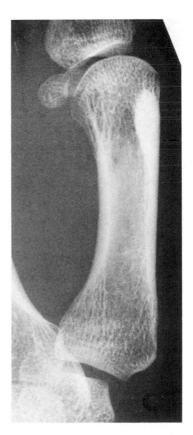

Figure 6–10. Asymptomatic area of sclerosis in the first metacarpal.

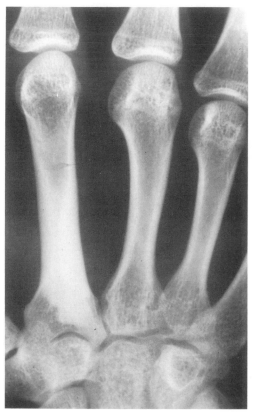

Figure 6–11. Asymptomatic area of bone sclerosis in the second metacarpal. (Courtesy Dr. D. Corbett, Detroit, Michigan.)

epiphysis and cone epiphysis. Many of these changes have little clinical significance. Occasionally the cone epiphysis and pseudoepiphysis may be clinically significant when they involve a large number of bones or when they involve specific bones.

Dense or Ivory Epiphyses

Dense or ivory epiphyses are relatively common normal variants (Fig. 6–14). The exact incidence of this anomaly depends somewhat on the definition. One uses the term only for the dense nontrabeculated epiphyses (that is, those large enough to show trabeculation). The incidence was 0.35 per cent of 8536 children between $2\frac{1}{2}$ and 13 years of age studied in the 10 State Nutrition Survey. On the other hand, de Itturzia and Tanner[2] found that 8.4 per cent of boys and 4.4 per cent of girls had dense epiphyses. However, they did not define what features the word "dense" included.

Ivory epiphyses normally occur only in the distal phalanges and in the fifth middle phalanx. The distribution found in the series of Kuhns et al.[3] is illustrated in Figure 6–15; they are most common in the second and fifth distal phalanges.

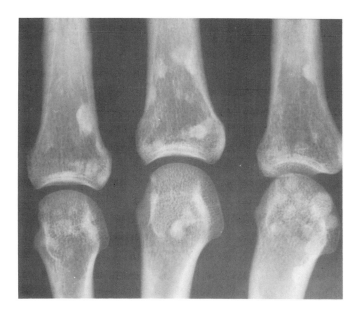

Figure 6–12. Osteopoikilosis. Multiple sclerotic areas are seen throughout the hand bones.

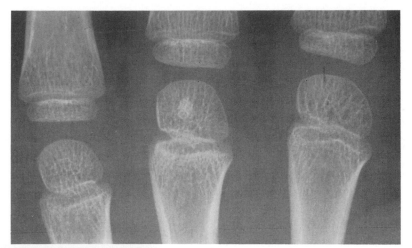

Figure 6–13. Bone island in the metacarpal head. This type of density is sometimes difficult to differentiate from a sesamoid bone.

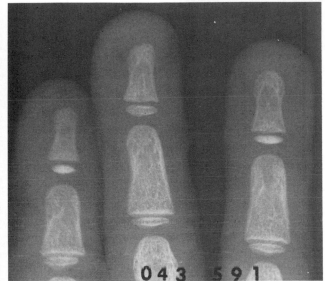

Figure 6–14. Ivory epiphyses. Extra-dense sclerotic epiphyses are seen in the distal phalanges of the index and ring fingers. These are nonspecific and are associated with conditions which retard growth. This child had associated chronic renal disease.

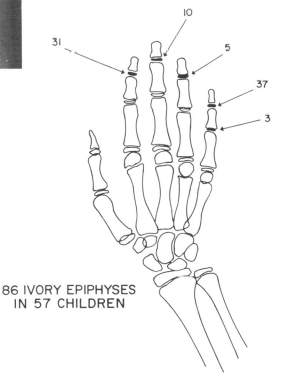

86 IVORY EPIPHYSES
IN 57 CHILDREN

Figure 6–15. Distribution of ivory epiphyses in the 10 State Nutrition Survey. (From Kuhns, L. R., et al.: *Radiology*, 109:643, 1973.)

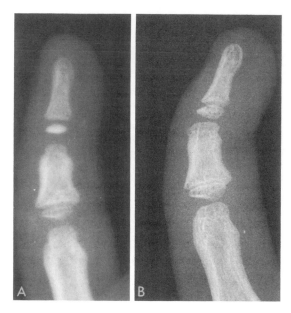

Figure 6–16. Disappearance of ivory epiphysis with time in Cockayne's syndrome. Films taken at ages 9 (*A*) and 13 (*B*).

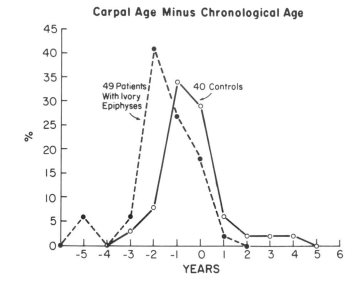

Carpal Age Minus Chronological Age

Figure 6–17. Ivory epiphyses and maturation in the 10 State Nutrition Survey. (From Kuhns, L. R., et al.: *Radiology,* 109:643, 1973.)

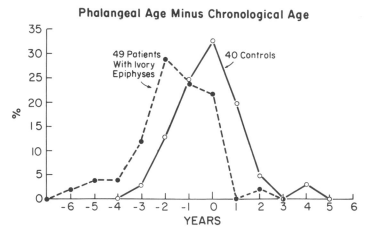

Phalangeal Age Minus Chronological Age

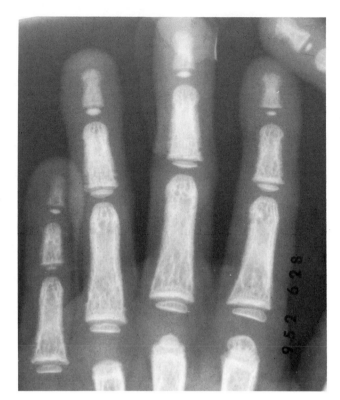

Figure 6–18. Dense epiphyses in renal osteodystrophy.

Ivory epiphyses are smaller in size than the corresponding normal epiphyses, and eventually become normal in appearance before they fuse with the shaft (Fig. 6–16).[1,4] Individuals with dense epiphyses are most likely to have some retardation of skeletal maturation (Fig. 6–17).[3] Dense epiphyses of the type seen in normal individuals are also seen in the tricho-rhino-phalangeal syndrome and in Cockayne's syndrome. They may also be seen in conditions associated with retardation of maturation, and in renal osteodystrophy (Fig. 6–18).

Dense epiphyses at other sites are usually not of the ivory type and have some trabeculation within them. Their presence frequently suggests some additional abnormality. Such dense epiphyses may be seen in hypothyroidism, in the epiphyseal dysplasias and in spondyloepiphyseal dysplasia.

REFERENCES

1. Brailsford, J. F.: *The Radiology of Bones and Joints,* 4th Ed. The Williams & Wilkins Co., Baltimore, 1948.

2. de Iturriza, J. R., and Tanner, J. M.: Cone-shaped Epiphyses and other Minor Anomalies in the Hands of Normal British Children. *J. Pediat.,* 75:265–272, 1969.
3. Kuhns, L. R., Poznanski, A. K., Harper, H. A. S., and Garn, S. M.: Ivory Epiphyses. *Radiology,* 109:643, 1973.
4. Staples, O. S.: Osteochondritis of the Epiphysis of the Terminal Phalanx of a finger. Report of a Case. *J. Bone Joint Surg.,* 25:917–920, 1943.

Pseudoepiphyses

Epiphyses normally occur at the proximal ends of the phalanges and at the distal ends of the metacarpals. An exception to this rule is the thumb, where the normal epiphysis is located at the proximal end of the first metacarpal. Pseudoepiphyses and tranverse notches are defined as epiphyses or attempts at formation of epiphyses located at the ends of the bones that do not normally contain them (Figs. 6–19 and 6–20). They are most commonly found at the base of the second metacarpal (Fig. 6–19). Again, the incidence figures for this normal variation are confusing, since they are somewhat dependent on what is defined as a significant notch and an insignifi-

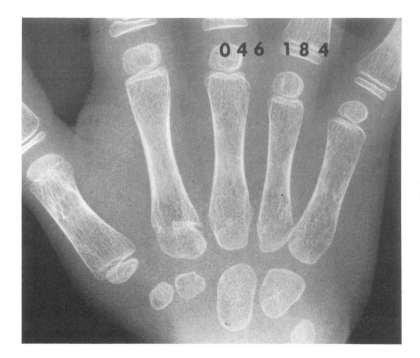

Figure 6–19. Notch in the base of the second metacarpal. This is a common anatomic variant.

cant notch. Longitudinal studies of children[3] show that pseudoepiphyses or notches are more common than would be expected in cross-sectional surveys, since they are so age-dependent and may appear only transiently. In their longitudinal studies, Lee and Garn[3] found notches in the second metacarpal in 28.4 per cent of boys and

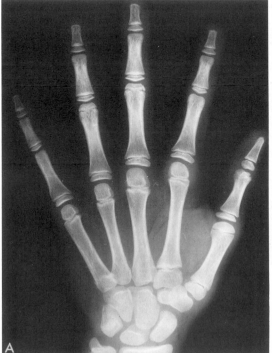

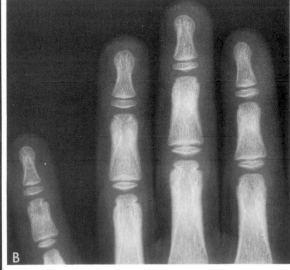

Figure 6–20 A, Pseudoepiphyses in all of the proximal phalanges and metacarpals. This is a very rare normal variant. (Courtesy Dr. Stanley Garn, 10 State Nutrition Survey.)

B, Pseudoepiphyses and notches in the proximal and middle phalanges. They are more marked on the ulnar than on the radial side. In the index finger the notches are just barely visible. This degree of notching is uncommon.

31.4 per cent of girls. In the fifth metacarpal a radial notch was seen in 88.8 per cent of girls and 87.3 per cent of boys. Occasionally in the base of the second metacarpal there is evidence of a supernumerary epiphysis that is completely separate from the rest of the bone. Such was seen in one boy and four girls in Lee and Garn's study (of 116 boys and 118 girls). Supernumerary epiphyses were seen in 1.4 per cent of boys by de Iturriza and Tanner,[2] and no cases were found in girls. Thus, completely separate epiphyses are relatively rare in a normal population.

There have been some attempts to relate pseudoepiphyses to various conditions causing skeletal retardation, poor nutrition and other abnormalities.[1, 6] The increase in incidence of these findings in retarded children is probably related to the fact that the slower they grow, the greater the probability of seeing one of these developmental features. Lee, Garn and Rohmann[4] were unable to observe any relationship between notching or pseudoepiphysis and stature or nutritional status. There does appear to be some familial tendency in notching. Lee and Garn noted an increased number of notches in siblings of children who had notches and also found that there is a similarity in the appearance of the notch in different siblings.

Rarely, pseudoepiphyses may occur in other bones of the hand as well (Fig. 6–20). Pseudoepiphyses in other bones are also seen in a number of pathologic conditions. Bizarre extra epiphyses may occur in cleidocranial dysostosis and in brachydactyly type C. Multiple pseudoepiphyses are commonly seen in Wolf's syndrome (4P-syndrome), and they are more common in spondyloepiphyseal dysplasia.

REFERENCES

1. Dreizen, S., Spirakis, C. N., and Stone, R. E.: The Distribution and Disposition of Anomalous Notches in the Non-epiphyseal Ends of Human Metacarpal Shafts. *Am. J. Phys. Anthropol.*, 23:181–188, 1965.
2. de Iturriza, J. R., and Tanner, J. M.: Cone-shaped Epiphyses and Other Minor Anomalies in the Hands of Normal British Children. *J. Pediat.*, 75:265–272, 1969.
3. Lee, M. M. C., and Garn, S. M.: Pseudoepiphyses or Notches in the Non-epiphyseal End of Metacarpal Bones in Healthy Children. *Anat. Rec.*, 159:263–272, 1967.
4. Lee, M. M. C., Garn, S. M., and Rohmann, C. G.: Relation of Metacarpal Notching to Stature and Maturational Status of Normal Children. *Invest. Radiol.*, 3:96–102, 1968.
5. Levine, E.: Notches in the Non-epiphyseal Ends of the Metacarpals and Phalanges in Children of Four South African Populations. *Am. J. Phys. Anthropol.*, 36:407–416, 1972.
6. Snodgrasse, R. M., Dreizen, S., Currie, C., Parker, G. S., and Spies, T. D.: The Association Between Anomalous Ossification Centers in the Hand Skeleton, Nutritional Status and Rate of Skeletal Maturation in Children Five to Fourteen Years of Age. *Am. J. Roentgenol.*, 74:1037–1047, 1955.
7. Snodgrasse, R. M., Dreizen, S., Parker, G. S., and Spies, T. D.: Serial Sequential Development of Anomalous Metacarpal and Phalangeal Ossification Centers in the Human Hand. *Growth*, 19:307–322, 1955.
8. Weinert, P.: Ein Beitrag zur Frage der Pseudoepiphysen. *Anat. Anz.*, 99:1–18, 1952.

Multiple Epiphyseal Centers

Although most epiphyses form as one ossification center, the occurrence of multiple foci, particularly early in the ossification of epiphyses, is common (Fig. 6–21). In a longitudinal study of 60 boys, Roche and Sutherland found that 46 had multiple centers in the proximal phalanx of the thumb, 13 had multiple centers in the first metacarpal and 11 had multiple centers in the fifth proximal phalanx. Multiple centers in other sites were less common. However, multiple centers were found in all of the bones except the distal phalanx of the thumb. In 60 girls, on the other hand, many fewer multiple epiphyseal centers were found. Twelve girls had multiple epiphyses in the proximal phalanx of the thumb, two had them in the proximal phalanx of the fifth finger and one each had multiple epiphyseal centers in seven of the other bones of the hands. The number of centers of ossification in each of these cases was quite variable. Usually only two ossification centers were present instead of the usual one, but in occasional cases, particularly in the proximal phalanx of the thumb, as many as five separate ossification centers were encountered. Eventually these multiple epiphyseal centers coalesce into one.

Thus, visualization of multiple epiphyseal centers, particularly in the proximal phalanx of the thumb, the first metacarpal and the fifth proximal phalanx, is normal. When other bones of the hand are involved,

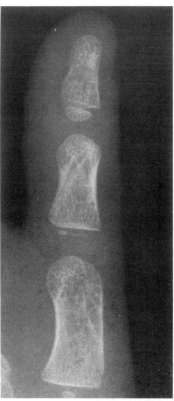

Figure 6–21. Multiple epiphyseal centers in the proximal phalanx of the thumb. This is an extremely common normal variant, particularly in males.

or when multiple bones are involved, the possibility of underlying abnormality should be considered. Multiple epiphyseal centers may be seen in hypothyroidism and in some epiphyseal dysplasias.

REFERENCE

1. Roche, A. F., and Sutherland, S.: Multiple Ossification Centres in the Epiphyses of the Long Bones of the Human Hand and Foot. *J. Bone Joint Surg.*, 41B:375–383, 1959.

Cone-Shaped Epiphyses

A cone-shaped epiphyses is defined as one which has a projection in its center extending toward the metaphysis. There is usually a corresponding indentation in the adjacent metaphysis. Cone epiphyses are usually seen very early in their ossification. In fact, the indentation in the shaft

of the bone may be seen even before the ossification of the epiphysis is visible. The cones may vary considerably in shape and size and, as in many variants, there is a continuum between what can be termed cone epiphysis and a normal flat epiphysis. Since there is a somewhat arbitrary definition of what is and what isn't a cone, incidence figures may be not very meaningful.

There is considerable variation in the incidence of cone epiphysis in different populations (Table 6–1). Cones are much more common in Japan than in Central America, and less common in the United States. Cones are significantly more common in girls than in boys in virtually all populations.[2, 5, 6]

The site of cone epiphyses has some diagnostic value. Differences exist in healthy and in sick children and between various population groups (Fig. 6–22). In the United States and Switzerland, cones in normal children are most common in the distal phalanx of the thumb (Fig. 6–23), and next most common in the middle phalanx of the fifth finger (Fig. 6–24). In Japan this relationship is reversed, while in Central America the incidence in these two anatomic regions may be equal. Cones at other sites are significantly less common (Figs. 6–25 and 6–26). As in Giedion's series, Hertzog et al.[5] found that the next most common cone in normal children was in the distal phalanx of the third finger, with an incidence of only 0.08 per cent. In the Japanese study quoted by Hertzog et al.,[5] there was some correlation between the presence of cones in the distal phalanx of the thumb and in the middle phalanx of the fifth finger. Moreover, in most of the children with cones in the middle phalanx of the second finger, there were also cones in the middle phalanx of the fifth finger.

TABLE 6–1. Cone Epiphyses*

POPULATION	SEX	MP5	DP1
Ohio	F	1.12	2.25
Ohio	M	0.77	1.15
El Salvador	F	4.26	5.26
El Salvador	M	1.43	2.68
Guatemala	F	8.71	5.51
Guatemala	M	2.38	2.17
Hiroshima	F	30.0	4.6
Hiroshima	M	13.1	5.3

*Data from Hertzog et al.: *Invest. Radiol.*, 3:433–441, 1968.

Figure 6-22. Distribution of cone-shaped epiphyses of the hands (CSEH) in normal and abnormal children. A line under the roman numeral refers to the distal phalanx of a digit; a line above and below the numeral refers to the middle phalanx; and a line on top of the numeral refers to the proximal phalanx. Thus we can see that cone epiphyses in the distal phalanx of the thumb and the middle phalanx of the fifth finger are commonly seen in normal, healthy children rather than in abnormal children. On the other hand, cones of some of the more unusual normal places, such as the fourth middle phalanx, the third middle phalanx, the first proximal phalanx and the fifth distal phalanx, have been seen only in abnormal children. (From Giedion, A.: *Ann. Radiol.*, 10: 322–329, 1967.)

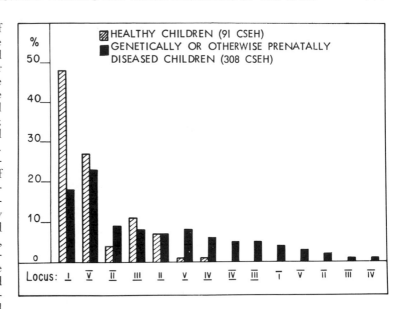

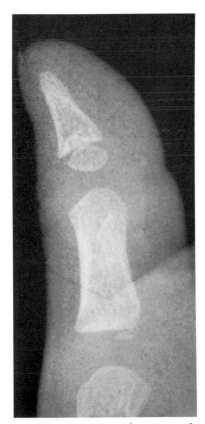

Figure 6-23. Cone epiphyses in the distal phalanx of the thumb in an otherwise normal individual. (Courtesy Dr. Stanley Garn, 10 State Nutrition Survey.)

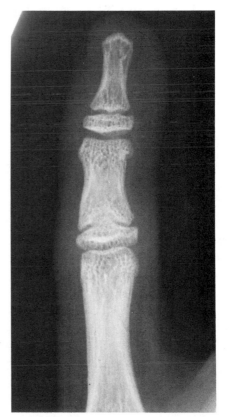

Figure 6-24. Cone epiphysis of the middle phalanx of the fifth finger. This is a common site for cone epiphyses in normal individuals and is often associated with clinodactyly.

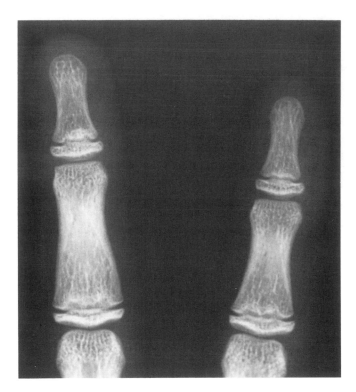

Figure 6–25. Minimal indentations on the diaphyses, involving many phalanges. These minimal types of changes can be classified as cones and may be seen in normal individuals. (Courtesy Dr. Stanley Garn, 10 State Nutrition Survey.)

There is some relationship between shortening of the hand bones and the presence of cone epiphyses. Cones were seen in some of the brachydactyly syndromes, and Garn et al.[1] have shown a relationship between brachydactyly of the fifth finger and cones. It appears that brachydactyly with cones is inherited differently from brachydactyly without cones (see brachydactyly A3, page 160). It also appears that shortening of the phalanx may actually occur prior to the formation of the cone.[5] The cone may, however, be precocious in its ossification.

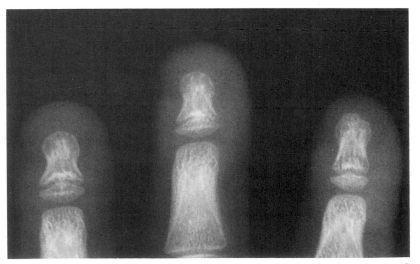

Figure 6–26. Distal cones of unknown cause associated with brachydactyly. We have seen several individuals with brachydactyly of the distal phalanges in the 10 State Nutrition Survey who had associated cones. Whether this is the result of an injury or of a congenital defect is not known. This type of cone was not seen in otherwise normal children by Giedion et al.

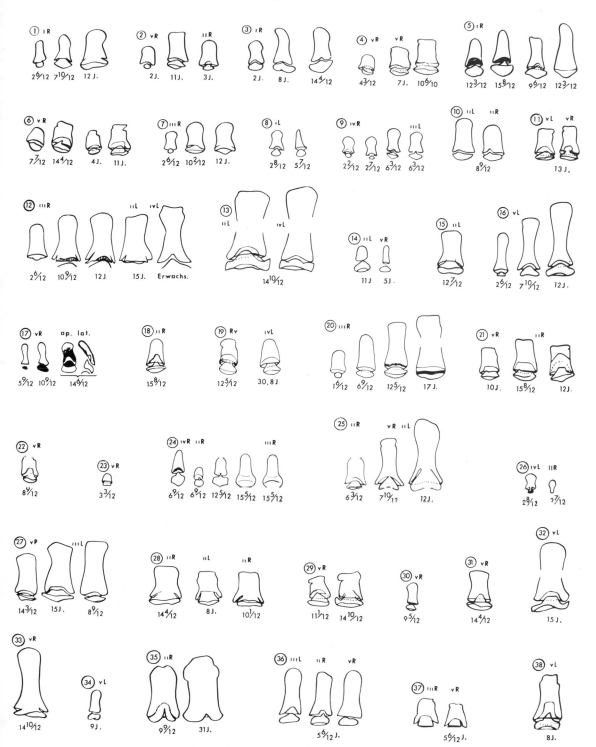

Figure 6–27. Giedion classification of cone epiphyses. Some of the types of epiphyses are commonly seen in normals, while others are pathognomonic of certain congenital malformation syndromes. The roman numerals indicate the position of the digit illustrated, using the same system as occurs in Figure 6–22. The age is listed below each figure. (From Giedion, A.: *Ann Radiol.*, 10:322–329, 1967.)

TABLE 6–2. Conditions Associated with
Cone Epiphyses

CONGENITAL
    Achondroplasia
    Acrodysostosis
    Chondroectodermal dysplasia (Ellis–van Creveld)
        (type 37 – middles)
    Cleidocranial dysostosis
        (type 19 or 20 mid, 24 distal)
    Kaschin-Beck disease
    Oro-facio-digital syndrome
    Oto-palato-digital syndrome (type 14)
    Peripheral dysostosis
    Thoracic-pelvic-phalangeal syndrome
    Tricho-rhino-phalangeal syndrome (type 12)
    Saldino-Mainzer syndrome

ACQUIRED
    Frostbite
    Infection
    Infarction – sickle cell
    Trauma

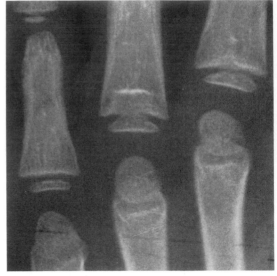

Figure 6–28. Deep cone in the proximal phalanx of the middle finger in a black male seen in the 10 State Nutrition Survey. This type of cone is the one associated with infarction and sickle cell disease. No definite clinical evidence of this was found, although it could have been missed.

The shape of the cone is also of some diagnostic value. Giedion has classified cones into 38 different types (Fig. 6–27).[3, 4] Some of these are seen in normal individuals whereas others are seen only in pathologic conditions and may actually be specific for these conditions. For example, Giedion found that type 24 in the distal phalanges and types 19 and 20 in the middle phalanges are pathognomonic and obligatory for cleidocranial dysostosis. Type 37 cones in the middle row are probably pathognomonic for the Ellis-van Creveld syndrome, while type 12 cones are seen in the tricho-rhino-phalangeal syndrome. Specific cone abnormalities are also seen in acrodysostosis and in the oto-palato-digital syndrome. Other conditions with cone-shaped epiphyses are listed in Table 6–2. See also Figures 6–28 to 6–31.

Thus, cone-shaped epiphyses must be

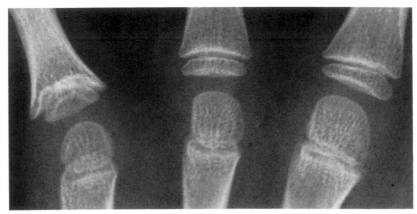

Figure 6–29. Unusual cone epiphysis localized to a single digit. The flaring of the bone and the cone is not usually the type seen in normals. This most likely represents some form of old trauma. (Courtesy Dr. Stanley Garn, 10 State Nutrition Survey.)

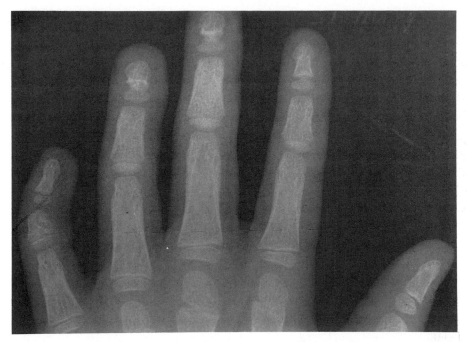

Figure 6–30. Bizarre distal cones somewhat suggestive of type 24 Giedion. No definite information about associated abnormalities was available on this patient. There is also shortening and irregularity of the middle phalanx of the fifth finger. (Courtesy Dr. Stanley Garn, 10 State Nutrition Survey.)

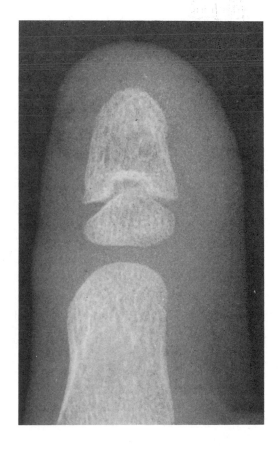

Figure 6–31. Cone epiphysis in the distal phalanx of the thumb in the oto-palato-digital syndrome. This type of coning in the thumb is commonly seen in children with this disorder.

considered abnormal it they are of an unusual type or at an unusual location.

REFERENCES

1. Garn, S. M., Poznanski, A. K., Nagy, J. M., and McCann, M. B.: Independence of Brachymesophalangia-5 from Brachymesophalangia-5 with Cone Mid-5. *Am. J. Phys. Anthropol.,* 36:295–298, 1972.
2. Giedion, A.: Cone-Shaped Epiphyses (CSE). *Ann Radiol.,* 8:135–145, 1965.
3. Giedion, A.: Cone-Shaped Epiphyses of the Hands and their Diagnostic Value. The Tricho-Rhino-Phalangeal Syndrome. *Ann. Radiol.,* 10:322–329, 1967.
4. Giedion, A.: Zapfenepiphysen. Naturgeschichte und diagnostiche Bedeutung einer Störung des enchondralen Wachst ums: *In* Glauner, R., Rüttimann, A., Thurn, P., and Vogler, E. (Eds.): *Ergebnisse der medizinische Radiologie.* Georg Thieme Verlag, Stuttgart, 1968, Vol. 1.
5. Hertzog, K. P., Garn, S. M., and Church, S. F.: Cone-shaped Epiphyses in the Hand. Population Frequencies, Anatomic Distribution and Developmental Stages. *Invest. Radiol.,* 3:433–441, 1968.
6. de Iturriza, J. R., and Tanner, J. M.: Cone-shaped Epiphyses and other Minor Anomalies in the Hands of Normal British Children. *J. Pediat.,* 75:265–272, 1969.
7. Saldino, R. M., and Mainzer, F.: Cone-Shaped Epiphyses (CSE) in Siblings with Hereditary Renal Disease and Retinitis Pigmentosa. *Radiology,* 98:39–45, 1971.
8. Takamori, T.: *Kaschin-Beck's Disease.* Professor Tokio Takamori Foundation, Gifu University School of Medicine, Japan, 1968, Vols. I and II.

SESAMOID BONE VARIATIONS

Sesamoid bones may occur adjacent to many of the joints of the hand.[1,2] Degen[2] showed two sesamoid bones adjacent to the metacarpophalangeal joint of the thumb in 100 per cent of patients, at the interphalangeal joint of the thumb in 72.9 per cent of cases and at the metacarpophalangeal joint of the fifth finger in 82.5 per cent of cases. Additional sesamoids are also seen over the metacarpal heads and at the distal interphalangeal joints of the second, fourth and fifth fingers, but sesamoids at these locations are considerably less common than at those sites previously mentioned (Fig. 6–32).

The sesamoids are variable in size and appearance, and some of the small ones may appear so dense as to be confused with bone islands when they are projected over the finger bones. The larger sesamoids are usually well trabeculated and clearly defined. The size of the sesamoids may be of value in the diagnosis of acromegaly (Chapter 2). The sesamoid may be double or multiple and this may make differentiation from fracture difficult.[5] Sometimes fractures are crescent-shaped, while the partitioned sesamoids are usually more linear. Fractures may be transverse, however, in which case differentiation may be more difficult. The usual criterion of looking

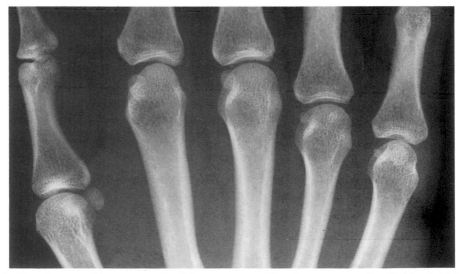

Figure 6–32. Sesamoid bones on all of the metacarpal heads in a normal individual. Although this large a number of sesamoids is uncommon, it has no particular diagnostic significance.

for definite cortical margins, as well as correlation with clinical signs and symptoms, is useful in differentiating these entities.

A rare problem with sesamoid bones is that they can become entrapped in metacarpophalangeal dislocations, causing problems in reduction. Nutter[3] and Sweterlitsch et al.[4] reported such cases.

REFERENCES

1. Bizarro, A. H.: On Sesamoid and Supernumerary Bones of the Limbs. *J. Anat.*, 55:256–268, 1921.
2. Degen, S.: Ueber das Auftreten der Knochenkern am Handskelett von der Geburt bis zur Reife. Mit einem Hinweis auf die Sesambeine der Hand. *Med. Klin.*, 46:1330–1332, 1951.
3. Nutter, P. D.: Interposition of Sesamoids in Metacarpophalangeal Dislocations. *J. Bone Joint Surg.*, 22:730–734, 1940.
4. Sweterlitsch, P. R., Torg, J. S., and Pollack, H.: Entrapment of a Sesamoid in the Index Metacarpophalangeal Joint. *J. Bone Joint Surg.*, 51A:995–998, 1969.
5. Voluter, G., and Calame, A.: Contribution a L'Etude Radiologique et Clinique des Fractures du Sesamoide Radial du Pouce. *J. Radiol. Electrol. Med. Nucl.*, 29:569–572, 1948.

VARIATION IN SHAPE OF THE PHALANGES AND METACARPALS

The size of the tufts of the distal phalanges is very variable (Fig. 6–33).[5] Males have larger phalangeal tufts than females. Those doing heavy manual labor have heavier tufts than those who use their hands less. The tuft itself may be smooth or round or have a very irregular margin. In some individuals, particularly among the elderly, small, proximally directed projections may be evident on each side of the tuft. In the lateral view they are usually directed toward the volar aspect (Fig. 6–34). The tufts increase in size in acromegaly, and have a drumstick-like appearance in Turner's syndrome.

Acroosteolysis of the tuft may be seen as a familial condition (Cheney's syndrome), or the tufts may be eroded in a large variety

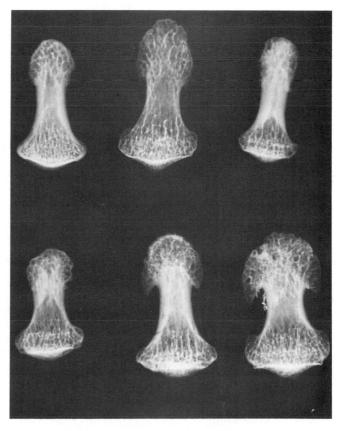

Figure 6–33. Assorted distal phalanges. Anatomic specimens. Note the variation in the shape and configuration of the tuft, the thickness of the cortex and the degree of ossification within it. Note variation in small spurs extending from tufts.

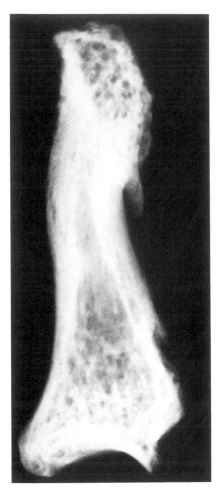

Figure 6–34. Lateral view of distal phalanx with spurs. Note volar direction of the small spurs.

cysts (Chapter 15). Defects in the distal phalanges may also be seen in tuberous sclerosis.

Kirner's deformity includes curving of the distal phalanx of the fifth finger and is further described in Chapter 10. It is associated with deformity of the epiphysis of that phalanx and on occasion can involve other fingers.

Another variation sometimes seen is a bulge in the midportion of the middle phalanges (Fig. 6–36). The exact significance of this is not clear. A number of these cases were seen in the 10 State Nutrition Survey. In some cases this has been associated with shortening of the middle phalanges with a length reduction pattern similar to that of the tricho-rhino-phalangeal syndrome. However, no cone epiphyses characteristic of the latter condition were seen. Char reported bulging of the middle phalanges in the Noonan syndrome.[1] Broad middle phalanges are also seen in frontometaphyseal dysplasia.

Decrease in size or lack of medullary cavities is sometimes seen in the metacarpals. This is termed medullary stenosis (Fig. 6–37). It may be an isolated normal

of disorders, including scleroderma, pyknodysostosis, leprosy, chemical exposure and other neurotrophic disorders.

The amount of cortical bone in the distal phalanx is also very variable (Fig. 6–33). It may be well defined with a definite cortex or it may be invisible. In some normal older individuals, particularly women, increased endosteal sclerosis may be evident.[3] We have seen very dense sclerotic tufts in a patient with hypoparathyroidism (Fig. 6–35).[4, 6] This has also been considered by some as a sign of collagen disease.[4, 6]

Lucencies in the distal phalanx may be due to a nutrient foramina as well as to a variety of other lesions, such as glomus tumors, epidermoid tumors and inclusion

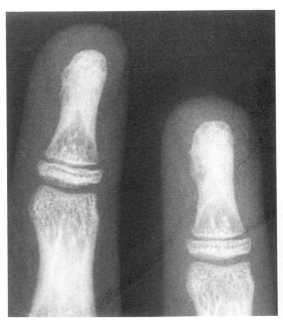

Figure 6–35. Endosteal sclerosis of phalanges in a teen-aged girl with idiopathic hypoparathyroidism.

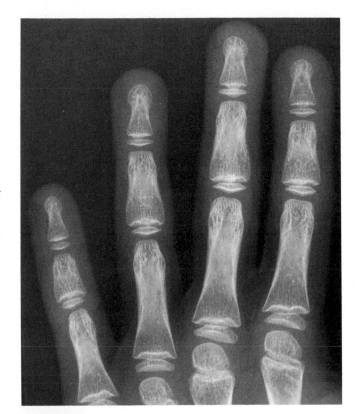

Figure 6–36. Broad middle phalanges. There is an unusual bulging of the middle phalanges. This variant has been seen in a proportion of the normal population and its significance is not clear.

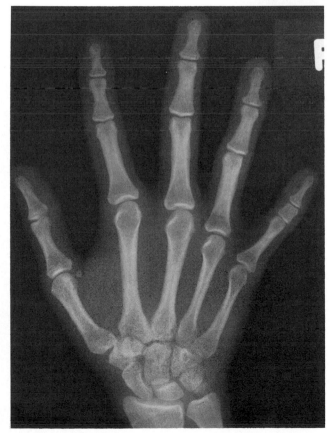

Figure 6–37. Medullary stenosis. This is a 4'9" tall, 17 year old girl who has been short all of her life. Note the almost complete absence of the medullary cavity. There is shortening of the middle phalanx of the fifth finger.

variant, or it may be associated with short-ness of stature and with the Caffey-Kenny syndrome.

There is also much variation in the ap-pearance of the styloid process of the sec-ond and third metacarpals. The third meta-carpal styloid process may be absent and in its place there may be a separate ossicle, the os styloideum or cape bossu (Chapter 8).

REFERENCES

1. Char, F., Rodriquez-Fernandez, H. L., Scott, C. I., Borgaonkar, D. S., Bell, B. B., and Rowe, R. D. The Noonan Syndrome. A Clinical Study of Forty-Five Cases. *Birth Defects, Original Article Series*, Part XV, Vol. 8, No. 5, 1972, pp. 100–118.
2. Cheney, W. D.: Acroosteolysis. *Am. J. Roentgenol.*, 94:595–607, 1965.
3. Deak, P.: Die Akroosteosklerose. *Fortschr. Geb. Roentgenstr.* Nuklearmed., 89:59–66, 1958.
4. Goodman, N.: The Significance of Terminal Pha-langeal Osteosclerosis. *Radiology*, 89:709–712, 1967.
5. Kohler, A., and Zimmer, E. A.: *Borderlands of the Normal and Early Pathologic in Skeletal Roent-genology*, 3rd Ed. Grune & Stratton, Inc., New York, 1968.
6. Podkaminsky, N. A.: Acrosclerosis Hyperplastica Intraossea. *Am. J. Roentgenol.*, 38:889–892, 1937.
7. Sugiura, Y., and Nakazawa, O.: *Bone Age, Roentgen Diagnosis of Skeletal Development*. Chugai-Igaku Company, Tokyo, 1968, p. 291.

Chapter 7

ANOMALIES OF THE HAND – GENERAL CONSIDERATIONS

HISTORICAL FACETS
NOMENCLATURE OF THE CONGENITAL LIMB
  DEFORMITIES
GLOSSARY OF TERMS USED TO DESCRIBE
  HAND ABNORMALITIES AND VARIANTS

CAUSES OF CONGENITAL MALFORMATIONS
INCIDENCE OF CONGENITAL MALFORMATIONS

HISTORICAL FACETS

Anomalies of the hands and feet have long interested both layman and physician. Many individuals with hand anomalies were exhibited in circuses. Even pre-Columbian sculptures show limb anomalies.[34] Artists have depicted many of the minor variations of the hand. Bruno[4] lists some paintings by the great masters which show clinodactyly, arachnodactyly and camptodactyly, although the presence of the latter is somewhat dubious since it could have been positional. Historical data on many hand anomalies are illustrated in Gould and Pyle's[15] book *Anomalies and Curiosities in Medicine*, published in 1900. Amelia and phocomelia were apparently described by Paré in the 16th century. There is a particular wealth of information on polydactyly and double hands which dates back to the Bible,[2] in which a giant with six fingers and six toes bilaterally is described. Burman[5] reviewed some of the cases of polydactyly in the 16th and 17th centuries, including a patient of Paré in 1575, who had double hands and forearms.

NOMENCLATURE OF THE CONGENITAL LIMB DEFORMITIES

The terminology for the various limb malformations has been somewhat confusing. Different terms for the same entity are used in different countries. Anatomists, geneticists, surgeons and radiologists use a different approach to nomenclature. No truly radiologic terminology has been described, except to define which anatomic parts are absent and which are present.

The original terminology for the various congenital anomalies was introduced by Isidore Geoffrey Saint-Hilaire[14] in 1837. He used the terms phocomèle, hemimèle and ectromèle. Phocomèle, which literally means seal limbs, referred to hands and feet of usual size supported by extremely short limbs. In hemimèle, part of the limb, i.e., the hand or foot, was missing. Ectromèle was characterized by complete absence of one of the imperfect digits and included three types: either a stump, a completely absent extremity or an extremity ending in one or more imperfect digits.

Since there was much confusion in the

usage of these terms, the Subcommittee on Children's Prosthetics of the National Academy of Science—National Research Council adopted a modification of the Frantz–O'Rahilly classification.[6] There was dissatisfaction with the term hemimelia because in some ways it implied absence of half of a limb while in many situations only a portion of it was missing. It thus dropped the term hemimelia. Also, terms like peromelia, ectromelia and phocomelia were dropped. It used only the terms amelia or meromelia, amelia being the absence of a limb and meromelia (a new term derived from the Greek words *meros*, meaning partial, and *melos*, meaning limb) being partial absence of a limb. Meromelia was then described in regard to its location, whether terminal or intercalary, and each of these categories was grouped as to whether it occurred along the transverse or the longitudinal axis.

The term meromelia, although convenient, has not been widely adopted; but the concept of the defect as terminal or intercalary and as transverse or longitudinal appears useful (Fig. 7–1). Partially because

of the persistent confusion in terminology and partially because of the lack of international acceptance of any of these terms, radiologic descriptions should include which parts are present, which are absent and which are deformed. Another classification of limb malformations has been developed by Swanson, Barsky and Entin,[32] and has been adopted for trial by the American Society of Surgery of the Hand. This is a more complete classification than the previous one in that it includes all abnormalities, not only the limb deficiencies. The portions relating to the hand are as follows:

1. Failure of differentiation of parts
   a. Syndactyly
   b. Contractures secondary to muscle, including camptodactyly
   c. Lateral deviation of digits, i.e., clinodactyly
2. Arrest of development of parts
   a. Transverse; includes aphalangia to amelia
   b. Intermediate, i.e., phocomelia

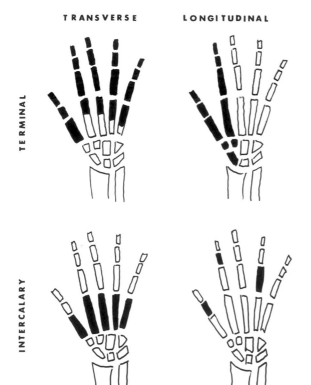

Figure 7–1. Classification of defects as terminal or intercalary, and as transverse or longitudinal.

c. Longitudinal
   (1) Radial defect
   (2) Central defect
   (3) Ulnar defect
3. Duplications, ranging from polydactyly to dicheiria
4. Overgrowth, including megalodactyly
5. Congenital circular constrictions—Streeter's bands
6. Generalized skeletal defects, such as in the bone dysplasias

Temtamy and McKusick[33] have classified the hand malformations into seven main groups on the basis of anatomic and genetic characteristics. The groups are

1. Absence deformities
2. Brachydactyly
3. Syndactyly
4. Polydactyly
5. Contracture deformities
6. Symphalangism
7. Hand malformations with congenital ring constrictions

Each of these groups is then divided into two categories: those that occur as isolated findings and those that are associated with other anomalies.

Although the previously described classifications are useful on clinical grounds, from the radiologic description point-of-view we shall consider malformations in subsequent chapters in terms of their location.

GLOSSARY OF TERMS USED TO DESCRIBE HAND ABNORMALITIES AND VARIANTS[6, 25, 33]

Some of the terms listed below can be used for other portions of the body as well as for the hand. However, the descriptions will refer mainly to the hand. The detailed description of most of these defects will be presented in the subsequent three chapters.

Acheiria—absence of the hand (also achiria).

Adactyly—absence of all the fingers.

Amelia—absence of limbs.

Amputation—absence of a distal part of a limb.

Brachydactyly—short fingers (usually refers to short phalanges).

Brachymetacarpalia—short metacarpals.

Brachymesophalangism—short middle phalanx.

Camptodactyly—curvature of a finger in the plane of flexion of the hand.

Central defect—absence of one or more of the central rays of the hand, either the second, third or fourth, or any combination thereof.

Clinodactyly—deviation of a finger in the plane of the hand, most commonly involving the fifth finger.

Dicheiria—double hand.

Dimelia—double limb.

Ectrodactyly—total or partial absence of fingers or hand. This is a confusing term which is used by different authors for a wide range of anomalies. Some authors even include split hand in this entity.

Hemimelia—absence of part of a limb. In the Frantz-O'Rahilly classification, this term is modified by the part that is missing, i.e., in radial hemimelia the radial portion is missing. Since the prefix hemi means a half, and since the term was confusing because it did not include amputations, the term meromelia was introduced to replace it.[6]

Hyperphalangism—the presence of accessory phalanges. This is most commonly present in the thumb.

Hypodactyly—decreased number of fingers; also called oligodactyly.

Hypophalangism—decreased number of phalanges.

Intercalary deficiency—absence of a middle portion of a limb while the proximal and distal portions are present.

Longitudinal deficiency—absence of a portion of the limb extending parallel to the long axis of the limb, such as a radial absence. It may be preaxial (on radial side), postaxial (on ulnar side) or central.

Macrodactyly—hyperplasia of the digit.

Megalodactyly—hyperplasia of the digit.

Meromelia—partial absence of a limb.

Micromelia—short limbs without absence of bone elements.

Oligodactyly—absence of some of the fingers.

Perodactyly—deformed fingers

Peromelia—used by some authors, particularly by the Germans, to denote hemimelia, but particularly for those cases of hands ending in a stump.

Phocomelia—partial absence of any proximal region of the limb. It usually refers to normal-sized hands supported by excessively short limbs.

Polydactyly—increased number of digits. May be preaxial, i.e., involving the radial side of the hand, or postaxial, on the ulnar side of the hand.

Postaxial—ulnar side of the hand.

Preaxial—thumb or radial side of the hand.

Split hand—includes hands with lobster-claw deformity (absence of central rays) and single digit types.

Symphalangism—congenital fusion of two phalanges in the same digit.

Syndactyly—fusion of adjacent digits. May be cutaneous or osseous.

Terminal deficiency—absence of bones which are distal to the proximal limit of the deficiency. This defect may be either transverse or longitudinal.

Transverse deficiency—absence of a portion of the limb going across the width of the limb.

CAUSES OF CONGENITAL MALFORMATIONS[9, 10, 11, 21, 34]

Only a minority of malformations have a major environmental cause or a major genetic cause. Most malformations result from complicated interactions between genetic predisposition and subtle factors in the environment.[9]

The environmental factors responsible for congenital defects of the extremities include various teratogens, the best known of which is thalidomide.[21] This is responsible in man for many anomalies of the upper extremity, ranging from hypoplasia of the thenar eminence to radial defects and absence of the extremities. Triphalangeal finger-like thumbs are the defects most commonly seen, and the legs are occasionally affected. Anomalies of other systems are also seen. The sensitive period is between the 34th and 50th day of gestation. Ear anomalies occur between 34 and 38 days; amelia occurs between 39 and 44 days and phocomelia occurs before 42 days. Triphalangism is associated with drug ingestion at about the 50th day. Dilantin and phenobarbital have also been implicated in producing digital hypoplasias (Figs. 9–3C and 9–16).[23]

The teratogenic action of other drugs in man is more questionable. Isolated reports of hand deformity have been reported with a variety of drugs,[34] including changes in a child whose mother took LSD,[1] but these may be purely coincidental. Fused carpals and a short forearm have been reported in a case due to aminopterin.[28] There has been much experimental evidence of limb abnormalities having been produced by many agents,[11] including vitamin deficiency (A, riboflavin, pantothenic acid); vitamin antagonists (including aminopterin), vitamin A excess, nucleic acid antagonists, alkylating agents (including nitrogen mustard and chlorambucil), physical agents (x-rays and hypothermia) and antibiotics (tetracycline and penicillin) as well as other drugs, including caffeine, salicylates and nicotine. The ability of these drugs to produce anomalies in animals may have little significance in man. Fraser[10] states that much of the experimental data in animals are not pertinent to man, since "one cannot reliably predict from the teratogenic behavior of a drug in one species, what it will do in another." Many species appear to be sensitive to certain drugs. With most of these drugs no evidence of human malformation has been seen. For example, there has been evidence that the use of insulin in chicks produces deformity of the extremities, whereas deformities from this cause have not occurred in man.

The mutagenic effects of radiation on limb anomalies are probably minor or nonexistent. Plummer,[27] in 1952, in follow-up studies of the offspring of pregnant women exposed to atom bombs at Hiroshima, found some increase in microcephaly but no significant change in the incidence of skeletal anomalies.

Intrauterine factors that may produce congenital defects include the amniotic bands, which may cause ring constrictions or amputations (Streeter's bands). Although experimentally these can be produced, there is little evidence to suggest that amniotic bands are responsible for most of these defects in man. Streeter has doubted this relationship.[31] However, there is evidence that these constrictions are related to amniotic rupture (p. 191).

Congenital malformations may be sporadic or genetically determined. Those of genetic origin may be inherited as either dominant or recessive traits. The majority of these malformations are sporadic, however. For example, cases of amputation amelia and many cases of ectrodactyly and cleft hands occur sporadically, although in the latter group there have been cases reported with dominant inheritance. Most of the brachydactyly syndromes are genetically determined, usually as a dominant. Polydactyly can be sporadic or genetically determined. Many of the syndrome-associated hand anomalies follow the inheritance pattern for that particular syndrome. The genetics of the various malformations will be given in further detail later, with the discussion of the individual syndromes. A confusing aspect of the pattern of inheritance of hand anomalies is that in many cases there is considerable variation in the expression of the trait and there may even be some crossover between different deformities. For example, in studying some of the families with clinodactyly, it was found that occasional members had camptodactyly. Similarly, in the Holt-Oram syndrome, in the same family the defects have varied from phocomelia with absent thumb, to triphalangeal thumb.

There is a higher incidence of hand abnormalities associated with certain defects, particularly cleft palate and those defects affecting the heart. The radial defects of the hand have been especially commonly associated with these.[3] Whether the association is related to the timing of the production of the defect is not clear.

In some cases acquired disorders mimic congenital abnormalities. For example, infarcts from sickle-cell disease can cause acquired brachydactyly or brachymetacarpelia similar to congenital forms due to other causes, except that the pattern of shortening is unusual. Other postnatal defects—an example is rheumatoid arthritis—can affect the growth of an epiphyseal plate and cause relative shortening of an extremity. Damage to the epiphysis from other causes, such as infection or trauma, may result in growth abnormality of the digits.

INCIDENCE OF CONGENITAL MALFORMATIONS

The incidence of congenital malformations of the hand is difficult to determine in most series, since many hand changes are minor and, unless specifically sought, can easily be missed. This is particularly true in reviews of birth certificates, where minor hand anomalies are usually omitted. The incidence of these anomalies is also very dependent on the population chosen. Some pertinent incidence data are listed in Table 7–1.

From birth certificate data, the most common anomaly appears to be polydactyly, which may be because it is a more obvious entity than other hand anomalies. The incidence of this defect in Pennsylvania birth certificates was 0.66 per 1000 births.[16] When broken down by race, its incidence was only 0.27 per 1000 in whites and 5.04 in non-whites.[17] International variations in this anomaly are considerable.[30] The lowest incidence was reported from Madrid, with approximately 0.05 per 1000, while the highest, from Pretoria (in Bantus), was 4.79 per 1000. The incidence of syndactyly from the birth certificate data was 0.76 per 1000 in Pennsylvania[16] and 0.40 per 1000 in Missouri.[29] A similar incidence of 0.42 per 1000 was found in Sweden,[18] but if the children who had other anomalies are not counted, the incidence is only 0.28.

However, some minor anomalies cannot be fully evaluated by this method. For example, clinodactyly is probably not described in birth certificates. Marden,[24] in an examination of 4322 infants with no major anomaly, found the incidence of clinodactyly to be 9.9 per 1000, while in the 90 babies that had other major anomalies the incidence of clinodactyly was 122 per 1000. Some of the other incidences of anomalies are listed in Table 7–1.

Some anomalies are not evident except on radiography. This is particularly true for the changes in the carpals. Triquetrum-lunate fusion, for example, cannot be clinically evaluated. In a study of 7500 subjects of African origin,[13] the incidence of triquetrum-lunate fusion was 1.6 per cent, while it was only 0.1 per cent in 11,663 persons of European origin.

The incidence of phocomelia and radial defects showed an upsurge in many countries during the thalidomide era, so that studies such as the one of Lock include these figures. Further details on the incidence of the various anomalies will be listed in subsequent chapters.

TABLE 7-1. Incidence of Some Hand Anomalies—Selected Data

DEFECT	INCIDENCE PER 1000	RACE	LOCATION OF POPULATION	POPULATION SIZE	TYPE OF DATA	REFERENCE
Polydactyly	0.27	white	Pennsylvania	962,853	birth certificate	Ivy[17]
"	5.04	nonwhite	"	126,842	"	Stevenson et al.[30]
Ulnar polydactyly	0.05		Madrid	19,967	"	" "
"	4.79	Bantu	Pretoria	10,224	"	" "
Radial polydactyly	0.025		Bombay	39,993	"	" "
"	0.91		Hong Kong	10,001	"	" "
Reduction deformities	0.05		Calcutta	19,465	"	" "
"	1.78		São Paulo	14,634	"	" "
"	0.45		Sweden	159,500	births with no other anomalies	Källen and Winberg[18]
Radial defects	0.83		Birmingham	159,500	births, all	Leck[20]
"	0.13		Denmark	256,234	mixed	Birch-Jensen[3]
Ulnar defects	0.018		Denmark	4,024,000	whole population	" "
Amelia	0.005					Leck[20]
"	0.01		Birmingham	256,324	1950–1962 combined methods	" "
Phocomelia—whole arm	0.04				"	" "
Terminal transverse above wrist	0.06				"	" "
Terminal transverse below or at wrist	0.09				"	" "
Amputation of hand	0.013		Denmark	4,024,000	entire population	Birch-Jensen[3]
Split hands	0.014				"	" "
Ectrodactyly	0.01				"	" "
Syndactyly	0.076	mixed	Pennsylvania	1,240,540	births with no other anomalies	Ivy[16]
"	0.28		Sweden	159,500	births, all	Källen and Winberg[18]
Clinodactyly	0.42		United States	4322	examined newborns with no anomalies	Marden et al.[24]
"	9.9		United States	90	examined newborns with other anomalies	" "
Brachymesophalangism[5]	122.0					Garn et al.[24]
"	6.0		Ohio	647	S.W. Ohio adults outpatients	" "
"	50.0		Hong Kong	247	recruits	" "
Triphalangism syndrome	0.04	whites	Unites States	75,000	recruits	Lapidus et al.[19]
Triquetrum-lunate fusion	1.0	whites	United States	11,663	10-state national nutrition survey	Garn et al.[13]
"	15.8	blacks	United States	7543	"	" "
"	89.0	Hausa (blacks)	Nigeria	500	radiologic survey	Cockshott[7]

REFERENCES

1. Assemany, S. R., Neu, R. L., and Gardner, L. I.: Deformities in a Child Whose Mother Took L.S.D. *Lancet*, 1:1290, 1970.
2. *The Bible*. 2 Samuel 21:20.
3. Birch-Jensen, A.: *Congenital Deformities of the Upper Extremities*. Andelsbogtrykkeriet, Odense, Denmark, 1949.
4. Bruno, G.: Malformazioni delle Dita della Mano nella Patologia e nell'Arte. *Minerva Med.*, 50:3685–3691, 1959.
5. Burman, M.: An Historical Perspective of Double Hands and Double Feet: The Survey of the Cases Reported in the 16th and 17th Centuries. *Bull. Hosp. Joint Dis.*, 29:241–254, 1968.
6. Burtch, R. L.: Classification Nomenclature of Congenital Skeletal Limb Deficiencies. *In*

Swinyard, C. A. (Ed.): *Limb Development and Deformity: Problems of Evaluation and Rehabilitation.* Charles C Thomas, Publisher, Springfield, Illinois, 1969, pp. 505–524.

7. Cockshott, W. P.: Carpal Fusions. *Am. J. Roentgenol.,* 89:1260–1271, 1963.

8. Frantz, C. H., and O'Rahilly, R.: Congenital Skeletal Limb Deficiencies. *J. Bone Joint Surg.,* 43A:1202–1224, 1961.

9. Fraser, F. C.: Causes of Congenital Malformations in Human Beings. *J. Chron. Dis.,* 10:97–110, 1959.

10. Fraser, F. C.: *Experimental Teratogenesis in Relation to Congenital Malformations in Man.* 2nd International Conference on Congenital Malformations. International Medical Congress, New York, 1964, pp. 277–287.

11. Freire-Maia, N.: Congenital Skeletal Limb Deficiencies—A General View. *Birth Defects, Original Article Series,* 5:7–13, 1969.

12. Garn, S. M., Fels, S. L., and Israel, H.: Brachymesophalangia of Digit Five in Ten Populations. *Am. J. Phys. Anthropol.,* 27:205–209, 1967.

13. Garn, S. M., Frisancho, A. R., Poznanski, A. K., Schweitzer, J., and McCann, M. B.: Analysis of Triquetral-Lunate Fusion. *Am. J. Phys. Anthropol.,* 34:431–433, 1971.

14. Geoffrey Saint-Hilaire, I.: *Histoire Générale et Particulière des Anomalies de l'Organisation chez d'Homme et les Animaux, Ouvrage . . . , avec Atlas.* 4 vols. J.-B. Baillière, Paris, 1832–1837.

15. Gould, G. M., and Pyle, W. L.: *Anomalies and Curiosities of Medicine . . .* (popular ed.). W. B. Saunders Company, Philadelphia, 1900, pp. 263–277, 350–352.

16. Ivy, R. H.: Congenital Anomalies as Recorded on Birth Certificates in the Division of Vital Statistics of the Pennsylvania Department of Health, for the Period of 1956 to 1960, Inclusive. *Plast. Reconstr. Surg.,* 32:361–367, 1963.

17. Ivy, R. H.: Congenital Deformities Recorded on Birth Certificates in Pennsylvania, 1961–1965 with Special Reference to Racial Influence on Incidence. *Plastic Reconstr. Surg.,* 41:50–53, 1968.

18. Källen, B., and Winberg, J.: A Swedish Register of Congenital Malformations: Experience with Continuous Registration during 2 Years with Special Reference to Multiple Malformations. *Pediatrics,* 41:765–776, 1968.

19. Lapidus, P. W., Guidotti, F. P., and Coletti, C. J.: Triphalangeal Thumb: Report of Six Cases. *Surg. Gynec. Obstet.,* 77:178–186, 1943.

20. Leck, I.: The Incidence of Limb Deficiencies in Recent Years. *In* Swinyard, C. A. (Ed.): *Limb Development and Deformity: Problems of Evaluation and Rehabilitation.* Charles C Thomas, Publisher, Springfield, Illinois, 1969, pp. 248–268.

21. Lenz, M. W.: Chemicals and Malformations in Man. In *Congenital Malformation: Papers and Discussions Presented at the Second International Congress, Session VI.* The International Medical Congress, Ltd., New York, 1964, pp. 263–276.

22. Lilienfeld, A. M.: Population differences in Frequency of Malformations at Birth. In *Congenital Malformations, Proceedings of the Third International Conference: Birth Defects—1969.* Excerpta Medica, The Hague, 7–13, September, 1969, pp. 251–263.

23. Loughnan, P. M., Gold, H., and Vance, J. C.: Phenytoin Teratogenicity in Man. *Lancet,* 1:70–72, 1973.

24. Marden, P. M., Smith, D. W., and McDonald, M. J.: Congenital Anomalies in the Newborn Infant, Including Minor Variations: A Study of 4,412 Babies by Surface Examination for Anomalies and Buccal Smear for Sex Chromatin. *J. Pediat.,* 64:357–371, 1964.

25. O'Rahilly, R.: Morphological Patterns in Limb Deficiencies and Duplications. *Am. J. Anat.,* 89:135–187, 1951.

26. O'Rahilly, R.: The Nomenclature and Classification of Limb Anomalies. *Birth Defects, Original Article Series,* 5:14–17, 1969.

27. Plummer, G.: Anomalies Occurring in Children Exposed *in Utero* to the Atomic Bomb in Hiroshima. *Pediatrics,* 10:687–693, 1952.

28. Shaw, E. B., and Steinbach, H. L.: Aminopterin-Induced Fetal Malformation: Survival of Infant After Attempted Abortion. *Am. J. Dis. Child.,* 115:477–482, 1968.

29. Silberg, S. L., Marienfeld, C. J., Wright, H., and Arnold, R. C.: Surveillance of Congenital Anomalies in Missouri, 1953–1964: A Preliminary Report. *Arch. Environ. Health,* 13:641–644, 1966.

30. Stevenson, A. C., Johnston, H. A., Stewart, M. I. P., and Golding, D. R.: Congenital Malformations: A Report of a Study of Series of Consecutive Births in 24 Centres. *World Health Organization Bulletin,* Supplement to 34:58–65, 1966.

31. Streeter, G. L.: Focal Deficiencies in Fetal Tissues and Their Relation to Intra-Uterine Amputation. In *Contributions to Embryology,* No. 126. Carnegie Institute of Washington, 22:1–44, 1930.

32. Swanson, A. B., Barsky, A. J., and Entin, M. A.: Classification of Limb Malformations on the Basis of Embryological Failures. *Surg. Clin. North Am.,* 48:1169–1179, 1968.

33. Temtamy, S., and McKusick, V. A.: Synopsis of Hand Malformations with Particular Emphasis on Genetic Factors: *Birth Defects, Original Article Series,* 5:125–184, 1969.

34. Warkany, J.: *Congenital Malformations.* Year Book Medical Publishers, Inc., Chicago, 1971.

35. Warkany, J.: Congenital Malformations in the Past. *J. Chron. Dis.,* 10:84–96, 1959.

Chapter 8

NORMAL VARIATION AND CONGENITAL ANOMALIES OF THE WRIST

The human carpus normally consists of eight small bones which, according to the *Nomina Anatomica* terminology, should be called the scaphoid, lunate, triquetrum, pisiform, trapezium, trapezoid, capitate and hamate.[2] The carpals begin to ossify shortly after birth. The first centers to appear are the capitate and hamate, while the pisiform is the last carpal bone to ossify. Normal values for the onset of ossification of the various carpals are given in Table 3–1.

VARIABILITY IN THE SHAPE OF THE CARPALS

The size and configuration of the carpals, as well as their relative position to each

other, often vary considerably among individuals. This variability is probably the greatest in the scaphoid, lunate and trapezium. Part of the variability is more apparent than real, being simply a manifestation of differences in position of the wrist during filming. Variation in apparent size of the carpus can also occur on the basis of relative delays in maturation. Disturbances in ossification, such as small bone islands (Fig. 8–1), and osteopoikilosis (Fig. 8–2) may be found in the carpals as in any other bone. Larger areas of sclerosis in the carpal bones may be seen in aseptic necrosis, particularly Kienböck's disease of the lunate (Chapter 21).

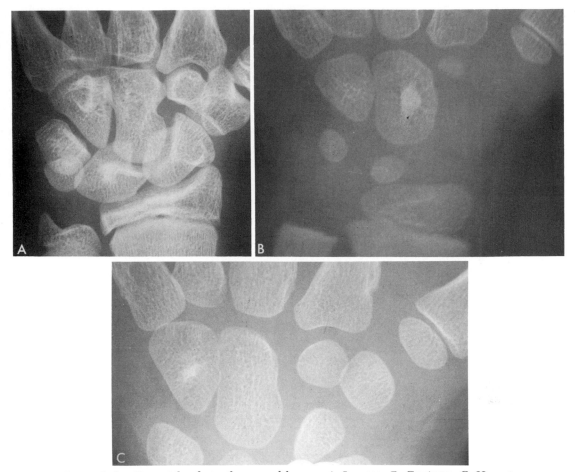

Figure 8–1. Bone islands in the carpal bones: *A*, Lunate. *B*, Capitate. *C*, Hamate.

Figure 8–2. Osteopoikilosis of the carpus. Adult male with multiple areas of increased density in the carpals.

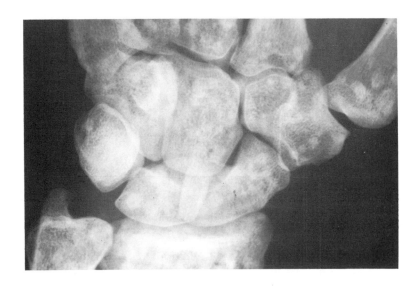

REFERENCES

1. Kohler, A., and Zimmer, E. A.: *Borderlands of the Normal and Early Pathologic in Skeletal Roentgenology,* 11th Ed. Grune & Stratton, Inc., New York, 1968.
2. O'Rahilly, R.: Developmental Deviations in Carpus and Tarsus. *Clin. Orthop.,* 10:9–18, 1957.
3. Poznanski, A. K., and Holt, J. F.: The Carpals in Congenital Malformation Syndromes. *Am. J. Roentgenol.,* 112:443–459, 1971.

CYSTS AND PSEUDOCYSTS OF THE CARPALS

Small radiolucencies in the carpal bones are common normal variants and may be seen at any age. They are, however, more common in late adulthood. They are most common in the capitate (Fig. 8–3A, B) and next most common in the lunate (Fig. 8–5), but may be seen in any of the carpals.[1] They are sometimes multiple. These cyst-like lesions were noted by Bugnion in 34.7 to 50.8 per cent (depending on the observer) of 600 cadaver wrists. When one radiographs dried capitates, a number of these radiolucencies appear to communicate with small linear canals that arise on the surface of the bone (Fig. 8–3C–G). These communications can be outlined with radiopaque material (Fig. 8–3E).

The nature of these lucent defects is not clear. Because of their communication with the vascular canals Ravelli[3] felt that these represented vascular channels. On the other hand, Bugnion[1] in detailed histologic studies showed that several different pathologic processes may be responsible. He felt that the cysts were of three types: those due to capsular herniation, "necrobiotic pseudocysts" due to vascular disturbances, and marginal arthrotic types. He felt that the ones seen normally in children were of the capsular herniation type. Scholder[4] felt that most of the cases were due to invagination of periarticular tissues along vascular channels.

Most of the cases studied by Bugnion were not related to occupation; however, occupational effects seem to be present, particularly in individuals who work with vibrating tools.[2] Cysts in these patients can be distinguished from the normal in that they are almost entirely subchondral in distribution. They would fit Bugnion's marginal arthrotic type.

REFERENCES

1. Bugnion, J.-P.: Lesions Nouvelles du Poignet. Pseudokystes Necrobiotiques. Kystes par Herniations Capsulaires. Arthrite Chronique Degenerative par Osteochondrose Marginale. *Acta Radiol.,* Supplement 90, Stockholm, 1951.
2. Horvath, F., and Kakosy, T.: Über strukturelle Veränderungen der Handwurzelknochen von Motorsägebedienern. *Z. Orthop.,* 107:482–494, 1970.
3. Ravelli, A.: Anatomisch-röntgenologische Handgelenkstudien. *Z. Orthop.,* 86:70–89, 1955.
4. Scholder, P.: Vascularisation Osseuse et Pseudokystes du Poignet. *Rev. Chir. Orthop.,* 39:1–56, 1953.

Figure 8–3. Capitate "cysts" or vascular channels. A normal variant.

A, Patient with "cyst" in the capitate in a typical location. Note also the normal notch in the radial aspect of the scaphoid.

B, Multiple carpal "cysts" in capitate, hamate and lunate.

C and D, Dry capitate in two different projections. A cyst-like lesion is well seen in the interior portion of the bone, and a channel from the cyst to the outer cortex can be seen in D. Several other cystic lesions are seen superiorly.

E, Tantalum powder was injected in a small foramen on the surface of the capitate shown in parts C and D. This fills the cavity.

F and G, Photograph of both sides of the dried capitate shown in parts C to E. Multiple small openings can be visualized at the surface of this bone. The indicated small opening (*arrow*) was the one that communicated with the large cavity within.

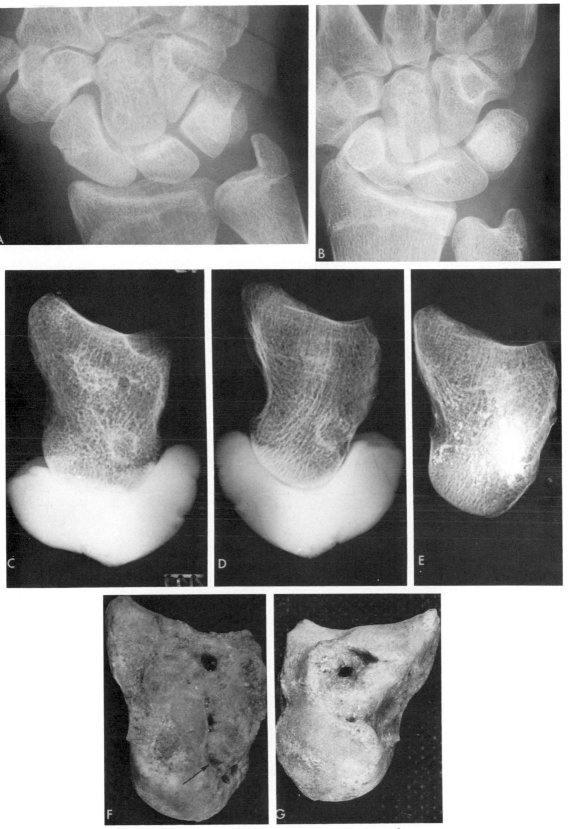

Figure 8–3. *See opposite page for legend.*

ALTERATIONS OF INDIVIDUAL CARPALS

Gross alterations in the structure, shape and configuration of the carpals may be seen in any condition that affects ossification; alterations are particularly severe in the mucopolysaccharidoses and the epiphyseal dysplasias and will be further discussed in subsequent chapters. Disappearance of the carpal bones may occur in familial osteolysis.

Scaphoid (Navicular)

The great variability in shape of the scaphoid makes it difficult to determine the limits of normal.[5] Its shape is particularly affected by radiographic position (Fig. 8–4). It can have a wide variety of bumps or notches along its contour. A notch along the ulnar side of the scaphoid may represent the site of fusion of the embryonal os centrale. A more common variation is a notch on the radial side of the scaphoid (Fig. 8–3A), which occurs in about 32 per cent of individuals after 50 years of age.[9] This notch has a cortical margin which is well defined and can thus be distinguished from notches due to bone erosion in rheumatoid arthritis and other conditions.[9] The notch may be produced by pressure of the radial styloid during radial deviation of the wrist.[9]

Even greater variability in the shape of the scaphoid is seen in a wide variety of

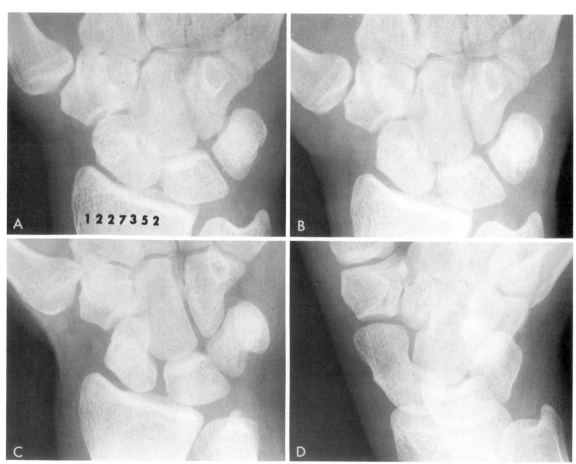

Figure 8–4. Variation in the shape of the scaphoid in different wrist positions. *A,* PA with thumb adducted. *B,* PA with thumb abducted. *C,* AP. *D,* Oblique. The scaphoid changes remarkably in shape in these views. Note the little bump on the radial side of the scaphoid in the oblique view. This is a common finding.

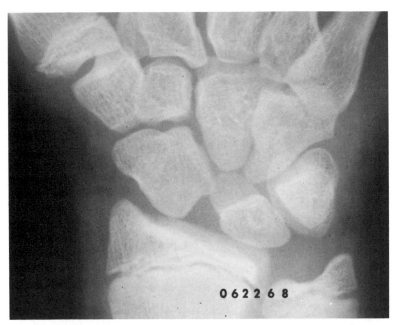

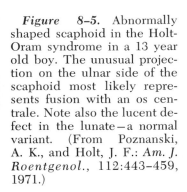

Figure 8–5. Abnormally shaped scaphoid in the Holt-Oram syndrome in a 13 year old boy. The unusual projection on the ulnar side of the scaphoid most likely represents fusion with an os centrale. Note also the lucent defect in the lunate—a normal variant. (From Poznanski, A. K., and Holt, J. F.: *Am. J. Roentgenol.*, 112:443–459, 1971.)

syndromes but particularly in the Holt-Oram, where some abnormality of the scaphoid was present in almost 100 per cent of cases.[7] Abnormally shaped scaphoids are present also in the hand-foot-uterus syndrome and in any condition where there is a tendency for persistent os centrale. Sometimes there is fusion of the os centrale with the scaphoid (Fig. 8–5).

The scaphoid may ossify from multiple centers (Figs. 8–6 and 8–7). Although this type of ossification may occur in otherwise normal individuals, it is commonly seen in association with marked delays in maturation, particularly in hypothyroidism. As maturation proceeds, these multiple ossicles coalesce into a single ossification center. It is likely that these separate centers are simply separate loci of calcification located within one cartilaginous bone.

A bipartite scaphoid may be seen in adults.[1, 3, 8] It is not clear how many of these are congenital and how many are the result of an old fracture. Some differential points include the fact that the bipartite scaphoid is often bilateral, or that there is a waist-like indentation in the scaphoid of the other hand. The joint space between the two portions may be lined with cartilage[8] or simply be smooth eburnated bone.[3] In either case the margins

are smooth on the radiograph and have a cortical margin as compared to the more irregular ill-defined edges of an old fracture. Generally, the space between the fragments is greater in the bipartite scaphoid than in an old fracture. Occasionally, an os centrale may be associated with the bipartite scaphoid.[3] In spite of these differences, differentiation from old fracture, particularly in unilateral cases, may not be possible without history.

Hypoplasia or absence of the scaphoid is often associated with radial defects (Fig. 8–8),[2, 7] including hypoplastic or absent thumbs or radii. The radial defects associated with hypoplasia of the carpals include both the isolated forms and those associated with various malformation syndromes, particularly Fanconi's anemia, Juberg-Hayward syndrome and Holt-Oram syndrome. In addition to absence of the scaphoid in these disorders, there may be hypoplasia or absence of the trapezium or the trapezoid. In the child, hypoplasia or absence of the scaphoid may be simply a manifestation of delayed maturation of this bone as compared to the other carpals. This type of dysharmonic maturation may exist in otherwise normal individuals. Delay in maturation may also be due to secondary factors, such as trauma or infection.

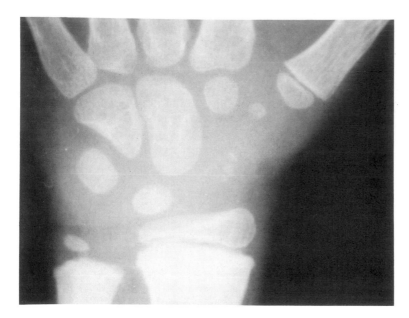

Figure 8–6. Tripartite scaphoid. Three separate ossification centers are seen in the scaphoid. (Courtesy Dr. S. M. Garn, 10 State Nutrition Survey, Ann Arbor, Michigan.)

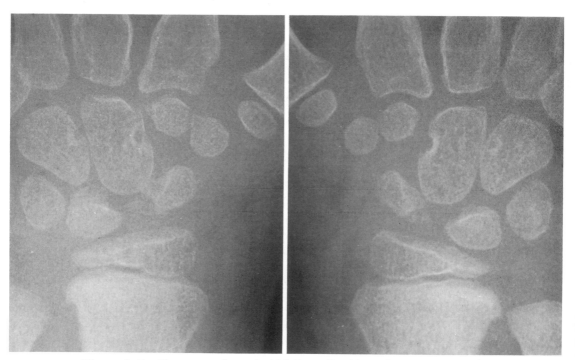

Figure 8–7. Fragmented scaphoid bilaterally. Note also capitate notch.

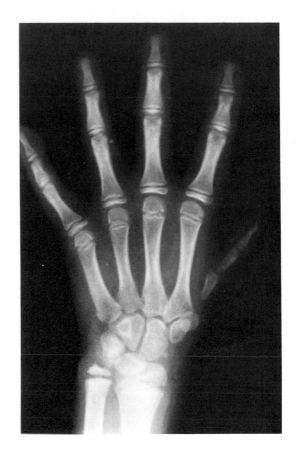

Figure 8–8. Hypoplastic scaphoid associated with hypoplastic thumb. This 10 year old girl had hypoplasia of the thumb as well as Klippel-Feil deformity, ventricular septal defect and mental retardation. The scaphoid is markedly underdeveloped. The trapezium is also hypoplastic. (From Poznanski, A. K., and Holt, J. F.: *Am. J. Roentgenol.*, 112:443–459, 1971.)

REFERENCES

1. Baciu, Cl., Gorun, N., and Roventza, N.: Le Scaph-oïde Carpien Bipartite. *Acta Orthop. Belg.*, 32:920–925, 1966.
2. Birch-Jensen, A.: *Congenital Deformities of the Upper Extremities.* Andelsbogtrykkeriet, Odense, Denmark, 1949.
3. Boyd, G. I.: Bipartite Carpal Navicular Bone. *Brit. J. Surg.*, 20:455–458, 1933.
4. Davison, E. P.: Congenital Hypoplasia of the Carpal-Scaphoid Bone. *J. Bone Joint Surg.*, 44B:816–827, 1962.
5. Kohler, A., and Zimmer, E. A.: *Borderlands of the Normal and Early Pathologic in Skeletal Roentgenology*, 11th Ed. Grune & Stratton, Inc., New York, 1968.
6. Poznanski, A. K., Garn, S. M., and Holt, J. F.: The Thumb in the Congenital Malformation Syndromes. *Radiology*, 100:115–129, 1971.
7. Poznanski, A. K., and Holt, J. F.: The Carpals in Congenital Malformation Syndromes. *Am. J. Roentgenol.*, 112:443–459, 1971.
8. Sherwin, J. M., Nagel, D. A., and Wouthwick, W. O.: Bipartite Carpal Navicular and the Diagnostic Problem of Bone Partition: A Case Report. *J. Trauma*, 11:440–443, 1971.
9. Swezey, R. L., and Alexander, S. J.: Notching of Carpal Navicular *Ann. Rheum. Dis.*, 28:45–48, 1969.

Lunate

The lunate is also a very variable bone both in terms of its shape and its onset of ossification. The 5th to 95th percentiles of onset for males are 1.53 to 6.77 years.[2] Ossification of the lunate may be delayed in onset in a wide variety of syndromes but particularly in the epiphyseal dysplasias and perhaps homocystinuria.[4] Absence of the lunate persisting into later life is most uncommon and may in some cases be related to previous infection or trauma.[5] Variations of shape may also be due to trauma, since the lunate is one of the more commonly dislocated bones of the wrist (see Chapter 15).

Double ossification centers for the lunate (Fig. 8–9) may be seen in normal individ-

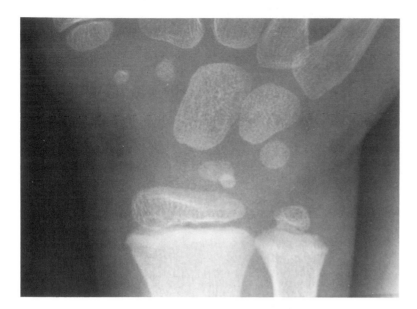

Figure 8–9. Double ossification center of the lunate. This nine year old boy has marked skeletal retardation due to hypothyroidism.

uals. They are relatively uncommon. There may be some familial tendency. Eggimann[1] described a double lunate center in a brother and sister. Bipartite lunates have also been seen in several malformation syndromes, particularly the oto-palato-digital (Fig. 8–10).

Increased density of the lunate is seen in Kienböck's disease (p. 570), which is probably related to trauma.

REFERENCES

1. Eggimann, V. P.: Zur Bipartition des Lunatum. *Radiol. Clin. Biol.*, 20:65–70, 1951.

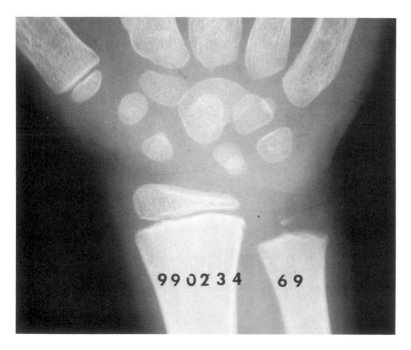

Figure 8–10. Wrist in the oto-palato-digital syndrome. This eight year old male has characteristic wrist findings of this disorder. There is a double ossification center of the lunate, the capitate is somewhat transverse in position, the scaphoid is hypoplastic for age and there is an accessory ossification center near the hamate. The trapezoid is somewhat unusual in shape and fits the broad base of the second metacarpal.

2. Garn, S. M., Rohmann, C. G., and Silverman, F. N.: Radiographic Standards for Postnatal Ossification and Tooth Calcification. *Med. Radiogr. Photogr.*, 43:45–66, 1967.
3. Gfeller, J., and Budliger, H.: Homocystinuria and Os Lunatum. *Lancet*, 2:548, 1966.
4. Morreels, C. L., Jr., Fletcher, B. D., Weilbaecher, R. G., and Dorst, J. P.: Roentgenographic Features of Homocystinuria. *Radiology*, 90:1150–1158, 1968.
5. Roche, A. F.: Absence of the Lunate. *Am. J. Roentgenol.*, 100:523–525, 1967.

Trapezium (Greater Multangular)

This bone is also very variable in its shape. It has a wide variety of protuberances. In some normal individuals it is markedly elongated.[1] This deformity may also be associated with abnormality of the first metacarpal and an elongated trapezium. Like any other carpal it may have several ossification centers (Fig. 8–11). Accessory ossicles adjacent to the trapezium may be seen (Fig. 8–12). An elongated trapezium has been found in some patients with the Holt-Oram syndrome. The trapezium is often absent or hypoplastic in cases of radial hypoplasia.

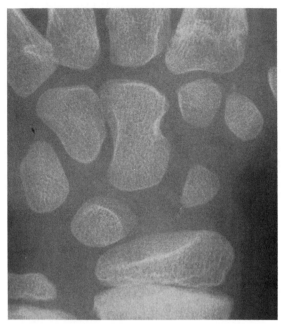

Figure 8–12. Notch in capitate is a common normal variant. This patient has a small ossicle adjacent to the trapezium.

REFERENCE

1. Rushforth, A. F.: A Congenital Abnormality of the Trapezium and First Metacarpal Bone. *J. Bone Joint Surg.*, 31B:543–546, 1949.

Trapezoid (Lesser Multangular)

This is a small bone which is partially overlapped by its neighbors. It may also be hypoplastic in association with severe radial defects. The most characteristic abnormality of this bone occurs in the oto-palato-digital syndrome, where it has the shape of a comma, which is related to the large pseudoepiphysis at the base of the second metacarpal (Fig. 8–10).

Capitate (Os Magnum)

This bone is a particularly common site for small cysts (Fig. 8–3). It often has a notch along its radial margin (Fig. 8–12). Absence of this bone is extremely rare and may be acquired. It can be deformed in the Holt-Oram syndrome. It has an unusual configuration in the oto-palato-digital syn-

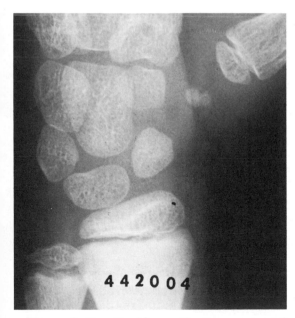

Figure 8–11. Double ossification center of the trapezium in an otherwise normal individual.

drome, where it assumes a somewhat transverse position (Fig. 8–10), particularly in young children. It may have a bizarre appearance in the Ellis-van Creveld syndrome, ranging from very slender to very wide, depending on whether it fuses with the adjacent carpal.

REFERENCE

1. Eraltug, U.: An Unusual Variety of Partial Carpal Agenesis. *Int. Surg.*, 46:594–595, 1966.

Hamate

Small cyst-like lesions may also occur in this bone. A number of variations of the hook of the hamate may be seen with a variety of ossicles forming about it. These can sometimes be mistaken for fractures. Additional ossification centers in the region of the hamate have been seen in the oto-palato-digital syndrome, as well as in the Ellis-van Creveld syndrome. These may eventually fuse with the hamate, resulting in an unusual configuration, or they may fuse with the capitate.

Triquetrum (Triangular or Cuneiform Bone)

This bone has been seen in bipartite form. Small fragments of it are subject to avulsion, causing multiple small ossicles adjacent to it. These are particularly common. They are further discussed in the section on accessory ossicles.

Pisiform

This is the last bone to ossify. It is variable in shape and may ossify with multiple centers (Fig. 8–13). The size of this bone is also quite variable. It may be somewhat large in several of the malformation syndromes.

VARIATIONS IN POSITIONS OF THE CARPALS—THE CARPAL ANGLE

There is considerable variation in the relative position of the carpals to one an-

other. One important relationship is the arrangement of the three proximal carpal bones which determines the carpal angle. This angle as described by Kosowicz[2, 3] is defined as the angle between two lines, the first tangent to the proximal surfaces of the scaphoid and lunate, the second tangent to the proximal margins of the triquetrum and lunate (Fig. 8–14). The normal angle according to Kosowicz measures 131.5° with a standard deviation of 7.2°.[3] In our own series it was 130.3° in white females and 137.4° in black females. A similar difference between blacks and whites was also seen in the male. A more complete breakdown of the normal values is given in Chapter 2.

The carpal angle may be decreased or increased in various conditions. A decreased carpal angle is seen in Madelung's deformity (Fig. 8–15). When associated with dwarfism and other minor anomalies, Madelung's deformity is called dyschondrosteosis.[4] Other conditions causing alteration in carpal angle are listed in Table 8–1. Frequently, carpal shape is affected when the angle is abnormal; for example, in arthrogryposis, when there is an increase in carpal angle, there is often an associated hypoplasia of the scaphoid (Fig. 8–14). When the carpal angle is decreased, as in Made-

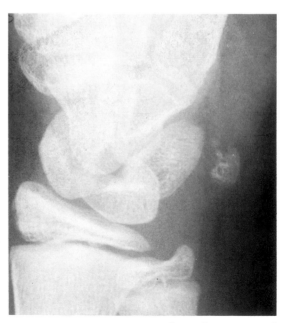

Figure 8–13. Fragmented pisiform, normal variation.

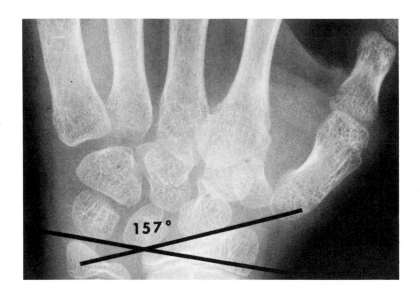

Figure 8–14. Carpal angle in arthrogryposis. The angle is elevated in this condition, measuring 157° in this patient. The proximal row of carpals forms less of a cup than usual. The hypoplastic scaphoid is commonly associated with this disease. (From Poznanski, A. K., and Holt, J. F.: *Am. J. Roentgenol.*, 112: 443–459, 1971.)

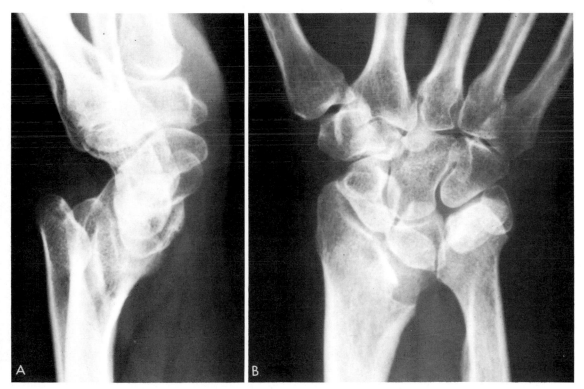

Figure 8–15. Madelung's deformity in a 33 year old female. The carpal bones form a deep cup with a marked decrease in the carpal angle (*B*). The ulna is displaced posteriorly (*A*).

TABLE 8–1. Syndromes Associated with Abnormality of the Carpal Angle

DECREASED
  Madelung's deformity
  Dyschondrosteosis
  Turner's syndrome
  Morquio's syndrome
  Hurler's syndrome

INCREASED
  Arthrogryposis
  Disastrophic dwarfism
  Epiphyseal dysplasias
  Frontometaphyseal dysplasia
  Oto-palato-digital syndrome
  Pfeiffer's syndrome
  Spondyloepiphyseal dysplasia
  Trisomy 21

per cent of individuals, while O'Rahilly[9] found them in 1.6 per cent.

Post-traumatic chip fragments are often difficult to differentiate from these ossicles. Although true ossicles have better defined cortical margins and are rounded and not associated with defects in adjacent bone, these signs may be identical to those of chip fractures, which over a period of many years can assume a smooth configuration. A rare entity which may be considered an accessory ossicle is tenosynovial chondrometaplasia;[6] however, the character of these calcifications and their location should allow differentiation.

The nomenclature of the accessory ossicles has been quite confusing. Different authors have used different terms for the same bone. In this book the terms sug-

lung's deformity (Fig. 8–15), again the scaphoid is the carpal most frequently altered in shape.

Some acquired conditions can also alter the relationship of the carpals to each other. Trauma with dislocation (Chapter 15), and rheumatoid arthritis particularly can cause significant disarrangements.

REFERENCES

1. Collins, L. C., Lidsky, M. D., Sharp, J. T., and Moreland J.: Malposition of Carpal Bones in Rheumatoid Arthritis. *Radiology*, 103:95–98, 1972.
2. Kosowicz, J.: Carpal sign in Gonadal Dysgenesis. *J. Clin. Endocrinol. Metab.*, 22:949–952, 1962.
3. Kosowicz, J.: Roentgen Appearance of Hand and Wrist in Gonadal Dysgenesis. *Am. J. Roentgenol.*, 93:354–361, 1965.
4. Langer, L. O., Jr.: Dyschondrosteosis; Hereditable Bone Dysplasia with Characteristic Roentgenographic Features. *Am. J. Roentgenol.*, 95: 178–188, 1965.

ACCESSORY CARPALS AND OTHER OSSICLES

Besides the eight normal carpal bones, a number of other ossicles about the wrist have been described.[5, 8, 9] These are illustrated in Figures 8–16 to 8–20. Most of the ossicles are of no clinical significance except that they must be differentiated from chip fractures. These ossicles are relatively common. Bogart[2] found them in about 0.3

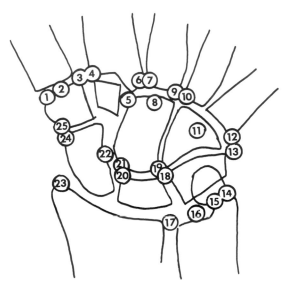

Figure 8–16. Accessory ossicles of the carpus using the terminology of O'Rahilly. The location of the ossicles is according to O'Rahilly, Kohler and Zimmer. *1*, Os paratrapezium; *2*, os praetrapezium; *3*, os trapezium secundarium; *4*, os trapezoideum secundarium; *5*, os metastyloideum; *6*, os parastyloideum; *7*, os styloideum; *8*, os subcapitatum; *9*, os capitatum secundarium; *10*, os Gruberi; *11*, os hamuli proprium; *12*, os Vesalianum; *13*, os ulnare externum; *14*, os ulnostyloideum; *15*, os pisiforme secundarium; *16*, os triangulare; *17*, small radioulnar ossicle; *18*, os epitriquetrum; *19*, os hypotriquetrum; *20*, os hypolunatum; *21*, os epilunatum; *22*, os centrale; *23*, os radiostyloideum; *24*, os radiale externum; *25*, os epitrapezium.

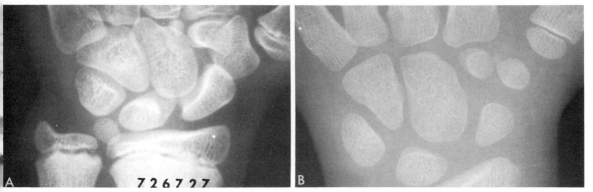

Figure 8–17. A, Accessory ossicle between the trapezoid, capitate and metacarpals, probably an os styloideum.

B, Accessory ossicle between the trapezium and trapezoid, probably an os trapezium secundarium.

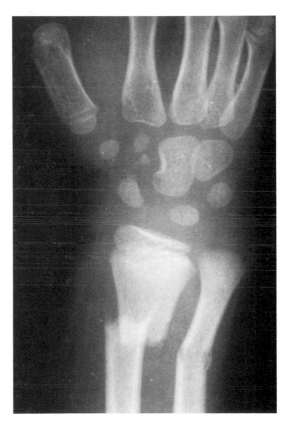

Figure 8–18. Os centrale in an otherwise normal child. There is a notch in the capitate, which is frequently associated with the os centrale. (From Poznanski, A. K., and Holt, J. F.: Am. J. Roentgenol., 112:443–459, 1971.)

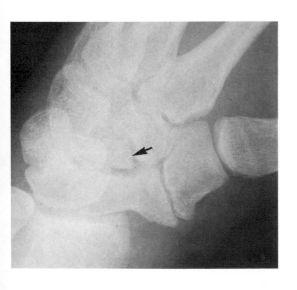

Figure 8–19. Os centrale in the Holt-Oram syndrome. The ossicle (*arrow*) lies between the capitate and the scaphoid in this adult male. The trapezium-scaphoid joint is also considerably narrowed and the trapezium has a somewhat unusual configuration.

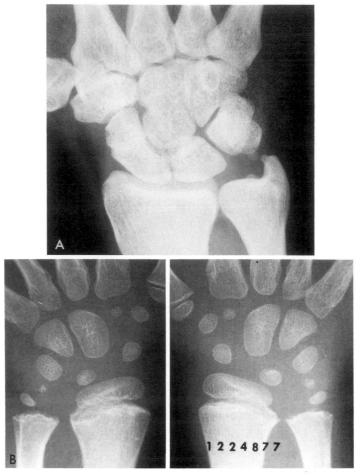

Figure 8–20. *A*, Os triangulare and an additional ossicle in an otherwise normal individual. A small ossicle overlying the ulna is the os triangulare. The other ossicle near the ulnar styloid may be termed either os ulnostyloideum or pisiforme secundarium. (From Poznanski, A. K., and Holt, J. F.: *Am. J. Roentgenol.*, 112:443–459, 1971.)

B, Bilateral os triangulare in a child.

Illustration continued on opposite page.

gested by O'Rahilly will be used. These are based mostly on the location of the bone. Actually, knowledge of the names of these ossicles is probably of little importance since they have so little significance. The first accessory ossicles were probably described by Vesalius in 1543, and one of these bears his name. Pfitzner,[10] in detailed anatomic studies, reported many of these ossicles. Most of the ossicles seem to have no known embryologic derivation except for the os centrale and the os triangulare, which are present in the developing embryo and disappear before birth. Interestingly enough, these two ossicles are particularly common in several of the congenital malformation syndromes (Table 8–2).

TABLE 8–2. Malformation Syndromes Associated with Accessory Carpal Ossicles

IN DISTAL ROW
  Diastrophic dwarfism
  Ellis-van Creveld syndrome
  Larsen's syndrome
  Oto-palato-digital syndrome
  Brachydactyly A–1

OS CENTRALE—REMNANTS OF CENTRAL ROW
  Hand-foot-uterus syndrome
  Holt-Oram syndrome
  Oto-palato-digital syndrome
  Gorlin-Schlorf-Paparella[4]
  Larsen's syndrome

OTHER
  Larsen's syndrome
  Ulnar dimelia

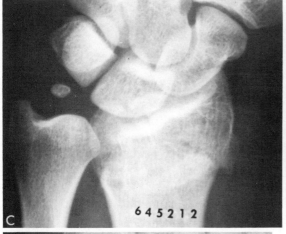

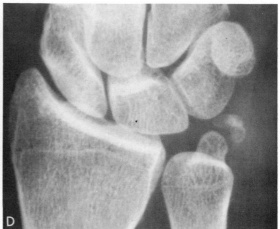

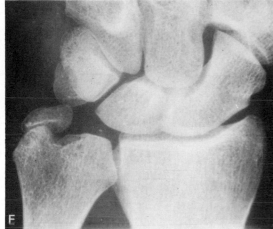

Figure 8–20. Continued. C to E, Ulnar ossicles of varying type may occur near the ulnar styloid. These ossicles can assume a variety of shapes. Occasionally they may be the result of old trauma.

A cartilaginous os centrale is usually present in the developing embryo at about six weeks' gestation, and it subsequently fuses with the scaphoid, forming part of the distal ulnar portion (see Chapter 1). Sometimes a lump or projection can be seen in the scaphoid at the site of this fusion. Occasionally these bones can fuse with the capitate or the trapezoid.[4] A notch of the capitate seen in some children may be the result of an indentation from an os centrale. The os centrale may be present in normal individuals (Fig. 8–18), but it is rather rare. On example was seen in 26,000 normal individuals in the 10 State Nutrition Survey. It is more commonly associated with a number of congenital malformation syndromes (Table 8–3). It thus may serve as a useful sign that one is

dealing with a malformation syndrome, particularly since several of these conditions associated with an os centrale have mild clinical findings and may be otherwise unsuspected. The os centrale associated with the Holt-Oram syndrome (Fig. 8–19) may be in its classic position between the capitate and the scaphoid or it may extend to the radial side of the wrist, resulting in a short scaphoid. Two such accessory ossicles between the proximal and distal rows were seen in 5 of 23 hands of patients with the Holt-Oram syndrome.[10] An os centrale has also been seen in other less well-defined syndromes, such as the one described by Gorlin et al.,[4] which also included cleft palate, stapes fixation and oligodontia.

Ossicles near the ulnar styloid are par-

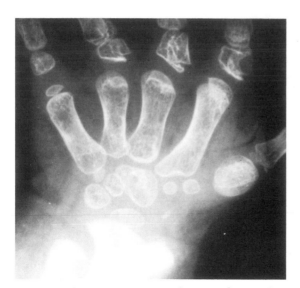

Figure 8–21. Extra carpals in a diastrophic dwarf. There is an additional carpal in the distal row along the ulnar side. The capitate is somewhat transverse in position. The thumb is hypoplastic. Phalangeal changes of diastrophic dwarfism are also seen. (From Poznanski, A. K., and Holt, J. F.: *Am. J. Roentgenol.*, 112:443–459, 1971.)

Besides the previously mentioned accessory ossicles a number of additional carpal bones may be seen in a variety of malformation syndromes (Table 8–3). Ossicles between the distal carpals and metacarpals are seen in Bell's type A-1 brachydactyly (Chapter 9). An increased number of distal carpals along the ulnar side of the wrist occurs in the oto-palato-digital syndrome (Fig. 8–10) and in some patients with diastrophic dwarfism (Fig. 8–21). Similarly, in the Ellis-van Creveld syndrome there is the formation of three bones in place of the hamate and capitate. In Larsen's syndrome the bones are arranged in an almost random fashion, and their number can be considerably increased (Fig. 8–22). An increased number of carpal bones is also seen in ulnar dimelia, where there is mirror duplication of the hand and wrist. Usually it is the bones on the ulnar side which are duplicated, particularly the hamate, capitate, triquetrum and lunate, while there is absence of the bones on the radial side. This is a rare entity and is usually not associated with malformation syndromes.[8]

ticularly common (Fig. 8–20). These bear different names, the most common of which is os triangulare, which is a more common normal variant than the os centrale. Bogart[2] found two such ossicles in 1425 individuals. This ossicle is also sometimes present in the fetal carpus in close relationship to the radioulnar joint, but it usually disappears at birth. A similar ossicle occurs in the carpus of the gibbon and is related to the meniscus which separates the ulna from the carpus. The occurrence of this ossicle in some of the congenital malformations is of less significance than the os centrale, since it is a more common entity.

One ossicle is worth mentioning, since it may be associated with symptoms. It is the os styloideum (Fig. 8–17A). This ossicle may be seen instead of the styloid process of the third metacarpal (in 2 per cent of patients according to O'Rahilly[9]). Occasionally it may be seen together with the styloid process. The ossicle may project posteriorly between the capitate and trapezoid and be easily traumatized. This disorder has been called carpe bossu or the hunchback carpal bone.[1, 3, 7]

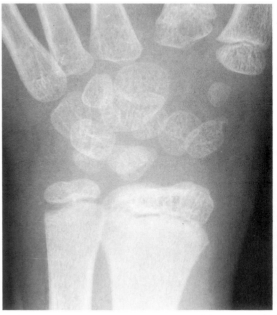

Figure 8–22. Carpals in probable Larsen's syndrome. The bizarre arrangement of carpals with unusual shape and increased number is characteristic of this disorder. (Courtesy Dr. John Carr and Dr. Stewart Reuter, Eloise, Michigan.)

REFERENCES

1. Bassöe, E., and Bassöe, H. H.: The Styloid Bone and Carpe Bossu Disease. *Am. J. Roentgenol.*, 74:886–888, 1955.
2. Bogart, F. B.: Variations of Bones of Wrist. *Am. J. Roentgenol.*, 28:638–646, 1932.
3. Curtiss, P. H., Jr.: The Hunchback Carpal Bone. *J. Bone Joint Surg.*, 43A:392–394, 1961.
4. Gorlin, R. J., Schlorf, R. A., and Paparella, M. M.: Cleft Palate, Stapes Fixation and Oligodontia —A New Autosomal Recessively Inherited Syndrome. *Birth Defects, Original Article Series*, 7:87–88, 1971.
5. Kohler, A., and Zimmer, E. A.: Borderlands of the Normal and Early Pathologic in Skeletal Roentgenology, 3rd Ed. Grune & Stratton, Inc., New York, 1968.
6. Lynn, M. D., and Lee, J.: Periarticular Tenosynovial Chondrometaplasia: Report of a Case at the Wrist. *J. Bone Joint Surg.*, 54A: 648–652, 1972.
7. Metz, C. W., and McIvor, R. T.: Carpe Bossu Disease. *U.S. Armed Forces Med. J.*, 9:277–280, 1958.
8. O'Rahilly, R.: Developmental Deviations in Carpus and Tarsus. *Clin. Orthop.*, 10:9–18, 1957.
9. O'Rahilly, R.: Survey of Carpal and Tarsal Anomalies. *J. Bone Joint Surg.*, 35A:626–642, 1953.
10. Pfitzner, W.: Beiträge zur Kenntniss des menschlichen Extremitätenskelets. *Z. Morphol. Anthropol.*, 2:77–157, 1900.
11. Pirie, A. H.: Extra Bones in the Wrist and Ankle Found by Roentgen Rays. *Am. J. Roentgenol.*, 8:569–573, 1921.
12. Poznanski, A. K., Gall, J. C., Jr., and Stern, A. M.: Skeletal Manifestations of the Holt-Oram Syndrome. *Radiology*, 94:45–53, 1970.
13. Poznanski, A. K., and Holt, J. F.: The Carpals in Congenital Malformation Syndromes. *Am. J. Roentgenol.*, 112:443–459, 1971.

CARPAL FUSIONS

Carpal fusions may occur as isolated anomalies or be associated with congenital malformation syndromes. The isolated fusions usually involve bones of the same row, such as triquetrum-lunate, capitate-hamate or trapezium-trapezoid, while syndrome-related fusions often go across rows, i.e., trapezium-scaphoid.

The most common isolated fusion is between the triquetrum and lunate (Figs. 8–23 and 8–24). It was present in 0.1 per cent of 11,663 white Americans and 1.6 per cent of 7543 black Americans.[10] It was twice as common in males as in females. It is much more common in Nigeria, where an incidence of 8 per cent has been reported. In a United States population, one case of triquetrum-lunate fusion was seen in 302 Puerto Ricans and one in 1589 Mexican Americans.[9] Triquetrum-lunate fusion has little or no clinical significance and has very little effect on wrist motion.[5]

Capitate-hamate fusion (Fig. 8–25) is the most common type of isolated carpal fusion. It is significantly less common than triquetrum-lunate fusion and somewhat more common in blacks than in whites. Garn[9] found four such fusions in 11,663 whites, six in 7543 blacks and one in 618 American Indians. This type of fusion is also more common in Africa. Smitham[23] found an incidence of 0.75 per cent. Cockshott[3] reported a higher incidence of capitate-hamate

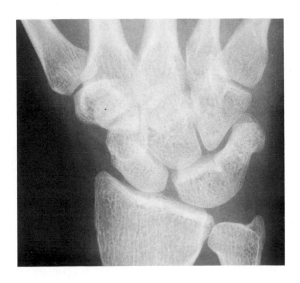

Figure 8–23. Triquetrum-lunate fusion in a girl without other congenital anomalies. A notch remains at the site of the fusion.

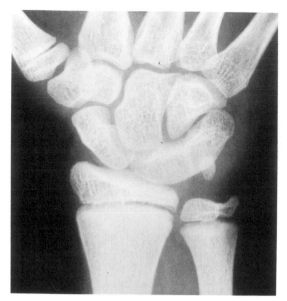

Figure 8–24. Triquetrum-lunate fusion from the 10 State Nutrition Survey. The site of the fusion is less evident than in Figure 8–23. (Courtesy Dr. Stanley Garn, 10 State Nutrition Survey, Ann Arbor, Michigan.)

fusion associated with triquetrum-lunate fusion.

Other isolated fusions are even rarer. The next most common is trapezium-trapezoid, which was found by Garn in three of 11,663 whites and two of 7543 blacks. One case of triquetrum-lunate fu-

sion was also seen in the group of blacks. Trapezium-trapezoid fusion is often difficult to ascertain, and unless one is careful, factitious fusion may be misdiagnosed (Fig. 8–26). In the Garn et al. series, only definite fusions with clear crossing of trabeculae between the two bones were included. Oblique films will easily resolve this problem of differentiation, but they are often not available in survey studies. Capitate-trapezoid fusion is extremely rare (Fig. 8–27). Pisiform-hamate fusion (Fig. 8–28) has been reported from Africa by Cockshott[4] but was not seen in Garn's series.

Although there have been occasional reports of isolated fusion across rows, i.e., trapezium-scaphoid,[15] this must be exceedingly rare. No cases of fusion from proximal to distal row were found in the more than 25,000 hand films examined by Garn et al. Thus, when this type of fusion is present, associated anomalies should be suspected.

Generally speaking, subjects of European ancestry have distal-row fusions rather than proximal-row fusions, while American Negroes have an excess of proximal-row fusions as compared to distal row fusions.

Fusions involving multiple carpals are rare without other associated anomalies, as are fusions of the carpals to the radius and ulna.[16, 17]

Carpal fusions are usually not symptomatic. They rarely interfere with function—

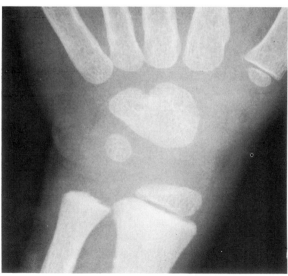
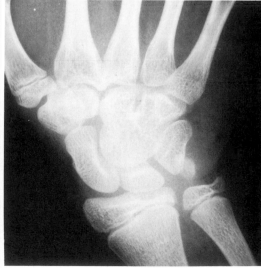

Figure 8–25. Capitate-hamate fusion in two patients. This is the second most common type of fusion. (Courtesy Dr. Stanley Garn, 10 State Nutrition Survey, Ann Arbor, Michigan.)

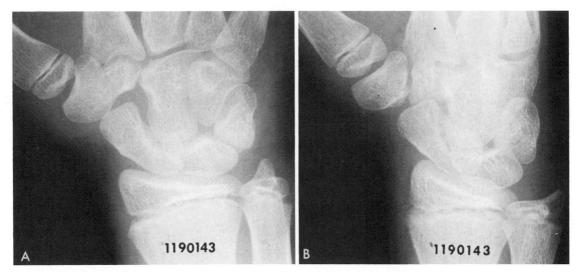

Figure 8–26. Factitious trapezium-trapezoid fusion. There is an illusion of trapezium-trapezoid fusion in the AP film (*A*) because of overlap of these bones. However, the oblique film (*B*) shows that the bones are indeed separate.

Figure 8–27. Capitate-trapezoid fusion. This is a rare type of fusion. (Courtesy Dr. Stanley Garn, 10 State Nutrition Survey, Ann Arbor, Michigan.)

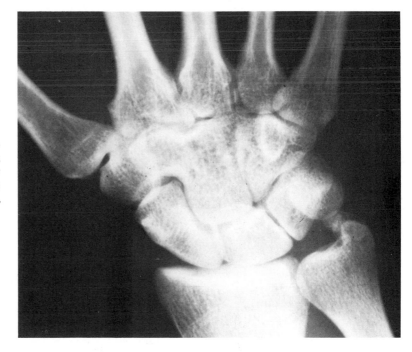

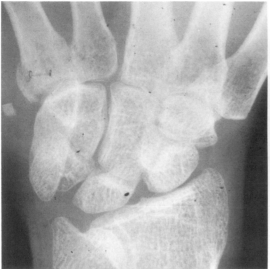

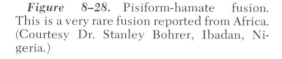

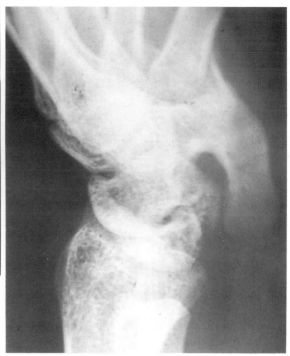

Figure 8–28. Pisiform-hamate fusion. This is a very rare fusion reported from Africa. (Courtesy Dr. Stanley Bohrer, Ibadan, Nigeria.)

a case of bilateral fusion was described in a championship golfer![12]

The term *carpal fusion* is probably a misnomer, since the anomaly actually represents a failure of segmentation of the primitive cartilaginous carpals with absence of joint formation. Cockshott[3] found support for this concept in the fact that he discovered six examples of lunate-triquetrum fusion in the dissection of stillborn infants. In reviewing sections of embryos, we also found an example of this (Fig. 8–29). The carpal fusions radiographically appear progressive.[5, 16] In reality there is only one cartilaginous center that comprises the two bones, but each of the bones has a separate ossification center which, with progressive ossification, eventually expands and coalesces. Whether the same process occurs in the other congenital malformations has not been proved. Newcombe et al.[19] raised some doubts about this in the dissection of arthrogrypotic wrists. The age at which these centers coalesce is variable, ranging from six to 15 years.[3] Sometimes a notch remains at the site of fusion (Fig. 7–23). Capitate-hamate fusion may occur considerably earlier in the Ellis-van Creveld syndrome, where it may be apparent shortly after the onset of ossification in these centers.

Carpal fusions associated with other malformations (Fig. 8–30 to 8–33) can involve almost any of the carpals. They may involve the same row or go between rows, such as trapezium-scaphoid (Fig. 8–32) or triquetrum-hamate,[2] or they may involve multiple carpals.[7] Sometimes the only associated abnormality is tarsal fusion, but often a different type of malformation may be present. Some of these, the hand-foot-uterus syndrome for example (Chapter 12), are relatively subtle and may not be detectable except on thorough examination. Carpal fusions associated with other anoma-

TABLE 8–3. Malformations and Syndromes Associated with Carpal Fusion

Acropectorovertebral dysplasia
Acrocephalosyndactyly syndrome
Arthrogryposis
Cleft hand and foot
Diastrophic dwarfism
Dyschondrosteosis
Ellis-van Creveld syndrome
Hand-foot-uterus syndrome
Holt-Oram syndrome
Liebenberg syndrome
Oto-palato-digital syndrome
Polydactyly
Symphalangism
Tarsal fusion
Turner's syndrome
Ulnar dimelia

lies are in some instances familial.[17] The abnormalities associated with carpal fusions are listed in Table 8–3. They include well-defined syndromes which will be described in greater detail in Chapter 12, in addition to a number of ill-defined combinations of malformations. A multitude of these reports have been published, and only a few will be listed here as examples. Sandrow et al.[22] described a patient with carpal fusions associated with hereditary ulnar and fibular dimelia, polydactyly and peculiar facies. Forney et al.[7] described a family with a syndrome which, besides carpal and tarsal fusions, included congenital insufficiency, conductive deafness, shortness of stature, extensive freckles and cervical spine fusion. This syndrome may be somewhat related to the lentigines syndrome. Hanley et al.[13] described a syndrome of osteochondritis dissecans associated with capitate-trapezium fusion in one of his patients. The syndrome consisted of osteochondritis dissecans and numerous devel-

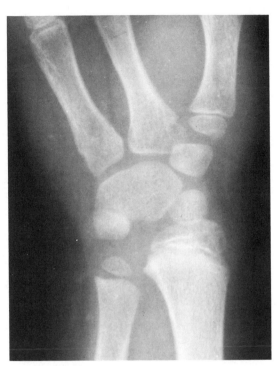

Figure 8–30. Fusion of carpal bones associated with cleft hand and ulnar hypoplasia. There is fusion of the capitate and hamate, and there is absence of some of the other carpal bones. (From Poznanski, A. K., and Holt, J. F.: *Am. J. Roentgenol.*, 112:443–459, 1971.)

opmental anomalies, including striking facial appearance, ptosis of the eyelids, peculiar thinning of the manubrium sterni and osseous fusion of the manubrium-sternal joint. There was also evidence of pectus excavatum, cryptorchidism and short little fingers and fifth toes. Carpal fusions which occur in association with congenital disorders also appear to be progressive, as they do in the isolated form. The most dramatic progression has been seen in arthrogryposis[21] where, in the adult, most of the carpals may be fused.

Although carpal fusions are often congenital, care must be taken not to confuse these with fusions due to acquired disease. Old inflammatory lesions, trauma, rheumatoid arthritis (Fig. 8–34) and even familial carpal necrosis (Fig. 8–35) can result in carpal fusion. Surgical intercarpal fusion may also be seen. This procedure is sometimes used for relieving the symptoms resulting from degenerative changes, fractures, nonunion, avascular necrosis and other conditions.[20]

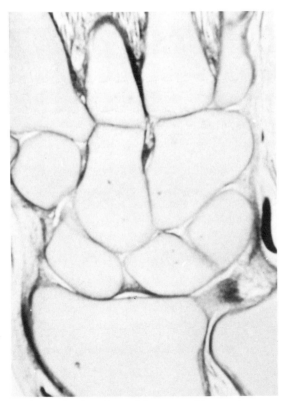

Figure 8–29. Carpal fusion in 60 mm. (crown-rump length) embryo (10.5 weeks' gestation). Early triquetrum-lunate fusion is seen. (Courtesy Dr. Alphonse Burdi, Ann Arbor, Michigan.)

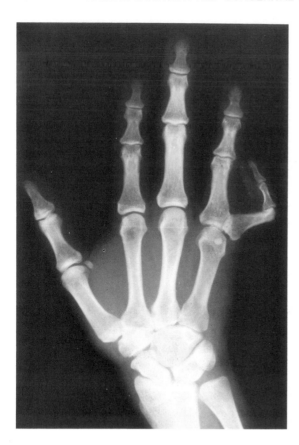

Figure 8–31. Fifth finger arising from fourth metacarpophalangeal joint. There is fusion of the capitate and hamate and of the triquetrum and lunate.

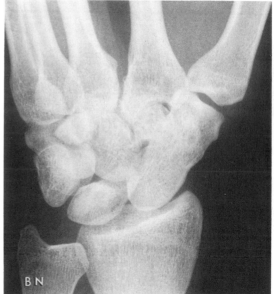

Figure 8–32. Trapezium-scaphoid fusion in the oto-palato-digital syndrome. This type of fusion is usually seen only in individuals with multiple other abnormalities.

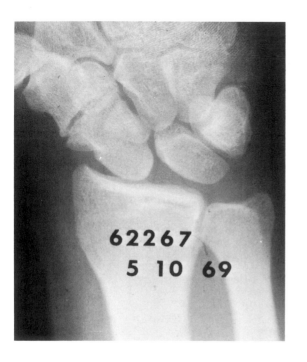
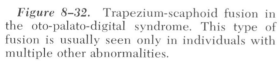

Figure 8–33. Incomplete trapezium-scaphoid fusion in the Holt-Oram syndrome. The narrowing of the joint between these two bones is evidence of attempt at fusion. This was a young man with no other arthritic changes. There is also an os centrale present. (From Poznanski, A. K., and Holt, J. F.: *Am. J. Roentgenol.*, 112:443–459, 1971.)

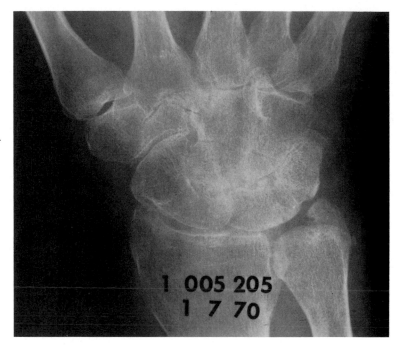

Figure 8-34. Acquired fusion in rheumatoid arthritis. Other stigmata of rheumatoid arthritis are present, including bony demineralization and irregularity in the joint spaces.

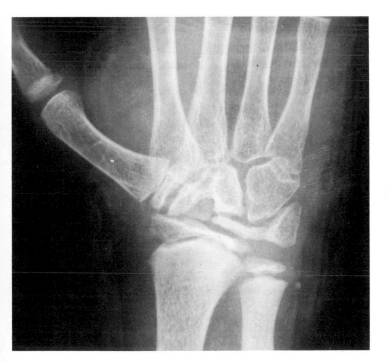

Figure 8-35. Familial carpal necrosis. Markedly distorted carpals. (Courtesy Dr. Don Babbitt, Milwaukee, Wisconsin.)

REFERENCES

1. Albrecht, R.: Beiträg zum Vorkommen der Synostosen am Hand- und Fusswurzelskelett. *Z. Orthop.*, 105:215–235, 1968.
2. Brøbeck, O.: Congenital Bilateral Synosteosis of the Calcaneus and Cuboid and of the Triquetral and Hamate Bones: Report of a Case. *Acta Orthop. Scand.*, 26:217–221, 1957.
3. Cockshott, W. P.: Carpal Fusions. *Am. J. Roentgenol.*, 89:1260–1271, 1963.
4. Cockshott, W. P.: Pisiform Hamate Fusion. *J. Bone Joint Surg.*, 51A:778–780, 1969.
5. Dean, R. F. A., and Jones, P. R. M.: Fusion of Triquetral and Lunate Bones Shown in Serial Radiographs. *Am. J. Phys. Anthrop.*, 17:279–288, 1959.
6. Dreiack, D., and Holland, C.: Synostosen im Handwurzelbereich, Angeboren oder Erworben? *Z. Orthop.*, 108:461–468, 1970.
7. Forney, W. R., Robinson, S. J., and Pascoe, D. J.: Congenital Heart Disease, Deafness, and Skeletal Malformations: A New Syndrome? *J. Pediat.*, 68:14–26, 1966.
8. Gall, J. C., Stern, A. M., Poznanski, A. K., Garn, S. M., Weinstein, E. D., and Hayward, J. R.: Oto-Palato-Digital Syndrome: Comparison of Clinical and Radiographic Manifestations in Males and Females. *Am. J. Hum. Genet.*, 24:24–36, 1972.
9. Garn, S. M.: Unpublished data—carpals.
10. Garn, S. M., Frisancho, A. R., Poznanski, A. K., Schweitzer, J., and McCann, M. B.: Analysis of Triquetral-Lunate Fusion, *Am. J. Phys. Anthropol.*, 34:431–434, 1971.
11. Geelhoed, G., Neel, J. V., and Davidson, R. T.: Symphalangism and Tarsal Coalitions: Hereditary Syndrome; Report on Two Families. *J. Bone Joint Surg.*, 51B:278–289, 1969.
12. Graham, C. E., and Mehta, M. C.: Bilateral Congenital Carpal Fusion in a Champion Golfer. A Case Report. *Clin. Orthop.*, 83:70–72, 1972.
13. Hanley, W. B., McKusick, V. A., and Barranco, F. T.: Osteochondritis Dissecans with Associated Malformations in Two Brothers: A Review of Familial Aspects. *J. Bone Joint Surg.*, 49A:925–937, 1967.
14. Harle, T. S., and Stevenson, J. R.: Hereditary Symphalangism Associated with Carpal and Tarsal Fusions. *Radiology*, 89:91–94, 1967.
15. Henry, M. G.: Anomalous Fusion of the Scaphoid and the Greater Multangular Bone. *Arch. Surg.*, 50:240–241, 1945.
16. Hughes, P. C. R., and Tanner, J. M.: Development of Carpal Bone Fusion as Seen in Serial Radiographs. *Brit. J. Radiol.*, 39:943–949, 1966.
17. Kewesch, E. L.: Über hereditäre Verschmelzung der Hand– und Fusswurzelknochen. *Fortschr. Geb. Roentgenstr. Nuklearmed.*, 50:550–556, 1934.
18. Levine, E.: Carpal Fusions in Children of Four South African Populations. *Am. J. Phys. Anthropol.*, 37:75–84, 1972.
19. Newcombe, D. S., Abbott, J. L., Munsie, W. J., and Keats, T. E.: Arthrogryposis Multiplex Congenita and Spontaneous Carpal Fusion. *Arthritis Rheum.*, 12:345–354, 1969.
20. Peterson, H. A., and Lipscomb, P. R.: Intercarpal Arthrodesis. *Arch. Surg.*, 95:127–134, 1967.
21. Poznanski, A. K., and La Rowe, P. C.: Radiographic Manifestations of the Arthrogryposis Syndrome. *Radiology*, 95:353–358, 1970.
22. Sandrow, R. E., Sullivan, P. D., and Steel, H. H.: Hereditary Ulnar and Fibular Dimelia with Peculiar Facies; Case Report. *J. Bone Joint Surg.*, 52A:367–370, 1970.
23. Smitham, J. H.: Some Observations on Certain Congenital Abnormalities of the Hand in African Natives. *Br. J. Radiol.*, 21:513–518, 1948.

Chapter 9

SHORTENING OR ABSENCE OF PORTIONS OF THE HANDS AND DIGITS
Brachydactylies, Radial and Ulnar Defects, Amputations

Short or absent fingers include a broad spectrum of abnormalities, ranging from minimal decrease in size of the middle phalanx of the fifth finger to complete ab-

sence of the hand. Deficiencies of the hand can be isolated or may be associated with similar anomalies in the feet, or the hand changes may be only one anomaly of an extensive congenital malformation complex. A number of these malformations have been noted in animals as well as in man.[2]

Various classifications of hand deficiencies have been used. General categories describing the defect as transverse or longitudinal and as terminal or intercalary have been discussed in Chapter 7, as was the Temtamy classification. Bell[1] in 1951 classified the brachydactylous syndromes into various groups on anatomic and genetic grounds (Fig. 9–1). Her classification has found considerable acceptance in the literature, but there are a significant number of cases which do not fit into this classification. There is also some overlap with the classification based on terminal or longitudinal defects. For example, hypoplasia of the distal phalanx of the thumb is included in both groups.

In this chapter a radiologic-anatomic classification will be used. Conditions will be considered according to whether they affect the row or the ray, and according to

which portion of the row or ray is involved. As with the previous classifications, there will be some overlap among the various groups.

1. Affecting rows
   a. Distal phalanges
   b. Middle phalanges
   c. Proximal phalanges
   d. Metacarpals
   e. Multiple rows
2. Affecting rays
   a. Radial
   b. Ulnar
   c. Central
3. Transverse defects
   a. Terminal transverse defects
   b. Streeter's bands

In this framework the various forms of Bell's brachydactyly will be included. Each type of aplasia or hypoplasia will be discussed from two points of view: the anomaly as it relates to the hand only, and the anomaly as it is found associated with other malformations.

Although in this chapter the concern will be primarily with congenital causes of shortening of the digits, the acquired conditions must always be considered. Any disorder which will close an epiphysis will result in shortening of that digit. This includes trauma of all types. Frostbite, for example, results in closure of the epiphyses of the distal phalanges but usually spares the thumb. Sickle cell disease may cause a wide variety of patterns of diminution of phalangeal or metacarpal size as a result of damage to the epiphysis from infarction during the hand-foot syndrome. Some of the arthritides may result in epiphyseal fusion and consequent diminution in size. Severe arthritic erosions may also cause shortening of the digits, whereas the hyperemia of arthritis may cause enlargement. Tumors, particularly exostoses, when located near the epiphysis can result in various forms of brachydactyly. A useful criterion in differentiating the acquired from congenital brachydactylies is that in the acquired forms involvement of the various bones is usually more random and asymmetric, while in the congenital form a more definite pattern and symmetry are evident.

Although many cases of relative shortening of the bone are severe enough to be

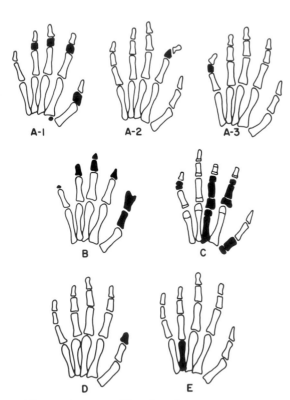

Figure 9–1. Bell's classification of brachydactyly. The black bones are those affected. See text for further description.

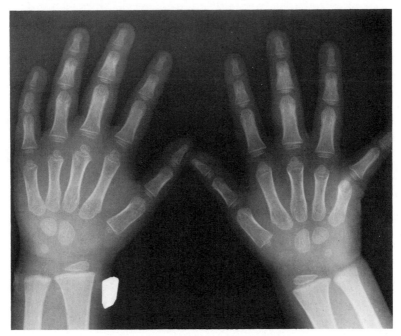

Figure 9–2. Pseudobrachydactyly. Shortening may be due to elevation of the finger from the table. A clue that the shortening of the second to fifth metacarpals on the right is not real is that their epiphyses overlie the shafts.

obvious to simple inspection, some subtle cases require measurement. The method of pattern-profile analysis[3] described in Chapter 2 lends itself well to the detection of finer degrees of shortening or lengthening that are not evident on visual inspection. Care has to be taken in positioning the hand, for if the hand bones are not in contact with the film a factitious shortening will occur (Fig. 9–2).

REFERENCES

1. Bell, J.: On Brachydactyly and Symphalangism. *In* Penrose, L. S.: *The Treasury of Human Inheritance.* University Press, Cambridge, England, 1951, Vol. 5, Part 1, pp. 1–31.
2. Morris, L. N.: Spontaneous Congenital Limb Malformations in Nonhuman Primates: A Review of the Literature. *Teratology,* 4:335–341, 1971.
3. Poznanski, A. K., Garn, S. M., Nagy, J. M., and Gall, J. C.: Metacarpophalangeal Pattern Profiles in the Evaluation of Skeletal Malformations. *Radiology,* 104:1–11, 1972.
4. Temtamy, S. A.: Genetic Factors in Hand Malformations. Thesis. Johns Hopkins University, Baltimore, Maryland, 1966.

DIMINUTION IN SIZE OF THE DISTAL PHALANGES (BRACHYTELEPHALANGY)

In normal individuals the distal phalanges show the widest range of variation in size of any of the bones of the hand except the middle phalanx of the fifth finger of females.[2] The tufts of the phalanges are also quite variable in size. Shortening of the distal phalanges occurs in several conditions and may be associated with underlying hypoplasia or absence of fingernails.[4] However, not all cases of hypoplastic nails are associated with hypoplasia of the distal phalanges. Short distal phalanges are also associated with cone-shaped epiphysis and may be the result of early fusion (Fig. 9–3A). Familial cases have also been reported.[1] Dermatoglyphic patterns are abnormal in patients with short distal phalanges and include a high incidence of dermal arches in the fingers.[7]

A number of syndromes may be associated with short distal phalanges (Fig. 9–3B).[3, 5] These are listed in Table 9–1. Some of these conditions are well known

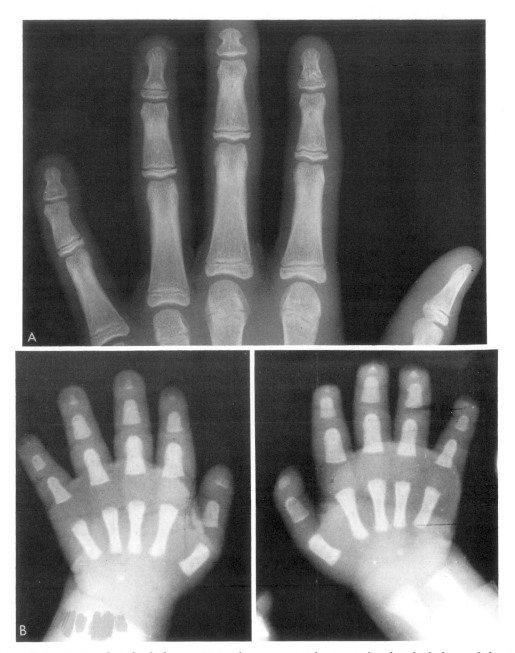

Figure 9–3. A, Brachytelephalangy. Note the cone epiphysis at the distal phalanx of the index finger, and the fused epiphysis at the third and fifth distal phalanges. (Courtesy Dr. Stanley Garn, 10 State Nutrition Survey.)

B, Brachytelephalangy in an infant with associated imperforate anus and bilateral cleft palate. Similar findings were seen in the feet. (The infant's mother received Librium during pregnancy, which may be unrelated.)

Illustration continued on opposite page.

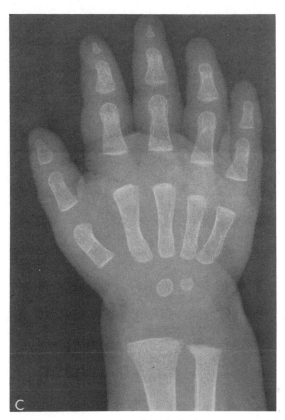

Figure 9–3 Continued. C, Hypoplasia of the distal phalanges associated with maternal usage of Dilantin and other anticonvulsants. The nails were also hypoplastic.

TABLE 9–1. Short Distal Phalanges

	THUMB ONLY	THUMB ONLY	ANY PHALANX	
	Short, broad	*Generally hypoplastic*	*Hypoplastic*	*Tuft Erosion*
Limited to distal phalanx	Brachydactyly D		In association with hypoplastic nails	
Affecting also other portions of the hand			Brachydactyly B	Brachydactyly B
Associated syndromes	Apert Carpenter Diastrophic dwarf Hand-foot-uterus Oto-palato-digital Rubinstein-Taybi	Christian Cornelia de Lange Cryptogenic brachymeta- carpalia Fanconi Holt-Oram Myositis ossificans Trisomy 18	Asphyxiating thoracic dysplasia Cleidocranial dysostosis Coffin-Siris Dilantin (maternal use) Keutel Liebenberg Rüdiger Trisomy 13 Trisomy 18 Zimmerman-Laband	Familial acroosteolysis Mandibuloacral dysplasia Porphyria Progeria Pseudoxanthoma elas- ticum Pycnodysostosis Rothmund
Acquired			Frostbite Trauma	Buerger's disease Burns Chemical acroosteoly- sis Congenital insensi- tivity to pain Frostbite Leprosy Neurotropic Psoriasis Raynaud's disease

and are further described in Chapters 12 and 13. Others are rarer. Keutel[3] described a recessive syndrome for brachytelephalangy with associated multiple peripheral pulmonary stenosis, inner ear deafness and ossification or calcification of the cartilages. Short distal phalanges have been associated with maternal usage of anticonvulsants, particularly Dilantin (Figs. 9–3C and 9–16).

Hypoplasia of all of the distal phalanges may also occur in a number of acquired diseases, particularly in association with acroosteolysis (see Table 9–1).

REFERENCES

1. Burrows, H. J.: Developmental Abbreviation of Terminal Phalanges. *Brit. J. Radiol.*, 11:165–176, 1938.
2. Garn, S. M., Hertzog, K. P., Poznanski, A. K., and Nagy, J. M.: Metacarpophalangeal Length in the Evaluation of Skeletal Malformation. *Radiology*, 105:375–381, 1972.
3. Keutel, J., Jörgensen, G., and Gabriel, P.: Ein Neues Autosomal-Rezessiv Vererbbares Syndrom. *Dtsch. Med. Wochenschr.*, 96:1676–1681, 1971.
4. Kohler, A., and Zimmer, E. A.: *Borderlands of the Normal and Early Pathologic in Skeletal Roentgenology*, 3rd Ed. Grune & Stratton, Inc., New York, 1968.
5. Loughnan, P. M., Gold, H., and Vance, J. C.: Phenytoin Teratogenicity in Man. *Lancet*, 1:70–72, 1973.
6. Qazi, Q. H., and Smithwick, E. M.: Triphalangy of Thumbs and Great Toes. *Am. J. Dis. Child.*, 120:255–257, 1970.
7. Robinow, M., and Johnson, G. F.: Dermatoglyphics in Distal Phalangeal Hypoplasia. *Am. J. Dis. Child.*, 124:860–863, 1972.

Short Distal Phalanx of the Thumb (Bell's Brachydactyly D, Potter's Thumb, Stub Thumb, Murderer's Thumb)

The short broad distal phalanx of the thumb may occur as an isolated finding (Fig. 9–4). It was first described by Breitenbecher[1] in 1923 and then by Thomsen[6] in 1928. The anomaly is relatively common and varies with racial origin and with sex. It is more common in females than in males (0.66 per cent vs. 0.17 per cent in the United States).[4] In the United States it has been seen in 0.41 per cent of whites and 0.1 per cent of blacks.[4] In Israel it has been described in 1.6 per cent of Jews and in 3.0 per cent of Arabs.[2] A high incidence is also

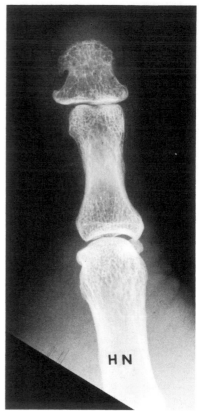

Figure 9–4. Stub thumb (brachydactyly D). The anomaly was an isolated finding in this adult female. The distal phalanx is broad. The same clinical finding was evident on a photograph of the patient's grandmother.

evident in the Japanese.[5] Stub thumbs can be either unilateral or bilateral.

The trait is transmitted as an autosomal dominant with incomplete penetrance. Members of the same family may have either unilateral or bilateral involvement, but when unilateral in a family it affects the same hand in all members.[2] Goodman reported the association of a short fourth toe. Although a short distal phalanx is sometimes associated with early closure of its epiphysis,[4] it sometimes may be present at birth.

The distal phalanx of the thumb may be hypoplastic in other forms of brachydactyly, and may be slender rather than wide. A wide short distal phalanx is also seen in brachydactyly B, where sometimes it is even split longitudinally.

Many congenital disorders are associated with a short, broad thumb similar to the isolated stub thumb. These are listed in

Table 9–1. There are also a number of congenital conditions in which the distal phalanx of the thumb is hypoplastic and slender (Table 9–1). This is particularly true in most of the radial hypoplasia syndromes.

REFERENCES

1. Breitenbecher, J. K.: Hereditary Shortness of Thumbs. *J. Hered.*, 14:15–22, 1923.
2. Goodman, R. M., Adam, A., and Sheba, C.: A Genetic Study of Stub Thumbs among Various Ethnic Groups in Israel. *J. Med. Genet.*, 2: 116–121, 1965.
3. Köhler, A., and Zimmer, E. A.: *Borderlands of the Normal and Early Pathologic in Skeletal Roentgenology*, 3rd Ed. Grune & Stratton, Inc., New York, 1968.
4. Stecher, R. M.: The Physical Characteristics and Heredity of Short Thumbs. *Acta Genet.*, 7: 217–222, 1957.
5. Sugiura, Y., Tajima, Y., Sugiura, I., Muramoto, K., and Wu, W. D.: Roentgenologic Study on the Skeletal Variant in the Hand and Foot Observed Among Shizuoka School Children. *Jap. J. Hum. Genet.*, 7:67–77, 1962.
6. Thomsen, O.: Hereditary Growth Anomaly of the Thumb. *Hereditas*, 10:261–273, 1928.

HYPOPLASIA OF THE MIDDLE PHALANGES (BRACHYMESOPHALANGY)

The various conditions with shortening of the middle phalanges have been called type A brachydactyly by Bell. A listing of the different types is found in Table 9–2. The various types are not always distinct entities and large intrafamilial variations may be seen.

TABLE 9–2. Short Middle Phalanges

	MP 5	MP 2	OTHER
Limited to middle phalanges	Brachydactyly A-3	Brachydactyly A-2	McKusick brachydactyly A-4
Affecting also other portions of the hand	Symphalangism		Brachydactyly A-1 Brachydactyly B Brachydactyly C
Associated syndromes	*Chromosomal* trisomy 21 XXXXY XXXXX ? trisomy 18	Sclerosteosis	Acrocephalosyndactyly Apert Carpenter
	Craniofacial ankyloglossia superior oculo-dento-digital oto-palato-digital Treacher Collins		Hermann-Opitz Poland's syndactyly Tricho-rhino-phalangeal
	Other Bloom Cornelia de Lange Goltz Holt-Oram myositis ossificans progressiva Noonan Poland Popliteal pterygium Silver Thrombocytopenia–absent radius syndrome		
Acquired			Arthritis Infection Neoplasm Sickle cell disease Trauma

Brachymesophalangy-5 (Bell's A-3 Brachydactyly)

This is the most common phalangeal shortening and is also the most common hand anomaly (Fig. 9–5). The middle phalanx of the fifth finger is the most variable in length of any of the hand bones in females; and almost the most variable in males.[2] The incidence of shortening of the fifth middle phalanx varies significantly in different populations.[5] Garn,[1] in his study of 10 population groups, found an incidence varying from 0.6 per cent in southwest Ohio adults to 5.0 per cent in Hong Kong and Peru. A study by Sugiura et al. of Japanese children revealed an incidence of 15 per cent in males and 24.5 per cent in females.

The short fifth middle phalanx is usually inherited as a Mendelian dominant trait with 50 to 60 per cent penetrance.[8]

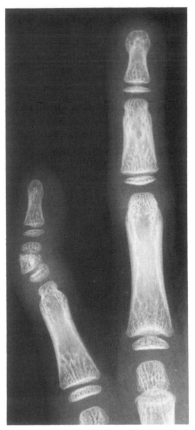

Figure 9–6. Brachymesophalangy-5 with cone epiphysis and pseudoepiphysis. (Courtesy Dr. Stanley M. Garn, 10 State Nutrition Survey.)

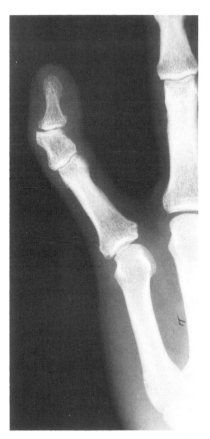

Figure 9–5. Brachymesophalangy-5 (Bell's A-1 brachydactyly in a normal adult). There is associated clinodactyly.

Short middle phalanges may in some cases be associated with cone epiphysis (Fig. 9–6). It appears that brachymesophalangy alone (without cones) is separately inherited, without apparent sex bias, while brachymesophalangy-5 with cone epiphysis at mid-5, and cone epiphysis at mid-5 alone are both inherited as a complex; with a marked increased incidence in females over males.[4]

A short middle phalanx is often shorter on its radial than on its ulnar side, resulting in radial clinodactyly. In some cases, however, the finger is straight (Fig. 9–7). The shortening of this phalanx can be quite marked. The short middle phalanx of the fifth finger is seen in increased frequency in individuals who are short in stature. According to Garn et al.,[3] this may represent a selective advantage in adaptation to situations where food is scarce, inasmuch as smaller individuals have a lower protein

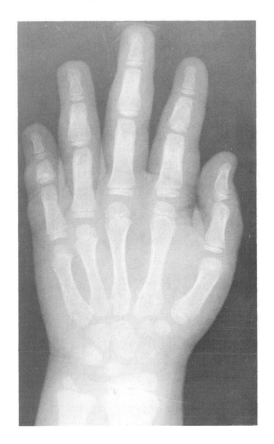

Figure 9-7. Brachymesophalangy-5 with cone epiphysis without clinodactyly. This child had acanthosis nigricans and mental deficiency.

requirement and consequently thrive better.

Many syndromes are associated with brachydactyly affecting the fifth middle phalanges; the most common and well known of these is trisomy 21. It is interesting that the Down's syndrome children with a short fifth middle phalanx are also shorter in stature than the Down's syndrome children without a short fifth middle phalanx. Other conditions with short middle phalanges of the fifth finger are listed in Table 9-2.

REFERENCES

1. Garn, S. M., Fels, S. L., and Israel, H.: Brachymesophalangia of Digit Five in Ten Populations. *Am. J. Phys. Anthropol.*, 27:205–209, 1967.
2. Garn, S. M., Hertzog, K. P., Poznanski, A. K., and Nagy, J. M.: Metacarpophalangeal Length in the Evaluation of Skeletal Malformation. *Radiology*, 105:375–381, 1972.
3. Garn, S. M., Nagy, J. M., Poznanski, A. K., and Mc-Cann, M. B.: Size Reduction Associated with Brachymesophalangia-5: A Possible Selective Advantage. *Am. J. Phys. Anthropol.*, 37: 267–270, 1972.
4. Garn, S. M., Poznanski, A. K., Nagy, J. M., and McCann, M. B.: Independence of Brachymesophalangia-5 from Brachymesophalangia-5 with Cone Mid-5. *Am. J. Phys. Anthropol.*, 36:295–298, 1972.
5. Hertzog, K. P.: Shortened Fifth Medial Phalanges. *Am. J. Phys. Anthropol.*, 27:113–118, 1967.
6. Poznanski, A. K., Pratt, G. B., Manson, G., and Weiss, L.: Clinodactyly, Camptodactyly, Kirner's Deformity, and Other Crooked Fingers. *Radiology*, 93:573–582, 1969.
7. Sugiura, Y., Tajima, Y., Sugiura, I., Muramoto, K., and Wu, W. D.: Roentgenologic Study on the Skeletal Variant in the Hand and Foot Observed Among Shizuoka School Children. *Jap. J. Hum. Genet.*, 7:67-77, 1962.
8. Temtamy, S. A.: Genetic Factors in Hand Malformations. Thesis. Johns Hopkins University, Baltimore, Maryland, 1966.

Brachymesophalangy-2 (Bell's A-2 Brachydactyly; Short Middle Phalanx, Index Finger)

This is a very rare disorder; only four families have been reported in the litera-

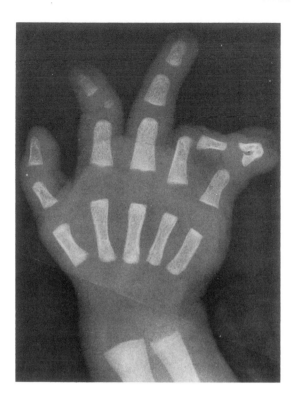

Figure 9-8. Brachydactyly A-2 and syndactyly. This was a bilateral anomaly, and family history was positive for it.

Figure 9-9. Brachymesophalangy-5 and -2. The distal phalanges of 2 and 5 are also hypoplastic. In this 2½ year old girl there was an associated imperforate anus, absent sacrum, and urethral stricture.

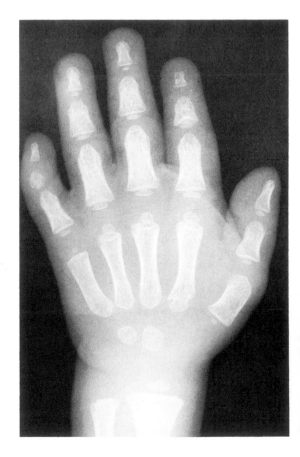

ture.[5] The genetic pattern of this disorder is not clear and there is a wide range of expression.

The characteristic appearance of the condition is that of a short rudimentary middle phalanx of the second finger. This phalanx may be triangular in shape, which results in radial deviation. It often lacks an epiphysis, perhaps because of early fusion. There is some variation in these cases. Our case had associated syndactyly of the fourth and fifth fingers (Fig. 9–8).

In a case of Temtamy and McKusick[5] there were typical findings in the propositus, but the father of the propositus had more severe changes: an unusual double ossification center with a longitudinal split between the two fragments, instead of a proximal phalanx and a very broad distal phalanx. There was also shortening of the middle phalanx of the fourth finger.

There is a somewhat higher incidence of shortening of the middle phalanx of the index finger in association with shortening of the middle phalanx of the fifth finger. This combination has been termed by McKusick[3] as brachydactyly type A-4, an addition to Bell's classification (Fig. 9–9). Shortening of the middle phalanx of the second finger (Bell's A-2) has been seen in sclerosteosis.[2, 6]

REFERENCES

1. Bell, J.: On Brachydactyly and Symphalangism. *In* Penrose, L. S.: The Treasury of Human Inheritance. University Press, Cambridge, England, 1951, Vol. 5, Part 1, pp. 1–31.
2. Gorlin, R. J., Spranger, J., and Koszalka, M. F.: Genetic Craniotubular Bone Dysplasias and Hyperostosis. A Critical Analysis. *Birth Defects, Original Article Series*, Vol. 5, No. 4, pp. 79–85, 1969.
3. McKusick, V. A.: *Mendelian Inheritance in Man. Catalogs of Autosomal Dominant, Autosomal Recessive and X-Linked Phenotypes*, 3rd Ed. The Johns Hopkins Press, Baltimore, 1971.
4. Mohr, O. L., and Wriedt, C.: *A New Type of Hereditary Brachyphalangy in Man.* Carnegie Institution of Washington, Washington, 1919, pp. 5–64.
5. Temtamy, S. A., and McKusick, V. A.: Synopsis of Hand Malformations with Particular Emphasis on Genetic Factors. *Birth Defects, Original Article Series*, Vol. 5, No. 3, 1969.
6. Truswell, A. S.: Osteopetrosis with Syndactyly. A Morphological Variant of Albers-Schönberg's Disease. *J. Bone Joint Surg.*, 40B:208–218, 1958.

SHORTENING OF ALL MIDDLE PHALANGES AND THE PROXIMAL PHALANX OF THE THUMB (BELL'S A-1 BRACHYDACTYLY)

The incidence of this condition is not known. Bell[1] reviewed 23 pedigrees of this disorder and Temtamy[6] has reviewed the literature to date and added some further cases. Type A-1 brachydactyly was probably the first human trait interpreted in terms of Mendelian dominant inheritance by Farabee in 1903.[6]

In Bell's A-1 brachydactyly, all the middle phalanges are short and may be fused to the terminal phalanges. Ultimately the middle phalanges may be absent (Fig. 9–10). All of the fingers and toes are involved. There is an associated shortening of the proximal phalanx of the thumb and of the great toe. Generally speaking, the little finger and index finger are the most affected, illustrating the greater sensitivity of these two digits to shortening.

In some brachydactylous families belonging to type A-1, the manifestations are widespread and involve all of the bones of the skeleton. Drinkwater[2] cites several of these and showed reduction in stature of affected individuals. In other individuals, particularly some of those described by Farabee, manifestations are mild. Temtamy[6] suggests calling the severe cases the Drinkwater type and the mild cases the Farabee type of brachydactyly A-1, although the distinction is somewhat artificial since both types can occur in the same family (Fig. 9–10).

In the severe cases the metacarpals may also be short, particularly the fourth and fifth.[5] The shortening of the middle phalanges in this disorder is probably related to the absence or early fusion of the epiphysis of the middle phalanges. In some patients there may also be minimal involvement of the proximal phalanges, in which case there may be some overlap with type C brachydactyly. In one of Hoefnagel and Gerald's[4] patients, the appearance suggested type C while the other members of the family had a typical type A-1 brachy-

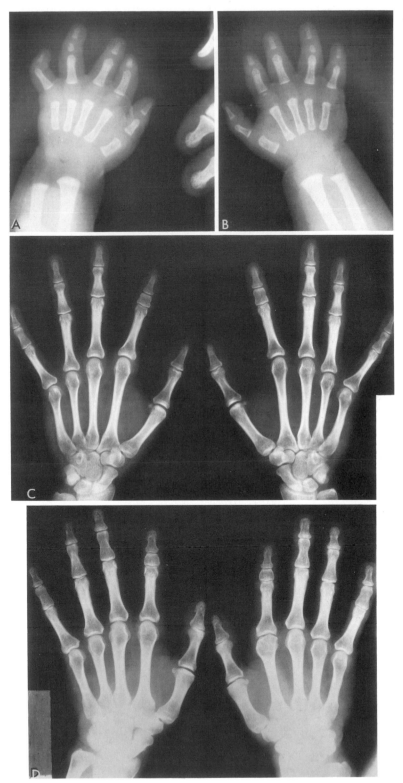

Figure 9–10. Three generations of a family with A-1 brachydactyly. The young child (A) has typical findings of absence and marked hypoplasia of the middle phalanges, while the adults (B and C) show mainly shortening of the middle phalanges of 5 and 2 and would fit better into the A-4 type brachydactyly. (Courtesy Dr. Leonard Swischuk, Galveston, Texas.)

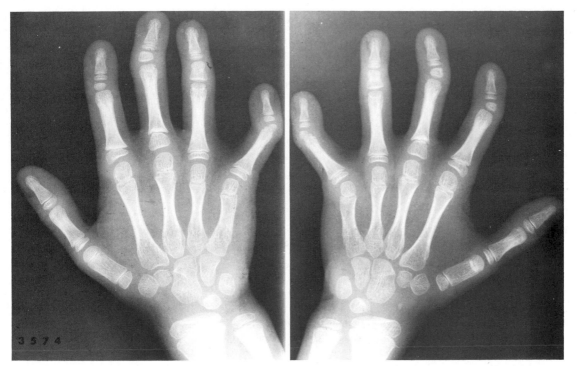

Figure 9–11. Shortening of middle phalanges, suggesting A-1 brachydactyly, but with some involvement of the proximal phalanges suggesting type C.

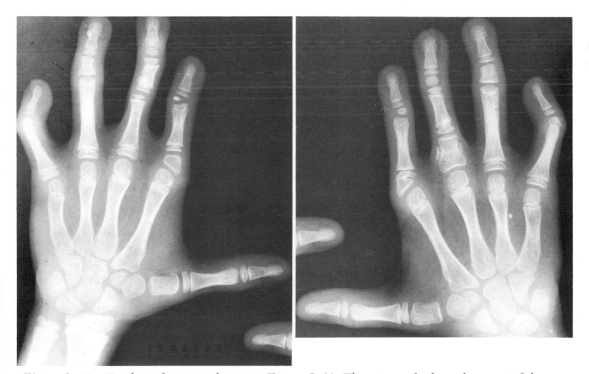

Figure 9–12. Brother of patient shown in Figure 9–11. There is marked involvement of the proximal and middle phalanges. The appearance is much more typical of type C brachydactyly.

dactyly. Two brothers that I saw also illustrated the variability of this condition. One had a fairly typical type A-1 brachydactyly (Fig. 9–11) with only minimal involvement of the proximal phalanges, while the other (Fig. 9–12) had a typical type C brachydactyly with gross involvement of the proximal phalanges. These boys illustrate the difficulty that sometimes exists in separating type A-1 from type C.

An interesting additional anomaly seen in A-1 brachydactyly is the presence of accessory carpal bones in the distal row of carpals adjacent to the metacarpal bases. This was seen in several of the reported cases and is best documented in Nissen's family.[5] It was also present in Hoefnagel's[4] and in Temtamy's[6] cases.

The bones of the foot are usually also involved. The main finding is the absence of the middle phalanges of the toes and short proximal phalanges of the great toes, resulting in bilateral shortening of this digit. There may also be shortening of other long bones.

Shortening of the middle phalanges is not limited to A-1 brachydactyly. It may occur also in some other forms of brachydactyly, particularly types B and C.

Shortening of the middle phalanges of the digits is seen in a number of malformation syndromes (Table 9–2), particularly in the various forms of acrocephalosyndactyly and in the tricho-rhino-phalangeal syndrome. Unilateral short middle phalanges in association with syndactyly are seen in Poland's syndrome.

REFERENCES

1. Bell, J.: On Brachydactyly and Symphalangism. In Penrose, L. S.: *The Treasury of Human Inheritance.* University Press, Cambridge, England, 1951, Vol. 5, Part 1, pp. 1–31.
2. Drinkwater, H.: Account of a Family Showing Minor-Brachydactyly. *J. Genet.*, 2:21–40, 1912.
3. Haws, D. V., and McKusick, V. A.: Farabee's Brachydactylous Kindred Revisited. *Johns Hopkins Med. J.*, 113:20–30, 1963.
4. Hoefnagel, D., and Gerald, P. S.: Hereditary Brachydactyly. *Ann. Hum. Genet.*, 29:377–382, 1966.
5. Nissen, K. I.: A Study in Inherited Brachydactyly. *Ann. Eugen.*, 5:281–301, 1933.
6. Temtamy, S. A.: Genetic Factors in Hand Malformations. Thesis. Johns Hopkins University, Baltimore, Maryland, 1966.

SHORT PROXIMAL PHALANGES

Shortening of the proximal phalanges does not seem to occur as an isolated finding but in association with shortening of the other hand bones, particularly in Bell's type C brachydactyly. There is sometimes shortening of the proximal phalanx of the thumb in type A-1 brachydactyly, and in many conditions the proximal phalanx of the thumb behaves in a manner similar to that of the middle phalanges of the other fingers.

Shortening of the proximal phalanx of the thumb occurs in a number of malformation syndromes, including the Apert and the Rubinstein-Taybi syndromes. Multiple proximal phalangeal shortenings can be seen in diastrophic dwarfism. (See Table 9–3.)

SHORT METACARPALS (BRACHYMETACARPALIA)

Short first metacarpals occur in many conditions associated with radial hypoplasia and are further discussed on page 176. They may be isolated or be associated with a large number of other anomalies as well as with a number of congenital malformation syndromes (Table 9–4).[2]

Short Fourth Metacarpals (Bell's Brachydactyly E)

Shortening of the fourth and sometimes associated shortening of the third and fifth metacarpals are common anomalies (Fig. 9–13) often inherited as a Mendelian dominant trait. In contradistinction to the other forms of brachydactyly which are usually evident at birth, the short metacarpals are often not noticed until later in childhood. This suggests that the condition is probably related to early closure of the epiphysis. It is often difficult to determine whether a case of short fourth metacarpal is isolated or associated with a mild syndrome such as pseudohypoparathyroidism (see Chapter 19), since in the latter condition the clinical stigmata may be so mild that they are not noticeable and family

TABLE 9–3. Short Proximal Phalanges

Limited to proximal phalanges		
Affecting also other parts of the hand	Brachydactyly A-1	Brachydactyly C
Associated syndromes	Acrocephalosyndactyly Rubinstein-Taybi	Diastrophic dwarf
	Occasional diastrophic dwarf hand-foot-uterus myositis ossificans nevoid basal cell carcinoma trisomy 18	
Acquired		Arthritides Infection Neoplasm Sickle cell disease Trauma

TABLE 9–4. Short Metacarpals

	MET 1	MET 3,4,5
Limited to metacarpals	Isolated	Brachydactyly E
Affecting also other parts of the hand	Brachydactyly C Radial hypoplasias	Brachydactyly A-1 (sometimes) Brachydactyly C
Associated syndromes	*Thin, Short* Fanconi Juberg-Hayward radial hypoplasia	Basal cell nevus syndrome Beckwith-Wiedemann Biedmond Bixler Cri du chat
	Normal Width, Short Cornelia de Lange Christian diastrophic dwarf hand-foot-uterus myositis ossificans progressiva	Cryptodontic brachymetacarpalia Epiphyseal dysplasia Pseudohypopara- thyroidism Ru valcaba Silver (5th) Tricho-rhino-phalangeal Turner Others
Acquired		Arthritis Infection Neoplasm Sickle cell disease Trauma

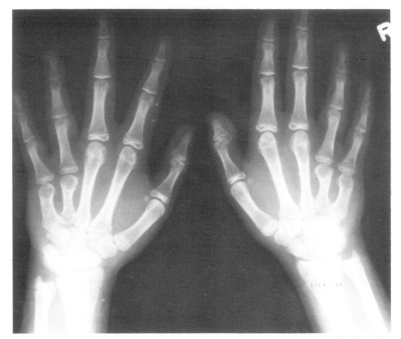

Figure 9–13. Brachymetacarpalia (brachydactyly E of Bell); also brachydactyly D (stub thumb) on the right. This obese female of normal height had a rapid growth rate.

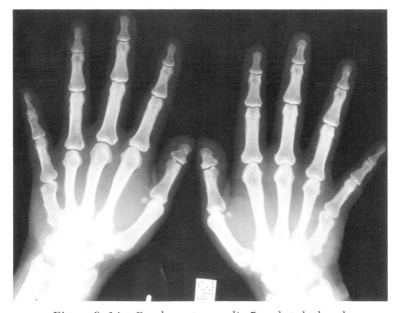

Figure 9–14. Brachymetacarpalia-5 and stub thumb.

history may be vague. In clear-cut cases of pseudohypoparathyroidism there is often associated shortening of other metacarpals, particularly the third and the fifth. A number of syndromes are associated with short metacarpals, and these are listed in Table 9–4.

Other Short Metacarpals

Shortening of the fifth metacarpal may occur without significant shortening of the fourth (Fig. 9–14). This probably should not be termed brachydactyly E. Shortening of the fifth metacarpal also occurs in the cri du chat syndrome.

Shortening of the second metacarpal has been described in a mother and her daughter.[3] The second metacarpals were composed of two bony fragments. There was slight associated shortening of the phalanges so that this condition could also be considered a form of central hypoplasia.

REFERENCES

1. Bell, J.: On Brachydactyly and Symphalangism. *In* Penrose, L. S.: *The Treasury of Human Inheritance.* University Press, Cambridge, England, 1951, Vol. 5, Part 1, pp. 1–31.
2. Biemond, A.: Brachydactylie, Nystagmus en Cerebellaire Ataxie als Familiair Syndroom. *Ned. Tijdschr. Verloskd Gynaecol.*, 78:1423–31, 1934.
3. Holmes, L. B., and Remensynder, J. P.: Hypoplasia of the Second Metacarpal in Mother and Daughter. *J. Pediat.*, 81:1165–1167, 1972.
4. Temtamy, S. A.: Genetic Factors in Hand Malformations. Thesis. Johns Hopkins University, Baltimore, Maryland, 1966.

SHORTENING AFFECTING BONES IN SEVERAL ROWS

Two well-defined syndromes affecting more than one row have been named types B and C by Bell.

Brachydactyly Type B (Apical Dystrophy, Symbrachydactyly)

Bell defined this group to include those patients in which the middle phalanx is short or rudimentary and where the terminal phalanx is also involved and may be completely absent (Fig. 9–15). The fingers and toes are reduced to short stumps with perhaps a single interphalangeal joint and no nail. There is great variation in this group with regard to completeness of the anomaly and to the number of fingers and toes involved. Often the thumbs and big toes of individuals of this group are normal. The condition has been termed apical dystrophy by MacArthur and McCullough[4] and has also been called symbrachydactyly, since mild syndactyly is commonly associated with these findings. The absence of nails appears to be a variable manifestation. The nails are absent when the distal phalangeal anomaly is severe. This is consistent with other conditions with hypoplasia of the distal phalanges which are associated with absent nails. McKusick[5] classified some cases as type A-5, particularly those described by Bass.[1] However, many of the manifestations fit well with the B type and probably should be included in this group.

Although the thumb may be normal, thumb abnormalities are relatively common in this condition. In some of the patients the distal phalanx of the thumb is somewhat flattened and splayed and may even be bifid, sometimes with a double nail. According to Bell,[2] the anomaly of the thumbs in members of a group tends to be uniform within the family but varies from one family to another.

The motion of the hand in these patients is remarkably good. There is usually good flexibility and the patients adapt well to the deformity. In one family we studied (Fig. 9–15), several of the members were able to play the piano in spite of the very short digits.

Sorsby[6] described a type B brachydactyly in a family in association with macular colobomas, and this type has been seen in association with congenital heart disease.

Findings somewhat similar to those of brachydactyly B may be seen in infants whose mothers used Dilantin (Fig. 9–16) (see also p. 158).

REFERENCES

1. Bass, H. N.: Familial Absence of Middle Phalanges with Nail Dysplasia: A New Syndrome. *Pediatrics*, 42:318–323, 1968.
2. Bell, J.: On Brachydactyly and Symphalangism. *In* Penrose, L. S.: *The Treasury of Human Inheritance.* University Press, Cambridge, England, 1951, Vol. 5, Part 1, pp. 1–31.

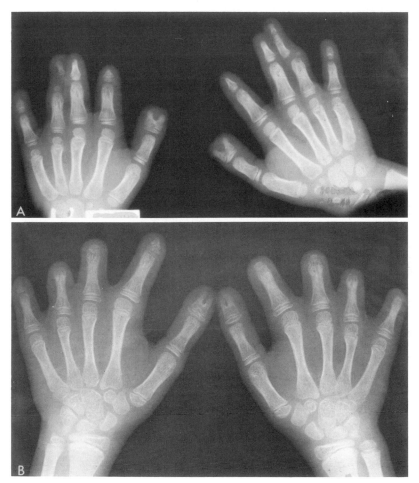

Figure 9–15. Brachydactyly B (apical dystrophy in one family). *A,* 5 year old female. *B,* 9 year old female.

Illustration continued on opposite page.

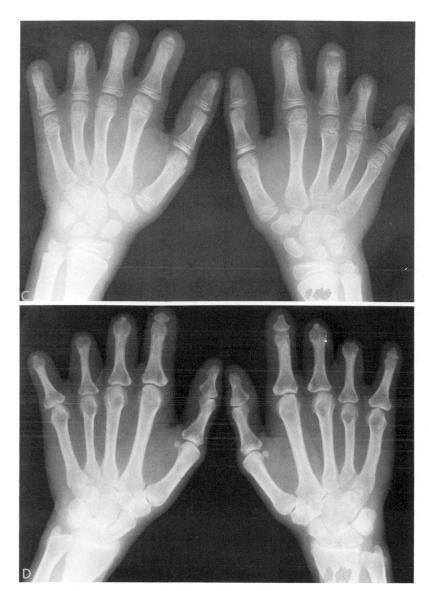

Figure 9–15 Continued. C, 13 year old male. D, 31 year old female. Three siblings and the mother are affected. The distal phalanges are absent or rudimentary. The middle phalanges are hypoplastic. In many of the patients the thumbs are bifid. These individuals have reasonably good use of their hands and have no other anomalies.

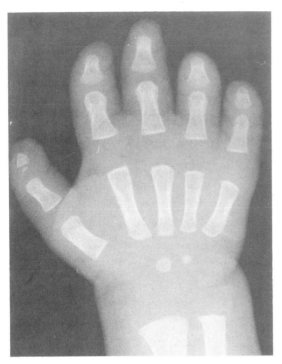

Figure 9–16. Hand similar to brachydactyly B. Patient's mother received Dilantin with Phenobarbital, and other drugs. The appearance could be difficult to distinguish from the dominantly inherited brachydactyly B.

3. Cuevas-Sosa, A., and Garcia-Segur, F.: Brachydactyly with Absence of Middle Phalanges and Hypoplastic Nails. A New Hereditary Syndrome. *J. Bone Joint Surg.*, 53B:101–105, 1971.
4. MacArthur, J. W., and McCullough, E.: Apical Dystrophy: An Inherited Defect of Hands and Feet. *Hum. Biol.*, 4:179–207, 1932.
5. McKusick, V. A.: *Mendelian Inheritance in Man: Catalogs of Autosomal Dominant, Autosomal Recessive and X-Linked Phenotype*, 3rd Ed. The Johns Hopkins Press, Baltimore, 1971.
6. Sorsby, A.: Congenital Coloboma of the Macula: Together with an Account of the Familial Occurrence of Bilateral Macular Coloboma in Association with Apical Dystrophy of Hands and Feet. *Brit. J. Ophthalmol.*, 19:65–90, 1935.
7. Temtamy, S. A.: Genetic Factors in Hand Malformations. Thesis. Johns Hopkins University, Baltimore, Maryland, 1966.

Brachydactyly Type C (Involvement Primarily of the Middle and Proximal Phalanges)

According to Bell,[1] this group of conditions includes cases presenting a more complex anomaly, differing markedly from one finger to another, with no resemblance between its manifestation in the fingers and toes. The distinguishing feature in the fingers is a defect of the middle and proximal phalanges of certain digits combined with relatively normal terminal phalanges (Figs. 9–11, 9–12 and 9–17). In these cases the thumbs may be normal. The index finger has a normal terminal phalanx with a very short middle phalanx. In some cases there is a small additional wedge-shaped ossification center at the base of the proximal phalanx which subsequently fuses with this digit, giving it a characteristic ulnar flexion. The middle finger also has a normal terminal phalanx in many cases, and a short middle phalanx. In some of these individuals the fourth finger is relatively normal and projects considerably beyond the other digits (Fig. 9–17). This is also a variable manifestation which may not be present in all members.

The extra ossicles at the base of the proximal phalanges represent large, bizarre pseudoepiphyses, and these eventually fuse with the bone. In the adult the only sign that may remain of these pseudoepiphyses is some deformity, particularly at the base of the second and third proximal phalanges. The middle phalanx of the fifth finger is frequently short and may be deviated radially. The thumb is affected in a significant percentage of cases with shortening of the first metacarpal.[4] The incidence of this condition is not known, but some large family groups have been described, particularly by Haws,[1] who reported an affected Mormon kindred in which 86 of 600 family members were affected. Instances occur in which there may be similarity to A-1 type brachydactyly in some members, whereas others have typical type C brachydactyly (Figs. 9–11 and 9–12).

REFERENCES

1. Bell, J.: On Brachydactyly and Symphalangism. *In* Penrose, L. S.: *The Treasury of Human Inheritance*. University Press, Cambridge, England, 1951, Vol. 5, Part 1, pp. 1–31.
2. Drinkwater, H.: Hereditary Abnormal Segmentation of the Index and Middle Fingers, *J. Anat. & Physiol.*, 50:177–188, 1916.
3. Gnamey, D., Walbaum, R., Saint-Aubert, P., and Fontaine, G.: Brachydactylie Hereditaire de Type C: Etude Clinique et Genetique de 3 Familles. *Ann. Pediat.*, 18:438–449, 1971.

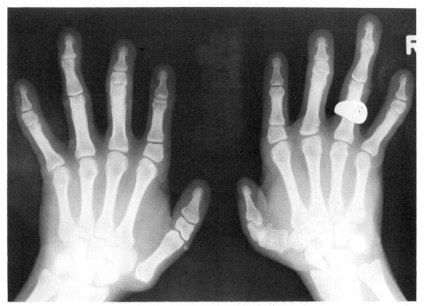

Figure 9–17. Brachydactyly C. There is shortening of middle phalanges, abnormal proximal phalanx of the second digit and abnormal thumbs. The ring finger is not affected in this patient. It is commonly spared in this disorder.

4. Haws, D. V.: Inherited Brachydactyly and Hypoplasia of the Bones of the Extremities. *Ann. Hum. Genet.*, 26:201–212, 1963.
5. Rennell, C., and Steinbach, H. L.: Epiphyseal Dysostosis without Dwarfism. *Amer. J. Roentgenol.*, 108:481–487, 1970.

ATYPICAL BRACHYDACTYLIES

Not all of the brachydactyly syndromes fit into the patterns described by Bell. Kanavel[4] and Schinz and coworkers[5] list

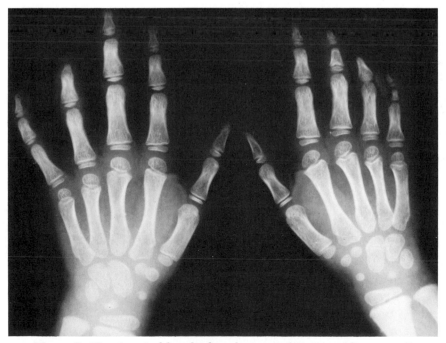

Figure 9–18. Atypical brachydactyly somewhat resembling type B.

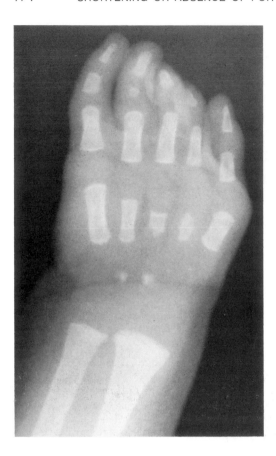

Figure 9–19. Atypical brachydactyly. This does not fit any known pattern; it is unilateral and no other anomaly was present. This could also be considered a type of central hypoplasia.

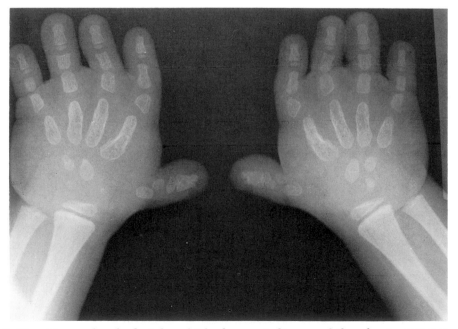

Figure 9–20. Bizarre brachydactyly which does not fit any of the classic patterns. (Courtesy Dr. Richard Schreiber and Dr. G. I. Sugarman, Los Angeles, California.)

other patterns. Bell[2] herself had a sizable group that she could not classify. The distal phalangeal brachydactylies, for example, have never been well classified. Some bear a slight resemblance to one of the well-defined syndromes (Fig. 9–18). Others are completely atypical (Figs. 9–19 and 9–20) and do not resemble any of the others. I have seen a familial unilateral brachy-dactyly involving distal and middle phalanges (Fig. 9–21).

The syndrome of acrodysostosis, which is described further in Chapter 12, is associated with a generalized form of brachydactyly that does not fit the available classifications. Arkless and Graham[1] described a case of an unusual brachydactyly which may have been another example of this.

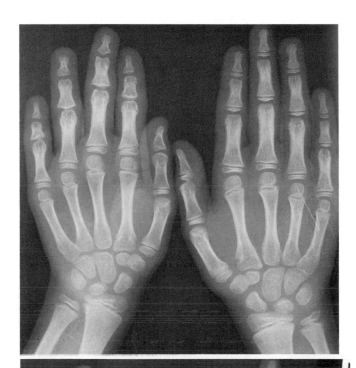

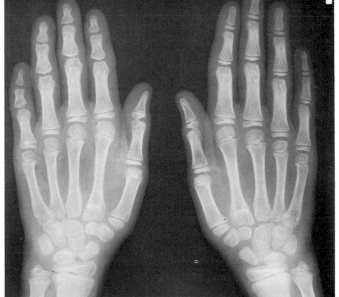

Figure 9–21. Familial brachydactyly resembling frostbite. These are two brothers. There is unusual brachydactyly with fusion of distal and middle epiphyses unilaterally.

Unusual patterns of shortening of various phalanges have also been seen in diastrophic dwarfism, but other abnormalities clearly differentiate this condition. Shortening of various segments of the hand has also been seen in many of the acrocephalosyndactyly syndromes, but again the presence of syndactyly and other findings usually clearly differentiates them. An exception is Carpenter's syndrome, which shows mainly shortening of the middle phalanges and could be confused with one of the brachydactylies if the associated polydactyly is not recognized. A variety of other ill-defined syndromes have been reported with unusual forms of brachydactyly, such as vaginal duplications with camptobrachydactyly.[3]

REFERENCES

1. Arkless, R., and Graham, C. B.: An Unusual Case of Brachydactyly: Peripheral Dysostosis? Pseudo-Pseudo-Hypoparathyroidism? Cone Epiphyses? *Am. J. Roentgenol.*, 99:724–735, 1967.
2. Bell, J.: On Brachydactyly and Symphalangism. *In* Penrose, L. S.: *The Treasury of Human Inheritance.* University Press, Cambridge, England, 1951, Vol. 5, Part 1, pp. 1–31.
3. Edwards, J. A., and Gale, R. P.: Camptobrachydactyly: A New Autosomal Dominant Trait with Two Probable Homozygotes. *Am. J. Hum. Genet.*, 24:464–474, 1972.
4. Kanavel, A. B.: Congenital Malformations of the Hands. *Arch. Surg.*, 25:282–320, 1932.
5. Schinz, H. R., Baensch, W. E., Friedl, E., and Uehlinger, E.: *Roentgen-Diagnostics* (James T. Case, Trans and Ed.). Grune & Stratton, Inc., New York, 1951, Vol. 1, *Skeleton*, Part 1.
6. Temtamy, S. A.: Genetic Factors in Hand Malformations. Thesis. Johns Hopkins University, Baltimore, Maryland, 1966.

HYPOPLASIAS OR DEFECTS OF THE HAND INVOLVING MAINLY RAYS

Radial Defects (Radial Hemimelia, Radial Club Hand, Radial Meromelia, Radial Dysplasia)

In 1924, Kato,[3] in an extensive review of radial absence, credited Petit (1733) with the first reported case of this disorder. There have been many reviews of the subject since that time.[1, 2, 6] Birch-Jensen[1] reported the incidence of this entity to be 1 in 30,000.

Most cases of this condition are sporadic, although a few cases with autosomal dominant inheritance have been reported.[8] Since a large number of malformation syndromes have been associated with radial defects and since many of these have been reported only recently, one cannot be certain from the literature whether the cases

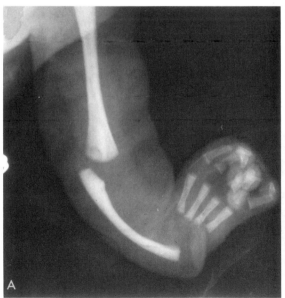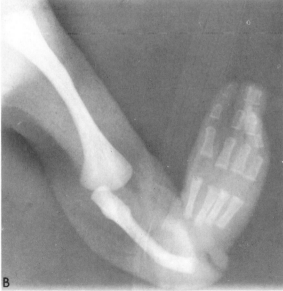

Figure 9–22. *A*, Radial aplasia with club hand and absent thumb. The forearm is shortened. *B*, Radial absence in patient with sirenomelia. The thumb is absent.

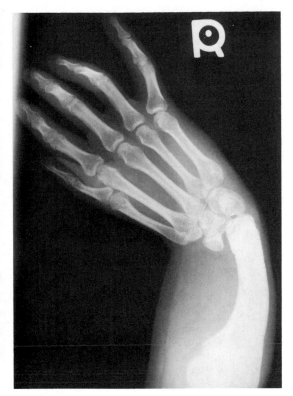

Figure 9-23. Absence of radius with persistence of thumb in a normal adult male. This is an unusual situation which should suggest the thrombocytopenia–absent radius (TAR) syndrome. There are numerous anomalies of the carpals.

reported were indeed isolated or whether they were part of some of the presently known malformation syndromes. Thus, the true incidence of the isolated form of the defect is difficult to determine.

The spectrum of radial hypoplasia is large, ranging from minimal hypoplasia of the thumb with a somewhat small metacarpal, to partial or complete absence of the radius and thumb. There is usually an associated absence of the radially placed carpals, particularly the scaphoid and the trapezium.

When there is total aplasia (Figs. 9–22 and 9–25 *A*), the hand appears clubbed and deviated radially and the thumb is usually absent. Rarely the thumb may be present (Fig. 9–23), but usually in this situation it is hypoplastic. When the radius is completely absent, the forearm is invariably shortened on the side of the radial aplasia. In one-third of cases the arm is also shortened.[2]

According to Heikel,[2] differentiation between total and partial aplasia cannot be made in the first few years of life since the initial films may show no sign of the radius whereas it is evident on follow-up films. The ulna is usually curved in association with radial aplasia and there is a tendency toward delayed onset of the distal ulnar epiphysis.[2]

When the radius is hypoplastic, the thumb is also usually hypoplastic or absent (Figs. 9–24 and 9–25 *B*). With hypoplasia of the thumb there is usually some hypoplasia of its metacarpal. In about one-half of the cases of hypoplasia of the first metacarpal, the epiphysis of the metacarpal is present in the distal rather than in the proximal portion (Fig. 9–26 *A*). The scaphoid and the trapezium are absent in almost all cases in which the bones of the thumb are absent (Fig. 9–26 *B*), and there may be absence of some of the other carpal bones as well. Carpal fusion may be evident in some patients.

As expected, muscular defects and joint

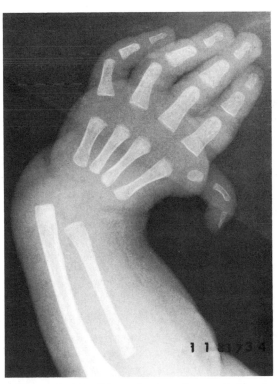

Figure 9-24. Hypoplastic radius and thumb. Patient with multiple spine and rib anomalies. The first metacarpal is markedly hypoplastic.

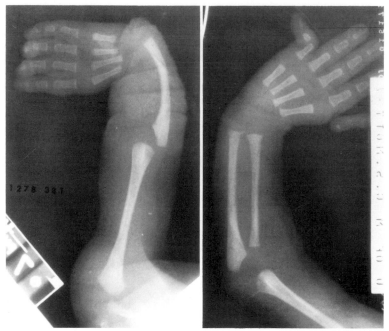

Figure 9–25. Radial absence (A) and hypoplasia (B) associated with esophageal atresia. The thumb is absent when the radius is absent, and it is hypoplastic when the radius is hypoplastic.

limitations also occur in this disease. A good description of the anatomic defects of muscles, nerves and joints has been given by Skerik.[8] There is limitation of motion of the elbow joint in many of these patients, particularly in cases of total aplasia. In most cases of hypoplasia, motion was normal. There is limitation of motion of the wrist and of the finger joints, including the index finger.

The incidence of associated anomalies is high in patients with radial defects. In a review of 85 cases from the literature, Birch-Jensen[1] found 40 per cent had some associated anomaly. Congenital heart disease was the most common with 10.6 per cent, while spina bifida, cleft palate or jaw and renal defects each had an incidence of 4.7 per cent. A multitude of other isolated anomalies was also seen. In a more recent review by Simcha[7] of 61 patients with radial clubbed hand, the incidence of congenital heart disease was 13 per cent. There was a somewhat different distribution of other anomalies. The two groups reviewed contain different populations. The more recent study includes cases

from the era of thalidomide, which was responsible for a number of cases of radial defect.

Radial hypoplasia may also be associated with polydactyly, triphalangism and syndactyly.[1, 9]

An association of radial dysplasia with anal atresia, tracheoesophageal fistula and hand anomalies has been termed the Vater association.[6] Some of the congenital malformations associated with radial defects are listed in Table 9–5.

As previously mentioned, radial defects may be unilateral or bilateral. Generally speaking, this is a useful sign in differentiating the isolated form from that associated with syndromes. It appears that most of the patients with unilateral radial dysplasia cannot be easily classified as having the well-defined inherited syndromes, even though they do have associated abnormalities.[4, 5] On the other hand, cases associated with familial malformation syndromes usually have bilateral involvement. A good example of this is in the combination of congenital heart disease with radial defects. In the Holt-Oram syndrome the findings

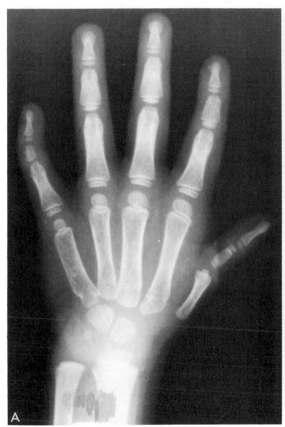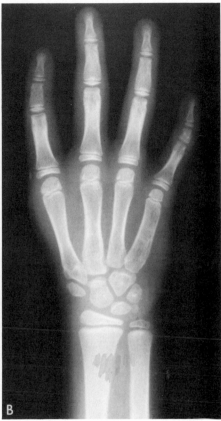

Figure 9–26. Hypoplastic thumbs in patient with tracheoesophageal fistula. *A,* The epiphysis is seen in the distal rather than in the proximal end of the metacarpal. There is also a short middle phalanx of the little finger.

B, This patient had a small appendage of a thumb, which was amputated. Note the absence of the scaphoid and trapezium, which is commonly associated with absent thumbs.

TABLE 9–5. Congenital Malformations and Malformation Syndromes Associated with Radial Defects (Partial List)

MALFORMATIONS
Cleft lip, jaw or palate
Congenital heart disease
Ear abnormalities
Esophageal atresia
Klippel-Feil deformity
Renal anomalies
Spina bifida

MALFORMATION SYNDROMES
Craniosynostosis
Ectodermal dysplasia
Fanconi
Holt-Oram
Nager's acrofacial dysostosis
Pseudothalidomide
Ring D
Thrombocytopenia–absent radius
Thalidomide
Trisomy 18

are almost universally bilateral, although different degrees of severity may be present on each side. The heart defect in these cases is almost invariably an atrial or ventricular defect. Unilateral radial defects are also associated with congenital heart disease, but they usually occur sporadically and the type of cardiac anomaly may be different from that occurring in the Holt-Oram syndrome. Similarly, cases of radial defect associated with Klippel-Feil deformity or cleft lip are often unilateral and sporadic.

Some of the syndromes associated with radial defects tend to produce a specific type of abnormality. For example, in thalidomide embryopathy there is frequently a triphalangeal thumb. This abnormality may be present in radial defects from other causes, but it is less common. The thrombocytopenia–absent radius (TAR) syndrome is characterized by the fact that the thumb is present even though the radius is absent. This is contrary to most other situations with an absent radius. In most of the malformation syndromes associated with radial defects, the severity of the anomaly can be quite variable, ranging from slight hypoplasia of the thumb to phocomelia in the same family. This wide range is particularly well illustrated in the Holt-Oram syndrome and in the thrombocytopenia–absent radius syndrome (TAR). Table 9–5 lists some of the malformation syndromes associated with radial defects.

REFERENCES

1. Birch-Jensen, A.: *Congenital Deformities of the Upper Extremities.* Andelsbogtrykkeriet, Odense, Denmark, 1949.
2. Heikel, H. V. A.: Aplasia and Hypoplasia of the Radius. *Acta Orthop. Scand.,* 39:1–155, 1959.
3. Kato, K.: Congenital Absence of the Radius with Review of Literature and Report of Three Cases. *J. Bone Joint Surg.,* 6:589–626, 1924.
4. Poznanski, A. K., Garn, S. M., and Holt, J. F.: The Thumb in the Congenital Malformation Syndromes. *Radiology,* 100:115–129, 1971.
5. Poznanski, A. K., Stern, A., and Gall, J.: Letter to the Editor, *Am. J. Dis. Child.,* 125:622–623, 1973.
6. Quan, L., and Smith, D. W.: The Vater Association. <u>V</u>ertebral Defects, <u>A</u>nal Atresia, <u>T-E</u> Fistula with Esophageal Atresia, <u>R</u>adial and <u>R</u>enal Dysplasia: A Spectrum of Associated Defects. *J. Pediat.,* 82:104–107, 1973.
7. Simcha, A.: Congenital Heart Disease in Radial Clubbed Hand Syndrome. *Arch. Dis. Child.,* 46:345–349, 1971.
8. Skerik, S. K., and Flatt, A. E.: The Anatomy of Congenital Radial Dysplasia. Its Surgical and Functional Implications. *Clin. Orthop.,* 66:125–143, 1969.
9. Temtamy, S. A.: Genetic Factors in Hand Malformations. Thesis. Johns Hopkins University, Baltimore, Maryland, 1966.

Ulnar Hypoplasia

This is a considerably rarer abnormality than absence of the radius. In an extensive review of the literature, Birch-Jensen[1]

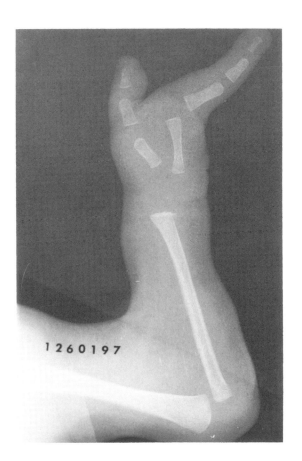

Figure 9–27. Unilateral ulnar absence. Only the thumb and index finger are present. This child had no other anomalies.

1 2 6 0 1 9 7

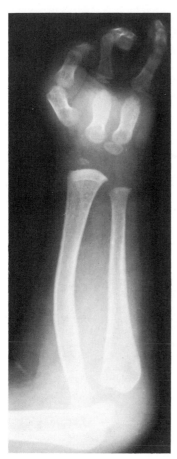

Figure 9-28. Hypoplasia of the ulna with associated absence of the fourth and fifth digits.

and humeral-radial synostosis (Fig. 9-28).[3] When digits are absent or hypoplastic, usually the fourth and fifth fingers are involved (Fig. 9-29). The corresponding carpals are also absent. Most commonly the pisiform and hamate are absent,[3] but sometimes also the triquetrum or capitate. In some cases carpal fusion may be seen (Fig. 9-31). In very mild cases there may be only hypoplasia of the phalanges of the fifth finger (Fig. 9-30). Occasionally only the metacarpal may be absent (Fig. 9-31).

In some patients radial and ulnar defects coexist (Fig. 9-32). Among 70 cases of ulnar defects reviewed by Lausecker[2] in 1954, 48 cases were unilateral and 22 were bilateral.

Birch-Jensen found a lesser frequency of associated abnormalities with ulnar defects than with radial defects. There is some overlap between split-hand deformity and ulnar defect. Symphalangism has been associated with ulnar defects, as has Nievergelt's

found only one case of total ulnar aplasia. The number of patients with partial ulnar hypoplasia was also considerably lower than that of partial radial hypoplasia. Temtamy[3] has reviewed the literature and similarly found only a few cases.

Most cases of ulnar defects are sporadic, although when associated with other malformations can be inherited in a Mendelian pattern. For example, split hand and ulnar deformity has been inherited as a dominant trait, while micromelic dwarfism with deficiency of the ulna and fibula has been inherited as a recessive.[3]

As in absence of the radius, ulnar defects range from a slight hypoplasia of some of the ulnar digits to complete absence of the ulna (Fig. 9-27). In the severe form there may be dislocation of the head of the radius

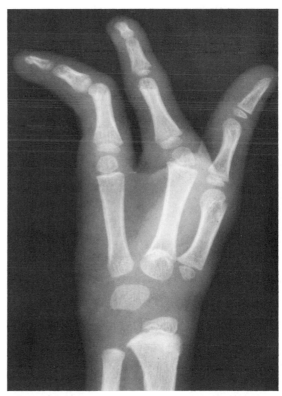

Figure 9-29. Absence of the fourth and fifth digits with a single carpal. This is a form of ulnar hypoplasia. The patient's mother underwent surgery for fibroids when two months pregnant.

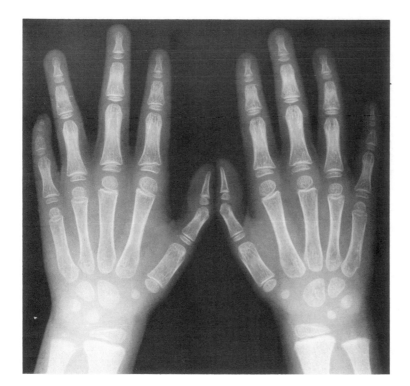

Figure 9–30. Minor hypoplasia of the middle and distal phalanges of both fifth fingers. There was also minimal syndactyly between the fourth and fifth fingers. Similar hypoplasia of the fifth digits was also present in the feet. The nails were not affected. This girl had a congenital heart defect.

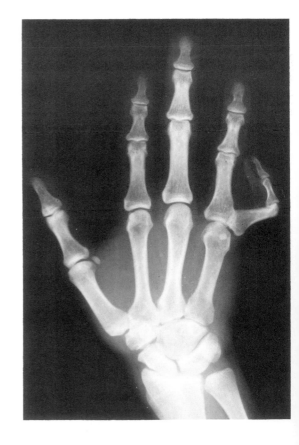

Figure 9–31. Unusual hypoplasia of the fifth digit. The mother of this child had multiple congenital anomalies.

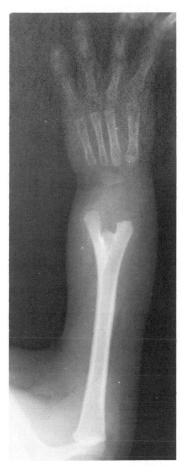

Figure 9–32. Ulnar absence and radial absence. This may be termed phocomelia. The hand has the appearance of radial absence with an absent thumb. The opposite upper extremity showed radial hypoplasia. The child was mentally retarded.

syndrome. Defects in the ulnar area are also seen in Weyers's oligodactyly syndrome[4] and in the Cornelia de Lange syndrome. (See Table 9–6.)

TABLE 9–6. Malformation Syndromes Associated with Ulnar Defects and with Split Hand

---

SYNDROMES ASSOCIATED WITH ULNAR DEFECTS
  Cornelia de Lange
  Nievergelt
  Symphalangism
  Weyers's oligodactyly

SYNDROMES ASSOCIATED WITH SPLIT HAND
  Anonychia
  Congenital nystagmus and fundal changes
  Wildervanck (1963) (with associated deafness)

REFERENCES

1. Birch-Jensen, A.: *Congenital Deformities of the Upper Extremities.* Andelsbogtrykkeriet, Odense, Denmark, 1949.
2. Lausecker, H.: Der angeborene Defekt der Ulna. *Virchows Arch.,* 325:211–226, 1954.
3. Temtamy, S. A.: *Genetic Factors in Hand Malformations.* Thesis. Johns Hopkins University, Baltimore, Maryland, 1966.
4. Weyers, H.: Das Oligodactylie-Syndrom des Menschen und seine Parallelmutation bei der Hausmaus. Ein Anomaliekomplex mit Ulnaaplasie, Reduktion der ulnaren Randstrahlen, Zwischenkiefer-, Sternum-, Nieren- und Milzanomalien. *Ann. Padiat.,* 189:351–370, 1957.

Central Hypoplasia—Split Hand (Lobster Claws, "Ectrodactyly," Oligodactyly)

The terminology for this entity is somewhat confusing. Although some authors call the split hand "ectrodactyly,"[9] this term is probably best used for transverse defects of the hand. Other terms used for split hand have been "perodactyly," "hypodactyly" and "oligodactyly." The condition is really a periaxial or longitudinal terminal deficiency of rays which is often associated with syndactyly. The condition has been known for many years. Perhaps the earliest report was a description by Paré of a boy with a split-hand deformity in one hand associated with absence deformity of the long bones of the legs.[7] A good review of the history of this defect is given by Temtamy.

The entity of split hand is not limited to man. Pearson[5] in 1931 described it in the chimpanzee and the rhesus monkey. Searle[6] reported a similar abnormality in the domestic cat, in which the condition was also inherited as an autosomal dominant trait. Hypodactyly was reported in mice also as a heritable disorder.[7]

Birch-Jensen[1] described two different types of this deformity in man. The first is the lobster-claw deformity; the second is monodactyly. The incidence of the typical split hand is given by Birch-Jensen as one in 90,000 at birth. However, according to Temtamy,[7] the distinction between lobster claw deformity and monodactyly is not valid on a genetic basis, since either type may occur in the same family or in different limbs of the same person (Fig. 9–36).

The genetics of this abnormality is not

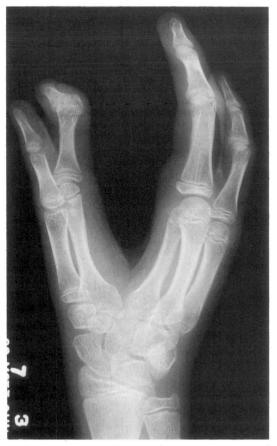

Figure 9–33. Split hand in a patient with cleft palate.

defects and the split hand, since hypoplasia of the ulnar rays may be present in cases of families with typical split hand. In these cases a study of family history may be useful in determining the type of abnormality that is expected.

The radiologic manifestations of cleft hand are variable, ranging from a simple cleft (Fig. 9–33) to a two-digit hand (Fig. 9–34) to monodactyly (Fig. 9–36). The manifestations may be unilateral (Fig. 9–35) or asymmetric (Fig. 9–36). Sometimes only a single ray may be hypoplastic, as in the family reported by Holmes and Remensnyder.[2] In the less severe form the carpals are unaffected, but when the defect is severe carpals may be fused or absent (Figs. 9–34 and 9–36) (see also Chapter 8). Bizarre changes in the digits may be asso-

clear. Some patients transmit the disease with typical dominant inheritance. In other cases there is lack of penetrance with skipped generations. The skipping of generations has been seen by several authors and may be the result of gonadal mosaicism.[7]

Temtamy felt that the typical split-hand deformity represents a genetically heterogeneous group. She was able to identify four categories of this trait on study of various pedigrees: (1) Pedigrees with a trait segregating as a regular autosomal dominant with constant involvement of the feet and wide variability in involvement of the hands; (2) pedigrees of more or less constant involvement of the feet but with irregular inheritance; (3) pedigrees with extensive involvement of the lower limbs with absence of long bones with irregular inheritance; and (4) pedigrees with no involvement of the lower limbs and with very irregular inheritance.

There is some overlap between ulnar

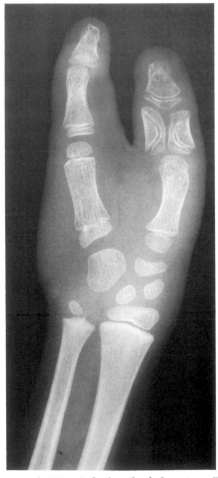

Figure 9–34. Split-hand deformity. There is bizarre duplication of the proximal phalanx of the thumb. (Courtesy Dr. Michael Ozonoff, Newington, Connecticut.)

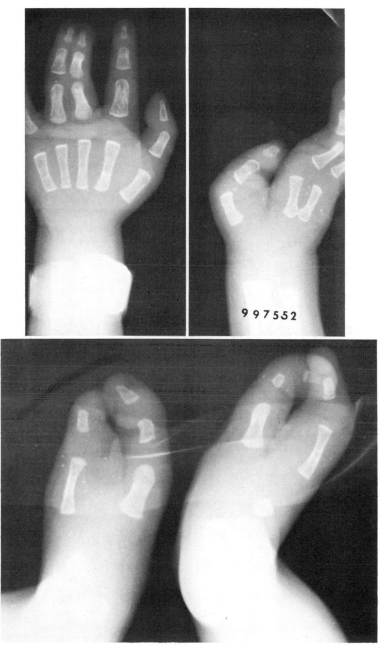

Figure 9–35. Cleft hand and feet in patient with pulmonary stenosis. There is syndactyly of the third and fourth fingers of the left hand.

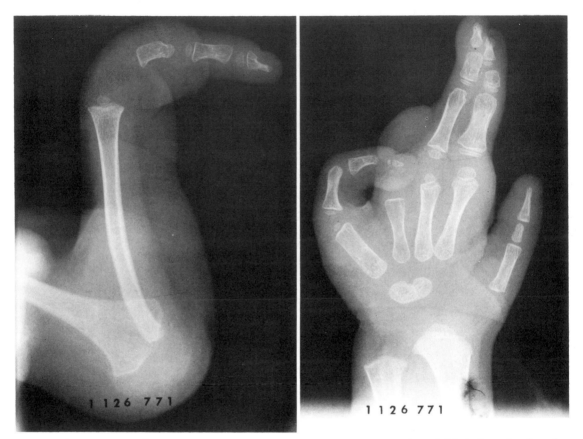

Figure 9–36. Monodactyly and cleft hand in the same patient. The child had multiple other anomalies, including cleft palate, microphthalmia, colobomas, and esotropia. The asymmetry of the findings suggests that monodactyly and cleft hand may be related.

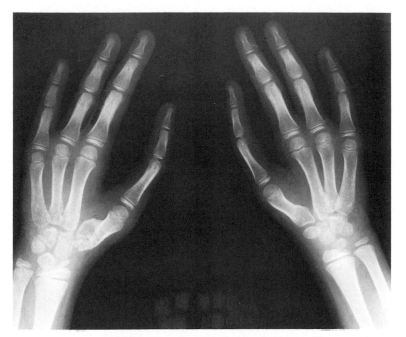

Figure 9–37.   Pseudocleft hand. This was the result of previous pollicization surgery for absence of thumb.

ciated with a cleft hand, and these include absence of the segments, duplications and so forth (Figs. 9–34 and 9–36).

An appearance similar to cleft hand may be due to previous pollicization, where the index finger is shifted to act as a thumb in patients with radial aplasia (Fig. 9–37).

A number of anomalies have been associated with split hand (Table 9–6). These have included various anomalies of the face, particularly cleft lip and palate, mandibulofacial dysostosis, deafness, congenital nystagmus, cataract[7] and anonychia. Warkany[9] quotes other conditions associated with split hand, including cyclopia, congenital heart disease and imperforate anus.

REFERENCES

1. Birch-Jensen, A.: *Congenital Deformities of the Upper Extremities.* Andelsbogtrykkeriet, Odense, Denmark, 1949.
2. Holmes, L. B., and Remensnyder, J. P.: Hypoplasia of the Second Metacarpal in Mother and Daughter. *J. Pediat.,* 81:1165–1167, 1972.
3. Lees, D. H., Lawler, S. D., Renwick, J. H., and Thoday, J. M.: Anonychia with Ectrodactyly: Clinical and Linkage Data. *Ann. Hum. Genet.,* 22:69–79, 1957.
4. Maisels, D. O.: Lobster-Claw Deformities of the Hands and Feet. *Brit. J. Plast. Surg.,* 23:269–282, 1970.
5. Pearson, K.: On the Existence of the Digital Deformity—So-called "Lobster Claw"—in the Apes. *Ann. Eugen.,* 4:339–340, 1931.
6. Searle, A. G.: Hereditary 'Split-Hand' in the Domestic Cat. *Ann. Eugen.,* 17:279–282, 1953.
7. Temtamy, S. A.: Genetic Factors in Hand Malformations. Thesis. Johns Hopkins University, Baltimore, Maryland, 1966.
8. Walker, J. C., and Clodius, L.: The Syndromes of Cleft Lip, Cleft Palate and Lobster-Claw Deformities of Hands and Feet. *Plast. Reconstr. Surg.,* 32:627–636, 1963.
9. Warkany, J.: *Congenital Malformations: Notes and Comments.* Year Book Medical Publishers, Chicago, 1971.

TERMINAL TRANSVERSE DEFECTS (ECTRODACTYLY, APHALANGISM, ADACTYLY, ACHEIRIA)

In this group of defects the distal portion of the upper extremity is missing. When only the phalanges are affected it is called aphalangism; when the digits are involved it is adactyly (Figs. 9–38 and 9–39); when the full hand is affected it is called acheiria (Figs. 9–40, 9–41 and 9–42). When both

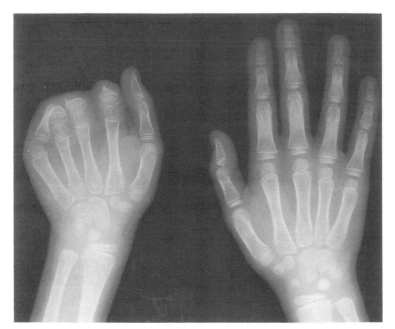

Figure 9–38. Adactyly in a patient with cleft palate and colobomas.

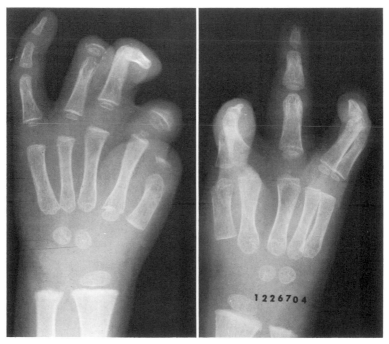

Figure 9–39. Absence of digits in a patient with cleft lip and palate. Syndactyly is also present.

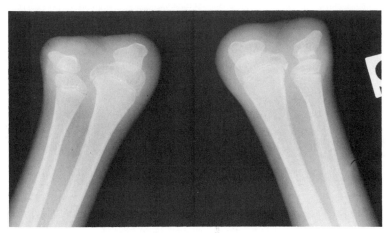

Figure 9–40. Acheiria, bilateral. This patient also had partial absence of the left foot. No bands were seen and no other anomalies were present.

hand and foot are absent the condition is called acheiropodia. The term "ectro-dactyly" (*ektroma* meaning abortion and *daktylos* meaning finger) has also been used for this deformity, although the term is somewhat confusing since St. Hillaire initially introduced the term to mean a split-hand deformity. Probably the term ecterodactyly should be eliminated to de-crease confusion. The term "amputation" is also misleading and should probably not be used for the various conditions with stump formations, since these limbs, rather than being amputated, were never formed.

In the Birch-Jensen series the incidence at birth of absence of the distal forearm and hand was 1:22,000, and absence of the hand (acheiria) was 1:65,000. Warkany reported

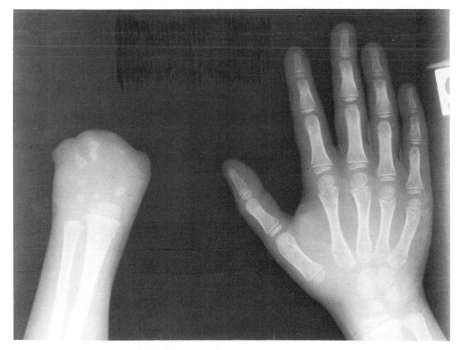

Figure 9–41. Acheiria, unilateral. The patient had a nevus flammeus of the face. There is no family history and no other abnormality.

that acheiria accounted for about 12 per cent of cases seen in child amputee centers.

Most of the cases of terminal transverse defects in the hand are sporadic.[3] Birch-Jensen[1] observed only occasionally such malformations in the families of patients.

The roentgen appearance of these transverse defects varies from only minimal aphalangia (Fig. 9–38) to more complicated lesions. The defects may involve the whole hand (Fig. 9–40) or even the entire forearm or arm. The defects are usually unilateral (Figs. 9–38 and 9–41), although bilateral symmetric lesions may occasionally be seen (Fig. 9–40). In Hall's series of amelia, 99 cases were unilateral while 4 were bilateral. According to Warkany, acheiria is more common on the left than on the right.

The distal end of the terminal defect in bone may have a pointed, tapered appear-

TABLE 9–7.	Congenital Malformations Associated with Absence of Digits

Aglossia-adactyly
Ankyloglossia superior
Cornelia de Lange syndrome
Hanhart's syndrome
Möbius's syndrome

ance (Fig. 9–38) or may be well defined and flat (Fig. 9–40). The terminal bones are often deformed and may not be identifiable as normal components (Figs. 9–40 and 9–41). Occasionally, soft tissue calcifications may be seen at the distal end (Fig. 9–42). Syndactyly may be sometimes associated with a terminal deficiency (Fig. 9–39).

Some cases of transverse defects can be confused with "Streeter's bands." In this condition, ring-like constrictions are usually seen in the soft tissues. These are not present in the cases of congenital aplasia.

A number of syndromes are associated with transverse defects of the fingers and hand. These include the aglossia-adactyly syndrome, ankyloglossia superior and micrognathia (Hanhart's syndrome). (See Table 9–7.)

REFERENCES

1. Birch-Jensen, A.: *Congenital Deformities of the Upper Extremities.* Andelsbogtrykkeriet, Odense, Denmark, 1949.
2. Hall, J. G., Levin, J., Kuhn, J. P., Ottenheimer, E. J., Van Berkum, K. A. P., and McKusick, V. A.: Thrombocytopenia with Absent Radius (TAR). *Medicine,* 48:411–439, 1969.
3. Temtamy, S. A.: Genetic Factors in Hand Malformations. Thesis. Johns Hopkins University, Baltimore, Maryland, 1966.
4. Warkany, J.: *Congenital Malformations: Notes and Comments.* Year Book Medical Publishers, Chicago, 1971.

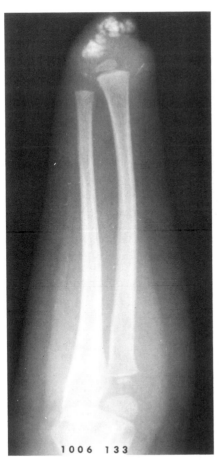

1006 133

Figure 9–42. Acheiria, unilateral, with amorphous calcification in the distal portion. No other anomalies were present.

Streeter's Bands (Congenital Amputations, Intrauterine Amputations, Amniotic Bands, Congenital Constricting Bands)

Congenital constriction rings are soft tissue grooves or depressions of any portion of the limbs or digits. They most frequently involve the fingers.

The etiology of the condition is disputed. Streeter[6] proposed a defect, or an extrinsic insult to the fetus, at the time of differentiation of the limb buds, while according to Torpin[7] this is the result of early rupture of the amnion, producing raw surfaces and strings which attach the fetus to it. Diamond[3] feels that these two theories are not exclusive, since an insult could result in both of these mechanisms. There is evidence that the condition is not caused by true bands or umbilical cord in an intact amnion. Bleeding in the third trimester is commonly associated with this condition.

The incidence of these rings was 1:10,000 births in Baker and Rudolph's series[1] and 1:45,000 in Birch-Jensen's series.[2] The rings are always sporadic. No familial cases have been seen. In a study of 83 cases Birch-Jensen showed no affected siblings and none of the 23 offspring of 10 affected individuals had the disease.

Clinically the lesions are usually epithelialized at the time of birth, but occasionally black eschars may be seen. To make the diagnosis one needs to see scarred rings circling a limb or digit. A useful clinical finding is the interruption of normal skin whorls at stumps of amputation. When whorls are present at the tips of nondigital stumps, primary agenesis is suggested.[3]

Radiologically the rings may be visible in the soft tissue (Fig. 9–43). If the rings are not visualized on the film, radiologic differentiation from congenital defects may be difficult. The bones distal to the ring are usually poorly developed or absent.

The rings are often multiple, but they are characteristically asymmetric (Fig. 9–43). The ring is quite variable in depth and may on occasion contact the bone. Distal to the constriction there may be distention of the finger due to lymphedema, or there may be a large quantity of fat. Fenestrated syndactyly is commonly associated with this abnormality and sometimes may be severe (Fig. 9–44). In some cases complete amputation occurs in utero. The severity of the changes in the bones of the hand does not always correspond to the depth of the constriction. The rings may extend across the forearm (Fig. 9–45) or even across the arm.

Occasionally some other anomaly may be seen in association with Streeter's bands.

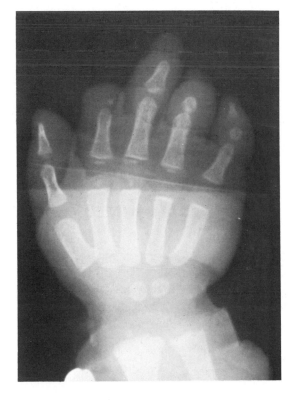

Figure 9–43. Constriction bands (Streeter's). Characteristic constrictions are noted.

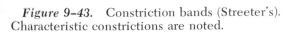

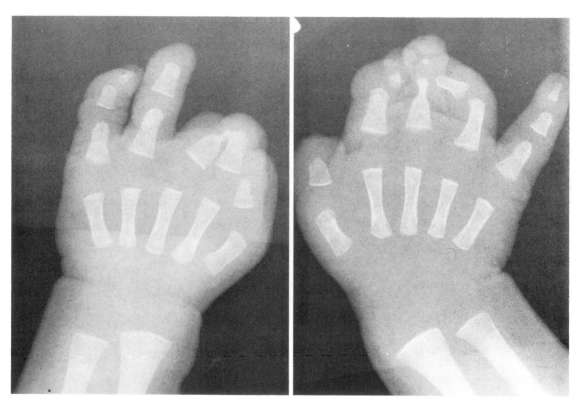

Figure 9–44. Constriction bands (Streeter's), bilateral. There is syndactyly distal to the bands. Another constricting ring was evident in the left leg. The right foot was clubbed.

Patterson[5] found some associated anomalies in 14 of 52 patients with rings. The most common were club feet in 9 cases and cleft lip and palate in 4.

Acquired rings may also occur. We have seen constriction of the finger associated only with soft tissue changes in a girl who left an elastic band on her finger for a prolonged time (Fig. 9–46).

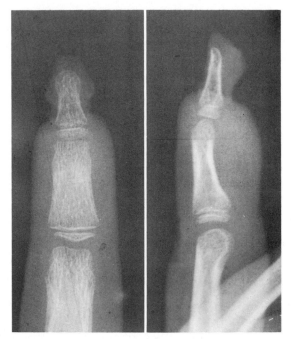

Figure 9–46. Acquired constriction ring due to soft tissue atrophy secondary to leaving an elastic band on the finger for a prolonged period of time. (Courtesy Ming Ting, M.D., Wayne County General Hospital, Eloise, Michigan.)

REFERENCES

1. Baker, C. J., and Rudolph, A. J.: Congenital Ring Constrictions and Intrauterine Amputations. *Am. J. Dis. Child.*, 121:393–400, 1971.
2. Birch Jensen, A.: *Congenital Deformities of the Upper Extremities.* Andelsbogtrykkeriet, Odense, Denmark, 1949.
3. Diamond, L. S.: Ring Constrictions. *In:* Bergsma, D.: *Birth Defects Atlas and Compendium.* The Williams & Wilkins Company, Baltimore, 1973, p. 795.
4. Kohler, H. G.: Congenital Transverse Defects of Limbs and Digits (Intrauterine Amputation). *Arch. Dis. Child.*, 37:263–276, 1962.
5. Patterson, T. J. S.: Congenital Ring-Constrictions. *Brit. J. Plast. Surg.*, 14:1–31, 1961.
6. Streeter, G. L.: Focal Deficiencies in Fetal Tissues and Their Relation to Intra-Uterine Amputation. *Contribution to Embryology.*, Vol. 22, No. 126. Publication No. 414. Carnegie Institution of Washington, 1930.
7. Torpin, R.: Amniochorionic Mesoblastic Fibrous Strings and Amnionic Bands. *Am. J. Obstet. Gynec.*, 91.65–75, 1965.

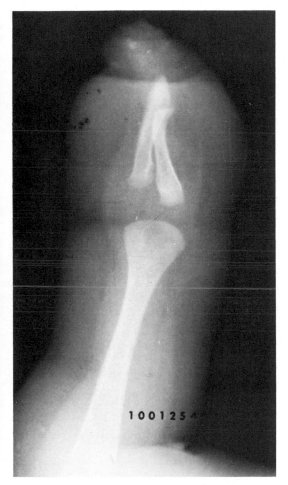

Figure 9–45. Constriction bands above wrist with acheiria. From the film alone it is impossible to be certain whether this represents a constricting band or a transverse amputation.

Chapter 10

OTHER ANOMALIES OF THE HAND
Hyperphalangism, Polydactyly, Syndactyly, Crooked Fingers, Symphalangism and Macrodactyly

Anomalies of the wrist and the various conditions which cause diminution of the hand bones have been discussed in Chapters 8 and 9. In this chapter we will discuss the remaining anomalies of the hand, including increased number of phalanges, increased digits (polydactyly), syndactyly, focal enlargement of the fingers and crooked fingers.

HYPERPHALANGISM

In some animals different numbers of phalanges may normally occur in each digit. In man, however, the usual arrangement of two phalanges in the thumb and three phalanges in the other fingers is rarely altered. The only documented true extra phalanges in man have occurred in the thumb. There are a number of conditions in which very large and abnormal pseudoepiphyses may exist at the base of some of the phalanges,[2, 5] and in the past these have been called accessory phalanges. This is particularly true in brachydactyly C. These accessory phalanges, however, usually fuse with the bone below them, and there is not a separate joint between the two bones. Manzke[5] described an accessory ossicle between the proximal phalanx and the metacarpal. Although from his study it is uncertain whether this represents a separate bone or a pseudoepiphysis, a later film in his case suggests that it is indeed an accessory epiphysis.

Triphalangeal Thumb

This is a rare normal variant. Only one case was seen in 25,000 hand radiographs in the 10 State Nutrition Survey.[8] Similarly, Lapidus et al.[4] found three cases in 75,000 recruits examined clinically. In one of these patients there was also absence of the pectoral muscle. Triphalangism may be familial. The additional phalanx may vary from a small nodule to a normally shaped accessory bone. In general, the individuals with small ossicles have normally opposing thumbs, but when the additional bone is large, apposition is usually impossible.[9] Triphalangeal thumbs may be associated with duplication of the thumb, either on the same side as the triphalangeal thumb or on the opposite hand (Fig. 10–1). This suggests that the two entities may have a common embryologic derivation. A similar association of triphalangeal thumb and duplication of the thumb is seen in a number of malformation syndromes, particularly Fanconi's anemia. Alternately, triphalangeal thumb may be associated with absence of the opposite thumb (Fig. 10–2). Both triphalangeal thumb and absence of the thumb may be seen in the Holt-Oram syndrome (Fig. 10–3).

In most cases of triphalangeal thumb the first metacarpal is relatively long and the

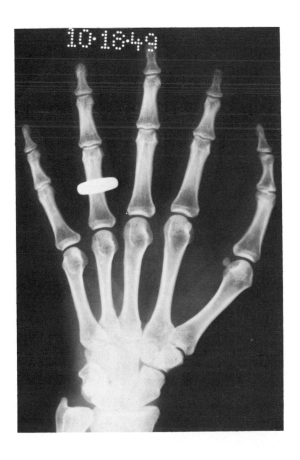

Figure 10–1. Triphalangeal thumb. This patient also had a duplication, as well as a triphalangeal thumb, on the opposite side. The triphalangeal thumb is somewhat finger-like in appearance.

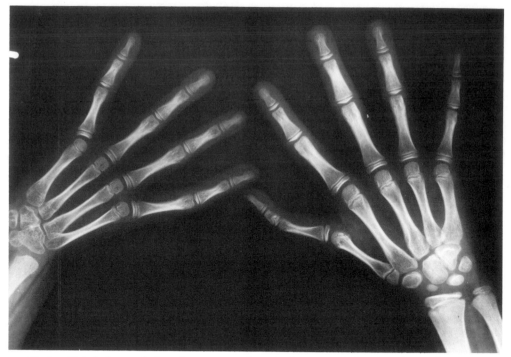

Figure 10–2. Triphalangeal thumb associated with absence of the thumb on the opposite hand. There is associated hypoplasia of the carpals. This patient had no associated congenital heart disease.

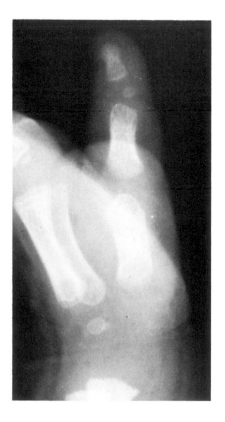

Figure 10–3. Triphalangeal thumb with a simple ossicle in the Holt-Oram syndrome. In this disorder the triphalangeal thumb can vary from a finger-like condition to a minute ossicle such as in this patient. For further description see Chapter 13.

TABLE 10–1. Syndromes and Other
Anomalies Associated
with Triphalangeal Thumb

SYNDROMES
Blackfan-Diamond anemia
Cardiomelic (Holt-Oram)
Juberg-Hayward
Thalidomide
Trisomy 13–15 (occasionally)

OTHER ASSOCIATED ANOMALIES
Absent pectoral muscle[4]*
Absent tibia[6, 9]
Duplication of great toe[3]
Imperforate anus, deafness
Lobster-claw hand[7]
Preaxial polydactyly[7]
Polydactyly, 5th toe[1]

*Superscripts indicate references below.

distal phalanx of the thumb is usually short when compared to the second metacarpal.

A number of congenital malformation syndromes have been associated with triphalangeal thumb and these are listed in Table 10–1.

REFERENCES

1. Abramowitz, M. B.: Triphalangeal Thumb. A Case Report and Evaluation of its Importance in the Morphology and Function of the Thumb. S. Afr. Med. J., 41:104–106, 1967.
2. Holthusen, W.: The Pierre Robin Syndrome: Unusual Associated Developmental Defects. Ann. Radiol., 15:253–262, 1972.
3. Komai, T., Ozaki, Y., and Inokuma, W.: A Japanese Kindred of Hyperphalangism of Thumbs and Duplication of Thumbs and Big-Toes. Folia Hered. Path., 2:307–312, 1953.
4. Lapidus, P. W., Guidotti, F. P., and Coletti, C. J.: Triphalangeal Thumb. Report of Six Cases. Surg. Gynec. & Obstet., 77:178–186, 1943.
5. Manzke, H.: Symmetrische Hyperphalangie des zweiten Fingers durch ein akzessorisches Metacarpale. Fortschr. Geb. Roentgenstr. Nuklearmed., 105:425–427, 1966.
6. Pashayan, H., Fraser, F. C., McIntyre, J. M., and Dunbar, J. S.: Bilateral Aplasia of the Tibia, Polydactyly and Absent Thumb in Father and Daughter. J. Bone Joint Surg., 53B:495–499, 1971.
7. Phillips, R. S.: Congenital Split Foot (Lobster Claw) and Triphalangeal Thumb. J. Bone Joint Surg., 53B:247–257, 1971.
8. Poznanski, A. K., Garn, S. M., and Holt, J. F.: The Thumb in the Congenital Malformation Syndromes. Radiology, 100:115–129, 1971.
9. Swanson, A. B., and Brown, K. S.: Hereditary Triphalangeal Thumb. J. Hered., 53:259–265, 1962.

POLYDACTYLY

Polydactyly refers to an increased number of digits. When the anomaly is on the ulnar side of the hand it is termed postaxial polydactyly, and when it is on the radial side it is called preaxial polydactyly. Uncommonly, it can involve the second, third or fourth digits. Polydactyly also occurs in other animals, where certain strains may have a number of digits which is greater than usual for the species. For example, polydactyly has been described in mice[31] and in fowl.[1]

Since polydactyly is an obvious clinical manifestation, it has been noticed since antiquity. Probably the earliest reference is in the *Old Testament:* "And there was again war at Gath, where there was a man of great stature, who had six fingers on each hand, and six toes on each foot." (2 Sam., 21:15–22.) It is believed that Anne Boleyn had postaxial polydactyly.[24] Polydactyly also has been seen in almost all of the inhabitants of several small isolated villages. It was found in Cervera de Buitrago in Spain[7] and in the village of Izeaux in France.[13] In Izeaux, interestingly enough, the incidence of polydactyly markedly decreased following the time the first train line ran through the village. Perhaps the first comprehensive paper dealing with polydactyly and using radiographs to illustrate it was published by Boinet in 1898.[3] In it he commented on an Arab tribe in which polydactyly was so common that infants who did not have six digits were immediately killed.

Polydactyly is recognized in most population groups, but there are great differences in both incidence and type.[27] Polydactyly is much more common in blacks than in whites. In fact, it is probably the most common hand anomaly in blacks. Mellin[17] in New York found an incidence of 10.7 per thousand in blacks and 1.6 per thousand in whites. In his series, polydactyly was twice as common in males as in females. In Uganda the incidence of postaxial polydactyly in African newborns was 14.0 per thousand.[26] Almost all of these abnormalities were small, pedunculated, extra digits attached to the fifth finger. Woolf and Woolf[34] in Salt Lake City and Wood in Iowa,[33] as well as other authors studying mainly white populations, have found preaxial polydactyly to be more common than postaxial. Preaxial polydactyly is also common in China. Handforth[11] found an incidence of 2.4 per thousand among Chinese prisoners in Hong Kong. Polydactyly was 19 times more common in embryos studied by Nishimura et al.[18] than in a similar population at birth.

Different types of polydactyly may have different modes of inheritance. Temtamy[29] feels that the inheritance of postaxial polydactyly is usually an irregular autosomal dominant pattern, although recessive patterns have also been known to occur. Woolf and Woolf,[34] in the study of 56 propositi with polydactyly who came for surgical intervention, found that 33 of these cases were preaxial and 19 were postaxial (four cases were undefined). Of the 33 preaxial cases, only two had a positive family history and one of these had triphalangeal thumbs. In the 19 postaxial cases dominant inheritance was postulated in seven (37 per cent). Fifteen of the propositi had a history of some other finger anomaly in a close relative. Temtamy[29] studied seven cases of polydactyly of the thumb and all were sporadic. The hereditary cases of thumb polydactyly were usually those associated with triphalangeal thumb, such as Manoiloff's case[15] and one of Woolf and Woolf's

cases.[34] Further descriptions of specific types of polydactyly will be discussed under subsequent headings.

Types of Polydactyly (Temtamy Classification)[29]

1. Postaxial (from the ulnar side)
   a. Type A: fully developed extra digits
   b. Type B: rudimentary extra digits or pedunculated postminimi
2. Preaxial (from the radial side)
   a. Thumb polydactyly
   b. Polydactyly of a triphalangeal thumb
   c. Polydactyly of an index finger
   d. Polysyndactyly
3. High degrees of duplication of parts of the upper limb

Postaxial Polydactyly

Temtamy[29] follows Sverdrup's[28] suggestion of classifying postaxial polydactyly into two groups, A and B, because of genetic differences. Type A individuals (with well-formed extra digits) (Fig. 10–4) produce children with either type A or B,

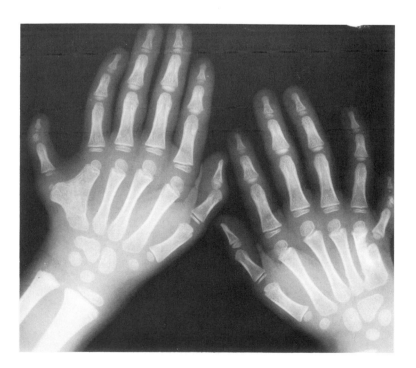

Figure 10–4. Postaxial polydactyly (type A). There is an attempt at duplication of the fifth metacarpal with a complete accessory phalanx bilaterally. The hamate on both sides appears enlarged.

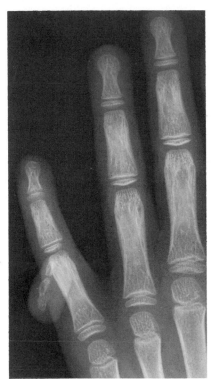

Figure 10-5. Postaxial polydactyly in a black female. A small, pedunculated accessory phalanx (type B) such as in this patient is a common anomaly, particularly in blacks.

while individuals with type B (small or pedunculated postminimi) (Figs. 10-5 and 10-6) produce children only with type B.

Often in association with type A there is some shortening of the associated metacarpal or phalanx.[28] In type B the rest of the hand is usually unremarkable. The fifth metacarpal may be duplicated in type A or the entire extra set of phalanges may arise from the fifth metacarpal. The carpals are often unaffected if the metacarpals are not duplicated. With duplication of the metacarpals, particularly in the syndromes, accessory carpals or carpal fusion may be present. It is generally type B, or postminimi, polydactyly which is common in blacks. In some individuals with polydactyly, the feet may be affected. In most cases, when polydactyly is preaxial in the hand it is also preaxial in the foot. However, there are exceptions to this rule. Goodman reported a case with preaxial polydactyly in the hand and postaxial polydactyly in the foot.[9] Generally, polydactyly in the feet does not occur with type B polydactyly, but if it does it is usually minimal.[26, 29] However, on occasion a complete polydactyly of the feet may occur in association with pedunculated postminimi.[28]

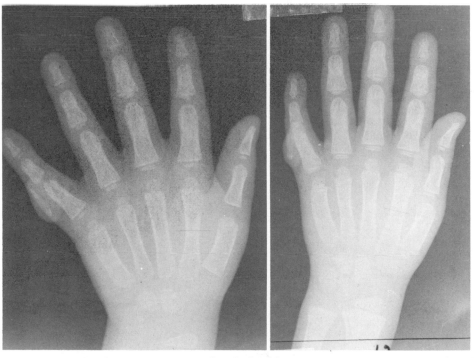

Figure 10-6. Two brothers with postaxial polydactyly, type B. (Courtesy Dr. Stanley Garn and 10 State Nutrition Survey.)

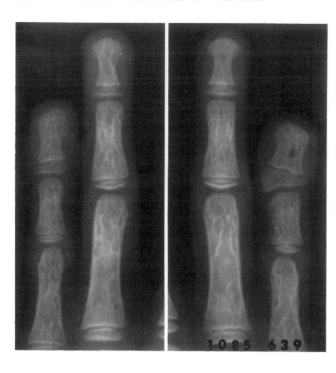

Figure 10-7. Incomplete postaxial polydactyly or megalodactyly involving the distal phalanges of the fifth fingers. This is a somewhat unusual appearance which in this patient was associated with sickle cell disease, as evidenced by the coarsened trabeculations.

Unusual forms of widening of the fingers may be considered a type of polydactyly (Fig. 10-7).

A number of malformation syndromes are seen in association with postaxial polydactyly. These are listed in Table 10-2. There are also a number of anomalies which may be seen in association with postaxial polydactyly that do not clearly fit into well-defined malformation syndromes. Polydactyly is commonly associated with some syndactyly. In this case it is probably genetically different from the usual form of polydactyly. The syndrome of gigantism and polydactyly alluded to in the *Bible* has not been recognized in present times, although Lucas[14] reported some tall individuals in a polydactylous family.

Preaxial Polydactyly

This is most likely a genetically heterogeneous group. It includes several conditions, which have been listed in the Temtamy classification.

TRUE THUMB POLYDACTYLY. In a white population this is the most common type of polydactyly. It is usually sporadic. It is variable in its manifestations (Figs. 10-8 to 10-11), ranging from a slight broadening of the thumb with a double

nail, to a split distal phalanx, to a double distal phalanx, to duplication of both phalanges, to two entirely separate thumbs, including metacarpals and phalanges, in its most severe form. Frequently one of the thumbs appears to be dominant while the other is hypoplastic, although on occasion both can be equal in size. As pre-

TABLE 10-2. Syndromes and Anomalies Associated with Postaxial Polydactyly

---

FREQUENTLY
    Biedmond II
    Chondroectodermal dysplasia (Ellis–van Creveld)
    Laurence-Moon-Biedl
    Meckel's[16]*
    Saldino dwarf
    Trisomy 13
    Ullrich-Feichtiger's[19]

OCCASIONALLY
    Asphyxiating thoracic dystrophy
    Goltz's focal dermal hypoplasia
    Mohr's[10]

OTHER ASSOCIATED ABNORMALITIES
    Hereditary hydrometrocolpos[8]
    Median cleft lip[29]
    Mental retardation[29]
    Neurocranial dysplasia[32]

---

*Superscripts indicate references on page 204.

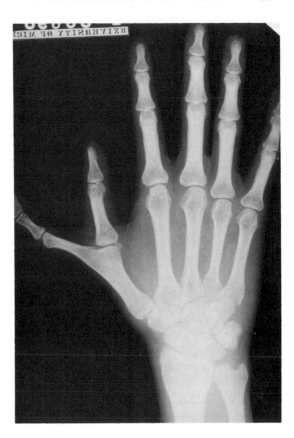

Figure 10–8. Preaxial polydactyly. Note the bizarre triphalangeal-like duplication with one phalanx fused with the first metacarpal.

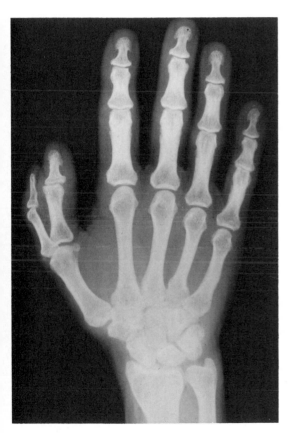

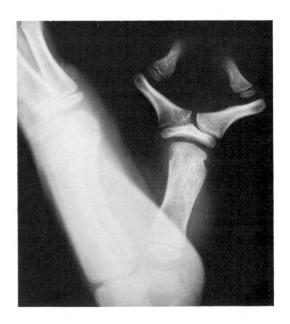

Figure 10–9. Duplication of the distal phalanges.

Figure 10–10. Delta-shaped epiphysis with duplication of two phalanges.

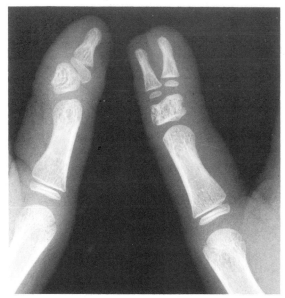

Figure 10-11. Duplication of distal phalanx of the thumb, associated with an extra ossicle. In essence this is a triphalangeal thumb. (Reproduced with permission. From Poznanski, A. K., et al.: *Radiology*, 100:115–129, 1971.)

viously mentioned, when associated with triphalangeal thumb, polydactyly of the thumb is probably a different entity, and familial cases have been reported.[29]

True thumb polydactyly is most usually unilateral. In Handforth's series[11] it was unilateral in 11 of 13 cases. Barsky[1] reported unilateral involvement in 24 of 25 cases.

Thumb polydactyly may also be seen in a number of syndromes, including particularly Fanconi's anemia and some of the acrocephalosyndactyly syndromes, as well as in association with other anomalies that do not fit well into a definite malformation syndrome (Table 10–3).

POLYDACTYLY OF TRIPHALANGEAL THUMB. Triphalangeal thumb has been described earlier in this chapter and may be seen in association with duplication.

POLYDACTYLY OF INDEX FINGER. This is a very uncommon form of polydactyly. It represented only 3.4 per cent of patients with polydactyly seen by Wood.[33] In his cases the polydactyly was associated with some syndactyly. Burman[6] found several such cases in the literature, including one in association with radioulnar synostosis. Temtamy[29] considers Manoiloff's[15] case to be an example of index finger polydactyly because, at least in the foot, there is duplication of the second digit. However, six

triphalangeal digits were seen in the hands and the two most radial ones acted together as a thumb. Thus, this may represent a different condition. An interesting facet about Manoiloff's case is that it may have been transmitted for at least 700 years.

POLYSYNDACTYLY. Temtamy[29] defines this as an autosomal dominant condition with associated preaxial polydactyly and syndactyly (Fig. 10–12). She classifies it as a form of polydactyly, because syndactyly does not occur in the absence of polydactyly in these families. In contradistinction, in synpolydactyly, polydactyly which affects the third and fourth fingers does not occur in the absence of syndactyly. Polysyndactyly has been seen in association with other abnormalities, particularly some of the craniofacial abnormalities. These include Carpenter's syndrome, Noack's syndrome and an additional syndrome recently reported by Hootnick and Holmes.[12]

Duplication of the Entire Hand

This is an extremely rare malformation. Paré described some cases of this type, and Burman[5] reviewed some of the ancient historical cases which were believed to have this anomaly. The most common situation is partial duplication of the ulna with an extra number of fingers. In this type of ulnar dimelia there is a mirror image of the hands with duplication of the ulnar por-

TABLE 10–3. Syndromes and Anomalies Associated with Preaxial Polydactyly

FREQUENTLY
    Acrocephalosyndactyly
      Noack's
      Carpenter's
    Acro-pectoro-vertebral dysplasia
    Blackfan-Diamond anemia
    Brachydactyly B

OCCASIONALLY
    Bloom's
    Cardiomelic (Holt-Oram) syndrome
    Mohr's
    Pancytopenia dysmelia (Fanconi's)

OTHER ASSOCIATED ANOMALIES
    Absent tibia[21]°
    Imperforate anus and vertebral anomalies[22, 23]

°Superscripts indicate references on page 204.

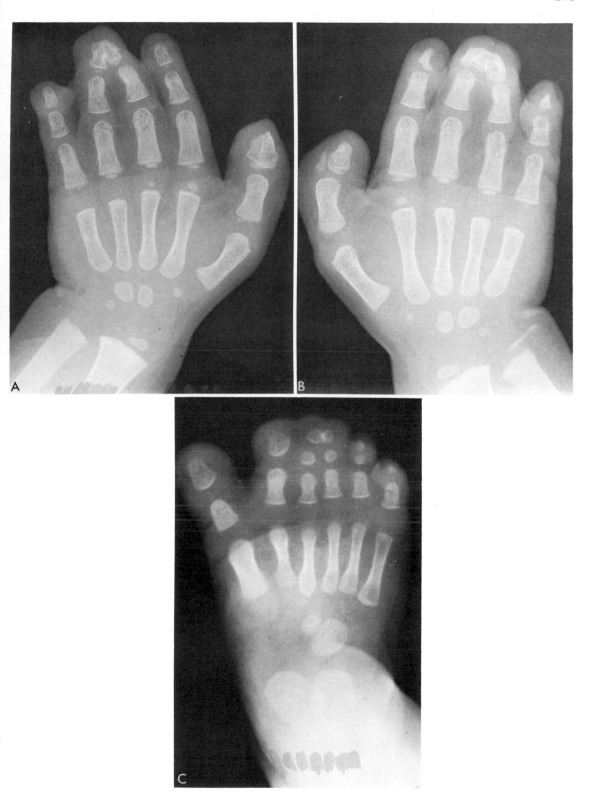

Figure 10–12. Familial polysyndactyly. *A* and *B*, There is typical right preaxial polydactyly associated with syndactyly. In *A* the distal phalanx of the thumb appears broad. *C*, The polydactyly is more evident in the foot.

Several individuals in this family were affected.

tion of the hands; duplication may include any number of fingers, and the most extreme cases have two separate hands. There is a corresponding duplication of the associated carpals. In some cases of ulnar dimelia there may be associated syndactyly.

REFERENCES

1. Barsky, A. J.: *Congenital Anomalies of the Hand and Their Surgical Treatment.* Charles C Thomas, Publisher, Springfield, 1958.
2. Baumann, L., and Landauer, W.: Polydactyly and Anterior or Horn Cells in Fowl. *J. Comp. Neurol.*, 79:153–163, 1943.
3. Boinet, E.: Polydactylie et Atavisme. *Rev. de Med.*, 19:316–328, 1898.
4. Bunge, R. G., and Bradbury, J. T.: Two Unilaterally Cryptorchid Boys with Spermatogenic Precocity in the Descended Testis, Hypertelorism and Polydactyly. *J. Clin. Endocrinol.*, 19:1103–1109, 1959.
5. Burman, M.: An Historical Perspective of Double Hands and Double Feet. The Survey of the Cases Reported in the 16th and 17th Centuries. *Bull. Hosp. Joint Dis.*, 29:241–254, 1968.
6. Burman, M.: Note on Duplication of the Index Finger. *J. Bone Joint Surg.*, 54A:884, 1972.
7. de Linares, L. G.: Collective Polydactylism in a Small Town. *J.A.M.A.*, 94:2080–2081, 1930.
8. Dungy, C. I., Aptekar, R. G., and Cann, H. M.: Hereditary Hydrometrocolpos with Polydactyly in Infancy. *Pediatrics*, 47:138–141, 1971.
9. Goodman, R. M.: A Family with Polysyndactyly and Other Anomalies. *J. Hered.*, 56:37–38, 1965.
10. Gustavson, K.-H., Kreuger, A., and Petersson, P. O.: Syndrome Characterized by Lingual Malformation, Polydactyly, Tachypnea, and Psychomotor Retardation (Mohr syndrome). *Clin. Genet.*, 2:261–266, 1971.
11. Handforth, J. F.: Polydactylism of the Hand in Southern Chinese. *Anat. Rec.*, 106:119–125, 1950.
12. Hootnick, D., and Holmes, L. B.: Familial Polysyndactyly and Craniofacial Anomalies. *Clin. Genet.*, 3:128–134, 1972.
13. Le Marec, B., and Coutel, Y.: La Polydactylie. Maladie ou Symptome? *Pediatrie*, 25:735–746, 1970.
14. Lucas, R. C.: On a Remarkable Instance of Hereditary Tendency to the Production of Supernumerary Digits. *Guy's Hosp. Rep.*, 25:417–419, 1881.
15. Manoiloff, E. O.: A Rare Case of Hereditary Hexadactylism. *Am. J. Phys. Anthropol.*, 15:503–508, 1931.
16. Mecke, S., and Passarge, E.: Encephalocele, Polycystic Kidneys, and Polydactyly as an Autosomal Recessive Trait Simulating Certain Other Disorders: The Meckel Syndrome. *Ann. Genet.*, 14:97–103, 1971.
17. Mellin, G. W.: The Frequency of Birth Defects. In Fishbein, M.: *Birth Defects.* J. B. Lippincott Co., Philadelphia, 1963, Chapter 1.
18. Nishimura, H., Takano, K., Tanimura, T., Yasuda, M., and Uchida, T.: High Incidence of Several Malformations in the Early Human Embryos as Compared with Infants. *Biol. Neonate,* 10:93–107, 1966.
19. Pfeiffer, R. A.: Associated Deformities of the Head and Hands. *Birth Defects, Original Article Series,* Part III, 5:18–34, 1969.
20. Pintilie, D., Hatmanu, D., Olaru, I., and Panoza, G.: Double Ulna with Symmetrical Polydactyly. Case Report. *J. Bone Joint Surg.,* 46B:89–93, 1964.
21. Reber, M.: Un Syndrome Osseux Peu Commun Associant Une Heptadactylie et Une Aplasie des Tibias. *J. Genet. Hum.*, 16:15–39, 1967–1968.
22. Say, B., Balci, S., Pirnar, T., and Tuncbilek, E.: A New Syndrome of Dysmorphogenesis: Imperforate-Anus Associated with Polyoligodactyly and Skeletal (Mainly Vertebral) Anomalies. *Acta Paediat. Scand.*, 60:197–202, 1971.
23. Say, B., and Gerald, P. S.: A New Polydactyly/Imperforate-Anus/Vertebral-Anomalies Syndrome? *Lancet*, 2:688, 1968.
24. Sergeant, P. W.: *The Life of Anne Boleyn.* D. Appleton & Co., New York, 1924.
25. Simopoulos, A. P., Brennan, G. G., Alwan, A., and Fidis, N.: Polycystic Kidneys, Internal Hydrocephalus and Polydactylism in Newborn Siblings. *Pediatrics*, 39:931–934, 1967.
26. Simpkiss, M., and Lowe, A.: Congenital Abnormalities in the African Newborn. *Arch. Dis. Child.*, 36:404–406, 1961.
27. Stevenson, A. C., Johnston, H. A., Stewart, M. I. P., and Golding, D. R.: Congenital Malformations. A Report of a Study of Series of Consecutive Births in 24 Centres. Supplement to Vol. 34, *Bull. WHO,* Geneva, 1966.
28. Sverdrup, A.: Postaxial Polydactylism in Six Generations of a Norwegian Family. *J. Genet.*, 12:217–240, 1922.
29. Temtamy, S. A.: Genetic Factors in Hand Malformations. Thesis. Johns Hopkins University, Baltimore, Maryland, 1966.
30. Townes, P. L., and Brocks, E. R.: Hereditary Syndrome of Imperforate Anus with Hand, Foot, and Ear Anomalies. *J. Pediat.*, 81:321–326, 1972.
31. Tsang, Y.: Ventral Horn Cells and Polydactyly in Mice. *J. Comp. Neurol.*, 70:1–8, 1939.
32. Walbaum, R., Dehaene, P., and Duthoit, F.: Polydactylie Familiale Avec Dysplasie Neuro-Cranienne. *Ann. Genet.*, 10:39–41, 1967.
33. Wood, V. E.: Duplication of the Index Finger. *J. Bone Joint Surg.*, 52A:569–573, 1970.
34. Woolf, C. M., and Woolf, R. M.: A Genetic Study of Polydactyly in Utah. *Am. J. Hum. Genet.*, 22:75–88, 1970.

SYNDACTYLY

This is defined by Warkany[5] as lack of differentiation between two or more digits. According to Warkany, syndactyly is not really a fusion, but it can be traced back to an early stage of development of mesenchymal tissue which has not properly differentiated. Syndactyly is a relatively common abnormality with an incidence between 1 in 2000 and 1 in 3000 births.[4] Syndactyly can involve only the soft tissues (Fig. 10–13) or it may involve the bones as well. Temtamy considers both these types as different degrees of the same malformation. Syndactyly is considered partial when it involves the proximal segments of the digits, and complete when it extends to the tips of the digits.

Syndactyly has been recognized for many centuries and, like many of the other malformations, comments were contained in the works of Paré.[4] Syndactyly is normally present in a number of animals, particularly marsupials, rodents and some primates.

Many classifications of syndactyly have been devised by various authors. These are reviewed by Temtamy.[4] None of the classifications is really ideal, but perhaps Temtamy's own classification has some value. The classes she describes are as follows:

TYPE I. Zygodactyly, in which there is syndactyly between the third and fourth fingers and the second and third toes (Figs. 10–14 and 10–15).

TYPE II. Synpolydactyly (Fig. 10–16). This is a syndactyly of the third and fourth

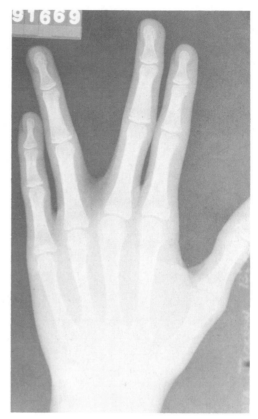

Figure 10–13. Cutaneous syndactyly. Only a web of skin is seen between the two digits. This is more a clinical than a radiologic diagnosis.

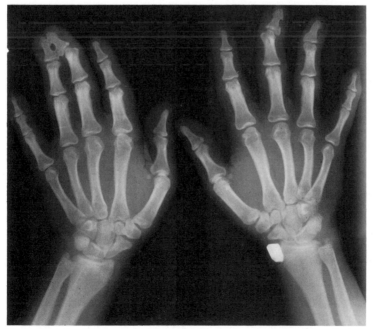

Figure 10–14. Zygodactyly. There was syndactyly of the third and fourth digits bilaterally, with osseous fusion distally. The right hand has been surgically corrected. This is a common form of syndactyly.

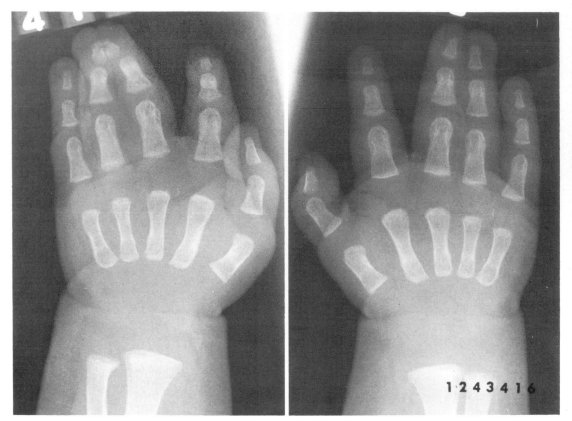

Figure 10–15. Familial zygodactyly. Bilateral fusion of the distal phalanges is evident. Several members of this family were affected.

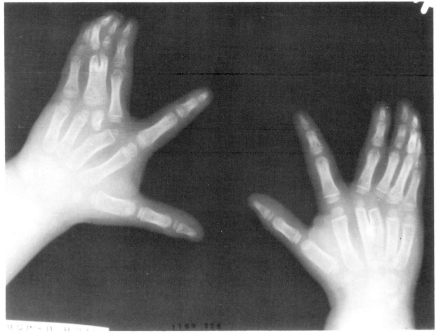

Figure 10–16. Synpolydactyly (type II syndactyly). There is syndactyly with an accessory digit in the region of the web.

fingers associated with partial duplication of the third or fourth finger in the web. A similar finding may be present in the foot.

TYPE III. Ring and little finger syndactyly. This is associated with a short fifth middle phalanx.

TYPE IV. Complete syndactyly of all the fingers.

TYPE V. Syndactyly associated with metacarpal and metatarsal synostosis (Fig. 10–17).[3, 4]

Fenestrated syndactyly is an additional type. It is associated with ring constrictions and has been described in the previous chapter (p. 190).

Most forms of syndactyly are inherited as an autosomal dominant, but sporadic cases are also seen. A significant sex difference is noted in most series. It appears that it is almost twice as frequent in males as in females.[4]

Syndactyly has been associated with a large number of miscellaneous anomalies, as well as with certain well-defined syndromes. Poland's syndrome, in which there

is syndactyly and absence of pectoral muscles, is an example of the latter (see Chapter 12). A number of other syndromes have also been associated with syndactyly, and these are listed in Table 10–4.

TABLE 10–4. Syndromes Associated with Hand Syndactyly

Aarskog°
Acrocephalosyndactyly—other°
Acro-pectoro-vertebral°
Aglossia-adactyly†
Ankyloglossia superior†
Apert's°
Bloom's‡
Brachydactyly B°
Carpenter's°
Conradi's‡
Cryptophthalmos‡
Cornelia de Lange‡
Fanconi's anemia‡
Goltz's focal dermal hypoplasia‡
Incontinentia pigmenti†
Laurence-Moon-Biedl‡
Lenz's microphthalmia‡
Möbius's†
Oculo-dento-digital°
Oro-facial-digital†
Pierre Robin†
Poland's°
Popliteal pterygium†
Rothmund-Thomson's†
Smith-Lemli-Opitz†
Thrombocytopenia–absent radius‡
Trisomy 13‡
Trisomy 18‡

°Common
†Incidence not known.
‡Occasional.

REFERENCES

1. Bell, J.: On Syndactyly and its Association with Polydactyly. In Penrose, L. S. (Ed.): The Treasury of Human Inheritance. Cambridge University Press, England, 1953, Vol. 5, Part II, pp. 33–43.
2. Cross, H. E., Lerberg, D. B., and McKusick, V. A.: Type II Syndactyly. Am. J. Hum. Genet., 20: 368–380, 1968.
3. Holmes, L. B., Wolf, E., and Miettinen, O. S.: Metacarpal 4-5 Fusion with X-Linked Recessive Inheritance. Am. J. Hum. Genet., 24: 562–568, 1972.
4. Temtamy, S. A.: Genetic Factors in Hand Malformations. Thesis. Johns Hopkins University, Baltimore, Maryland, 1966.
5. Warkany, J.: Congenital Malformations. Notes and Comments. Year Book Medical Publishers, Chicago, 1971.

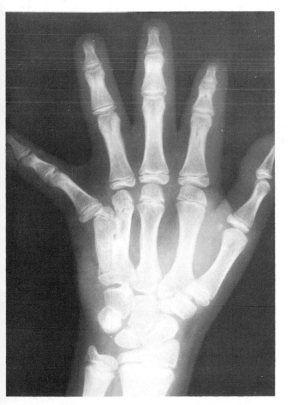

Figure 10–17. Type V syndactyly. There is fusion of the metacarpals.

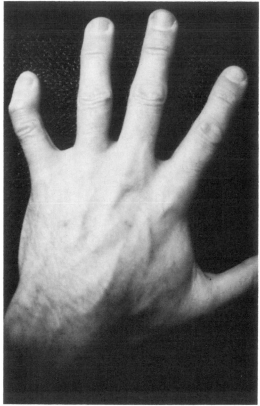

Figure 10–18. Clinical photograph of a patient with clinodactyly. He is an otherwise normal adult male.

CURVATURES OF THE FINGERS (CLINODACTYLY, CAMPTODACTYLY, KIRNER'S DEFORMITY)

Curvatures of the fingers are fairly common. Three main types are seen. Clinodactyly[5, 10, 13] refers to curvature of finger in a mediolateral plane (Figs. 10–18 to 10–20). This may be radial or ulnar in direction and may involve any finger, but it usually refers to radial deviation of the fifth finger at the distal interphalangeal joint. In this case it is usually associated with a short middle phalanx which is shorter on its radial than on its ulnar side (brachydactyly A-3).

Camptodactyly[4, 7, 8, 12, 15, 19] denotes a permanent flexion of one or more of the fingers (Figs. 10–21 to 10–23). This deformity is located usually at the proximal interphalangeal joint and also involves the fifth finger. The condition is probably related to a fascial abnormality and may be due to contracture of the flexor digitorum sublimis. Some authors use the term streblomicrodactyly to mean camptodactyly of the fifth finger.

Kirner's deformity (Fig. 10–24),[2, 11, 17, 18] also called dystelephalangy, is a palmar bending involving the shaft of the terminal phalanx at the epiphysis and often associated with some epiphyseal separation. It is usually bilateral.

There are other crooked-finger conditions, the best known of which perhaps is Dupuytren's contracture. Contracture of the thumb may also occur as a so-called congenital clasped thumb.[3] Crooked fingers may also be associated with a number of brachydactyly syndromes, aplasias, hypoplasias, cleft hands and so forth, which are discussed in Chapter 9.

Radiologic diagnosis of curvature of the fingers should be made with caution, since radiographic semblance of curvature can occur by faulty radiographic technique

(Text continued on page 212.)

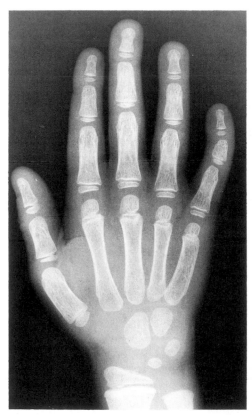

Figure 10–19. Clinodactyly associated with brachymesophalangy-5, but without a cone epiphysis.

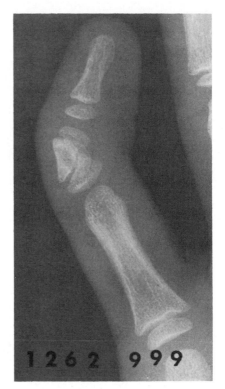

Figure 10–20. Severe clinodactyly with bizarre pseudo-epiphysis and cone and marked shortening of the middle phalanx. This boy was seen with recurrent dislocations but no other abnormality.

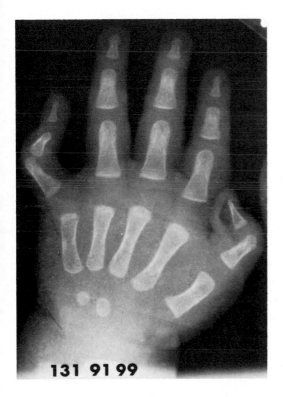

Figure 10–21. Typical camptodactyly. There is flexion of the proximal interphalangeal joint of the fifth finger. A rigid contraction was present in this case.

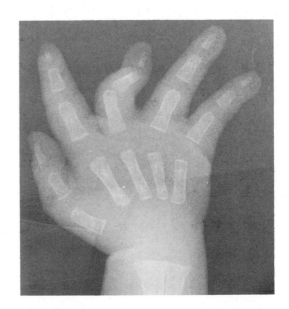

Figure 10–22. Camptodactyly of the middle finger. Permanent contracture was present. There was also a bone-in-bone appearance. This child had a chronic illness since birth.

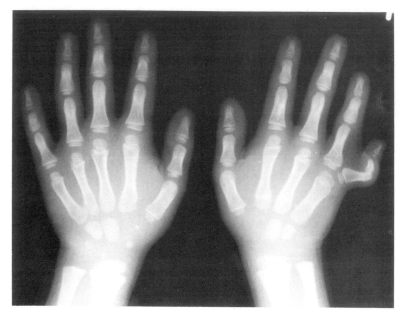

Figure 10–23. Ulnar hypoplasia associated with camptodactyly. There is absence of the fifth metacarpal, and the fifth finger has a permanent contracture.

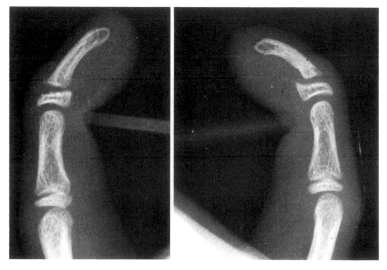

Figure 10–24. Kirner's deformity. There is bilateral deformity with palmar bending of the distal phalanx at the site of the epiphysis. (Reproduced with permission. Poznanski, A. K., et al.: *Radiology*, 93:573–582, 1969.)

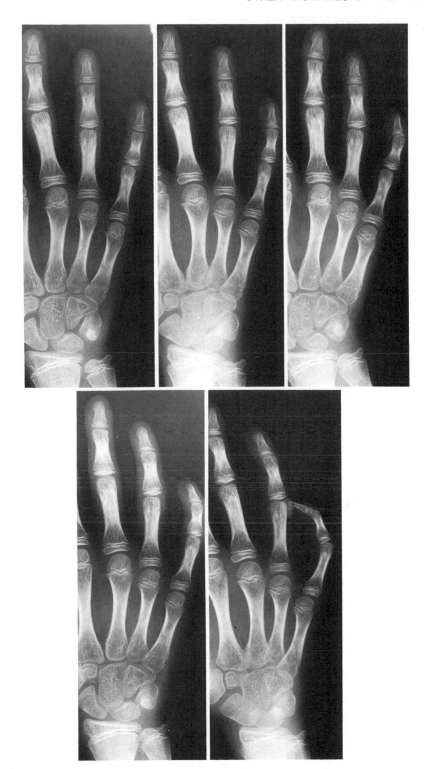

Figure 10–25. Factitious clinodactyly. The normal hand is positioned in different ways to simulate clinodactyly. Clinodactyly can be ruled out because of overlapping of the bones and bending of the adjacent digits, which indicate that this seeming abnormality is due to curvature rather than to deformity. Also, on bright light examination the soft tissues showed evidence of skin folds.

(Fig. 10–25). Camptodactyly particularly may be difficult to differentiate from simple flexion. Clinodactyly, however, can be differentiated from factitious deviation, since the presence of skin folds and the angulation of adjacent digits provide clues that the finger is simply deviated on the film (Fig. 10–25).

Isolated Clinodactyly

Most persons with clinodactyly are otherwise normal and the finding is an incidental feature. Most of the cases are associated with Bell's brachydactyly A-3 (short middle phalanx of the fifth finger). The incidence in different series is variable because of problems in definition. Some have suggested that an angle of 15° be used as a criterion. In a white population the incidence lies somewhere between 1.0 and 0.1 per cent. Like brachydactyly of the middle phalanges, clinodactyly is more common in nonwhites. Although cases of clinodactyly can be sporadic, many pedigrees of autosomal dominant inheritance have been reported.[5, 10, 13] Expressivity may be variable.

Isolated Camptodactyly

Many pedigrees of this trait have also been studied.[12] It is transmitted as an autosomal dominant with variable penetrance. In most cases this is not a radiologic diagnosis since it is necessary to determine that a rigid contracture is present and that it is not due simply to positioning. The incidence of this deformity is probably less than 1.0 per cent of the population. There is some relationship between camptodactyly and clinodactyly as illustrated by the fact that several members of a large family with camptodactyly described by Ashley[1] developed clinodactyly.

Isolated Kirner's Deformity

This abnormality may be sporadic or may be transmitted as an autosomal dominant. It is characterized by deflection of the distal phalanx at the epiphysis in a volar direction and is probably an epiphyseal abnormality, but the etiology is not clear in spite of some of the pathological studies by Kaufmann and Taillard.[11] Sugiura et al.[17] found this anomaly in 0.15 per cent of 6295 Japanese school children. Sugiura and Nakazawa[16] have also seen hereditary Kirner's deformity involving all of the fingers.

Syndromes Associated with Crooked Fingers

Curvatures of the fingers have been seen in a wide variety of syndromes. The most classic picture of clinodactyly occurs in Down's syndrome, where it has been recognized for many years, although it certainly does not occur in all Down's syndrome children. Only a partial specificity exists for the type of crooked fingers that may occur in certain syndromes. Some conditions, such as oculo-dento-digital syndrome, may be associated with either clinodactyly or camptodactyly, while others, such as Down's syndrome, usually have only clinodactyly. Silver's syndrome and the Cornelia de Lange syndrome are usually associated with clinodactyly but occasionally may show Kirner's deformity. Crooked fingers are also seen in many less well-defined syndromes, such as campto-brachydactyly,[6] which includes many other anomalies including biseptate vagina, syndactyly and polydactyly. Camptodactyly has also been noted in a syndrome consisting of inability to open the mouth fully[9] and in patients with radioulnar synostosis.[12] The presence of crooked fingers, although nonspecific, can thus be useful in diagnosis, particularly when considered in combination with other radiologic findings. (See Table 10–5.)

Crooked fingers may be seen in acquired disease as well as in congenital disease, particularly as the result of trauma (Figs. 10–26 and 10–27). Any process which affects the epiphysis will produce uneven growth and cause deviation of the fingers. Crooked fingers may also be seen in burns (Fig. 10–28) in association with exostoses. In addition, crooked fingers may be due to contractures from various causes, including various neurologic problems (Fig. 10–29).

(*Text continued on page 216.*)

TABLE 10–5. Crooked Fingers and Malformation Syndromes

	CLINODAC-TYLY 5	OTHER CLINO-DACTYLIES	CAMPTO-DACTYLY	KIRNER'S DEFORMITY	OTHER CURVATURES
HAND AND FOOT SYNDROMES					
Brachydactyly A-1	+	●			●
Brachydactyly A-2		●			
Brachydactyly A-3	●				
Brachydactyly B					●
Brachydactyly C	+	●			
Dupuytren's contracture					●
Symphalangism	+				
Chromosomal Disorders					
Trisomy 13			●		+
Trisomy 18	+	+			+
Trisomy 21	●				
XXXXY	●				
XXXXX	+				
Other Chromosomal	+		+		+
Craniofacial Syndromes					
Ankyloglossia superior	+	+	+		+
Oculo-dento-digital	●		●		
Oro-facio-digital	●		●		
Oto-palato-digital	●				
Treacher Collins	+				
Other Congenital Malformations					
Aarskog syndrome	●		●		●
Arthrogryposis	●				●
Bloom's syndrome	●				
Cardiomelic (Holt Oram) syndrome	●		+		
Cerebro-hepato-renal	+		●		
Cornelia de Lange syndrome	+			+	
Goltz's focal dermal hypoplasia syndrome	+		+		+
Lenz's microphthalmia syndrome	+				+
Leri's pleonosteosis	+				●
Marfan's syndrome	+		+		
Mucopolysaccharidosis	+				+
Myositis ossificans progressiva	+				
Myotonic dystrophy	+				+
Noonan's syndrome	●				
Osteo-onycho-dysplasia	+		+		
Pancytopenia dysmelia (Fanconi's)	+				
Poland's syndrome	+		+		
Popliteal pterygium syndrome	+		+		
Progeria					+
Seckel's syndrome	●				
Silver's syndrome	●			+	
Thrombocytopenia–absent radius syndrome	●				
Tricho-rhino-phalangeal syndrome	+	+	+		
Whistling face					●

● Common.
+ Occasional.

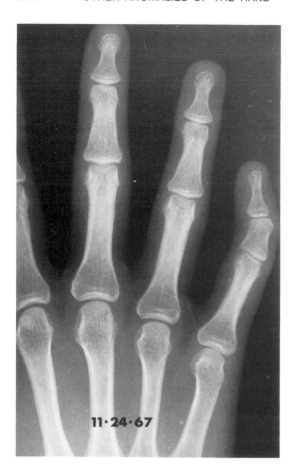

Figure 10–26. Traumatic clinodactyly. The patient had an injury in childhood resulting in this unilateral clinodactyly, which is indistinguishable from the congenital type.

Figure 10–27. Traumatic clinodactyly with fusion. This patient was injured previously on a grinder with resultant fusion across the proximal interphalangeal joint and clinodactyly. This is also in essence an acquired symphalangism.

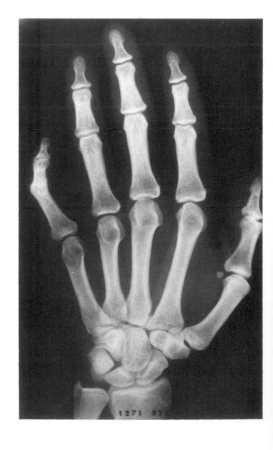

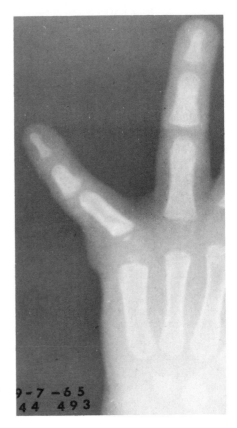

Figure 10-28. Damage to epiphysis from burn, with associated deviation of the fifth finger.

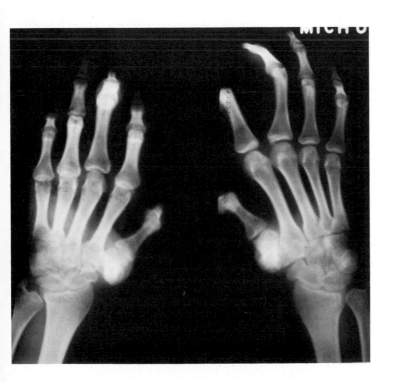

Figure 10-29. Contractures of the fingers associated with cervical meningocele.

REFERENCES

1. Ashley, L. M.: Inheritance of Streblomicrodactyly. *J. Hered.*, 38:93–96, 1947.
2. Blank, E., and Girdany, B. R.: Symmetric Bowing of the Terminal Phalanges of the Fifth Fingers in a Family (Kirner's Deformity). *Am. J. Roentgenol.*, 93:367–373, 1965.
3. Christian, J. C., Andrews, P. A., Conneally, P. M., and Muller, J.: The Adducted Thumbs Syndrome. An Autosomal Recessive Disease with Arthrogryposis, Dysmyelination, Craniostenosis, and Cleft Palate. *Clin. Genet.*, 2:95–103, 1971.
4. Currarino, G., and Waldman, I.: Camptodactyly. *Am. J. Roentgenol.*, 92:1312–1321, 1964.
5. Dutta, P.: The Inheritance of the Radially Curved Little Finger. *Acta Genet.*, 15:70–76, 1965.
6. Edwards, J. A., and Gale, R. P.: Camptobrachydactyly: A New Autosomal Dominant Trait with Two Probable Homozygotes. *Am. J. Hum. Genet.*, 24:464–474, 1972.
7. Goodman, R. M., Katznelson, M. B. M., and Manor, E.: Camptodactyly: Occurrence in Two New Genetic Syndromes and its Relationship to Other Syndromes. *J. Med. Genet.*, 9:203–212, 1972.
8. Gordon, H., Davies, D., and Berman, M.: Camptodactyly, Cleft Palate, and Club Foot: A Syndrome Showing the Autosomal-Dominant Pattern of Inheritance. *J. Med. Genet.*, 6:266–274, 1969.
9. Hecht, F., and Beals, R. K.: Inability to Open the Mouth Fully: An Autosomal Dominant Phenotype with Facultative Campylodactyly and Short Stature. Preliminary Note. *Birth Defects, Original Article Series*, Part III, 5:96–98, 1969.
10. Hersh, A. H., Dearinis, F., and Stecher, R. M.: On the Inheritance and Development of Clinodactyly. *Am. J. Hum. Genet.*, 5:257–268, 1953.
11. Kaufmann, H. J., and Taillard, W. F.: Bilateral Incurving of Terminal Phalanges of Fifth Fingers. *Am. J. Roentgenol.*, 86:490–495, 1961.
12. Littman, A., Yates, J. W., and Treger, A.: Camptodactyly. A Kindred Study. *J.A.M.A.*, 206:1565–1567, 1968.
13. Poznanski, A. K., Pratt, G. B., Manson, G., and Weiss, L.: Clinodactyly, Camptodactyly, Kirner's Deformity and Other Crooked Fingers. *Radiology*, 93:573–582, 1969.
14. Roche, A. F.: Clinodactyly and Brachymesophalangia of the Fifth Finger. *Acta Paediat.*, 50:387–391, 1961.
15. Smith, R. J., and Kaplan, E. B.: Camptodactyly and Similar Atraumatic Flexion Deformities of the Proximal Interphalangeal Joints of the Fingers. *J. Bone Joint Surg.*, 50A:1187–1204, 1968.
16. Sugiura, Y., and Nakazawa, O.: *Bone Age. Roentgen Diagnosis of Skeletal Development.* Chugai-Igaku Company, Tokyo, 1968.
17. Sugiura, Y., Ueda, T., Umezawa, K., Tajima, Y., and Sugiura, I.: Dystelephalangy of the Fifth Finger. Dystrophy of the Fifth Finger. *J. Jap. Orthop. Assoc.*, 34:1573–1579, 1961.
18. Taybi, H.: Bilateral Incurving of the Terminal Phalanges of the Fifth Fingers (Osteochondrosis?). *J. Pediat.*, 62:431–432, 1963.
19. Welch, J. P., and Temtamy, S. A.: Hereditary Contractures of the Fingers (Camptodactyly). *J. Med. Genet.*, 3:104–113, 1966.

SYMPHALANGISM

This is a condition in which there is fusion of one phalanx to another within the same digit (Figs. 10–30 to 10–32). This abnormality can exist as a simple isolated condition with changes only in the hands or feet, or it may be related to other congenital malformations. There has been some historical interest in symphalangism, in that it possibly existed in John Talbot, the first Earl of Shrewsbury, and was transmitted to present times. This has not been entirely substantiated.[2] Symphalangism is

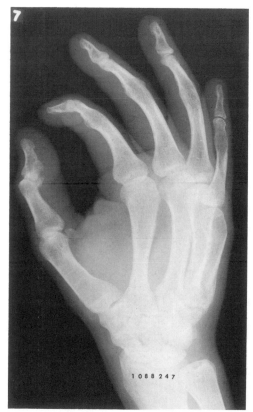

Figure 10–30. Familial symphalangism. Note the fusion of the proximal interphalangeal joints of the four fingers. There is also fusion of the scaphoid and trapezium.

There are some associated changes in the metacarpals, with shortening and flattening of the distal head of the first metacarpal in 6 of 25 cases. Carpal and tarsal fusions are common in this condition and there may be some deformities of the carpals as well. There are a number of other anomalies associated with symphalangism. Strasburger et al.[5] describe some cases of conductive deafness due to fusion of the stapes to the round window. A number of other minor anomalies have been reported[5] and include a short middle phalanx of the fifth finger, a short fifth metacarpal, absence of the first metacarpal, clubfoot, absent distal and middle phalanges in the fingers, fused humerus and ulna, a short first metacarpal, cutaneous syndactyly, Tower's skull, absent styloid process of the ulna and absent distal phalanges in the middle and ring finger with loss of nail. Wildervanck et al.[7] also reported symphalangism in association with accessory ossicles in the foot.

A number of syndromes have been seen in association with symphalangism. These include diastrophic dwarfism, Bell's brachydactyly types A and C, popliteal pterygium

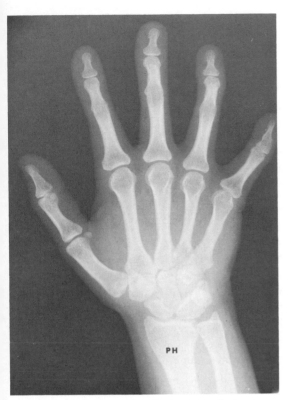

Figure 10-31. Familial symphalangism. Note again the interphalangeal fusions involving the proximal interphalangeal joints of the second to fourth fingers and the distal interphalangeal joint of the fifth finger.

usually inherited as a mendelian dominant trait.

The skin overlying the affected joint is smooth since no flexion occurs, and by this sign it can be clinically detected at birth. Radiologically, symphalangism is not evident at birth since the affected portion is not yet ossified. However, in children there is often hypoplasia of the joint with an abnormal epiphysis of the middle phalanx.[5] Most commonly, the proximal interphalangeal joint of the fingers and the distal interphalangeal joint of the toes are affected. Occasionally the distal interphalangeal joint of the fingers may be involved.[1] Strasburger et al.[5] reported some cases that involved the distal interphalangeal joint in the little finger, and in these cases there was proximal interphalangeal fusion as well. The incidence of involvement of various digits decreases from the fifth to the second digit. The thumb is usually not affected.[4]

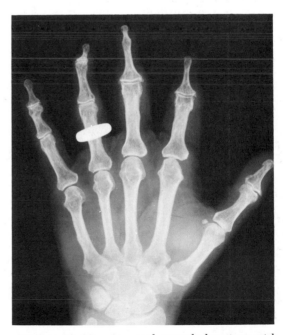

Figure 10-32. Atypical symphalangism with some hypoplasia of the distal phalanges. This may represent an example of type B brachydactyly. (Courtesy Dr. Stanley Garn, 10 State Nutrition Survey.)

syndrome and some of the acrocephalo-syndactyly syndromes.

REFERENCES

1. Daniel, G. H.: A Case of Hereditary Anarthrosis of the Index Finger, with Associated Abnormalities in the Proportions of the Fingers. *Ann. Eugen.*, 7:281–296, 1936.
2. Elkington, S. G., and Huntsman, R. G.: The Talbot Fingers: A Study in Symphalangism. *Br. Med. J.*, 1:407–411, 1967.
3. Geelhoed, G., Neel, J. V., and Davidson, R. T.: Symphalangism and Tarsal Coalitions: A Hereditary Syndrome. A Report on Two Families. *J. Bone Joint Surg.*, 51B:278–298, 1969.
4. Harle, T. S., and Stevenson, J. R.: Hereditary Symphalangism Associated with Carpal and Tarsal Fusions. *Radiology*, 89:91–94, 1967.
5. Strasburger, A. K., Hawkins, M. R., Eldridge, R., Hargrave, R. L., and McKusick, V. A.: Symphalangism: Genetic and Clinical Aspects. *Johns Hopkins Med. J.*, 117:108–127, 1965.

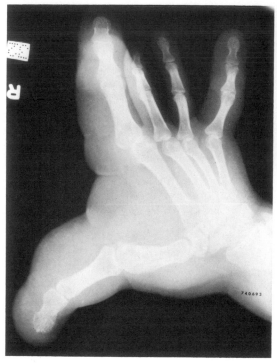

Figure 10–34. Macrodactyly involving mainly the thumb and index finger. This is a less common manifestation of localized gigantism. (Reproduced with permission. Poznanski, A. K., et al.: *Radiology*, 100:115–129, 1971.)

6. Walker, G.: Remarkable Cases of Hereditary Anchyloses, or Absence of Various Phalangeal Joints, with Defects of the Little and Ring Fingers. *Johns Hopkins Med. J.*, 12:129–133, 1901.
7. Wildervanck, L. S., Goedhard, G., and Meijer, S.: Proximal Symphalangism of Fingers Associated with Fusion of Os Naviculare and Talus and Occurrence of Two Accessory Bones in the Feet (Os Paranaviculare and Os Tibiale Externum) in an European-Indonesian-Chinese Family. *Acta Genet.*, 17:166–177, 1967.

MACRODACTYLY (MEGALODACTYLY)

Barsky[1] defined megalodactyly as a congenital malformation characterized by an increase in size of all of the elements of structures of a digit or digits (Figs. 10–33 to 10–35). There is enlargement of the phalanges, tendons, nerves, vessels, subcutaneous fat, fingernails and skin, but the metacarpals are usually not affected. Involvement may be unilateral or bilateral, and it may or may not be symmetrical. The fifth finger is very rarely involved. Barsky

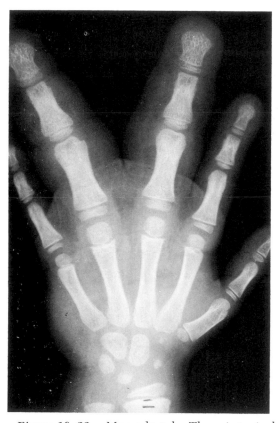

Figure 10–33. Macrodactyly. There is typical enlargement involving the distal portions of the finger. Both the bone and the soft tissues are enlarged. The metacarpals are only minimally involved.

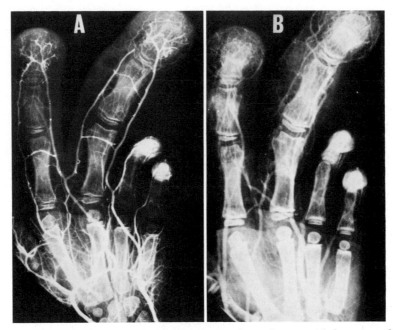

Figure 10–35. Macrodactyly. Angiogram. Large vessels at the site of the macrodactyly are seen. (Courtesy Dr. Peter Cockshott, McMaster University, Canada.)

was able to find only three cases in spite of 64 reported in the literature.

Barsky[1] classifies megalodactyly into two forms: (1) enlargement which is present at birth and in which the proportions do not change; (2) disproportionate growth type, in which the involved digits increase in size at a faster rate than can be attributed to normal growth alone. There is also overgrowth of the fatty tissues in the palm and dorsum of the hand and in the forearm.

The cause of the malformation is not clear. Barsky feels that somehow during fetal development some disturbance of the growth-limiting factors occurs in the local area affected, and because of this lack of inhibition the part continues to increase in size. Enlargement of the digits may also be secondary to other entities. It is seen in the Klippel-Trenaunay-Weber syndrome, where it may be associated with hemangiomas and arteriovenous malformations. It may be seen in association with lymphangioma (Fig. 10–36). Local gigantism of an extremity can also be seen in association with neurofibromatosis. Miscellaneous other abnormalities may be associated with it. Inglis[2] reported the association of osteochondromas with macrodactyly.

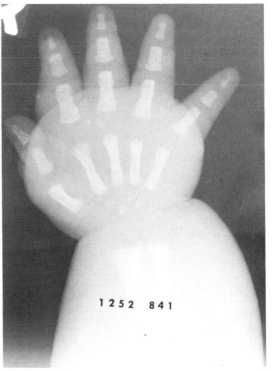

Figure 10–36. Congenital lymphedema. There is soft tissue swelling due to lymphedema. There was also evidence of lymphedema of the legs. The bones are relatively unremarkable.

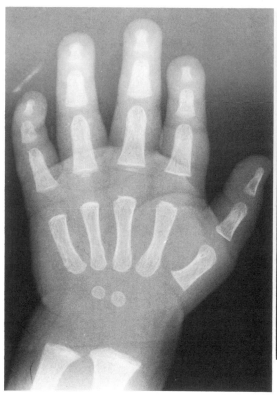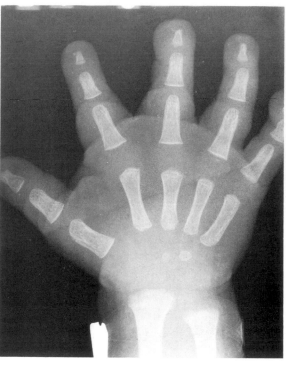

Figure 10–37. Hemihypertrophy. The left side is greater in size than the right. Maturation is more advanced on the left; phalangeal centers are beginning to occur on the left but not on the right, and the carpal centers are larger.

REFERENCES

1. Barsky, A. J.: Macrodactyly. *J. Bone Joint Surg.*, 49A:1255–1266, 1967.
2. Inglis, K.: Local Gigantism (A Manifestation of Neurofibromatosis): Its Relation to General Gigantism and to Acromegaly. Illustrating the Influence of Intrinsic Factors in Disease when Development of the Body is Abnormal. *Am. J. Pathol.*, 26:1059–1083, 1950.
3. Rechnagel, K.: Megalodactylism. Report of 7 Cases. *Acta Orthop. Scand.*, 38:57–66, 1967.
4. Thorne, F. L., Posch, J. L., and Mladick, R. A.: Megalodactyly. *Plast. Reconstr. Surg.*, 41: 232–239, 1968.

HEMIHYPERTROPHY

This is in essence another form of enlargement of an extremity. The enlargement is usually uniform (Fig. 10–37). It is associated with enlargement of other portions of the body as well. The enlarged size is usually advanced in maturation as compared to the uninvolved area.[1] Often both the soft tissues and the bones appear larger. Hemihypertrophy is associated with a number of tumors in children, particularly Wilms's tumor and, more rarely, tumors of the adrenal glands.

REFERENCE

1. Poznanski, A. K., Garn, S. M., Kuhns, L. R., and Sandusky, S. T.: Dysharmonic Maturation of the Hand in the Congenital Malformation Syndromes. *Am. J. Phys. Anthropol.*, 35:417–432, 1971.

Part III

THE HAND AS A MIRROR OF CONGENITAL MALFORMATIONS

THE CHROMOSOMAL DISORDERS

The hand is frequently affected in chromosomal disorders, both in the well-defined syndromes, such as Down's syndrome, and in rarer chromosomal abnormalities. The abnormalities of the hand can involve the length of the hand bones, the relationships of fingers to one another and changes in dermatoglyphic patterns. As is true with many of the clinical findings in the chromosomal disorders, the hand findings are not present in every case of a particular chromosomal syndrome but occur with varying frequency. Many of the radiologic signs of the chromosomal disorders may also occur as anatomic variants in normal individuals. The frequency in normal individuals, however, is usually considerably less than that in affected individuals. The significance of those radiologic signs is that when several of them are present together, the diagnosis of a chromosomal disorder can be suggested.

The cells of normal humans contain 23 pairs of chromosomes (total of 46). These have been grouped by gross, morphologic criteria of size and position of the centromere into seven autosomal groups (designated A to G) plus two sex chromosomes. The sex chromosomes are two Xs in the female and an X and a Y in the male. Radioautographic and fluorescent staining techniques allow for differentiation of the chromosomes in each group. The groups are A (1 to 3), B (4 and 5), C (6 to 12 and the X chromosome), D (13 to 15), E (16 to 18), F (19 and 20) and G (21 and 22).

Although there are many forms of morphologic chromosomal abnormalities that can be detected, there are three major types that are associated with radiologic findings. These are trisomies, deletions and translocations.

The trisomy conditions are some of the best known of the chromosomal disorders. In a trisomy condition there are three chromosomes of a certain type rather than the usual pair. In contrast, a monosomy exists when there is just one chromosome rather than a pair. Most of the autosomal trisomies are associated with severe clinical changes or are incompatible with life, in contrast to trisomies of the sex chromosomes, which produce less severe clinical and radiologic changes. The best known autosomal trisomy with longest longevity is Down's syndrome in which an extra number 21 chromosome is present (total of 47). This is designated as trisomy 21. Most trisomies are produced by meiotic nondisjunction. During meiosis, two haploid (23-chromosome) gametes are formed from a single diploid (46-chromosome) gametocyte. If one of the gametes receives either one chromosome too many or one too few, fertilization with a normal gamete will then form a zygote that is either trisomic or monosomic, respectively. Occasionally, particularly in some of the sex chromosome abnormalities, several extra chromosomes may be present, as in the XXXXY (a total of 49 chromosomes).

Deletions are a group of chromosomal abnormalities in which a portion of a chromosome is absent. When a deletion involves the short arm of a chromosome, it is designated as p—; when it involves the long arm it is called q—. Thus, a short arm deletion of the fourth chromosome is written 4p—. Ring chromosomes are believed to be caused by deletions in both long and short arms with subsequent joining of the broken ends.

Translocations are formed when there is an exchange of material between different chromosomes. If none of the chromosomal material is lost, it is a balanced translocation and the individual has normal physical and radiologic characteristics. However, a person with a chromosomally balanced translocation may have chromosomally abnormal children. Depending on the particular chromosome involved, the person with an unbalanced chromosome translocation will have characteristics that resemble those due to a partial deletion or a trisomy. This phenomenon is seen in about 3 per cent of Down's syndrome patients.

Not all of the cells in an individual need to be the same. The presence of two or more cell lines is referred to as mosaicism. When there is a normal and abnormal line, the clinical and radiologic findings can vary from normal to abnormal. The degree of involvement is not closely related to the percentage of cells affected, since only skin or leukocytes can be examined.

The most common autosomal disorders are trisomy 21, trisomy 18 and trisomy 13, while the most common sex chromosome abnormalities are the XO, the XXY and the XYY syndromes. Because of the large number of associated clinical and radiologic findings in these conditions, they cannot all be listed and only those pertaining to the hands will be discussed in detail. Some of the other significant clinical and radiologic changes will also be described.

The disorders which will be discussed are as follows:

1. Sex chromosomes
   a. Turner's syndrome (XO)
   b. XXXXY
   c. XYY
   d. other
2. Group G
   a. trisomy 21 (Down's syndrome)
   b. trisomy 22
   c. monosomy 21 (Monosomy G)
3. Group E
   a. trisomy 18
   b. other 18 abnormalities (18p—, 18q—, 18r)
4. Group D
   a. trisomy 13
   b. ring D, 13q—
5. Group C
   a. trisomy C
6. Group B
   a. 4p—(Wolf's syndrome)
   b. 5p— (cri-du-chat syndrome)
   c. ring B
7. Other
   a. Bloom's syndrome
   b. triploidy

SEX CHROMOSOME ABNORMALITIES

Turner's Syndrome

This is one of the most common of the chromosomal malformation syndromes with an incidence of about one in 5000 newborns. The karyotype is usually 45 XO, but in many cases there is mosaicism.

Patients have a female phenotype with a broad chest and wide spacing of the nipples, and they may have a web neck.

They are of short stature and may have lymphedema at birth. Other important clinical findings include coarctation of the aorta and, less commonly, other congenital heart defects.

RADIOLOGIC FINDINGS IN THE HAND. One of the most classic radiologic findings in the hand is the relative shortening of the fourth metacarpal, which was described by Archibald et al.[1] as the metacarpal sign. If a line is drawn through the heads of the fifth and fourth metacarpals, in normal patients it does not intersect the third. In Turner's syndrome in a significant percentage of cases, the third metacarpal is intersected (Fig. 11–1). This finding, however, is not universal and its reported incidence is variable. Baker et al.[2] found a much lower incidence of short fourth metacarpals than did Preger.[11] Part of this difference may be due to the age of the patients, since the shortening of the fourth metacarpal is sometimes associated with early fusion of the metacarpal head. Thus, in younger individuals the short fourth metacarpal may not yet be present. In some of the patients not only is the fourth meta-

carpal shortened but there is also shortening of the fifth and third (Fig. 11–2). Similar findings may occur in mosaic Turner's as well as in the pure XO syndrome. There are also other alterations in the length of the other hand bones that may not be seen on casual inspection but which are evident on pattern profile analysis (Fig. 11–3).[8] The proximal phalanges are relatively longer than the metacarpals. Also, the fourth metacarpal is not necessarily the shortest. In a mean profile for 14 patients, the fifth metacarpal was more involved.

The carpals in Turner's syndrome are often abnormal. The normal, gentle arch of the proximal bones becomes V-shaped, or in the most extreme form it has a Madelung deformity (Fig. 11–4). The quantitative evaluation of this arch was described by Kosowicz[7] in terms of a carpal angle. The method of measuring this angle as well as normal values of it are given in Chapter 2. In Kosowicz's series, in 55 per cent of patients with gonadal dysgenesis the carpal angle was more than 2 standard deviations below normal. Other authors found a somewhat smaller incidence of

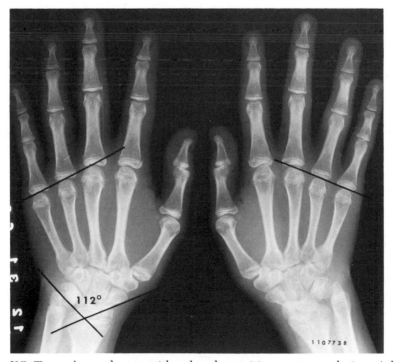

Figure 11–1. XO Turner's syndrome with a barely positive metacarpal sign. A line drawn tangential to the fourth and fifth metacarpals intersects the third. The carpal angle is also diminished (normal = 131°).

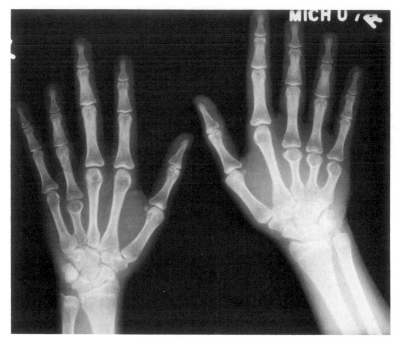

Figure 11–2. XO Turner with multiple metacarpal involvement. On the left the fourth metacarpal is markedly shortened. On the right, however, the third, fourth and fifth metacarpals are shortened. (From Poznanski, A. K., et al.: *Radiol. Clin. N. Amer.*, 9:435, 1971.)

this finding. This may be due to the fact that the abnormal carpal angle changes are not present in young children but become evident when the carpals become more mature. Some patients also have fusion of the carpal bones. Finby and Archibald[4]

reported two examples in 33 cases, and Preger et al.[11] had four examples in 40 patients.

Maturation is usually delayed in older patients with Turner's syndrome.[3, 7] It may be normal in early childhood.[7] While

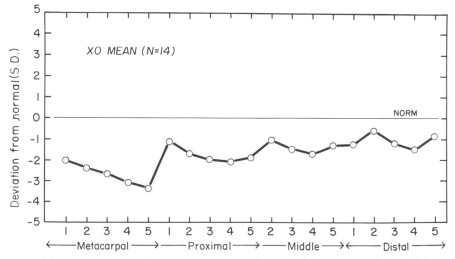

Figure 11–3. Mean pattern profile in Turner's syndrome. There is a gradient of shortening from the first to the fifth metacarpal. The proximal phalanges are relatively longer than the metacarpals.

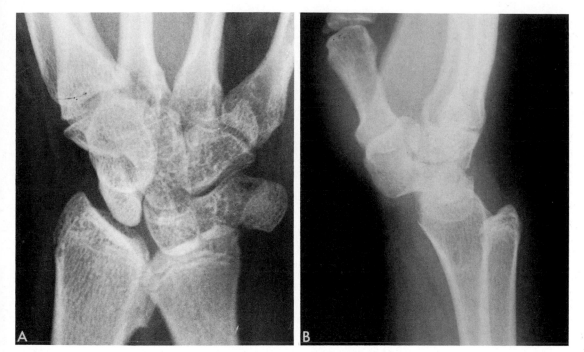

Figure 11-4. Mosaic Turner (XX–isoX) with Madelung deformity. *A*, Sharp V in the wrist with (*B*) modeling deformity seen in lateral view. (Part *B* from Poznanski, A. K., and Holt, J. F.: *Am. J. Roentgenol.*, 112:443, 1971.)

there is delay in ossification of the carpals, some localized acceleration of the maturation of the fourth metacarpal or the third, fourth and fifth metacarpals may occasionally be seen in association with shortening of these bones.

Osteoporosis is common in Turner's syndrome. There is decreased bone formation and increased bone loss.[6] Generally speaking, the total width of the bone is diminished, while the medullary width is increased. Thus, the cortical thickness and cortical area are both reduced, as is the percentage cortical area (Fig. 11–5).

The decreased shaft diameter was noted by Kosowicz, who showed that the ratio

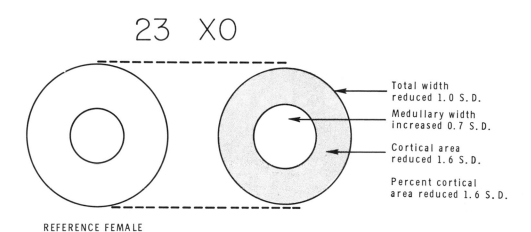

Figure 11-5. Turner's syndrome. Diagram of cortex in this disorder. Total width of the bone is diminished while the medullary width is increased. Thus, the cortical thickness and the cortical area are both reduced. (From Garn, S. M., et al.: *Radiology*, 100:509–518, 1971.)

of shaft length to width was increased in this disorder in most of the bones of the hand.[7] The distal phalanges have a drumstick appearance, partially as a result of this shaft thinness (Fig. 11–6). Kosowicz found the ratio of tuft width to shaft width to be 1.3 in normals with a standard deviation of 0.17.[7] In Turner's syndrome this ratio was 1.7. The tuft also appeared more rounded, although this subjective finding is often difficult to evaluate.

Clinodactyly is very rarely seen in this disorder. Most of the cases with clinodactyly are those of Noonan's syndrome rather than the XO phenotype, although occasional cases which are described may be due to the relatively high incidence of clinodactyly in the general population.

OTHER RADIOLOGIC FINDINGS. Renal anomalies, such as horseshoe kidney and duplication, are common. Generalized bone demineralization may be present. There may be a short fourth metatarsal. Cubitus valgus is often seen. In the older patients

with Turner's syndrome, small exostoses along the inferior margin of the medial tibial epiphysis are often present. In pneumopelvic studies the ovaries are usually aplastic. In the young patient, congenital lymphedema, particularly in the dorsum of the foot and the lower extremities, may be evident.

REFERENCES

1. Archibald, R. M., Finby, N., and De Vito, F.: Endocrine Significance of Short Metacarpals. J. Clin. Endocrinol., 19:1312–1322, 1959.
2. Baker, D. H., Berdon, W. E., Morishima, A., and Conte, F.: Turner's Syndrome and Pseudo-Turner's Syndrome. Am. J. Roentgenol., 100: 40–47, 1967.
3. Dalla Palma, L., Cavina, C., Giusti, G., and Borghi, A.: Skeletal Development in Gonadal Dysgenesis, Female in Phenotype. Am. J. Roentgenol., 101:876–883, 1967.
4. Finby, N., and Archibald, R. M.: Skeletal Abnormalities Associated with Gonadal Dysgenesis. Am. J. Roentgenol. 89:1222–1235, 1963.
5. Garn, S. M., Poznanski, A. K., Hertzog, K., Nagy, J. M., and Miller, R. L.: Metacarpophalangeal Ratios in the Evaluation of Skeletal Malformations, in press.
6. Garn, S. M., Poznanski, A. K., and Nagy, J. M.: Bone Measurement in the Differential Diagnosis of Osteopenia and Osteoporosis. Radiology, 100:509–518, 1971.
7. Kosowicz, J.: The Roentgen Appearance of the Hand and Wrist in Gonadal Dysgenesis. Am. J. Roentgenol., 93:354–361, 1965.
8. Poznanski, A. K., Garn, S. M., Nagy, J. M., and Gall, J. C., Jr.: Metacarpophalangeal Pattern Profiles in the Evaluation of Skeletal Malformations. Radiology, 104:1–11, 1972.
9. Poznanski, A. K., and Holt, J. F.: The Carpals in Congenital Malformation Syndromes. Am. J. Roentgenol., 112:443–459, 1971.
10. Poznanski, A. K., Stern, A. M., and Gall, J. C., Jr.: Skeletal Anomalies in Genetically Determined Congenital Heart Disease. Radiol. Clin. N. Am., 9:435–458, 1971.
11. Preger, L., Steinbach, H. L., Moskowitz, P., Scully, A. L., and Goldberg, M. B.: Roentgenographic Abnormalities in Phenotypic Females with Gonadal Dysgenesis. A Comparison of Chromatin Positive Patients and Chromatin Negative Patients. Am. J. Roentgenol., 104: 899–910, 1968.

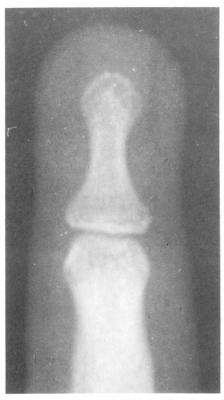

Figure 11–6. Drumstick-like distal phalanx in XO Turner. The ratio of the tuft to shaft is 1.6, which is much greater than normal. The tuft is also more rounded than in normal individuals.

XXXXY Syndrome

This abnormality consists primarily of hypogenitalism, frequent mental deficiency and lack of elbow pronation. It is the result of 49 chromosomes, of which three are extra X chromosomes.

RADIOLOGIC FINDINGS IN THE HAND.

Houston,[1] in a review of the cases in the literature, described elongation of the distal ulna in 89 per cent. Some pseudo-epiphyses were seen in 84 per cent (Fig. 11–7). These, of course, can occasionally be seen as normal variants. A short middle phalanx of the fifth finger with clinodactyly was seen in 56 per cent, while clinodactyly

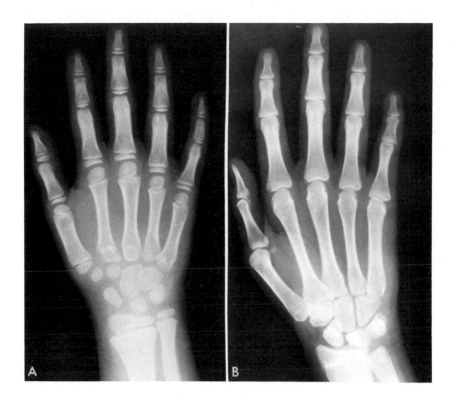

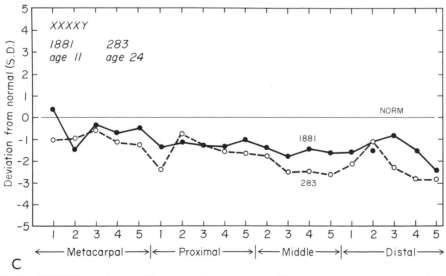

Figure 11-7. XXXXY syndrome. X-rays and pattern profiles on two patients with this syndrome. The child (A) shows pseudoepiphyses in the proximal metacarpals and in the distal first metacarpal. There is no significant clinodactyly present. There is, however, considerable similarity in the patterns of both pattern profile analyses, and both of these cases were also quite similar to those described by Houston. (From Poznanski, A. K., et al.: *Radiology*, 104:1–11, 1972.)

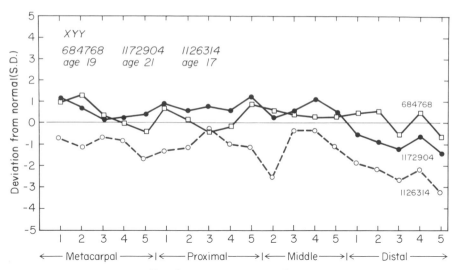

Figure 11–8. XYY. Pattern profile showing some similarities between patients with the XYY karyotype. These similarities are not great except between the 17 year old and the 21 year old.

was seen in 84 per cent. The bone age was retarded in almost all cases.

Alteration in length of the hand bones has also been noted in our cases. There is probably a characteristic pattern. There was considerable similarity in pattern profile between two unrelated cases that we had an opportunity to see and those published by Houston (Fig. 11–7).

OTHER RADIOLOGIC FINDINGS. The most characteristic other radiologic finding in this condition is radioulnar synostosis or other elbow abnormality. Although the radioulnar synostosis was seen in only 32 per cent of cases, 100 per cent showed some abnormality in the region of the elbow. Coxa valga was commonly present in almost half the cases, as well as narrow iliac wings. The distal femora have shallow intercondylar fossa. The feet have a gap between the first and second toes, with a short, somewhat wide distal phalanx of the great toe in the majority of cases. The skull findings are not particularly characteristic. Scoliosis and kyphosis are frequent. The sternum may be thick and lack segmentation.

Other Sex Chromosome Abnormalities

The other abnormalities of sex chromosomes also show relatively little radiographic change. No obvious radiologic findings are found in the hands of patients with the XYY syndrome. Pattern profiles do, however, show some similarities between the cases examined (Fig. 11–8). Clinodactyly has been reported in the XXXXX female, while short fingers have been described in the XXX.[1] Little detailed information is available on these. Sergovich et al.[3] reported some findings in XXXXX which were similar to those seen in the XXXXY. Their patient had an elongated distal ulna, pseudoepiphysis, clinodactyly, brachymesophalangy of the fifth digit, corner defect in the capitate, poor modeling of the fifth metacarpal and some elongation of the third metacarpal. Shortening of the fourth and fifth metacarpals has been reported by Dallapiccola (quoted by Sergovich[3]) in the XXXXX syndrome.

REFERENCES

1. Barr, M. L., Sergovich, F. R., Carr, D. H., and Shaver, E. L.: The Triple-X Female: An Appraisal Based on a Study of 12 Cases and a Review of the Literature. *Can. Med. Assoc. J.,* 101:247–258, 1969.

REFERENCE

1. Houston, C. S.: Roentgen Findings in the XXXXY Chromosome Anomaly. *J. Can. Assoc. Radiol.,* 18:258–267, 1967.

2. Di Cagno, L., and Franceschini, P.: Feeblemindedness and XXXX Karyotype. *J. Ment. Defic. Res.*, 12:226–236, 1968.
3. Sergovich, F., Uilenberg, C., and Pozsonyi, J.: The 49, XXXXX Chromosome Constitution: Similarities to the 49, XXXXY Condition. *J. Pediat.*, 78:285–290, 1971.

AUTOSOMAL DISORDERS

G Group

Down's Syndrome (Trisomy 21, Trisomy G, Mongolism)

This is probably the best known of the chromosomal disorders and was described in 1866 by Down, long before the advent of karyotypes. It is a relatively common condition, having an overall incidence of one in 660 births.

Down's syndrome is usually the result of an extra number 21 chromosome. A certain percentage of patients with Down's syndrome have a mosaic chromosomal pattern with a varying percentage of normal and trisomy 21 lines. The radiographic findings of these individuals range from those of classic Down's syndrome to no radiologic abnormality at all. In about 3 per cent of patients the number 21 chromosome is translocated to another chromosome. The usual places of the translocation are to the D and G groups and are signified as D/G and G/G translocations. The translocation types are important in that they account for many familial cases.

CLINICAL FINDINGS. Hypotonia, mental retardation, slanted palpebral fissures and relatively small stature are usually present. Other clinical findings include changes in the eyes with Brushfield spots and fine lens opacities. Congenital heart disease is common, with an incidence of somewhere between 40 per cent[20] and 60 per cent. The most common defect is atrioventricular canal defect, either with atrioventricularis communis or ostium primum. The next most common is ventricular septal defect. A multitude of other congenital abnormalities have also been noted. The hands are relatively small, often with a crooked fifth finger. The skin folds of the hands are often abnormal, with a simian crease in about half of the cases. Dermatoglyphic patterns may be characteristic, with a distal

position of the palmar axial triradius and an ulnar loop dermal ridge pattern on all digits.

RADIOLOGIC FINDINGS IN THE HAND. The short middle phalanx of the fifth digit (brachymesophalangy-5) and clinodactyly (Fig. 11–9) were probably the first radiologic signs described in Down's syndrome. They were noted by Smith in 1896![22] The incidence of clinodactyly was described as 43 per cent by Hefke[12] and as 55 per cent by Roche.[19] In our series of 437 Down's syndrome patients the incidence varied, depending on the criteria used. If only very definite clinodactyly was included, the incidence was 22 per cent, while if minimal degrees were considered, the incidence was 76 per cent. A definite short middle phalanx of the fifth digit is noted in 20 per cent of Down's patients.[8] Interestingly enough, the shortening of the fifth middle phalanx is not associated with cone-shaped epiphysis, which is

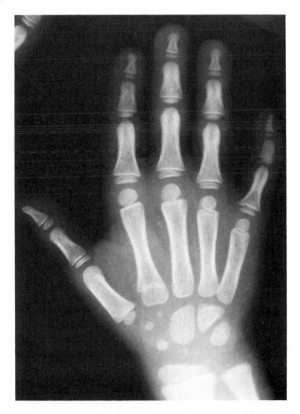

Figure 11–9. Down's syndrome child, 6.25 years old. Shortening of the middle phalanx of the fifth finger and clinodactyly are common findings in Down's syndrome but are not specific for this syndrome. Other alterations in length of the hand bones are difficult to perceive.

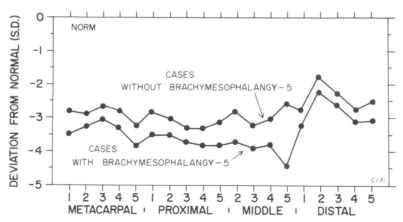

Figure 11–10. Pattern profile of Down's syndrome patients with and without short fifth middle phalanx. Both are characteristic Down's syndrome pattern profiles with relative shortening of the ulnar part of the hand, most evident in the fourth and fifth metacarpals and in the fourth and fifth distal phalanges. The patients without shortening of the middle phalanx of five are generally larger than those with the short middle phalanx, as evidenced by a higher position in the pattern profile plot. Otherwise, the plots are very similar. (From Poznanski, A. K., et al.: *Radiology*, 104:1–11, 1972.)

somewhat different from the general population, where cone-shaped epiphyses are commonly associated with a short middle phalanx.

Although it is the oldest sign, the reduction in size of the middle phalanx is not the only length alteration in the hand. Indeed, many other shortenings of the hand bones are common.[15] These are illustrated in Figure 11–10, which is a mean representation of pattern profiles of Down's syn-

drome patients. From the pattern profiles it is evident that the Down's patients with a short middle phalanx have hands which are overall shorter than those with normal phalanges (one plot lies significantly lower than the other). It has also been shown that the Down's patients with the short middle phalanx are shorter in stature than those with normal middle phalanges. Carpal alterations in Down's syndrome are also evident (Fig. 11–11). Generally the carpal

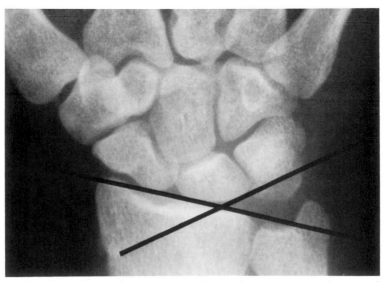

Figure 11–11. Adult Down's syndrome patient. Note the increase in the carpal angle (143°) and the relatively hypoplastic scaphoid and lunate bones.

angle is increased. The scaphoid is often small.

Mineralization of the skeleton is also reduced (Fig. 11–12).[7] There is loss of bone at both the subperiosteal and endosteal surfaces. During adolescence, however, endosteal surface apposition improves so that the percentage of cortical area is close to the adult norm. This is due to a greater than normal rate of apposition of both the subperiosteal and the endosteal surfaces.

Maturation in the patient with Down's syndrome is usually retarded. According to most authors the maturation of the younger Down's patients, when compared to the hand standards of Greulich and Pyle, is more retarded than that of the older Down's patients.[18, 19] An interesting finding in Down's patients is the rather large range of variations of maturation. This parallels the larger range of other normal variants in Down's patients. There is in essence a widening of the entire spectrum of normal variation in this condition. Roche[19] described the fact that the ulnar side of the hand is more retarded than the radial, particularly in females, and that the mean skeletal age of the fifth middle phalanx is retarded relative to the mean skeletal age of the hand-wrist area on the same side. Other evidence of dysharmonic maturation in Down's syndrome is the different sequence of carpal ossification that occurs more commonly in patients with Down's syndrome (Fig. 11–13). The trapezium ossifies before the lunate in 46.7 per cent of Down's patients, but in 5.0 per cent of normal white females and in 0.7 per cent of normal white males.[9]

Dermatoglyphic abnormality in Down's syndrome may also be demonstrated radiologically (Fig. 11–14). The simian crease is well seen on tantalum dermatography or sometimes even may be outlined by air

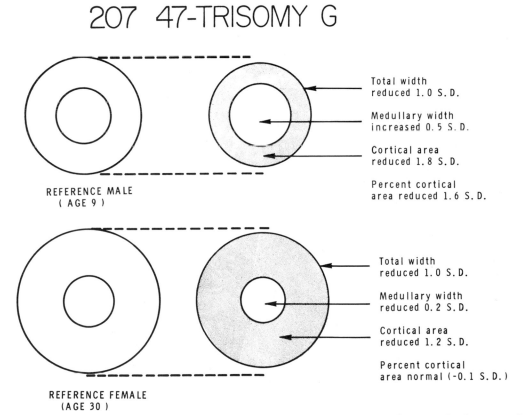

207 47-TRISOMY G

REFERENCE MALE
(AGE 9)

Total width
reduced 1.0 S.D.

Medullary width
increased 0.5 S.D.

Cortical area
reduced 1.8 S.D.

Percent cortical
area reduced 1.6 S.D.

REFERENCE FEMALE
(AGE 30)

Total width
reduced 1.0 S.D.

Medullary width
reduced 0.2 S.D.

Cortical area
reduced 1.2 S.D.

Percent cortical
area normal (-0.1 S.D.)

Figure 11–12. Diagrams of bone cortex in patients with Down's syndrome. The bone in these individuals is deficient at both surfaces. In the young Down's syndrome patient this loss of bone is most marked; some of the bone is regained in adolescence, bringing it close to the adult normal. (From Garn, S. M., et al.: *Radiology,* 100:509, 1971.)

on plain film. Other dermatoglyphic findings include a distally positioned palmar axial triradius.

OTHER RADIOLOGIC FINDINGS. The skull is relatively small and there is hypoplasia of the facial bones with absence of the frontal sinuses in 93 per cent of Down's syndrome patients.[23] There is hypotelorism[10] and shortening of the palate.[21] Cleft lip and palate are somewhat more common, occurring in 0.5 per cent of patients as compared to 0.14 to 0.18 per cent in the normal population.[5] In the spine of older patients there may be a subluxation of the atlantoaxial joint which may be associated with a third condyle.[14] There is a relative increase in height of the vertebrae in the lumbar region as compared to their anteroposterior diameter.[17] Eleven pairs of ribs are seen somewhat more commonly in Down's syndrome than in the normal population. A double ossification center of the manubrium occurs in 90 per cent of young patients.[4] Probably the most characteristic radiologic findings are those affecting the pelvis with the typical flattening of the acetabular slopes, large flared ilia and reduction of the iliac index. Tables for the numerical

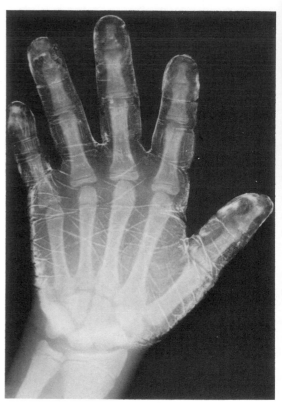

Figure 11–14. Radiodermatography in Down's syndrome. The skin folds can be demonstrated using tantalum powder opacification of the skin. This technique is useful mainly in correlating the length of the bones with the position of the skin folds. The single transverse crease is commonly seen.

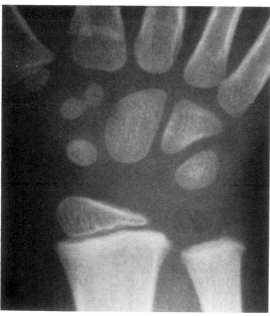

Figure 11–13. Disproportion in osseus maturation in 6.2 year old male with Down's syndrome. The lunate is late in onset, as it is in a large percentage of Down's syndrome patients. The same phenomenon may be seen in a normal population, but it is much less common.

values of these angles have been published by Caffey[3] and by Taybi and Kane.[24]

REFERENCES

1. Austin, J. H. M., Preger, L., Siris, E., and Taybi, H.: Short Hard Palate in Newborn: Roentgen Sign of Mongolism. *Radiology,* 92:775–776, 1969.
2. Beber, B. A., Litt, R. E., and Altman, D. H.: A New Radiographic Finding in Mongolism. *Radiology,* 86:332–333, 1966.
3. Caffey, J., and Ross, S.: Pelvic Bones in Infantile Mongoloidism. Roentgenographic Features. *Am. J. Roentgenol.,* 80:458–467, 1958.
4. Currarino, G., and Swanson, G. E.: A Developmental Variant of Ossification of the Manubrium Sterni in Mongolism. *Radiology,* 82: 916, 1964.
5. Fabia, J., and Drolette, M.: Malformations and Leukemia in Children with Down's Syndrome. *Pediatrics,* 45:60–70, 1970.
6. Garn, S. M., Gall, J. C., Jr., and Nagy, J. M.: Preliminary Radiogrammetric Analysis of the Bone Recovery Phase in Adolescents with Down's Syndrome, *Invest. Radiol.,* 7:97–101, 1972.

7. Garn, S. M., Poznanski, A. K., and Nagy, J. M.: Bone Measurement in the Differential Diagnosis of Osteopenia and Osteoporosis. *Radiology*, 100:509–518, 1971.

8. Garn, S. M., Poznanski, A. K., Nagy, J. M., and McCann, M. B.: Independence of Brachymesophalangia-5 from Brachymesophalangia-5 with Cone Mid-5. *Am. J. Phys. Anthropol.*, 36:295–298, 1972.

9. Garn, S. M., Sandusky, S. T., Miller, R. L., and Nagy, J. M.: Developmental Implications of Dichotomous Ossification Sequences in the Wrist Region. *Am. J. Phys. Anthropol.*, 37:111–116, 1972.

10. Gerald, B. E., and Silverman, F. N.: Normal and Abnormal Interorbital Distances, with Special Reference to Mongolism. *Am. J. Roentgenol.*, 95:154–161, 1965.

11. Hall, Bertil: Mongolism in Newborns. A Clinical and Cytogenic Study. *Acta Paediat.*, Supplement 154, pp. 41–105, 1964.

12. Hefke, H. W.: Roentgenologic Study of Anomalies of the Hands in One Hundred Cases of Mongolism. *Am. J. Dis. Child.*, 60:1319–1323, 1940.

13. Levinson, A., Friedman, A., and Stamps, F.: Variability of Mongolism. *Pediatrics*, 16: 43–54, 1955.

14. Martel, W., and Tishler, J. M.: Observations on the Spine in Mongoloidism. *Am. J. Roentgenol.*, 97:630–638, 1966.

15. Poznanski, A. K., Garn, S. M., Nagy, J. M., and Gall, J. C., Jr.: Metacarpophalangeal Pattern Profiles in the Evaluation of Skeletal Malformations. *Radiology*, 104:1–11, 1972.

16. Pozsonyi, J., Gibson, D., and Zarfas, D. E.: Skeletal Maturation in Mongolism (Down's Syndrome). *J. Pediat.*, 64:75–78, 1964.

17. Rabinowitz, J. G., and Moseley, J. E.: The Lateral Lumbar Spine in Down's Syndrome: A New Roentgen Feature. *Radiology*, 83:74–79, 1964.

18. Rarick, G. L., Rapaport, I. F., and Seefeldt, V.: Long Bone Growth in Down's Syndrome. *Am. J. Dis. Child.*, 112:566–571, 1966.

19. Roche, A. F.: Skeletal Maturation Rates in Mongolism. *Am. J. Roentgenol.*, 91:979–987, 1964.

20. Rowe, R. D., and Uchida, I. A.: Cardiac Malformation in Mongolism. A Prospective Study of 184 Mongoloid Children. *Am. J. Med.*, 31: 726–735, 1961.

21. Shapiro, B. L., Gorlin, R. J., Redman, R. S., and Bruhl, H. H.: The Palate and Down's Syndrome. *N. Engl. J. Med.*, 276:1460–1463, 1967.

22. Smith, T. T.: A Peculiarity in the Shape of the Hand in Idiots of the "Mongol" Type. *Pediatrics*, 2:315–320, 1896.

23. Spitzer, R., and Robinson, M. I.: Radiological Changes in Teeth and Skull in Mental Defectives. *Br. J. Radiol.*, 28:117–127, 1955.

24. Taybi, H., and Kane, P.: Small Acetabular and Iliac Angles and Associated Diseases. *Radiol. Clin. N. Am.*, 6:215–221, 1968.

Trisomy 22

This condition has different clinical manifestations from trisomy 21 and can be differentiated in karyotyping by the newer techniques. Hsu et al. described several cases with typical finger-like malapposed thumbs as well as other abnormalities.

REFERENCE

1. Hsu, L. Y. F., Shapiro, L. R., Gertner, M., Lieber, E., and Hirschhorn, K.: Trisomy 22: A Clinical Entity. *J. Pediat.*, 79:12–19, 1971.

Monosomy G or Antimongolism

Monosomy G or antimongolism may include two separate entities. The hand changes in some reported cases include low set thumbs or flex thumb.

REFERENCE

1. Challacombe, D. N., and Taylor, A.: Monosomy for a G Autosome. *Arch. Dis. Child.*, 44:113–119, 1969.

E Group

Trisomy 18 Syndrome (E Trisomy, Edwards's Syndrome)

These are generally small, poorly developed babies. The hand is frequently clenched with overlapping of the second over the third finger. The dermatoglyphic patterns are characteristic, with arches on three or more of the fingertips seen in 100 per cent of cases.[13] The infants are usually hypertonic after the neonatal period and fail to thrive. Most die within the first year of life. The head is elongated. The ears are low set and malformed. There is usually micrognathia. Foot deformities are common and the great toe is usually short and dorsiflexed. Congenital heart disease is seen in almost all cases,[13] with ventricular septal defects the most common finding (96 per cent of cases), although patent ductus arteriosus is also fairly common (69 per cent). Renal anomalies are also frequently found. A large number of other clinical findings may be present.

RADIOLOGIC FINDINGS IN THE HAND.[1, 3, 5, 6] When the hand of a patient with trisomy 18 is flattened out for filming, there is usually ulnar deviation of some or all of the fingers. There is often a gap between the second and third fingers (Fig. 11–15). This is usually seen at each filming but

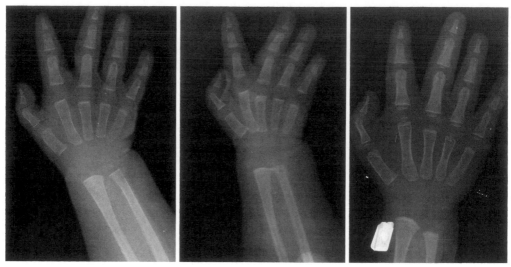

Figure 11–15. Trisomy 18. V-shaped deviation between the second and third fingers. These three radiographs were obtained at three different ages. On the last film (*C*), taken at age three, no carpal centers were yet present, while phalangeal epiphyses are evident. There is hypoplasia of the distal phalanges. (From Poznanski, A. K., et al.: *Radiol. Clin. N. Am.,* 9:435, 1971.)

is not a good radiologic sign, since a similar configuration can be due simply to faulty positions of the normal hand. There is sometimes more definite deviation of the second and third digits (Fig. 11–16). There is shortening of the fifth finger usually due to a short middle phalanx (Fig. 11–16) but also associated with a thin, hypoplastic distal phalanx. Clinodactyly is common.

The thumb is sometimes short with some hypoplasia of the first metacarpal. The distal phalanges of the fingers are small, slender and sometimes triangular in shape. Although maturation is markedly retarded in most cases, a case of mosaic trisomy 18 has been recorded with advanced maturation.[10] Other hand changes occasionally seen in trisomy 18 have been an association of radial hypoplasia and absence of the thumb,[9] or even more severe changes including phocomelia and absence of the thumb (Zellweger, et al).[15] The maturation of the hand is usually markedly retarded, but the carpals are significantly more retarded than the phalanges. If the patients survive long enough, phalangeal and metacarpal epiphyses ossify before the carpal ossification centers (Fig. 11–17).[7, 8]

OTHER RADIOLOGIC FINDINGS.[1, 5, 6] The skull is thin with a prominent occiput and

hypoplasia of the facial bones. Occasionally there is fusion of the cervical vertebrae. The ribs are thin and hypoplastic. Congenital heart defects are frequently

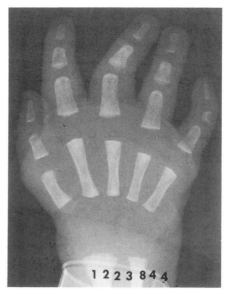

Figure 11–16. Trisomy 18. There is marked deviation of the third finger to the ulnar side. Shortening of the middle phalanx of the fifth finger and clinodactyly are often seen in this disorder. There is some hypoplasia of the distal phalanges, particularly of the fifth finger.

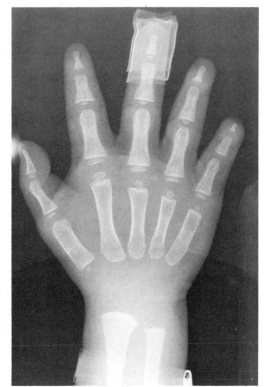

Figure 11–17. Dysharmonic maturation in trisomy 18. This is the same patient shown in Figure 11–15. Note the absence of carpal ossification centers while the phalangeal and metacarpal epiphyses are in most part already present. This abnormal pattern of maturation is not seen in normal individuals. Note also the relative slenderness of the distal phalanges of the digits, which is characteristic of this disorder; and in this particular individual the relative shortening of the distal phalanges on the ulnar side of the hand. (From Poznanski, A. K., et al.: *Am. J. Phys. Anthropol.,* 35:417–432, 1971.)

present. Foot deformities are also common and include rocker bottom foot, short great toe with triangular distal phalanges and some deviation of the toes. The sternum is frequently slender and unsegmented. Pelvic wings are anteriorly rotated and antimongoloid in appearance.

Skeletal maturation at birth is considerably delayed, particularly as evaluated by the knee ossification centers. Maturation of the teeth, however, is less retarded.[4] This disproportion between knee and tooth maturation is not specific for trisomy 18; it has been seen in many other congenital syndromes,[4] including other chromosomal disorders.

REFERENCES

1. Astley, R.: Trisomy 17/18. *Br. J. Radiol.,* 39:86–91, 1966.
2. Conen, P. E., and Erkman-Balis, B.: Frequency and Occurrence of Chromosomal Syndromes. I. D-Trisomy. II. E-Trisomy. *Am. J. Hum. Genet.,* 18:374–398, 1966.
3. James, A. E., Jr., Belcourt, C. L., Atkins, L., and Janower, M. L.: Trisomy 18. *Radiology,* 92: 37–43, 1969.
4. Kuhns, L. R., Sherman, M. P., and Poznanski, A. K.: Determination of Neonatal Maturation on the Chest Radiograph. *Radiology,* 102:597–603, 1972.
5. Moseley, J. E., Wolf, B. S., and Gottlieb, M. I.: The Trisomy 17-18 Syndrome. Roentgen Features. *Am. J. Roentgenol.* 89:905–913, 1963.
6. Ozonoff, M. B., Steinbach, H. L., and Mamunes, P.: The Trisomy 18 Syndrome. *Am. J. Roentgenol.* 91:618–628, 1964.
7. Poznanski, A. K., Garn, S. M., Kuhns, L. R., and Sandusky, S. T.: Dysharmonic Maturation of the Hand in the Congenital Malformation Syndromes. *Am. J. Phys. Anthropol.,* 35:417–432, 1971.
8. Poznanski, A. K., and Holt, J. F.: The Carpals in Congenital Malformation Syndromes. *Am. J. Roentgenol.,* 112:443–459, 1971.
9. Rabinowitz, J. G., Moseley, J. E., Mitty, H. A., and Hirschhorn, K.: Trisomy 18, Esophageal Atresia, Anomalies of the Radius, and Congenital Hypoplastic Thrombocytopenia. *Radiology,* 89:488–491, 1967.
10. Robinson, A. E., Parry W. H., and Blizard, E. B.: Mosaic Trisomy 18. A Case Report with Some Unusual Radiographic Features. *Radiology* 100:379–380, 1971
11. Smith, D. W., Patau, K., Therman, E., and Inhorn, S. L.: The No. 18 Trisomy Syndrome. *J. Pediat.,* 60:513–527, 1962.
12. Taylor, A. I.: Autosomal Trisomy Syndromes: A Detailed Study of 27 Cases of Edwards' Syndrome and 27 Cases of Patau's Syndrome. *J. Med. Genet.,* 5:227–252, 1968.
13. Taylor, A. I.: Patau's Edwards' and Cri du Chat Syndromes: A Tabulated Summary of Current Findings. *Dev. Med. Child. Neurol.,* 9:78–86, 1967.
14. Warkany, J., Passarge, E., and Smith, L. B.: Congenital Malformations in Autosomal Trisomy Syndromes. *Am. J. Dis. Child.,* 112:502–517, 1966.
15. Zellweger, H., Huff, D. S., and Abbo, G.: Phocomelia and Trisomy E. *Acta Genet. Med.,* 14: 164–173, 1965.

Other 18 Chromosome Abnormalities (18p–, 18q–, 18r)

Many of these have some hand abnormality but very little has been written about their radiographic appearance. A good summary of these anomalies is given by de Grouchy.[2]

Most cases of short arm deletion (18p–) have short fingers and clinodactyly of the fifth finger. Both of these findings are visible on published dermatoglyphic patterns. Abnormal thumb position has been reported by Gilgenkrantz et al.[5] Radiologic information on these conditions is sparse. Clinically the syndromes are better defined. The patients are of low birth weight, mentally retarded and have ocular and orbital malformations.

In the long arm deletion of 18 (18q–), the fingers have been described as fusiform, and a proximally implanted thumb is frequently seen. The palms appear long in relation to finger lengths due to the shortening of proximally implanted thumbs and flattening of the thenar and hypothenar eminences. Clinodactyly is common.

The clinical syndrome of long arm deletion is well defined. It includes mental retardation, microcephaly, facial abnormality related to midface aplasia, and abnormal ears.

The ring 18 (18r) chromosomal abnormality can sometimes mimic deletions of either the short arm or the long arm. Short fingers, tapering fingers and high set thumbs have been described, as well as abnormal flexion of the fingers.

D Group

Trisomy 13 (D Trisomy, Patau's Syndrome)

Characteristics of this syndrome are cleft lip and palate, polydactyly, developmental retardation and long hyperconvex fingernails. Microphthalmia is common, as are colobomas of the iris. Malformed ears are seen in most cases. Infants may be either hypertonic or hypotonic. Cardiac defects occur in most cases and are variable. There is usually microcephaly and scalp defects are common. In the hand there is commonly a simian crease (92 per cent).[6] The thumb is often retroflexible.

RADIOGRAPHIC FINDINGS IN THE HAND. Polydactyly in the hands or feet occurs in 76 per cent of cases (Fig. 11–18).[6] It is usu-

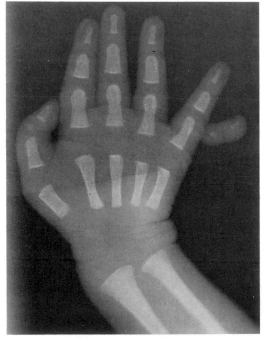

Figure 11-18. Trisomy 13. There is polydactyly with a rudimentary finger with two phalanges on the ulnar side of the hand. There is an extra ossicle in the region of the middle phalanx of the thumb. The extra ossicle is not a common finding in this syndrome. The distal phalanges of all the fingers are slender. (From Poznanski, A. K., et al.: *Radiology,* 100:115, 1971.)

REFERENCES

1. Curran, J. P., Al-Salihi, F. L., and Allderdice, P. W.: Partial Deletion of the Long Arm of Chromosome E-18. *Pediatrics,* 46:721–729, 1970.
2. de Grouchy, J.: The 18p–, 18q– and 18r Syndromes. *Birth Defects, Original Article Series,* 5:74–87, 1969.
3. de Grouchy, J., Bonnette, J., and Salmon, Ch.: Délétion du Bras Court du Chromosome 18. *Ann. Genet.,* 9:19–26, 1966.
4. Destine, M. L., Punnett, H. H., Thovichit, S., DiGeorge, A. M., and Weiss, L.: La Délétion Partielle du Bras Long du Chromosome 18 (Syndrome 18q–). Rapport de Deux Cas. *Ann. Genet.,* 10:65–69, 1967.
5. Gilgenkrantz, S., Marchal, C., and Neimann, N.: La Délétion du Bras Court du Chromosome 18 (Syndrome 18p–). A Propos D'Une Nouvelle Observation. *Ann. Genet.,* 11:17–21, 1968.
6. Weiss, L., and Mayeda, K.: Case Reports. A Patient with a Short Arm Deletion of Chromosome 18 (46, XY, 18p–). *J. Med. Genet.,* 6:216–219, 1969.
7. Wertelecki, W., and Gerald, P. S.: Clinical and Chromosomal Studies of the 18q– Syndrome. *J. Pediat.,* 78:44–52, 1971.

ally postaxial. Along the ulnar side the distal phalanges may be slender and are associated with hyperconvex nails. Triphalangism of the thumb may occur. It was seen in one of our cases, but otherwise its occurrence has not been described in the literature. Wilson[8] reported a case with several extra digits. Also occasionally the thumbs can be broad and mimic those of the Rubinstein-Taybi syndrome. Mosaic trisomy D has similar findings to those described.

OTHER RADIOLOGIC FINDINGS. Maturation is retarded as evidenced by the knee and foot standards. The tooth maturation is usually ahead of the knee maturation. The most significant clinical findings are in the head and neck and they are manifested radiologically by a small skull with a prominent occiput, hypotelorism and midline cleft deformities. The orbits are small. External auditory canals are hypoplastic. Roentgen findings of congenital heart disease are common. The heel is prominent and there may be polydactyly in the feet. Occasionally duplication of the vagina or uterus may be seen.

REFERENCES

1. Bowen, P., Lee, C. S. N., Shea, D. R., and Armstrong, H. B.: Polydactyly and Other Minor Stigmata Associated with 46,XX/47,XX,D+ Mosaicism. *Can. Med. Assoc. J.*, 102:49–51, 1970.
2. Conen, P. E., and Erkman-Balis, B.: Frequency and Occurrence of Chromosomal Syndromes. I. D-Trisomy. II. E-Trisomy. *Am. J. Hum. Genet.*, 18:374–398, 1966.
3. James, A. E., Jr., Belcourt, C. L., Atkins, L., and Janower, M. L.: Trisomy 13–15. *Radiology*, 92:44–49, 1969.
4. Neimann, N., Pierson, M., Gilgenkrantz, S., Olive, D., and Kahn, Cl.: La Trisomie 13–15. *Arch. Fr. Pediat.*, 21:661–686, 1964.
5. Taylor, A. I.: Autosomal Trisomy Syndromes: A Detailed Study of 27 Cases of Edwards' Syndrome and 27 Cases of Patau's Syndrome. *J. Med. Genet.* 5:227–252, 1968.
6. Taylor, A. I.: Patau's, Edwards' and Cri du Chat Syndromes: A Tabulated Summary of Current Findings. *Dev. Med. Child. Neurol.*, 9:78–86, 1967.
7. Warkany, J., Passarge, E., and Smith, L. B.: Congenital Malformations in Autosomal Trisomy Syndromes. *Am. J. Dis. Child.*, 112:502–517, 1966.
8. Wilson, M. G.: Rubinstein-Taybi and D₁ Trisomy Syndromes. *J. Pediat.*, 73:402–408, 1968.

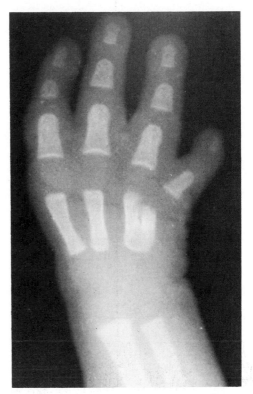

Figure 11–19. Ring D. This is a characteristic hand in this disorder, with absence of thumb and fusion of the fourth and fifth metacarpals. There is shortening and clinodactyly of the fifth finger with absence of ossification of the middle phalanx. The other middle phalanges are short. (From Juberg, R. C., et al.: *J. Med. Genet.*, 6:314, 1969.)

Ring D, 13q− Syndrome

This syndrome is radiologically characterized by specific hand abnormality. It is due to the deletion of the long arm of the 13th chromosome (13q−),[1] which may also be manifested as a ring (ring D, 13r). It is now felt that it is chromosome 13 in the D group that is responsible; 14q− and 15q− produce different syndromes.[3]

The characteristic radiologic findings in the hand (Fig. 11–19) are an absence or hypoplasia of the thumb. There is an osseous synostosis between the fourth and fifth metacarpals. There is a very short fifth middle phalanx, as well as marked shortening of the entire fifth digit. Various deviations of the phalanges are also seen. Carpal retardation is marked as compared to the phalanges, although both show evidence of retardation. Other radiographic findings include dislocation of the hips and spine anomalies.

REFERENCES

1. Allderdice, P. W., Davis, J. G., Miller, O. J., Klinger, H. P., Warburton, D., Miller, D. A., Allen, F. H., Jr., Abrams, C. A. L., and McGilvray, E.: The 13q— Deletion Syndrome. *Am. J. Hum. Genet.*, 21:499–512, 1969.
2. Juberg, R. C., Adams, M. S., Venema, W. J., and Hart, M. G.: Multiple Congenital Anomalies Associated with a Ring-D Chromosome. *J. Med. Genet.*, 6:314–321, 1969.
3. Laurent, C., Noel, B., and David, M.: Essai de Classification des Délétions du Bras Long D'un Chromosome du Groupe D. A Propos D'un Cas 15q–. *Ann. Genet.*, 14:33–40, 1971.
4. Sparkes, R. S., Carrel, R. E., and Wright, S. W.: Absent Thumbs with a Ring D2 Chromosome: A New Deletion Syndrome. *Am. J. Hum. Genet.*, 19:644–659, 1967.

C Group

Trisomy C

This is a group of poorly defined syndromes which without mosaicism are probably incompatible with life.[2] Numerous associated anomalies have been reported, including polycystic kidney and other genitourinary abnormalities. Hand deformities have been described with flexion deformities[5, 6] and deviation of digits. Other findings in the hand are bilateral clinodactyly and some shortening of the fourth metacarpal in the patient of Van Eys et al. Most of the findings were not specific. Van Eys'[5] case apparently showed some advancement of skeletal maturation at one year of age, which is somewhat unusual for the chromosomal disorder and which was not present in Higurashi's case.[1] Some of the children have absent patellae and iliac horns and mimic osteo-onchyo-dysplasia.[3]

REFERENCES

1. Higurashi, M., Naganuma, M., Matsui, I., and Kamoshita, S.: Case Report. Two Cases of Trisomy C6–12 Mosaicism with Multiple Congenital Malformations. *J. Med. Genet.*, 6:429–434, 1969.
2. Juberg, R. C., Gilbert, E. F., and Salisbury, R. S.: Trisomy C in an Infant with Polycystic Kidneys and Other Malformations. *J. Pediat.*, 76:598–603, 1970.
3. Lejeune, J., Dutrillaux, B., Rethore, M. O., Berger, R., Debray, H., Veron, P., Gorce, F., and Grossiord, A.: Sur Trois Cas de Trisomie C. *Ann. Genet.*, 12:28–35, 1969.
4. Oikawa, K., Kajii, T., Shimba, H., and Sasaki, M.: 46,XY/47,XY,C+ Mosaicism in a Male Infant with Multiple Anomalies. *Ann. Genet.*, 12:102–106, 1969.
5. Riccardi, V. M., Atkins, L., and Holmes, L. B.: Absent Patellae, Mild Mental Retardation, Skeletal and Genitourinary Anomalies, and C Group Mosaicism. *J. Pediat.*, 77:664–672, 1970.
6. van Eys, J., Nance, W. E., and Engel, E.: C Autosomal Trisomy with Mosaicism: A New Syndrome? *Pediatrics*, 45:665–671, 1970.

B Group

Wolf's Syndrome (Deletion of Short Arm of Chromosome 4, 4p—)

This syndrome represents a characteristic clinical and radiologic entity. As in many other congenital chromosomal syndromes a multitude of findings is present. The infants affected have a characteristic facial appearance with a prominent forehead, low set ears, marked mental retardation and misshaped nose. The radiologic findings in the hand have not been well documented since most published reports do not include a hand radiograph. A few films, however, have been published[2, 6] and show considerable similarity to a case seen by us (Fig. 11–20). Pseudoepiphyses are seen in all of the metacarpals and pseudoepiphyses or notches may occur in the phalanges as well. These signs, of course, are evident only in the older individual after the epiphyses have formed.

Clinodactyly and shortness of the fifth middle phalanx are common. Maturation is delayed and dysharmonic maturation is similar to that seen in Down's syndrome. The lunate is particularly delayed as compared to the other carpal bones.

OTHER RADIOLOGIC FINDINGS. These include microcephaly, hypertelorism, cleft palate, hydrocephalus and micrognathia. Abnormality of the pelvis may be seen with dislocation and increased iliac angle, although this may well be related to the fact that these children have poor mobility. Clubfoot deformity is commonly present.

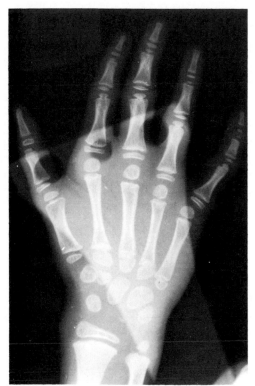

Jr.: Partial Deletion of the Short Arm of Chromosome No. 4 (4p–): Clinical Studies in Five Unrelated Patients. *J. Pediat.*, 77:792–801, 1970.

5. Poznanski, A. K., Garn, S. M., and Holt, J. F.: The Thumb in the Congenital Malformation Syndromes. *Radiology*, 100:115–129, 1971.

6. Reinwein, H., and Wolf, U.: Radiological Examinations of Patients with Autosomal Aberrations. *Ann. Radiol.*, 10:311–316, 1967.

Cri-du-Chat Syndrome (Partial Deletion of the Short Arm of Chromosome 5 (5p–)

These children have mental retardation and a peculiar cat-like cry which appears only in infancy, as well as other congenital malformations. The hand findings include shortening of the metacarpals.[3] Short fourth and fifth metacarpals were present in many of Breg's[1] patients (Fig. 11–21). In others the shortening was not as gross (Fig. 11–22), but still visible on pattern profile

Figure 11-20. Wolf's syndrome. Deletion of the short arm of the fourth chromosome. Note the multiple pseudoepiphyses in the distal portions of the proximal and middle phalanges and in the proximal portion of all of the metacarpals. Although these pseudoepiphyses can occasionally be seen as normal variants, this large number is most unusual. Note also the abnormality of the carpal ossification pattern, with a very delayed lunate. The entire maturation of this child is delayed. There is an increase in the carpal angle. There is also clinodactyly and brachymesophalangy of the fifth digit. The distal phalanges are slender with relatively poorly developed tufts. (From Poznanski, A. K., et al.: *Radiology*, 100:115, 1971.)

REFERENCES

1. Arias, D., Passarge, E., Engle, M. A., and German, J.: Human Chromosomal Deletion: Two Patients with the 4p– Syndrome. *J. Pediat.*, 76: 82–88, 1970.

2. Franceschini, P., Grassi, E., and Marchese, G. S.: Les Principaux Signes Radiologiques du Syndrome 4p–. *Ann. Radiol.*, 14:335–340, 1971.

3. Leao, J. C., Bargman, G. J., Neu, R. L., Kajii, T., and Gardner, L. I.: New Syndrome Associated with Partial Deletion of Short Arms of Chromosome No. 4. *J.A.M.A.* 202:434–437, 1967.

4. Miller, O. J., Breg, W. R., Warburton, D., Miller, D. A., deCapoa, A., Allderdice, P. W., Davis, J., Klinger, H. P., McGilvray, E., and Allen, F. H.,

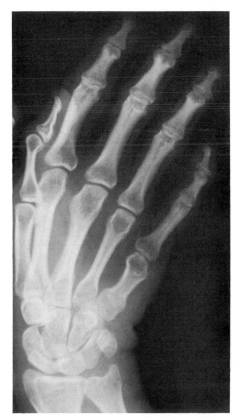

Figure 11-21. Adult with cri-du-chat syndrome. A short fifth metacarpal is common in this condition. (Courtesy Dr. W. R. Breg, Southbury Training School, Southbury, Connecticut.)

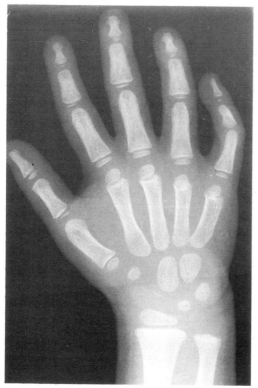

Figure 11–22. Two and a half year old with cri-du-chat syndrome. The shortening of the fourth and fifth metacarpals is not as evident on examination of the radiograph, but was clearly apparent on pattern profile analysis.

analysis (Fig. 11–23). Similar shortening of the lateral metatarsals was present.

REFERENCES

1. Breg, W. R., Steele, M. W., Miller, O. J., Warburton, D., deCapoa, A., and Allderdice, P. W.: The Cri-du-Chat Syndrome in Adolescents and Adults: Clinical Finding in 13 Older Patients with Partial Deletion of the Short Arm of Chromosome No. 5(5p–). *J. Pediat.*, 77:782–791, 1970.
2. James, A. E., Jr., Atkins, L., Feingold, M., and Janower, M. L.: The Cri du Chat Syndrome. *Radiology*, 92:50–52, 1969.
3. Reinwein, H., and Wolf, U.: Radiologic Examinations of Patients with Autosomal Aberrations. *Ann. Radiol.*, 10:311–316, 1967.

Ring B Chromosome

Ring B chromosome abnormality has been associated with thumb hypoplasia.

REFERENCES

1. Carter, R., Baker, E., and Hayman, D.: Case Reports. Congenital Malformations Associated with a Ring 4 Chromosome. *J. Med. Genet.*, 6:224–227, 1969.
2. Dallaire, L.: A Ring B Chromosome in a Female

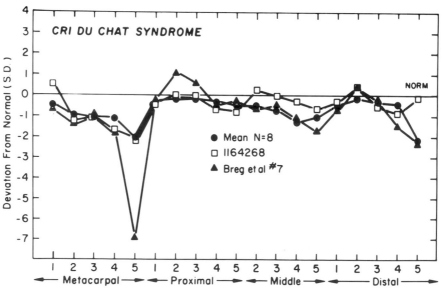

Figure 11–23. Pattern profile of patients with cri-du-chat syndrome. There is some similarity between the mean and our patient 1 164 268 (Fig. 11–22) and Breg's patient (Fig. 11–21).

with Multiple Skeletal Abnormalities. *Birth Defects, Original Article Series*, Part V, 5:114, 1969.

Other Autosomal Disorders

A variety of other autosomal chromosome abnormalities have been described, including double and triple trisomy lines and a variety of translocations, many of which are associated with hand abnormality. Many of these do not appear to form a specific syndrome. Interestingly enough in many of them there is shortening of the middle phalanx of the fifth finger, as well as clinodactyly. Some of the hand changes can be gross.

An increased number of chromosomal breaks is associated with Bloom's syndrome and Fanconi's anemia. In Bloom's syndrome[1] chromosome breaks are increased while the hand findings are mainly those of clinodactyly of the fifth finger, although syndactyly and double thumb have also been reported. The radiologic changes of Fanconi's anemia are described in the section of congenital malformation syndromes.

REFERENCE

1. German, J.: Bloom's Syndrome. I. Genetical and Clinical Observations in the First Twenty-Seven Patients. *Am. J. Hum. Genet.*, 21:196–227, 1969.

Triploidy

Most infants born with 69 chromosomes are stillborn. Schmickel et al. reported a live-born infant with 69 chromosomes. The characteristic hand findings are syndactyly of the third and fourth digits. This is evident radiologically (Fig. 11–24). Clinodactyly may also be present. Other clinical findings included coloboma, hypospadias and abnormal dermatoglyphic pattern. Other than the cutaneous syndactyly, the radiologic changes are unremarkable.

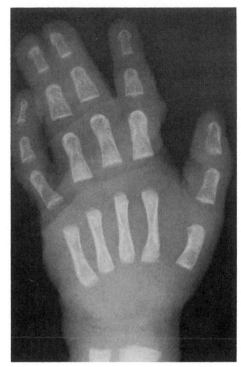

Figure 11–24. Triploidy. This infant was born with 69 chromosomes and died shortly after birth. Syndactyly of the third and fourth digits is commonly seen in this condition, as is clinodactyly of the fifth finger. The findings are nonspecific.

A patient with triploid-diploid mosaicism described by Book[1] had multiple hand anomalies, including flexure contracture of several digits and syndactyly, as well as shortening of the fingers, particularly the thumbs.

REFERENCES

1. Book, J. A.: Epidermal Ridge Configurations in a Boy with Triploid/Diploid Mosaicism. *Acta Genet. Med. Gemellol.*, 19:417–420, 1970.
2. Schmickel, R. D., Silverman, E. M., Floyd, A. D., Payne, F. E., Pooley, J. M., and Beck, M. L.: A Live-Born Infant with 69 Chromosomes. *J. Pediat.*, 79:97–103, 1971.

Chapter 12

THE CONGENITAL MALFORMATION SYNDROMES: AN INTRODUCTION

There are a large number of conditions with multiple malformations in which the hand is also involved. Of these the chromosomal disorders have been discussed separately in Chapter 11. The remaining group is heterogeneous and includes both generalized bone disorders as well as congenital malformations involving the hands. The group of generalized bone disorders consists of the bone dysplasias and certain disorders of bone metabolism with known biochemical defects, such as hypophosphatasia and the mucopolysaccharidoses. There are also many congenital disorders in which acquired hand manifestations may be seen.

DEFINITION

The term *congenital malformation syndrome* is not clearly defined. There are problems in the definition of all of its component words. The term *congenital* usually refers to being present since birth, although not all congenital conditions are

diagnosable at birth (for instance, many of the bone dysplasias). The term *malformation* is defined to mean a gross structural anomaly and, according to Warkany,[10] should not be used to include biochemical and other nonstructural changes. This limitation is not accepted by all authors. The term *syndrome* is even more difficult to define. Strictly speaking, any combination of anomalies in the patient may represent a syndrome. However, most authors consider a combination of anomalies to be a syndrome only if it is a relatively distinct combination, particularly if there is a familial tendency for this combination to occur or if the combination of findings is due to a single event during development or to a single biochemical cause. Obviously the distinction between the chance association of two or more anomalies and a syndrome is an artificial one.

It is well known that once an anomaly is present there is a significantly greater chance for another to exist. In a Swedish population, Källen and Winberg[4] found that the frequency of two malformations in a

244

single individual was 13 times the frequency expected from simple chance occurrence. The coincidental occurrence of three anomalies which occurred in a number of his patients is statistically even less likely. Even minor anomalies such as clinodactyly are more common in children who have other anomalies than in the general population.[6]

Birch-Jensen[2] has shown that radial aplasia is associated with a large number of other congenital abnormalities, including congenital heart disease, the Klippel-Feil deformity, esophageal atresia and cleft palate. The combination of radial aplasia and congenital heart disease is particularly common and thus could be considered a syndrome. Similarly, the association of radial aplasia and esophageal atresia could represent another syndrome, as could radial aplasia and the Klippel-Feil deformity. Obviously there are many combinations of two or more of these anomalies that could be considered to constitute separate congenital malformation syndromes. A syndrome nomenclature based on these associations would have little advantage because it would have no real genetic or etiologic meaning. Within this group, however, there is a heart–radial aplasia association which represents a more distinct syndrome, namely the Holt-Oram syndrome. It is inherited as an autosomal dominant and in many cases can be differentiated morphologically from simple radial aplasia and congenital heart disease.

VARIATIONS WITHIN THE CONGENITAL MALFORMATION SYNDROME

One of the problems in the definition of the congenital malformation syndromes is that there is variation within each entity and that similar entities may be due to different causes. The term "pleiotropism" is used to describe the varying phenotypic features, both radiologic and clinical, which may be due to one genetic factor, whereas the term "genetic heterogeneity" refers to similar phenotypes due to different causes.[5]

A good example of pleiotropism is the Holt-Oram syndrome, in which the manifestations may include an absent thumb, a hypoplastic thumb or even a triphalangeal thumb. In this situation, these are known to be variations within the same syndrome, since all three may occur in the same family and since different thumb manifestations may exist in the same patient. Another problem with the definition of the congenital malformation syndromes is that most of the clinical and radiologic signs are not present in 100 per cent of cases. This lack of uniformity is particularly bothersome when a syndrome is first described, since the so-called cardinal features may turn out not to be the most common ones once a larger group of patients is recognized. Again, a good example of this is the Holt-Oram syndrome in which the cardiac defect was originally thought to be an atrial shunt, but as more cases have been defined it has become apparent that ventricular defects may be as common and that some affected individuals have no shunt but may instead have pulmonary arterial hypertension or rhythmic disturbances.

GENETIC HETEROGENEITY

Because of the problems of pleiotropism it may be difficult to determine that a certain phenotype actually represents a single entity. The problem is particularly acute when no cause for the syndrome is known or when no clear-cut genetic pattern is evident. An example of the problem is in the definition of the Laurence-Moon-Biedl-Bardet syndrome. Some reports appeared in the literature describing congenital heart disease in this condition. It was only after Temtamy clearly defined the Carpenter syndrome that it was apparent that many of the cases with heart disease in the Laurence-Moon-Biedl-Bardet Syndrome were really examples of Carpenter's syndrome. Once this distinction was made, the two separate entities were much more clearly defined.

Often it is very difficult to define a syndrome simply on morphologic grounds, and genetic information is very helpful. An example of this is Hurler's disease, which was thought to include a broad spectrum of abnormality. When one form of the disorder was found to be X-linked in inheritance (Hunter's syndrome), it could then be separated from the group and its different clinical manifestations could then be identified. For example, in Hunter's syndrome no corneal clouding could be seen. Biochemical differences also allowed for further splitting of the Hurler-like group into different types (mucopolysaccharidoses I to VII). It was also found that some of these patients did not excrete mucopolysaccharides. These were eventually classified as various forms of the mucolipidoses. Although some differences in clinical phenotype were discovered before the biochemical changes were identified, it is only now that the biochemical changes are becoming known that the conditions are becoming more clearly delineated.

Not all disorders show distinct manifestations with distinct genetic forms of inheritance. The phenotypic manifestations may differ in severity. Generally speaking, the dominant form of a condition is less severe in its clinical manifestations than is the recessive form, while the X-linked form is usually intermediate.

SPLITTERS AND LUMPERS

There are two opposing trends in the nosology of the congenital malformation syndromes.[5] The "lumpers" try to find more things in common and put several entities in one large group, while the "splitters" tend to divide each entity into smaller and smaller fragments. Lumping appears logical because of the pleiotropism of many of the syndromes and because it is easier to find similarities than differences,[5] while splitting becomes necessary as genetic and biochemical heterogeneity becomes apparent.

Splitting into smaller groups is generally important when different genetic, etiologic or prognostic factors can be separated by this means. Splitting on purely morphologic grounds probably has little value, particularly when conditions are split so that each group contains only a few individuals or families.

PERCEPTIONS OF PATTERNS OF CONGENITAL ABNORMALITIES

Identification of a syndrome is a problem in pattern recognition, and it is complicated by the variation within each syndrome (pleiotropism) and by the common association of a variety of other abnormalities. As in all pattern recognition, once the pattern is known and becomes familiar it is easier to perceive.[3] Giedion's tricho-rhino-pha-

langeal syndrome illustrates this point. Children and adults with these abnormalities unquestionably were seen in a number of institutions prior to Giedion's description, but the association of an unusual nose, thin hair and certain characteristic roentgen changes in the hand had not been recognized. Once the pattern of abnormality was defined, many cases were found. For example, in our own files we were able to find three previously undiagnosed cases in which re-examination confirmed the classic clinical features of the nose and the hair of the tricho-rhino-phalangeal syndrome. Also, when a new patient appeared with both clinical and radiologic findings, he was quickly identified.

Since the congenital malformation syndromes are numerous and relatively rare, it is often difficult for anyone to remember many of the findings that make up the syndrome. Thus, reference texts are essential in diagnosis. A number of these have become available, some of which are listed at the end of this chapter.

CARDINAL FEATURES OF SYNDROMES

The definition of the important diagnostic signs or symptoms of a condition is very difficult because of the pleiotropism of many of these disorders. In the original description of a syndrome, the described cardinal features are limited somewhat by the interest of the observer. For example, an ophthalmologist may stress the eye changes while a radiologist may stress the bone manifestations. Also, in the early stages of description of a disease the cardinal features are defined from just a few cases and may not remain valid when a larger group is accumulated.

Probably no single sign should be considered essential in the diagnosis of a syndrome since in most cases no sign is present 100 per cent of the time. As Greenfield has stated, "A three-legged dog is still a dog." A problem in this regard occurs when an absent sign is included in the name of the syndrome. For example, in the oto-palato-digital syndrome, which was named for deafness, palatal defects and finger anomalies, we now find that some affected patients do not have deafness or palatal defects. They otherwise fit very well into the general syndrome and have relatives who have the more complete entity, while they themselves may only have the digital and spine findings. Similarly, in cleidocranial dysplasia we find no problem in accepting the diagnosis if the pelvic changes are absent; however, it is much more difficult to make the diagnosis when the clavicles are intact.

NOMENCLATURE AND CLASSIFICATION

The nomenclature of the malformation syndromes has been most confusing. A variety of approaches have been used to name these conditions. As a result, many of the disorders are each called by a number of names. Also, significant differences are evident in the terminology used in various countries.

Probably the oldest approach to naming the various congenital disorders has been the use of eponyms. This has the advantage that it does not assume what signs and symptoms are considered cardinal for the syndrome, nor what the etiologic or genetic considerations are. This is particularly important early in the description of a syndrome which may not yet be completely defined. One of the disadvantages of eponyms is that it is often difficult to determine whether it should be named after the individual who first described the condition, or after the individuals who better defined it. Various name combinations have been used, including the authors of an initial paper as in the Dyggve-Melchior-Clausen syndrome, or a list of names of people who contributed to the definition of the syndrome as in the Laurence-Moon-Biedl-Bardet syndrome. Although usually the last name of the author is used, occasionally the first name has been used as well, as in the Cornelia de Lange syndrome.

Another common approach to the nomenclature of syndromes has been the use of anatomic sites of involvement. Examples of this are the oto-palato-digital, the oculo-dento-digital and the hand-foot-uterus syndromes. In the bone dysplasias the conditions are often named after the portion of the bone that is affected; for example, diaphyseal dysplasia, metaphyseal chondrodysplasia and epiphyseal dysplasia. This approach is useful because it reminds one of the sites of abnormalities. One of the problems of this approach, however, is

that the findings are often not limited to the areas named in the syndrome and later it may turn out that other abnormalities are more commonly present or more significant. Also, the nomenclature may not be unique for the area described. For example, pyknodysostosis also has skull and clavicular changes and could therefore be considered a cleidocranial dysplasia.

Other more rarely used approaches to nomenclature have included the use of the patient's name for the disease, or names of cities in which the disease was discovered as in typus degenerativus Amstelodamensis — another name for the Cornelia de Lange syndrome.

Some conditions are named for biochemical manifestations, such as what is excreted in the urine, what the biochemical changes in the blood are or what the basic metabolic defect is. Examples of this include hyperuricosuria (the Lesch-Nyhan syndrome), homocystinuria and hypophosphatasia.

Other terminology is based on general clinical and pathologic findings. Many of the forms of dwarfism bear unusual names derived from Greek or Latin, such as diastrophic dwarfism, meaning crooked dwarfism, or metatropic dwarfism, meaning changing dwarfism.

An additional form of nomenclature of the syndromes has been used for splitting a syndrome when genetic heterogeneity has been discovered. An example of this is in the oro-facio-digital syndrome (OFD), in which an X-linked dominant and recessive form have been described which have some morphologic differences. These are now named the OFD I and OFD II syndromes. A similar split has been used in the nomenclature of the mucopolysaccharidoses, which are now known as types I through VII, although alternative eponymic names for the various forms also are used.

A STANDARD NOMENCLATURE

Because of multiple names used for each syndrome by various authors, some attempts have been made to devise a more uniform nomenclature. In 1970, a committee of the European Society of Pediatric Radiology, chaired by Maroteaux, described a nomenclature of intrinsic diseases of bone, reproduced in Table 12–1. This no-

TABLE 12-1. Constitutional (Intrinsic) Diseases of Bones*

CONSTITUTIONAL DISEASES OF BONES WITH UNKNOWN PATHOGENESIS

OSTEOCHONDRODYSPLASIA

(Abnomalities of cartilage and/or bone growth and development)

1) **Defects of growth of tubular bones and/or spine.**

A) *Manifested at birth.*
1 - Achondrogenesis.
2 - Thanatophoric dwarfism.
3 - Achondroplasia.
4 - Chondrodysplasia punctata (formerly stippled epiphysis), several forms.
5 - Metatropic dwarfism.
6 - Diastrophic dwarfism.
7 - Chondro-ectodermal dysplasia (ELLIS-VAN CREVELD).
8 - Asphyxiating thoracic dysplasia (JEUNE).
9 - Spondylo-epiphyseal dysplasia congenital.
10 - Mesomelic dwarfism, type NIEVERGELT, type LANGER.
11 - Cleido-cranial dysplasia (formerly cleido-cranial dysostosis).

B) *Manifested in later life.*
1 - Hypochondroplasia.
2 - Dyschondrosteosis.
3 - Metaphyseal chondro-dysplasia, type JANSEN.
4 - Metaphyseal chondro-dysplasia, type SCHMID.
5 - Metaphyseal chondro-dysplasia, type McKUSICK (formerly cartilage-hair hypoplasia).
6 - Metaphyseal chondro-dysplasia with malabsorption and neutropenia.
7 - Metaphyseal chondro-dysplasia with thymolymphopenia.
8 - Spondylo-metaphyseal dysplasia (KOZLOWSKI).
9 - Multiple epiphyseal dysplasia (several forms).
10 - Heriditary arthro-ophthalmopathy.
11 - Pseudo-achondroplasic dysplasia (formerly pseudo-achondroplasic type of spondylo-epiphyseal dysplasia).
12 - Spondylo-epiphyseal dysplasia tarda.
13 - Acrodysplasia :
   • Rhino-tricho-phalangeal syndrome (GIEDION) ;
   • epiphyseal (THIEMANN) ;
   • epiphyso-metaphyseal (BRAILSFORD).

2) **Disorganized development of cartilage and fibrous components of the skeleton.**

1 - Dysplasia epiphysealis hemimelica.
2 - Multiple cartilagenous exostoses.
3 - Enchondromatosis (OLLIER).
4 - Enchondromatosis with hemangioma (MAFFUCCI).
5 - Fibrous dysplasia (JAFFE-LICHTENSTEIN).
6 - Fibrous dysplasia with skin pigmentation and precocious puberty (McCUNE-ALBRIGHT).
7 - Cherubism.
8 - Multiple fibromatosis.

3) **Abnormalities of density, of cortical diaphyseal structure and/or of methaphyseal modeling.**

1 - Osteogenesis imperfecta congenita (VROLIK, PORAK-DURANTE).
2 - Osteogenesis imperfecta tarda (LOBSTEIN).
3 - Juvenile idiopathic osteoporosis.
4 - Osteopetrosis with precocious manifestations.
5 - Osteopetrosis with delayed manifestations.
6 - Pycnodysostosis.
7 - Osteopoikilosis.
8 - Melorheostosis.
9 - Diaphyseal dysplasia (CAMURATI-ENGELMANN).
10 - Cranio-diaphyseal dysplasia.
11 - Endosteal hyperostosis (VAN BUCHEM and other forms).
12 - Tubular stenosis (KENNY-CAFFEY).
13 - Osteodysplastia (MELNICK-NEEDLES).
14 - Pachydermoperiostosis.
15 - Osteo-ectasia with hyperphosphatasia.
16 - Metaphyseal dysplasia (PYLE).
17 - Cranio-metaphyseal dysplasia (several forms).
18 - Fronto-metaphyseal dysplasia.
19 - Oculo-dental-osseous dysplasia (formerly oculo-dento-digital syndrome).

DYSOSTOSES

(Malformation of individual bone, singly or in combination)

1) **Dysostoses with cranial and facial involvement.**

1 - Craniosynostosis, several forms.
2 - Cranio-facial dysostosis (CROUZON).
3 - Acrocephalo-syndactylia (APERT).
4 - Acrocephalo-polysyndactylia (CARPENTER).
5 - Mandibulo-facial dysostosis (TREACHER-COLLINS, FRANCESCHETTI and others).
6 - Mandibular hypoplasia (includes Pierre ROBIN Syndrome).
7 - Oculo-mandibulo-facial syndrome (HALLERMANN-STREIFF-FRANÇOIS).
8 - Nevoid basal cell carcinoma syndrome.

°From Maroteaux, P.: Nomenclature Internationale Des Maladies Osseuses Constitutionneles. *Ann. Radiol.,* 13:455–464, 1970.

TABLE 12–1. *Continued*

2) **Dysostoses with predominant axial involvement.**

1 - Vertebral segmentation defects (including KLIPPEL-FEIL).
2 - Cervico-oculo-acoustic syndrome (WILDER-VANCK).
3 - SPRENGEL deformity.

4 - Spondylo-costal dysostosis (several forms).

5 - Oculo-vertebral syndrome (WEYERS).
6 - Osteo-onychodysostosis (f o r m e r l y nail-patella-syndrome).

3) **Dysostoses with predominant involvement of extremities.**

1 - Amelia.
2 - Hemimelia (several types).
3 - Acheiria.
4 - Apodia.
5 - Adactylia and oligodactylia.
6 - Phocomelia.
7 - Aglossia-adactylia syndrome.
8 - Congenital bowing of long bones (several types).
9 - Familial radio-ulnar synostosis.
10 - Brachydactylia (several types).
11 - Symphalangism.
12 - Polydactylia (several types).
13 - Syndactylia (several types).
14 - Poly-syndactylia (several types).
15 - Camptodactylia.
16 - Clinodactylia.
17 - LAURENCE-MOON Syndrome.
18 - Popliteal pterygium syndrome.
19 - Pectoral aplasia-dysdactylia syndrome (POLAND).
20 - RUBINSTEIN-TAYBI syndrome.
21 - Pancytopenia-dysmelia syndrome (FANCONI).
22 - Thrombocytopenia-radial-aplasia syndrome.

23 - Oro-digito-facial syndrome (PAPILLON-LEAGE).
24 - Cardiomelic syndrome (HOLT-ORAM and others).

IDIOPATHIC OSTEOLYSES

1 - Acro-osteolysis :
 • Phalangeal type ;
 • Tarso-carpal form with or without nephropathy.
2 - Multicentric osteolysis.

PRIMARY DISTURBANCES OF GROWTH

1 - Primordial dwarfism (without associated malformation).
2 - CORNELIA DE LANGE's syndrome.
3 - Bird-headed dwarfism (VIRCHOW, SECKEL).

4 - Leprechaunism.

5 - RUSSELL-SILVER syndrome.
6 - Progeria.
7 - COCKAYNE's syndrome.
8 - BLOOM's syndrome.
9 - Geroderma osteodysplastica.
10 - Spherophakia-brachymorphia syndrome (WEILL-MARCHESANI).
11 - MARFAN's syndrome.

CONSTITUTIONAL DISEASES OF BONES
WITH KNOWN PATHOGENESIS

I. - CHROMOSOMAL ABERRATIONS

II. - PRIMARY METABOLIC ABNORMALITIES

1) **Calcium phosphorous metabolism.**

1 - Hypophosphatemic familial rickets.
2 - Pseudo-deficiency rickets (type ROYER, PRADER).
3 - Late rickets (type McCANCE).
4 - Idiopathic hypercalciuria.
5 - Hypophosphatasia (several forms).
6 - Idiopathic hypercalcemia.
7 - Pseudo-hypoparathyroïdism (n o r m o and hypercalcemic forms).

2) **Mucopolysaccharidosis.**

1 - Mucopolysaccharidosis I (HURLER).

2 - Mucopolysaccharidosis II (HUNTER).
3 - Mucopolysaccharidosis III (SANFILIPPO).
4 - Mucopolysaccharidosis IV (MORQUIO).
5 - Mucopolysaccharidosis V (ULLRICH-SCHEIE).
6 - Mucopolysaccharidosis VI (MAROTEAUX-LAMY).

3) **Mucolipidosis and lipidosis.**

1 - Mucolipidosis I (SPRANGER-WIEDEMANN).
2 - Mucolipidosis II (LEROY-OPITZ).
3 - Mucolipidosis III (Pseudo-polydystrophia).
4 - Fucosidosis.
5 - Mannosidosis.
6 - Generalised GM1 gangliosidosis (several forms).
7 - Sulfatidosis with mucopolysacchariduria (AUSTIN, THIEFFRY).
8 - Cerebrosidosis including GAUCHER's disease.

4) **Other metabolic extra-osseous disorders.**

BONY ABNORMALITIES
SECONDARY TO DISTURBANCES
OF EXTRA SKELETAL SYSTEMS

1 - Endocrine.
2 - Hematologic.
3 - Neurologic.
4 - Renal.
5 - Gastro-intestinal.
6 - Cardio-pulmonary.

menclature was subsequently approved by the Society of Pediatric Radiology in the United States and has been published in pediatric, orthopedic and radiologic journals. Although the list is as yet somewhat incomplete, it should serve as a useful basis for attaining the goal of a common terminology and will be used when possible in the subsequent chapter.

THE IMPORTANCE OF DIAGNOSIS OF THE MALFORMATION SYNDROMES

Since little more than symptomatic relief can usually be achieved therapeutically for most of the congenital malformation syndromes, the common reaction is "why bother to identify these conditions?" Unquestionably, the main importance of correct diagnosis is in genetic counseling. A good example of this is to be found in the short-limbed dwarfs, all of which were originally included in the category of achondroplasia. From this heterogeneous group many other conditions were isolated, including the presently distinct entities of achondroplasia, diastrophic dwarfism, metatropic dwarfism, thanatophoric dwarfism and achondrogenesis. Let us consider simply the importance of separating two of these conditions, achondroplasia, which has a dominant inheritance, and diastrophic dwarfism, which is recessive. Parents of a child with achondroplasia, if they are unaffected, are extremely unlikely to have another achondroplastic infant. The occurrence of achondroplasia must have been the result of a new mutation. Unaffected parents, on the other hand, who have a diastrophic dwarf have a 25 per cent chance of subsequent children being affected, since here we are dealing with a recessive gene.

Correct diagnosis is also important in advising the affected individual of his future genetic risk. Thus, the achondroplastic patient would have a 50 per cent chance of having an achondroplastic child with each birth if he or she marries a normal individual. The diastrophic dwarf, having a recessive condition, would with a normal spouse have very little chance of producing affected offspring.

Correct diagnosis may also be important in the medical care of the affected individual. If the patient is achondroplastic, knowing that he may be very prone to spinal cord compression will result in greater vigilance in detecting early signs and lead to more aggressive therapy of disc disease. Also, identification of some of the stigmata of the syndrome, like a thumb in the Holt-Oram syndrome, may lead to the detection of heart disease, both in the individual and in other members of the family.

THE HAND IN THE CONGENITAL MALFORMATION SYNDROMES

Abnormalities of the hand are common in various congenital malformation syndromes. In some of these the malformations are due to generalized bone disease and simply reflect the changes seen in other portions of the skeleton. Examples are osteopetrosis, metaphyseal chondrodysplasia and most of the other so-called bone dysplasias. In other conditions, however, various anomalies of the hand occur. Although many of these are nonspecific, some are characteristic of the disorder, as in the oto-palato-digital syndrome, where the combination of carpal and metacarpal changes is probably unique. In some of the other congenital malformation syndromes, acquired changes may occur in the hand bones and can be helpful in diagnosis. For example, the erosions of the phalanges in the Lesch-Nyhan syndrome are not diagnostic, but their presence indicates that we are dealing with a certain small group of disorders.

Patterns of Hand Abnormalities

The pattern of radiologic change in various hand anomalies can be diagnostically useful. For example, hypoplasia of the thumb can be due to a wide range of conditions, including the Holt-Oram syndrome, Fanconi's anemia, thalidomide embryopathy, myositis ossificans progressiva and diastrophic dwarfism. This large list of causes of small thumbs can be narrowed down considerably depending on which bones of the thumb are involved. For example, the small thumb may be due to a short distal phalanx as in the oto-palato-digital syndrome, or to a short metacarpal as in Fanconi's anemia. The short metacarpal may be thick as in Cornelia de Lange's syndrome, or thin as in Fanconi's anemia. Tables listing some of the causes of shortening and lengthening of the various hand bones are listed in Chapter 9.

Part of the pattern approach of the diagnosis of hand abnormalities also involves examining the remainder of the hand. The association of various anomalies in the hand, although in themselves not specific, may be diagnostic when combined. For example, hypoplasia of the thumb with hypoplasia of the entire fifth finger usually suggests the Cornelia de Lange syndrome, while hypoplasia of the thumb associated with multiple extra carpals, epiphyseal abnormalities and a hitchhiker's position of the thumb suggests diastrophic dwarfism.

Some of the minor normal variants of the hand may also be useful in diagnosis. Clinodactyly, which is present in a significant percentage of normal people, can be useful diagnostically if accompanied by other roentgen signs. For example, asymmetric growth, maturational retardation and clinodactyly usually suggest the diagnosis of Silver's syndrome. Even acquired changes in the hand which occur in some congenital conditions can be useful diagnostically. Tuft erosion and sclerosis of bone each can be seen in a number of entities, while when these two findings occur together the diagnosis of pyknodysostosis is likely. The tables in Chapters 6 through 10 list the conditions associated with the variants and anomalies of the hand.

Measurement of the Hand Bones

Alterations in length of the various hand bones are useful diagnostically, and when gross they can be easily perceived on simple examination of the hand radiograph. Subtle changes in length, however, may be not be evident even to the experienced examiner, and the use of other techniques, such as pattern profile analysis or ratios described in Chapter 2, may be useful in diagnosis. These methods are particularly important in conditions where the clinical manifestations are mild, they may be necessary to determine whether an individual is affected. For example, we have seen a case of Larsen's syndrome where the radiologic finding of an increased number of carpal bones was not present but in whom the clinical findings were very suggestive. On pattern profile analysis the similarity between the mean and the condition was dramatic (Fig. 13–81). We now have established pattern profile means for a number of conditions, and when available these will be discussed or illustrated in Chapter 13. In many syndromes, however, only a few cases have been reported, and the amount of clinical material available has not allowed us to depict an adequate mean at this time.

The hand obviously cannot be diagnostic in every condition, and a diagnosis should only be made by evaluation of the total patient, including clinical, radiologic, genetic and biochemical studies. However, it is remarkable how often the hand is the mirror of congenital malformation syndromes and how often much information can be gained from a simple hand radiograph.

In the next chapter we will consider a number of congenital malformation syndromes. Rather than grouping them into poorly defined categories, they will be listed in alphabetical order using the European Society's classification nomenclature when available. Certainly not all of the syndromes that have hand manifestations can be discussed; considered will be those in which the hand changes have some value in diagnosis, and those for which sufficient information is available regarding the roentgen findings in the hand.

REFERENCES

1. Allan, W.: Relation of Hereditary Pattern to Clinical Severity as Illustrated by Peroneal Atrophy. *Arch. Int. Med.*, 63:1123–1131, 1939.
2. Birch-Jensen A.: *Congenital Deformities of the Upper Extremities.* Andelsbogtrykkeriet, Odense, Denmark, 1949.
3. Hebb, D. O., and Favreau, O.: The Mechanism of Perception. *Radiol. Clin. N. Am.*, 7:393–401, 1969.
4. Källén, B., and Winberg, J.: A Swedish Register of Congenital Malformations. Experience with Continuous Registration During 2 Years with Special Reference to Multiple Malformations. *Pediatrics*, 41:765–776, 1968.
5. McKusick, V. A.: On Lumpers and Splitters, or the Nosology of Genetic Disease. *Perspect. Biol. Med.*, 12:298–312, 1969.

6. Marden, P. M., Smith, D. W., and McDonald, M. J.: Congenital Anomalies in the Newborn Infant, Including Minor Variations. A Study of 4,412 Babies by Surface Examination for Anomalies and Buccal Smear for Sex Chromatin. *J. Pediatr.*, 64:357–371, 1964.
7. Maroteaux, P.: Nomenclature Internationale Des Maladies Osseuses Constitutionnelles. *Ann. Radiol.*, 13:455–464, 1970.
8. Pinsky, L., and Fraser, F. C.: Atypical Malformation Syndromes. *J. Pediatr.*, 80:141–144, 1972.
9. Smith, D. W.: Recognizable Patterns of Malformation in Childhood. *Birth Defects: Original Article Series*, 5:255–272, 1969.
10. Warkany, J.: Syndromes. *Am. J. Dis. Child.*, 121: 365–370, 1971.

TEXTBOOKS ON THE CONGENITAL MALFORMATION SYNDROMES AND BONE DYSPLASIAS

Bailey, J. A.: *Disproportionate Short Stature. Diagnosis and Management*. W. B. Saunders Company, Philadelphia, 1973.

Birth Defects: Original Article Series. Many parts now available. The Williams and Wilkins Company, Baltimore.

Gellis, S. S., and Feingold, M.: *Atlas of Mental Retardation Syndromes. Visual Diagnosis of Facies and Physical Findings*. U. S. Department of Health, Education and Welfare, Washington, D.C., 1968.

Gorlin, R. J., and Pindborg, J. J.: *Syndromes of the Head and Neck*, McGraw-Hill Book Company, New York, 1964.

Holmes, L. B., Moser, H. W., Halldorsson, S., Mack, C., Pant, S. S., and Matzilevich, B.: *Mental Retardation. An Atlas of Diseases with Associated Physical Abnormalities*. The Macmillan Company, New York, 1972.

Kaufman, H. J. (Ed.): *Progress in Pediatric Radiology*. Vol. 4, *Intrinsic Diseases of Bones*. S. Karger, Basel, 1973.

McKusick, V. A.: *Heritable Disorders of Connective Tissue*. The C. V. Mosby Company, St. Louis, 1972.

McKusick, V. A.: *Mendelian Inheritance in Man. Catalogs of Autosomal Dominant, Autosomal Recessive, and X-Linked Phenotypes*, 3rd Ed. The Johns Hopkins Press, Baltimore, 1971.

Rubin, P.: *Dynamic Classification of Bone Dysplasias*. Year Book Medical Publishers, Inc., Chicago, 1964.

Smith, D. W.: *Recognizable Patterns of Human Malformation*. W. B. Saunders Company, Philadelphia, 1970.

Spranger, J. W., Langer, L., and Wiedemann, H.-R.: *Bone Dysplasias: An Atlas of Constitutional Disorders of Skeletal Development*. W. B. Saunders Company, Philadelphia, 1974.

Waardenburg, P. J., Franceschetti, A., and Klein, D.: *Genetics and Ophthalmology*. Royal VanGorcum Ltd., Assen, Netherlands, 1961.

Warkany, J.: *Congenital Malformations. Notes and Comments*. Year Book Medical Publishers, Inc., Chicago, 1971.

Chapter 13

SPECIFIC CONGENITAL MALFORMATION SYNDROMES

AARSKOG SYNDROME (AARSKOG-SCOTT SYNDROME, FACIO-DIGITO-GENITAL SYNDROME)
ACHONDROGENESIS (PARENTI DISEASE)
ACHONDROPLASIA (CHONDRODYSTROPHIA FETALIS)
ACROCEPHALOPOLYSYNDACTYLY (CARPENTER SYNDROME)
ACROCEPHALOSYNDACTYLY
   Acrocephalosyndactyly — Typical (Types I and II, Apert Syndrome, Apert-Crouzon Syndrome)
   Acrocephalosyndactyly — Other Types (Type II, Saethre-Chotzen; Type IV, Waardenburg; Type V, Pfeiffer; and Others)
ACRODYSOSTOSIS
ACROOSTEOLYSIS — CARPOTARSAL FORM
ACROOSTEOLYSIS — PHALANGEAL (CHENEY SYNDROME)
ACRO-PECTORO-VERTEBRAL DYSPLASIA (F-SYNDROME)
AGLOSSIA-ADACTYLY SYNDROME
ANKYLOGLOSSIA SUPERIOR (GLOSSOPALATINE ANKYLOSIS)
ARTHROGRYPOSIS
ARTHROOPHTHALMOPATHY (HEREDITARY PROGRESSIVE ARTHROOPHTHALMOPATHY, STICKLER SYNDROME)
ASPHYXIATING THORACIC DYSPLASIA (JEUNE DISEASE, THORACIC-PELVIC-PHALANGEAL DYSTROPHY)
BECKWITH-WIEDEMANN SYNDROME (EXOMPHALOS-MACROGLOSSIA-GIGANTISM SYNDROME, EMG SYNDROME, SYNDROME OF HYPERPLASTIC FETAL VISCEROMEGALY)
BIEDMOND SYNDROME I
BIEDMOND SYNDROME II
BLACKFAN-DIAMOND ANEMIA (CONGENITAL HYPOPLASTIC ANEMIA)
CEREBRAL GIGANTISM
CEREBRO-HEPATO-RENAL SYNDROME (CHRS, ZELLWEGER SYNDROME)
CHONDRODYSPLASIA PUNCTATA (CHONDRODYSTROPHIA CALCIFICANS CONGENITA, STIPPLED EPIPHYSES)
CHONDROECTODERMAL DYSPLASIA (ELLIS — VAN CREVELD SYNDROME)
CHRISTIAN BRACHYDACTYLY SYNDROME (DOMINANT PREAXIAL BRACHYDACTYLY)
CLEIDOCRANIAL DYSPLASIA (CLEIDOCRANIAL DYSOSTOSIS, MARIE-SAINTON SYNDROME, MUTATIONAL DYSOSTOSIS)
CLOVERLEAF SKULL (KLEEBLATTSCHÄDEL DEFORMITY SYNDROME)
COCKAYNE SYNDROME
COFFIN-SIRIS SYNDROME

COFFIN-SIRIS-WEGIENKA SYNDROME
CRANIOFACIAL DYSOSTOSIS (CROUZON DISEASE)
CRANIOMETAPHYSEAL DYSPLASIA (METAPHYSEAL DYSPLASIA, PYLE DISEASE)
CRYPTODONTIC BRACHYMETACARPALIA
CRYPTOPHTHALMOS SYNDROME
DE LANGE SYNDROME (BRACHMANN-DE LANGE SYNDROME, CORNELIA DE LANGE SYNDROME, TYPUS DEGENERATIVUS AMSTELODAMENSIS)
DIAPHYSEAL DYSPLASIA (ENGELMANN-CAMURATI DISEASE)
DIASTROPHIC DWARFISM
DYGGVE-MELCHIOR-CLAUSEN SYNDROME (MORQUIO-ULLRICH DISEASE)
DYSCHONDROSTEOSIS (LÉRI-WEILL SYNDROME)
DYSOSTEOSCLEROSIS
DYSPLASIA EPIPHYSEALIS HEMIMELICA
ECTODERMAL DYSPLASIA
ENCHONDROMATOSIS (OLLIER DISEASE, DYSCHONDROPLASIA)
ENCHONDROMATOSIS WITH HEMANGIOMA (MAFFUCCI SYNDROME)
ENDOSTEAL HYPEROSTOSIS (VAN BUCHEM DISEASE, HYPEROSTOSIS CORTICALIS GENERALISATA)
EPIDERMOLYSIS BULLOSA
EPIPHYSEAL DYSPLASIA (MULTIPLE EPIPHYSEAL DYSPLASIA, DYSPLASIA EPIPHYSEALIS MULTIPLEX, FAIRBANK DISEASE)
FARBER DISEASE (LIPOGRANULOMATOSIS)
FIBROUS DYSPLASIA (JAFFE-LICHTENSTEIN DISEASE, WITH SEXUAL PRECOCITY — THE McCUNE-ALBRIGHT SYNDROME)
FOCAL DERMAL HYPOPLASIA (GOLTZ SYNDROME)
FRONTODIGITAL SYNDROME
FRONTOMETAPHYSEAL DYSPLASIA
GM$_1$ GANGLIOSIDOSIS, TYPE I (NEUROVISCERAL STORAGE DISEASE, NEUROVISCERAL LIPIDOSIS, INFANTILE GENERALIZED GANGLIOSIDOSIS, PSEUDO-HURLER)
HAND-FOOT-UTERUS SYNDROME
HOLT-ORAM SYNDROME AND OTHER CARDIOMELIC SYNDROMES
HOMOCYSTINURIA
HYPERCALCEMIA — INFANTILE (HYPERCALCEMIA — SUPRAVALVULAR AORTIC STENOSIS SYNDROME)
HYPOCHONDROPLASIA
HYPOPHOSPHATASIA
INSENSITIVITY TO PAIN — CONGENITAL (CONGENITAL INDIFFERENCE TO PAIN, CONGENITAL ANALGIA)
JUBERG-HAYWARD SYNDROME
JUVENILE IDIOPATHIC OSTEOPOROSIS (JUVENILE OSTEOPOROSIS)

KASCHIN-BECK DISEASE
KEUTEL SYNDROME
KLIPPEL-TRENAUNAY-WEBER SYNDROME (PARKES WEBER SYNDROME, ANGIO-OSTEOHYPERTROPHIC SYNDROME, OSTEOHYPERTROPHIC-VARICOSE NEVUS SYNDROME)
KNIEST DWARFISM
LARSEN SYNDROME
LAURENCE-MOON-BIEDL-BARDET SYNDROME
LENTIGINES SYNDROME (LEOPARD SYNDROME)
LENZ MICROPHTHALMIA SYNDROME
LERI PLEONOSTEOSIS
LESCH-NYHAN SYNDROME (CONGENITAL HYPERURICOSURIA)
LIEBENBERG SYNDROME
LIPODYSTROPHY — CONGENITAL, TOTAL
MANDIBULOACRAL DYSPLASIA
MANDIBULOFACIAL DYSOSTOSIS (TREACHER COLLINS SYNDROME)
MARFAN SYNDROME
MARSHALL SYNDROME
MECKEL SYNDROME (DYSENCEPHALIA SPLANCHNOCYSTICA)
MELORHEOSTOSIS
MENKES SYNDROME (KINKY HAIR SYNDROME)
MESOMELIC DWARFISM — TYPE LANGER (MESOMELIC DWARFISM OF THE HYPOPLASTIC ULNA, FIBULA, MANDIBLE TYPE)
METAPHYSEAL CHONDRODYSPLASIA — TYPE JANSEN
METAPHYSEAL CHONDRODYSPLASIA (METAPHYSEAL DYSOSTOSIS) — OTHER TYPES
METATROPIC DWARFISM
MÖBIUS SYNDROME (CONGENITAL FACIAL DIPLEGIA)
MUCOLIPIDOSIS II (I-CELL DISEASE, LEROY DISEASE)
MUCOLIPIDOSIS III (PSEUDO-HURLER POLYDYSTROPHY)
MUCOPOLYSACCHARIDOSES (HURLER'S SYNDROME, HUNTER'S SYNDROME, SANFILIPPO SYNDROME, MAROTEAUX-LAMY)
MUCOPOLYSACCHARIDOSIS IV (MORQUIO DISEASE, MORQUIO-BRAILSFORD DISEASE)
MULTIPLE CARTILAGINOUS EXOSTOSES (DIAPHYSEAL ACLASIS, MULTIPLE OSTEOCHONDROMAS, CARTILAGINOUS EXOSTOSES, DEFORMING CHONDROPLASIA)
MULTIPLE FIBROMATOSIS (GENERALIZED HAMARTOMATOSIS, STOUT FIBROMATOSIS)
MYOSITIS OSSIFICANS PROGRESSIVA (FIBRODYSPLASIA OSSIFICANS PROGRESSIVA)
NEUROFIBROMATOSIS
NEVOID BASAL CELL CARCINOMA (BASAL CELL NEVUS SYNDROME)
NOONAN SYNDROME (MALE TURNER, TURNER PHENOTYPE)
OCULO-CEREBRO-RENAL SYNDROME (LOWE SYNDROME)
OCULO-DENTO-OSSEOUS DYSPLASIA (OCULO-DENTO-DIGITAL SYNDROME)
ORO-DIGITO-FACIAL SYNDROME, TYPE I (PAPILLON-LÉAGE AND PSAUME SYNDROME, ORO-FACIO-DIGITAL SYNDROME I, OFD I)
ORO-DIGITO-FACIAL SYNDROME, TYPE II (MOHR SYNDROME, ORO-FACIO-DIGITAL II, OFD II)

OSTEOECTASIA WITH HYPERPHOSPHATASIA
OSTEOGENESIS IMPERFECTA (CONGENITA FORM — VROLIK'S DISEASE, FRAGILITAS OSSIUM, OSTEOPSATHYROSIS; TARDA FORM — LOBSTEIN DISEASE)
OSTEO-ONYCHO-DYSOSTOSIS (NAIL-PATELLA SYNDROME, ONYCHO-OSTEO-ARTHRO-DYSPLASIA)
OSTEOPATHIA STRIATA
OSTEOPETROSIS (ALBERS-SCHÖNBERG DISEASE, MARBLE BONE DISEASE)
OTO-PALATO-DIGITAL SYNDROME (OPD SYNDROME, TAYBI SYNDROME)
PACHYDERMOPERIOSTOSIS (IDIOPATHIC HYPERTROPHIC OSTEOARTHROPATHY, FAMILIAL IDIOPATHIC OSTEOARTHROPATHY)
PANCYTOPENIA-DYSMELIA SYNDROME (FANCONI ANEMIA)
PARASTREMMATIC DWARFISM
PECTORAL APLASIA–DYSDACTYLY SYNDROME (POLAND SYNDROME, PECTORAL MUSCLE ABSENCE AND SYNDACTYLY SYNDROME)
POPLITEAL-PTERYGIUM SYNDROME (POPLITEAL WEB SYNDROME)
PORPHYRIA — CONGENITAL
PRADER-WILLI SYNDROME
PROGERIA (HUTCHINSON-GILFORD SYNDROME)
PSEUDOACHONDROPLASTIC DYSPLASIA (PSEUDOACHONDROPLASTIC SPONDYLOEPIPHYSEAL DYSPLASIA)
PSEUDOTHALIDOMIDE SYNDROME (SC SYNDROME)
PSEUDOXANTHOMA ELASTICUM (PXE)
PYCNODYSOSTOSIS (PYKNODYSOSTOSIS)
ROTHMUND SYNDROME (ROTHMUND-THOMSON SYNDROME)
RUBINSTEIN-TAYBI SYNDROME (BROAD THUMBS SYNDROME)
RUDIGER SYNDROME
RUVALCABA SYNDROME
SALDINO-NOONAN SYNDROME (SHORT-RIB POLYSYNDACTYLY, SALDINO-NOONAN TYPE)
SCALP DEFECTS AND HAND ANOMALIES
SCLEROSTEOSIS
SECKEL DWARFS (BIRD-HEADED DWARFS, VIRCHOW-SECKEL DWARFS)
SILVER SYNDROME (RUSSELL-SILVER DWARF)
SMITH-LEMLI-OPITZ SYNDROME
SPHEROPHAKIA BRACHYMORPHIA (MARCHESANI SYNDROME, WEILL-MARCHESANI SYNDROME, CONGENITAL MESODERMAL DYSMORPHODYSTROPHY)
SPONDYLOEPIPHYSEAL DYSPLASIA CONGENITA
SPONDYLOMETAPHYSEAL DYSPLASIA (KOZLOWSKI)
THANATOPHORIC DWARFISM
THIEMANN DISEASE (EPIPHYSEAL ACRODYSPLASIA — THIEMANN, OSTEOCHONDROPATHY OF THE FINGERS)
THROMBOCYTOPENIA–RADIAL APLASIA SYNDROME (THROMBOCYTOPENIA–RADIAL HYPOPLASIA SYNDROME, THROMBOCYTOPENIA–ABSENT RADIUS SYNDROME, TAR SYNDROME, THROMBOCYTOPENIA-PHOCOMELIA SYNDROME)
TRICHO-RHINO-PHALANGEAL SYNDROME (GIEDION SYNDROME, ACRODYSPLASIA)
TUBEROUS SCLEROSIS

TUBULAR STENOSIS (KENNY-CAFFEY SYNDROME, MEDULLARY STENOSIS SYNDROME)
UNILATERAL ECTROMELIA — ICHTHYOSIS SYNDROME
WERNER SYNDROME

WHISTLING FACE SYNDROME (FREEMAN-SHELDON SYNDROME, CRANIO-CARPO-TARSAL DYSPLASIA)
ZIMMERMANN-LABAND SYNDROME

AARSKOG SYNDROME (AARSKOG-SCOTT SYNDROME, FACIO-DIGITO-GENITAL SYNDROME)

This is a pattern of malformations that includes short stature, abnormal facies, hand and foot abnormalities and an unusual scrotal skin configuration that encircles the penis ventrally. The facial findings include a round face with hypertelorism, antimongoloid slanting of the palpebral fissures, maxillary hypoplasia and broadening of the nasal bridge with a short stubby nose and anteverted nostrils. The patients often have a widow's peak. The condition is inherited as an autosomal dominant with partial expression in affected women.

RADIOLOGIC FINDINGS IN THE HAND. A variety of hand abnormalities may be seen, among them mild syndactyly, clinodactyly, camptodactyly, simian creases and a peculiar positioning of the fingers. Sometimes a single crease is seen in a short fifth finger. According to Sugarman et al.,[4] the thumbs are usually short with limitation of abduction. Simian creases are common. The hands have an unusual profile when extended: the distal interphalangeal joints are flexed and the proximal interphalangeal joints are hyperextended.

OTHER RADIOLOGIC FINDINGS. Foot abnormalities have been described, including an appearance which apparently has been similar to that seen in the oto-palato-digital syndrome, although published radiographs are not available.[4] Scott's cases[3] showed some cervical spine abnormalities, with hypoplasia of the arch of C1 and abnormalities of the odontoid process.

REFERENCES

1. Aarskog, D.: A Familial Syndrome of Short Stature Associated with Facial Dysplasia and Genital Anomalies. *J. Pediatr.*, 77:856–861, 1970.
2. Furukawa, C. T., Hall, B. D., and Smith, D. W.: The Aarskog Syndrome. *J. Pediatr.*, 81:1117–1122, 1972.
3. Scott, C. I.: Unusual Facies, Joint Hypermobility, Genital Anomaly and Short Stature: A New Dysmorphic Syndrome. *Birth Defects, Original Article Series*, 7:240–246, 1971.
4. Sugarman, G. I., Rimoin, D. L., and Lachman, R. S.: The Facial-Digital-Genital (Aarskog) Syndrome. *Am. J. Dis. Child.*, 126:248–252, 1973.

ACHONDROGENESIS (PARENTI'S DISEASE)

This is a usually fatal form of neonatal dwarfism. The head is disproportionately

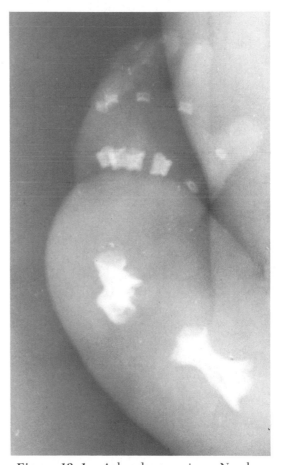

Figure 13–1. Achondrogenesis. Newborn. There is marked shortening of all of the bones in the upper extremity, including those of the hand. The bones are sharply cupped.

large, the extremities are very small and the trunk is diminished in size. It may be clinically difficult to differentiate from thanatophoric dwarfism. Another condition has also been called achondrogenesis (Grebe form),[3] but this is a different entity which is manifested by severe hypoplasia of the extremities and digits and which is incompatible with life. The genetics of achondrogenesis is not clear; however, Saldino reported two affected siblings and it is thus probably transmitted as autosomal recessive.

RADIOLOGIC FINDINGS IN THE HAND. There is very little ossification in the hand bones, which are very short and slightly cupped (Fig. 13-1). From the hand alone it may be difficult to differentiate achondrogenesis from thanatophoric dwarfism.

OTHER RADIOLOGIC FINDINGS. The spine changes of achondrogenesis are probably the most characteristic and allow differentiation from thanatophoric dwarfism. There is almost complete absence of ossification of the vertebral bodies. There is also a lack of sacral ossification, and the iliac bones are small. All of the long bones are markedly shortened. The skull is unremarkable.

REFERENCES

1. Fraccaro, M.: Contributo Allo Studio Delle Malattie Del Mesenchima Osteopoietico L'Acondrogenesi. *Folia Hered. Pathol.*, 1:190–207, 1952.
2. Freire-Maia, N., and Lenz, W. D.: Discussion. *Birth Defects, Original Article Series*, 5:14–16, 1969.
3. Grebe, H.: Die Achondrogenesis Ein Einfach Rezessives Erbmerkmal. *Folia Hered. Pathol.*, 2:23–29, 1952.
4. Houston, C. S., Awen C. F., and Kent, H. P.: Fatal Neonatal Dwarfism. *J. Can. Assoc, Radiol.*, 23:45–61, 1972.
5. Parenti, G. C.: La Anosteogenesi. (Una Varietà della Osteogenesi Imperfetta). *Pathologica*, 28:447–462, 1936.
6. Saldino, R. M.: Lethal Short-Limbed Dwarfism: Achondrogenesis and Thanatophoric Dwarfism. *Am. J. Roentgenol.*, 112:185–197, 1971.

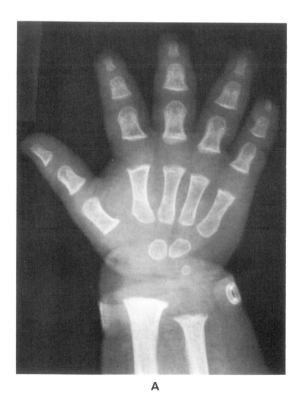

A

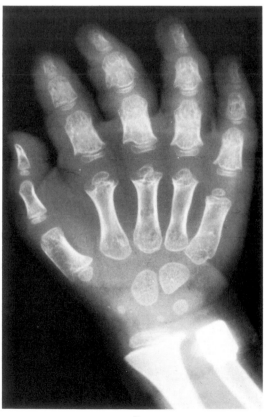

B

Figure 13–2. *A*, Achondroplasia. Infant at 11 months. The digits are short. The fingers are spread in a trident configuration. There is minimal irregularity of the bone ends.

B, There is metaphyseal irregularity and some cupping; these are less common manifestations of achondroplasia. (Courtesy Dr. William McAlistair, St. Louis, Missouri.)

ACHONDROPLASIA (CHONDRODYSTROPHIA FETALIS)

This is one of the most common and best known forms of short-limbed dwarfism. It is evident at birth. Although in the past most cases of short-limbed dwarfism were included under this term, it is now felt that achondroplasia is a distinct entity. The affected individuals usually have normal intelligence and normal activity. They have a typical facial appearance with a flat nasal bridge and a prominent forehead. Histologic studies by Rimoin et al.[3] have shown that the endochondral ossification is regular in achondroplasia and that the defect may be a quantitative decrease in the rate of endochondral ossification. The condition is inherited as an autosomal dominant.

RADIOLOGIC FINDINGS IN THE HAND. The hand may have a trident shape, particularly in infancy, and there is an inability to approximate the fingers in extension (Fig. 13–2A). There is shortening of the hand bones, particularly the second, third and fourth metacarpals and proximal phalanges, with a fairly consistent profile pattern (Fig. 13–4). Occasionally, in severe cases there is some cupping of the epiphyses and there may be metaphyseal irregularity as well (Fig. 13–2B). However, the appearance may be not very specific, and the diagnosis from the hand film alone may be difficult (Fig. 13–3). It may be difficult to differentiate this entity from hypochondroplasia, in which similar but even milder findings are present (Figs. 13–70 and 13–71), and the pattern profile is less specific.

The cortical thickness in achondroplasia

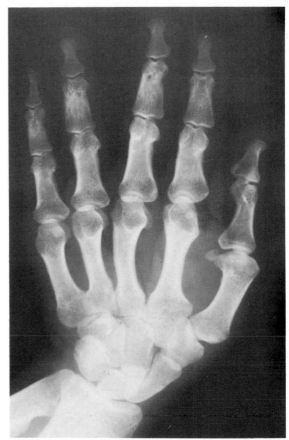

Figure 13–3. Achondroplasia. 33 year old. The tubular bones are short but well formed.

is slightly decreased when compared to normals. It was 1.27 standard deviations below the mean normal value in 68 patients, while the percentage of cortical area was 1.64 standard deviations below the mean.

OTHER RADIOLOGIC FINDINGS. The pelvic wings have a characteristic appear-

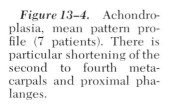

Figure 13–4. Achondroplasia, mean pattern profile (7 patients). There is particular shortening of the second to fourth metacarpals and proximal phalanges.

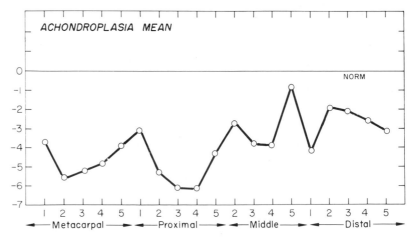

ance, particularly in infancy, with a flat acetabular angle and a squarish ilium with shortening of the distal portion; the appearance is that of a paddle without a handle. There is narrowing of the interpediculate distance from L1 to L5. There is some narrowing in the anteroposterior diameter of the chest. The shortening of the extremities is usually rhizomelic, with the humeri being relatively shorter than the bones of the forearm. The calvarium appears large, particularly in relation to the base of the skull.

REFERENCES

1. Bailey, J. A.: Orthopaedic Aspects of Achondroplasia. *J. Bone Joint Surg.*, 52A:1285–1301, 1970.
2. Langer, L. O., Jr., Baumann, P. A., and Gorlin, R. J.: Achondroplasia. *Am. J. Roentgenol.* 100:12–26, 1967.
3. Rimoin, D. L., Hughes, G. N., Kaufman, R. L., Rosenthal, R. E., McAlister, W. H., and Silberberg, R.: Endochondral Ossification in Achondroplastic Dwarfism. *N. Engl. J. Med.*, 283:728–735, 1970.
4. Silverman, F. N., and Brünner, S.: Errors in the Diagnosis of Achondroplasia. *Acta Radiol.*, 6:305–321, 1967.
5. Silverman, F. N.: Achondroplasia. *Progr. Pediatr. Radiol.*, 4:94–124, 1973. (*Intrinsic Diseases of Bones*, edited by H. J. Kaufmann, Karger, Basel.)

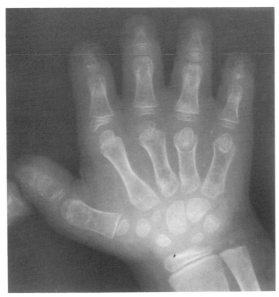

Figure 13–5. Acrocephalopolysyndactyly (Carpenter syndrome). Five year old male. There is a broad short thumb with a small ossicle adjacent to it. The middle phalanges of the fingers are severely shortened or absent. Cone epiphyses are seen in some of the metacarpals.

ACROCEPHALOPOLYSYNDACTYLY (CARPENTER SYNDROME)

This is a syndrome of acrocephaly, peculiar facies, mild syndactyly of the fingers, preaxial polydactyly, syndactyly of the toes, hypogenitalism, obesity, and mental retardation. Congenital heart disease is seen in a significant proportion of cases, as are abdominal hernias. This syndrome has previously been confused with Apert syndrome and with the Laurence-Moon-Biedl-Bardet syndrome. This condition is inherited as an autosomal recessive. A form of acrocephalopolysyndactyly with dominant inheritance has been reported by Noack, but this is probably a different condition.

RADIOLOGIC FINDINGS IN THE HAND. There is usually minimal soft tissue syndactyly, mainly between the third and fourth fingers. The phalanges are short, particularly the middle phalanges (Figs. 13–5 to 13–7). Curvature of the fingers is common. The thumb may be broad and in older individuals there may be a double ossification of the proximal phalanx (Fig. 13–6*B*). In some ways this extra ossicle could be considered a form of polydactyly, but a separate digit in the region of the thumb is usually not seen.

OTHER RADIOLOGIC FINDINGS. There is preaxial polydactyly of the feet, syndactyly of the toes and pes varus. The skull findings include coronal suture synostosis, but other sutures may also be affected. The skull findings are somewhat variable.

REFERENCES

1. Carpenter, G.: Two Sisters Showing Malformations of the Skull and Other Congenital Abnormalities. *Rep. Soc. Study Dis. Child.*, 1:110–118, 1900–1901.
2. McKusick, V. A.: *Mendelian Inheritance in Man. Catalogs of Autosomal Dominant, Autosomal Recessive, and X-Linked Phenotypes*, 3rd Ed. The Johns Hopkins Press, Baltimore, 1971.
3. Noack, M.: Ein Beitrag zum Krankheitsbild der Akrozephalosyndaktylie (Apert). *Arch. Kinderheilk.*, 160:168–171, 1959.
4. Palacios, E., and Schimke, R. N.: Craniosynostosis-Syndactylism. *Am. J. Roentgenol.*, 106:144–155, 1969.
5. Poznanski, A. K., Garn, S. M., and Holt, J. F.: The Thumb in the Congenital Malformation Syndromes. *Radiology*, 100:115–129, 1971.
6. Temtamy, S. A.: Carpenter's Syndrome: Acrocephalopolysyndactyly. An Autosomal Recessive Syndrome. *J. Pediatr.*, 69:111–120, 1960.

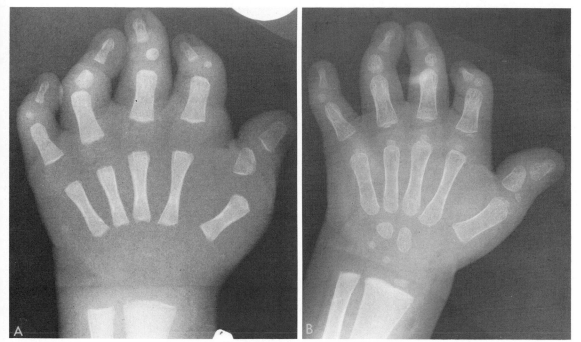

Figure 13–6. Acrocephalopolysyndactyly (Carpenter syndrome). *A,* One month old infant. Note hypoplasia of the middle phalanges and the unusual proximal phalanx of the thumb. There was polydactyly of the feet. (From Poznanski, A. K., et al.: *Radiology,* 100:115–129, 1971.)

B, Follow-up at 2½ years of age. There is now duplication of the proximal phalanx of the thumb.

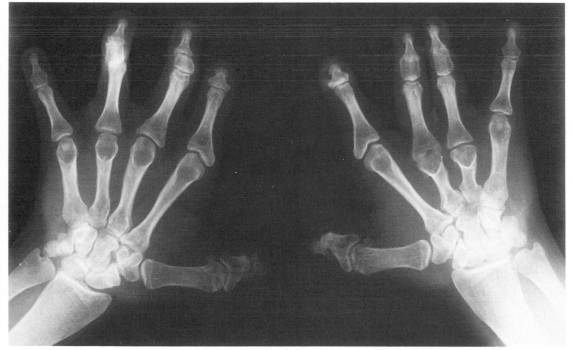

Figure 13–7. Atypical acrocephalopolysyndactyly (Carpenter syndrome). This patient had preaxial polydactyly in the feet. There is marked shortening of the right third and fourth metacarpals. The proximal phalanx of the thumb is short and broad. The middle phalanges of the fingers are also shortened.

ACROCEPHALOSYNDACTYLY

The classification of these conditions is very complex. There are a great number of variables in the appearance of the face and hands. The appearance ranges from that in the classic Apert syndrome, with a mitten hand and foot and severe changes in the skull, to that in very mild cases, in which hands could pass as normal and skulls show only minimal effects of craniosynostosis. Blank[1] classified these conditions into two types: typical Apert syndrome, and atypical groups. McKusick further subdivided them into five groups:

1. Type I, Apert, with severe brachycephaly and mitten hands and feet.

2. Type II, Apert-Crouzon or Vogt cephalodactyly, with mitten hands and feet, similar to Apert but changes in the face having more the appearance of Crouzon disease.

3. Type III, Saethre-Chotzen form, with skull asymmetry and mild syndactyly.

4. Type IV, Waardenburg type, with asymmetry, bifid digits and absence of the first metatarsals, as well as other anomalies.

5. Type V, Pfeiffer form, with mild face and hand changes and with broad thumbs.

Many cases may be seen with clinical and radiologic findings that do not fit well into any of these categories, and part of the distinction may be artificial. We shall discuss these conditions in two main groups: acrocephalosyndactyly—typical (types I and II), and acrocephalosyndactyly—other types (including types III, IV and V).

Acrocephalosyndactyly—Typical (Types I and II, Apert Syndrome, Apert-Crouzon Syndrome)

Apert's syndrome consists of craniosynostosis, usually of the coronal suture, flat facies, shallow orbits, hypertelorism and osseous and cutaneous syndactyly with short, broad thumbs. In some patients the maxilla is very hypoplastic and the facial appearance may resemble more that of Crouzon disease, in which case it should be included in the Vogt type. The hands and feet have a mitten configuration, often with a single nail in the middle portion of the hands and feet. The patients are often mentally retarded. The condition is transmitted as an autosomal dominant with most cases representing a fresh mutation. The average paternal age of the fathers of these children is higher than normal.

RADIOLOGIC FINDINGS IN THE HAND. The findings in the hand are usually symmetric. There is a mitten configuration with both cutaneous and osseous syndactyly affecting particularly the second, third and fourth digits (Fig. 13–8). The fifth finger may sometimes be free of the syndactyly and the thumb is often separate from it. The osseous syndactyly appears progressive. Symphalangism is common. The thumb in Apert syndrome is characteristically abnormal, with a short, broad distal phalanx, which is usually deviated laterally. The proximal phalanx is short or may be absent in a significant number of cases. Symphalangism, or fusion of two phalanges in the

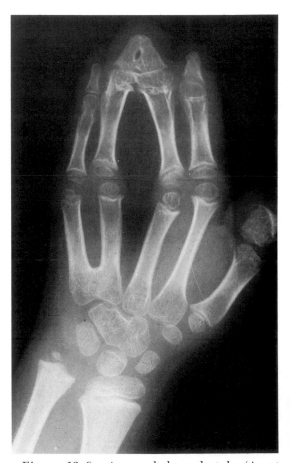

Figure 13–8. Acrocephalosyndactyly (Apert syndrome). There is a mitten hand with osseous as well as cutaneous syndactyly. The distal portions of the third and fourth phalanges are fused. Symphalangism is present in many of the digits. There is fusion between the base of the fourth and fifth metacarpals, and the capitate and hamate are fused. The thumb is broad and hypoplastic with only a single phalanx.

same digit, is common, with only two phalanges present in most fingers. The proximal phalanges are the ones that appear long and slender, suggesting that the fusion is between the proximal and the middle phalanges. The synostoses between the bones of different digits usually involve the distal phalanges; however, synostoses between the metacarpals have also been seen. Carpal fusion is occasionally noted in this condition and may involve the capitate and hamate.

OTHER RADIOLOGIC FINDINGS. Progressive fusion between the tarsal bones is common.[6] This may not be apparent in early childhood. These fusions, as do many syndrome-associated fusions, often affect the cuneiforms. Symphalangism of the toes is also common. The great toe is short due to a short first metatarsal and the presence of only one phalanx in many cases. There may be fusion between metatarsals, particularly the first and second. A large os peroneum has also been described. Fusions of the cervical spine are seen in older individuals. The skull has a characteristic appearance, with shortening in the anteroposterior diameter due to coronal suture synostosis.

REFERENCES

1. Blank, C. E.: Apert's syndrome (a Type of Acrocephalosyndactyly) — Observations on a British Series of Thirty-Nine Cases. *Ann. Hum. Genet.*, 24:151–164, 1960.
2. Cohen, M. M., Gorlin, R. J., Berkman, M. D., and Feingold, M.: Facial Variability in Apert Type Acrocephalosyndactyly. *Birth Defects: Original Article Series*, 7:143–146, 1971.
3. Hoover, G. H., Flatt, A. E., and Weiss, M. W.: The Hand and Apert's Syndrome. *J. Bone Joint Surg.*, 52A:878–895, 1970.
4. McKusick, V. A.: *Mendelian Inheritance in Man. Catalogs of Autosomal Dominant, Autosomal Recessive, and X-Linked Phenotypes*, 3rd Ed. The Johns Hopkins Press, Baltimore, 1971.
5. Palacios, E., and Schimke, R. N.: Craniosynostosis-Syndactylism. *Am. J. Roentgenol.*, 106:144–155, 1969.
6. Schauerte, E. W., and St.-Aubin, P. M.: Progressive Synosteosis in Apert's Syndrome (Acrocephalosyndactyly). With a Description of Roentgenographic Changes in the Feet. *Am. J. Roentgenol.*, 97:67–73, 1966.
7. Temtamy, S. A.: Genetic Factors in Hand Malformations. Thesis, The Johns Hopkins University, Baltimore, Maryland, 1966.
8. Vogt, A.: Dyskephalie (Dysostosis cranio-facialis, Maladie de Crouzon 1912) und eine neuartige Kombination dieser Krankheit mit Syndaktylie der 4 Extremitäten (Dyskephalodaktylie). *Klin. Monatsbl. Augenheilkd.*, 90:441–454, 1933.

Acrocephalosyndactyly — Other Types (Type III, Saethre-Chotzen; Type IV, Waardenburg; Type V, Pfeiffer; and Others)

In all of these conditions there are various degrees of mild syndactyly in the hand and mild changes in the skull. The skull may be flattened in appearance or in some cases scaphocephalic. Intelligence is normal more often in these patients than in the ones with the Apert or the Apert-Crouzon type of disorder. The inheritance of most of these conditions is autosomal dominant, although in several a clear pattern of inheritance cannot be determined since no offspring have been produced.

RADIOLOGIC FINDINGS IN THE HAND. The hand manifestations include mainly syndactyly and broad thumbs and are usually mild.

In the type III or Saethre-Chotzen form, the osseous changes may be absent and there may only be cutaneous syndactyly. The thumbs in this form appear normal.

In the type IV or Waardenburg form, mild syndactyly is also present. Some members of this group have bifid distal phalanges of the second and third digits.

The type V or Pfeiffer form is probably one of the most common in this large group. It is also heterogeneous in terms of its hand abnormalities. In Pfeiffer's original cases the proximal phalanges of the thumbs were grossly abnormal, having a triangular configuration, and commonly they were fused with the distal phalanges. Other cases which have been labeled Pfeiffer had considerably milder manifestations, as illustrated in the families reported by Saldino et al.,[12] in which the proximal phalanx had a much more normal configuration but in which fusion to the distal phalanx was present. Also in Saldino's group there was shortening of the middle phalanges, particularly involving the second to fifth, which resembles the findings in Carpenter syndrome. In a large family studied by Jackson,[5] some of the members of the family had such mild hand changes that they could not be easily detected on simple examination of the film.

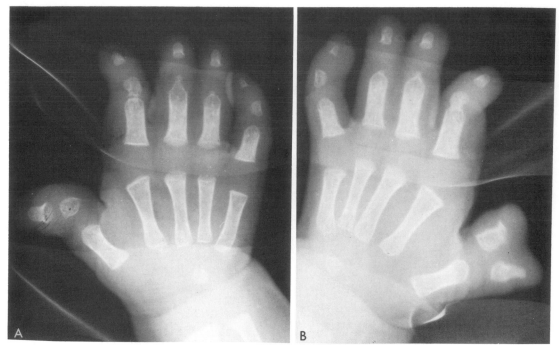

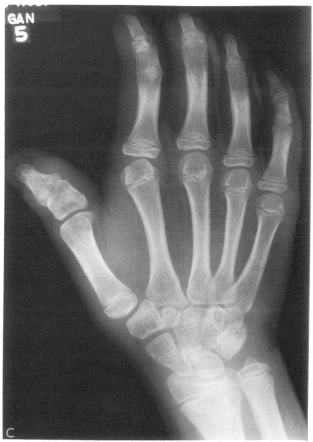

Figure 13–9. Acrocephalosyndactyly (type unknown). *A* and *B,* During infancy there is polydactyly of the thumb of the left hand, and a thumb more typical of acrocephalosyndactyly on the right. The middle phalanges are hypoplastic or absent.

C, Right hand at an older age. There is now symphalangism between the middle and proximal phalanges. The thumb is typical of the acrocephalosyndactyly syndrome, with a short middle phalanx. The carpals are unremarkable. This child had associated scaphocephaly due to sagittal suture synostosis.

Pattern profile analysis, however, did show some abnormality. A number of other types of hand anomalies have been seen and reported by many authors. The changes range from mild to those approaching the findings in Apert syndrome. Zippel and Schüler[16] reported a family having moderately severe hand changes with thumbs similar to those in Pfeiffer syndrome and with symphalangism between digits in the hand as well as in the thumb. This probably is a variant of Pfeiffer syndrome. We have seen some cases where a bifid thumb has been seen in association with these findings (Fig. 13–9). Whether this should be included as an unusual form of Carpenter syndrome or an unusual form of Pfeiffer is still not clear.

OTHER RADIOLOGIC FINDINGS. The skull manifestations vary and include a variety of suture synostoses. The coronal suture is most frequently involved although occasionally the sagittal may also be closed. Brachycephaly from coronal suture synostosis is the most common abnormality.

REFERENCES

1. Bartsocas, C. S., Weber, A. L., and Crawford, J. D.: Acrocephalosyndactyly Type III: Chotzen's Syndrome. J. Pediatr., 77:267–272, 1970.
2. Blank, C. E.: Apert's Syndrome (a Type of Acrocephalosyndactyly)—Observations on a British Series of Thirty-Nine Cases. Ann. Hum. Genet., 24:151–164, 1960.
3. Chotzen, F.: Eine eigenartige familiäre Entwicklungsstörung. (Akrocephalosyndaktylie, Dysostosis craniofacialis und Hypertelorismus). Monatsschr. Kinderheilkd., 55:97–122, 1932.
4. Hermann, J., and Opitz, J. M.: An Unusual Form of Acrocephalosyndactyly. Birth Defects, Original Article Series, 5:39–42, 1969.
5. Jackson, C. E.: Personal communication.
6. Kreiborg, S., Pruzansky, S., and Pashayan, H.: The Saethre-Chotzen Syndrome. Teratology, 6:287–294, 1972.
7. Martsolf, J. T., Cracco, J. B., Carpenter, G. G., and O'Hara, A. E.: Pfeiffer Syndrome. An Unusual Type of Acrocephalosyndactyly with Broad Thumbs and Great Toes. Am. J. Dis. Child., 121:257–262, 1971.
8. McKusick, V. A.: Mendelian Inheritance in Man. Catalogs of Autosomal Dominant, Autosomal Recessive, and X-Linked Phenotypes, 3rd Ed. The Johns Hopkins Press, Baltimore, 1971.
9. Palacios, E., and Schimke, R. N.: Craniosynostosis-Syndactylism. Am. J. Roentgenol., 106:144–155, 1969.
10. Pfeiffer, R. A.: Dominant erbliche Akrocephalosyndaktylie. Z. Kinderheilkd., 90:301–320, 1964.
11. Saethre, H.: Ein Beitrag zum Turmschädelproblem. (Pathogenese, Erblichkeit und Symptomatologie). Deutsche Zeitschrift fur Nervenheilkunde, 119:533–555, 1931.
12. Saldino, R. M., Steinbach, H. L., and Epstein, C. J.: Familial Acrocephalosyndactyly (Pfeiffer Syndrome). Am. J. Roentgenol., 116:609–622, 1972.
13. Summitt, R. L.: Recessive Acrocephalosyndactyly with Normal Intelligence. Birth Defects, Original Article Series, 5:35–38, 1969.
14. Waardenburg, P. J.: Ein merkwürdige Kombination von angeborenen Missbildungen: doppelseitiger Hydrophthalmus verbunden mit Akrokephalosyndaktylie, Herzfehler, Pseudohermaphroditismus und anderen Abweichungen. Klin. Monatsbl. Augenheilkd., 92:29–44, 1934.
15. Walsh, R. J.: Acrosyndactyly. A Study of Twenty-Seven Patients. Clin. Orthop., 71:99–111, 1970.
16. Zippel, H., and Schüler, K.-H.: Dominant Vererbte Akrozephalosyndaktylie (ACS). Fortschr. Geb. Roentgenstr. Nuklearmed., 110:234–245, 1969.

ACRODYSOSTOSIS

This is a syndrome of peripheral dysostosis, nasal hypoplasia and mental retardation. The nasal hypoplasia is a striking clinical feature: the entire nose appears flat and short and often has a dimple in its tip. The digits of the hands and feet are short and stubby. All cases so far have been sporadic.

RADIOLOGIC FINDINGS IN THE HAND. Cone-shaped epiphyses of the Giedion type 35 are seen in the phalanges. They fuse prematurely with their shafts. There is marked digital shortening without significant change in the width of the hand bones (Fig. 13–10). Skeletal maturation is markedly advanced both in terms of epiphyseal closure and in the maturation of the carpals. The association of marked shortening of the bones, the cone-shaped epiphysis and advanced maturation is characteristic of this condition; however, similar radiographic findings may be seen in severe cases of pseudohypoparathyroidism.

OTHER RADIOLOGIC FINDINGS. There is marked shortening of the digits of the toes, although the great toe is less affected. There may be fusion of the epiphyses around the elbow. Other portions of the body are only minimally affected.

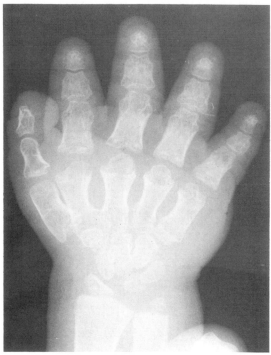

Figure 13-10. Acrodysostosis. Two year old girl. There is significant shortening of the bones of the hand. The epiphyses are cone shaped and are incorporated into the shafts of the bones. The bone age is markedly advanced in the entire hand.

REFERENCES

1. Maroteaux, P., and Malamut, G.: L'Acrodysostose. *Presse Med.,* 76:2189–2192, 1968.
2. Robinow, M., Pfeiffer, R. A., Gorlin, R. J., McKusick, V. A., Renuart, A. W., Johnson, G. F., and Summitt, R. L.: Acrodysostosis. *Am. J. Dis. Child.,* 121:195–203, 1971.

ACROOSTEOLYSIS— CARPOTARSAL FORM

This is a heterogeneous group of disorders in which there is lysis of the carpal and tarsal bones. The symptoms are those of an acute arthritis. Some forms are associated with renal disease and hypertension.[3] Both dominant and recessive forms of this disorder have been described.

RADIOLOGIC FINDINGS IN THE HAND. Destruction of the carpal bones occurs sometimes during childhood. The carpals diminish in size and become markedly distorted (Figs. 13–11 and 13–12). The intercarpal joints may be markedly narrowed. In some cases before this process occurs there is evidence of skeletal maturational advancement, probably resulting from the associated hyperemia. The disease often be-

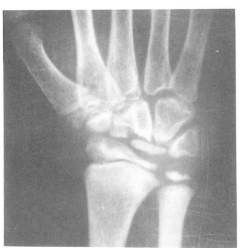
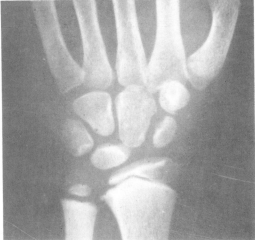

Figure 13-11. Acroosteolysis (carpals). There is marked loss of volume of the carpals, which appear irregular and deformed. This is a familial condition but is asymmetric in this patient. (Courtesy Dr. Don Babbitt, Milwaukee, Wisconsin.)

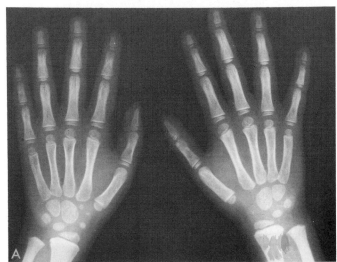

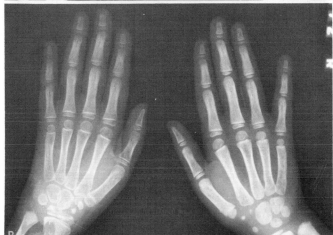

Figure 13–12. Acroosteolysis (carpals. Progressive changes. *a*, The initial film shows only some advancement of skeletal maturation in the carpals of the left hand.

B, Six months later destructive carpal changes are seen.

C, Seven years later the carpals are severely diminished in size and fused. (Courtesy Dr. Don Babbitt, Milwaukee, Wisconsin. This is the family reported in *Radiology*, 108:99–105, 1973.)

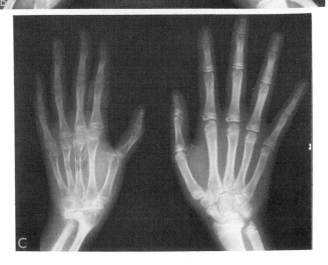

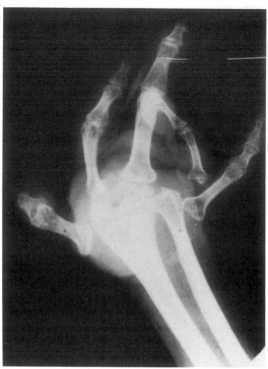

Figure 13–13. Acroosteolysis (carpals). Bizarre. There is marked destruction of bone. (Courtesy Dr. A. A. White, III, New Haven, Connecticut, and *J. Bone Joint Surg.*, 53B:303–309, 1971).

comes quiescent in adult life, but there is resultant deformity and scarring. Other bizarre forms of acroosteolysis may be seen in Figure 13–13.

OTHER RADIOLOGIC FINDINGS. Similar changes are seen in the feet. Osteoporosis may be noted. In one family there was a Marfan-like appearance, with scoliosis, pes cavus and micrognathia.

REFERENCES

1. Gluck, J., and Miller J. J.: Familial Osteolysis of the Carpal and Tarsal Bones. *J. Pediatr.*, 81:506–510, 1972.
2. Kohler, E., Babbitt, D., Huizenga, B., and Good, T. A.: Hereditary Osteolysis. A Clinical, Radiological and Chemical Study. *Radiology*, 108:99–105, 1973.
3. Macpherson, R. I., Walker, R. D., and Kowall, M. H.: Essential Osteolysis with Nephropathy. *J. Can. Assoc. Radiol.*, 24:98–103, 1973.
4. Shurtleff, D. B., Sparkes, R. S., Clawson, D. K., Guntheroth, W. G., and Mottet, N. K.: Hereditary Osteolysis with Hypertension and Nephropathy. *J.A.M.A.*, 188:363–368, 1964.
5. Thieffry, S., and Sorrel-Dejerine, J.: D'Osteolyse Essentielle Hereditaire et Familiale. A Stabilisation Spontanee, Survenant dans l'Enfance. *Presse Med.*, 66:1858–1863, 1958.
6. Torg, J. S., DiGeorge, A. M., Kirkpatrick, J. A., Jr., and Trujillo, M. M.: Hereditary Multicentric Osteolysis with Recessive Transmission: A New Syndrome. *J. Pediatr.*, 75: 243–252, 1969.

ACROOSTEOLYSIS – PHALANGEAL (CHENEY SYNDROME)

The clinical manifestations of this condition include somewhat short fingers that may be broad distally, slightly clubbed and often tender. Paresthesias have also been noted. The individuals usually have some joint hypermobility. The nails are usually intact. The condition is inherited as an autosomal dominant.

RADIOLOGIC FINDINGS IN THE HAND. Loss of a portion of the finger tufts may vary from slight erosions to loss of most of the tuft (Fig. 13–14). The appearance of the erosions is indistinguishable from that of

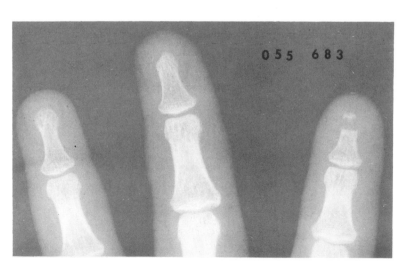

Figure 13–14. Acro-osteolysis (phalangeal). Destruction of the distal phalangeal tips varies from a minor defect, to a gross defect on the right with a small fragment that appears to be separate from the remainder of the phalanx. This patient was related to the family reported by Cheney.

erosions due to other causes of acroosteoly-sis, including acroosteolysis due to pycno-dysostosis, Rothmund syndrome and pseudoxanthoma elasticum, and acquired forms of acroosteolysis such as occurs in chemical workers and scleroderma.

OTHER RADIOLOGIC FINDINGS. Similar changes may be seen in the feet. There has been some skull deformity, bony de-mineralization in the spine and, in children, persistence of wormian bones.

REFERENCES

1. Cheney, W. D.: Acro-Osteolysis. *Am. J. Roent-genol.*, 94:595–607, 1965.
2. Herrmann, J., Zugibe, F. T., Gilbert, E. F., and Opitz, J. M.: Arthro-Dento-Osteo Dys-plasia (Hajdu-Cheney Syndrome). Review of a Genetic "Acro-Osteolysis" Syndrome. *Z. Kinderheilk.*, 114:93–110, 1973.

ACRO-PECTORO-VERTEBRAL DYSPLASIA (F-SYNDROME)

Grosse et al. reported eight patients with a disorder which included prominence of the sternum, with or without pectus ex-cavatum, spina bifida occulta and severe hand and foot changes. The patient had subnormal intelligence and the condition was inherited as an autosomal dominant with variable expressivity.

RADIOLOGIC FINDINGS IN THE HAND. The thumbs were invariably abnormal, appearing short and broad. There was often duplication of the thumb with a web between the thumb and the index finger. Accessory ossicles, which were sometimes seen in the web, may have been derived from thumb phalanges. In some of the cases the web between the thumb and the index finger was complete, while the third, fourth and fifth fingers were unremarkable. The capitate and hamate were fused in most of their cases.

OTHER RADIOLOGIC FINDINGS. The abnormalities in the toes were similar to those in the hand. There was webbing between the first and second toes, and accessory bones were seen between them. Extensive tarsal fusions were also noted.

REFERENCE

1. Grosse, F. R., Herrmann, J., and Opitz, J. M.: The F-Form of Acro-Pectoro-Vertebral Dysplasia: The F-Syndrome. *Birth Defects, Original Arti-cle Series*, 5:48–63, 1969.

AGLOSSIA-ADACTYLY SYNDROME

This is a rare syndrome that is probably not a single entity. There may be some over-lap with the ankyloglossia superior syn-drome. There is an associated hypoplasia of the tongue and digits. The tongue is rare-ly completely absent; usually at least a nub-bin exists. A variety of other anomalies have also been associated with this syn-drome.

The face is characteristically narrow with a narrow, receding chin. The aglossia-adactyly syndrome occurs sporadically and may be due to intrauterine factors.

RADIOLOGIC FINDINGS IN THE HAND. The broad spectrum of hand findings in-cludes a decrease in the number of digits, cleft hand, monodactyly, or total absence of the hand. In some cases partial amputations of the digits are present. Syndactyly is com-mon.

OTHER RADIOLOGIC FINDINGS. The mandible is hypoplastic. There may be ab-sence of the mandibular incisors.

REFERENCES

1. Cohen, M. M., Pantke, H., and Siris, E.: Noso-logic and Genetic Considerations in the Aglossy-Adactyly Syndrome. *Birth De-fects, Original Article Series*, 7:237–240, 1971.
2. Grislain, J., Mainard, R., De Berranger, P., Brelet, G., Cadudal, J. L., and Billet, J.: Aglossie-Adactylie et Syndrome d'Han-hardt. *Pediatrie*, 26:353–364, 1971.
3. Hall, B. D.: Aglossia-Adactylia. *Birth Defects, Original Article Series*, 7:233–236, 1971.
4. Kelln, E. E., Bennett, C. G., and Klingberg, W. G.: Aglossia-Adactylia Syndrome. *Amer. J. Dis. Child.*, 116:549–552, 1968.

ANKYLOGLOSSIA SUPERIOR (GLOSSOPALATINE ANKYLOSIS)

This syndrome of adherence of the tongue to the roof of the mouth is often as-sociated with hand abnormalities. The tongue may be ankylosed to the hard palate or to the upper alveolar ridge. It is frequent-ly associated with absence of the teeth, and cleft palate. There is usually no family his-tory.

RADIOLOGIC FINDINGS IN THE HAND. A variety of changes may occur, and they may be asymmetric. The findings include syn-dactyly, brachydactyly of various types, hypoplasia of digits, lobster-claw deformity and monodactyly.

OTHER RADIOLOGIC FINDINGS. There is hypoplasia of the mandible, and occasionally hypodontia may be present. In the foot there may be changes similar to those in the hand. Absence of the tarsal bones has also been described.

REFERENCES

1. Gorlin, R. J., and Pindborg, J. J.: *Syndromes of the Head and Neck.* McGraw-Hill Book Company, New York, 1964.
2. Wilson, R. A., Kliman, M. R., and Hardyment, A. F.: Ankyloglossia Superior (Palato-glossal Adhesion in the Newborn Infant). *Pediatrics,* 31:1051–1054, 1963.

ARTHROGRYPOSIS

This is a syndrome of multiple joint contractures associated with numerous bone anomalies. It is somewhat ill-defined and has diverse etiologies. Most cases are sporadic but a few familial cases have been reported.[3] The etiology may be related to abnormality of the anterior horn cells. The contractures are present at birth and are usually, but not always, symmetrical. There is usually limitation of active and passive motion. The distribution of the deformities is variable. The lower extremities are more frequently involved than the upper, but a large number of patients have involvement of both.[2,7]

RADIOLOGIC FINDINGS IN THE HAND. The usual wrist deformity is flexion and ulnar deviation. However, occasionally extension contractures may be present. The carpals assume a characteristic configuration—a linear arrangement with consequent increase in carpal angle (normal carpal angle is 131.5°). This carpal sign was present in 11 of 17 patients who had hand abnormalities and sufficiently ossified carpals. The increased carpal angle may be related to the ulnar deviation frequently seen in arthrogryposis (see Chapter 2). This carpal malalignment is followed by narrowing of the intercarpal joint spaces and subsequent fusion (Figs. 13–15 to 13–17). Fusions do not occur until after the age of 10 years and are progressive. Usually the fusion begins in the proximal row, but eventually all of the carpals are fused. Fusion across rows occurs in this condition and is different from the isolated fusion, where only the same row is usually affected.[6]

Other abnormalities in the hand include congenital amputations, syndactyly, camptodactyly and delayed maturation. Maturation is, however, difficult to evaluate because of the carpal abnormalities. A clasped thumb is frequently seen (Fig. 13–18).

OTHER RADIOLOGIC FINDINGS. The most common findings include diminished muscle mass and a relative increase in fat. The feet are commonly abnormal, with clubfoot the most common lesion, although vertical talus and rocker bottom foot have also been described. Congenital amputa-

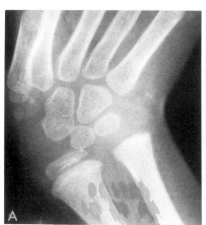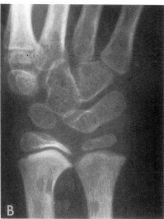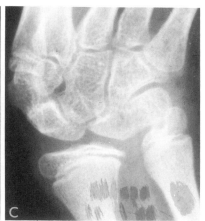

Figure 13–15. Arthrogryposis. Appearance of the wrist at 6, 8 and 12 years of age. There is progressive lunate-triquetrum fusion, and on the last film there is scaphoid-trapezium fusion. The carpal angle is increased. (From Poznanski, A. K., and La Rowe, P. C.: *Radiology,* 95:353–358, 1970.)

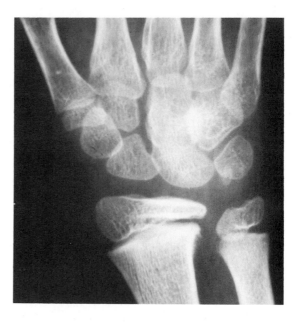

Figure 13–16. Arthrogryposis. Note carpal fusion and the accessory os triangularis near the pisiform. The carpal angle is markedly increased (161°). (From Poznanski, A. K., and Holt, J. F.: *Am. J. Roentgenol.* 112:443–459, 1971.)

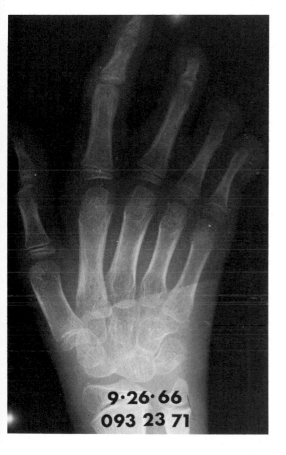

Figure 13–17. Arthrogryposis. Hypoplasia of the distal phalanges is seen occasionally in arthrogryposis. Similar findings were present in the feet. There is also extensive carpal fusion and increase in the carpal angle.

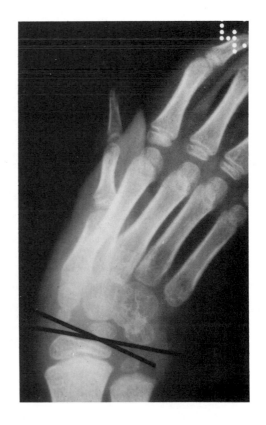

Figure 13–18. Arthrogryposis. Clasped thumb. Ulnar deviation and an increased carpal angle are also seen.

tion of the toes and tarsal fusions are occasionally seen. The hips are frequently dislocated and coxa vara or coxa valga may be present. The knees may be dislocated or show flexion contractures. Scoliosis is common in older individuals. Infants with the syndrome are prone to an increased incidence of fracture. The significant finding in the skull is ankylosis of the temporomandibular joint, which can significantly interfere with feeding. Brachycephaly, high-arched palate and hypoplastic mandible have also been described.

REFERENCES

1. Drachman, D. B., and Banker, B. Q.: Arthrogryposis Multiplex Congenita. Case Due to Disease of the Anterior Horn Cells. *Arch. Neurol.*, 5:77–93, 1961.
2. Friedlander, H. L., Westin, G. W., and Wood, W. L., Jr.: Arthrogryposis Multiplex Congenita. A Review of Forty-Five Cases. *J. Bone Joint Surg.*, 50A:89–112, 1968.
3. Lebenthal, E., Shochet, S. B., Adam, A., Seelenfreund, M., Fried, A., Najenson, T., Sandbank, U., and Y. Matoth.: Arthrogryposis Multiplex Congenita: Twenty-Three Cases in an Arab Kindred. *Pediatrics,* 46:891–899, 1970.
4. Newcombe, D. S., Abbott, J. L., Munsie, W. J., and Keats, T. E.: Arthrogryposis Multiplex Congenita and Spontaneous Carpal Fusion. *Arthritis Rheum.,* 12:345–354, 1969.
5. Orlin, H., and Alpert, M.: Carpal Coalition in Arthrogryposis Multiplex Congenita. *Brit. J. Radiol.* 40:220–222, 1967.
6. Poznanski, A. K., and Holt, J. F.: The Carpals in Congenital Malformation Syndromes. *Am. J. Roentgenol.*, 112:443–459, 1971.
7. Poznanski, A. K., and La Rowe, P. C.: Radiographic Manifestations of the Arthrogryposis Syndrome. *Radiology,* 95:353–358, 1970.

ARTHROOPHTHALMOPATHY (HEREDITARY PROGRESSIVE ARTHROOPHTHALMOPATHY, STICKLER SYNDROME)

Stickler described a familial syndrome consisting of progressive myopia beginning during the first decade of life, which resulted in retinal detachment and blindness. It may be associated with the Pierre Robin syndrome. There was associated evidence of premature degenerative changes in various joints, which could appear swollen and red. The condition is inherited as an autosomal dominant.

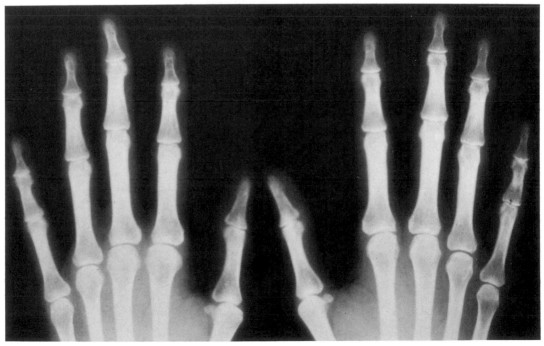

Figure 13–19. Arthro-ophthalmopathy (Stickler syndrome). 39 year old female. There is narrowing of the interphalangeal joints with relatively little sclerosis around them. (Courtesy Dr. William McAlister, St. Louis, Missouri.)

RADIOLOGIC FINDINGS IN THE HAND.
There is a broadening of the ends of the metacarpals with flattening of their articular surfaces,[1, 4] and joint narrowing with relatively little spurring (Fig. 13–19). According to Stickler et al.,[4] these changes do not appear to be due to degenerative joint disease but they lead to it. Knobloch and Layer[1] reported some cases with flexion deformities of the hands. One patient had an accessory carpal between the capitate and third metacarpal. Another had shortening of the third metacarpal associated with enchondroma. Curvature of the fingers, particularly clinodactyly, was seen by Spranger.[3]

OTHER RADIOLOGIC FINDINGS. These include changes of arthritis in the knees and hips, Scheuermann-like changes of the vertebrae and hypoplasia of the mandible. Probably the most typical finding is hypoplasia of the lateral portion of the distal tibial epiphysis.[2]

REFERENCES

1. Knobloch, W. H., and Layer, J. M.: Clefting Syndromes Associated with Retinal Detachment. *Am. J. Ophthalmol.*, 73:517–530, 1972.
2. Schreiner, R. L., McAlister, W. H., Marshall, R. E., and Shearer, W. T.: Stickler Syndrome in a Pedigree of Pierre Robin Syndrome. *Am. J. Dis. Child.*, 126:86–90, 1973.
3. Spranger, J.: Arthro-Ophthalmopathia Hereditaria. *Ann. Radiol.*, 11:359–364, 1967.
4. Stickler, G. B., Belau, P. G., Farrell, F. J., Jones, J. D., Pugh, D. G., Steinberg, A. G., and Ward, L. E.: Hereditary Progressive Arthro-Ophthalmopathy. *Mayo Clin. Proc.*, 40:433–455, 1965.
5. Stickler, G. B., and Pugh, D. G.: Hereditary Progressive Arthro-Ophthalmopathy. II. Additional Observations on Vertebral Abnormalities, A Hearing Defect, and A Report of A Similar Case. *Mayo Clin. Proc.*, 42:495–500, 1967.

ASPHYXIATING THORACIC DYSPLASIA (JEUNE DISEASE, THORACIC-PELVIC-PHALANGEAL DYSTROPHY)

This syndrome includes short extremities and a long narrow thorax which may be associated with difficulty in respiration. Renal disease is sometimes present. It is inherited as an autosomal recessive trait.

RADIOLOGIC FINDINGS IN THE HAND.
The tubular bones of the hand are short,

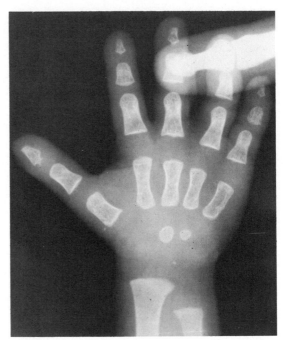

Figure 13–20. Asphyxiating thoracic dysplasia. The hand changes are only minimal, with short distal phalanges and unusual cone epiphyses, particularly in the thumb. The ulna is relatively short.

particularly the distal and middle phalanges (Fig. 13–20). When the epiphyses appear, they are usually cone shaped and fuse early with the metaphyses; again, the findings are most marked in the distal and middle phalanges. Postaxial polydactyly may be an occasional finding.[3]

OTHER RADIOLOGIC FINDINGS. The thoracic cage is small in both the anteroposterior and transverse diameters and may have a bell-shaped configuration. The pelvis is small. Foot findings are similar to those of the hand, with cone-shaped epiphysis, brachydactyly and occasionally polydactyly.

REFERENCES

1. Cremin, B. J.: Infantile Thoracic Dystrophy. *Br. J. Radiol.*, 43:199–204, 1970.
2. Herdman, R. C., and Langer, L. O.: The Thoracic Asphyxiant Dystrophy and Renal Disease. *Am. J. Dis. Child.*, 116:192–201, 1968.
3. Langer, L. O., Jr.: Thoracic-Pelvic-Phalangeal Dystrophy. Asphyxiating Thoracic Dystrophy of the Newborn, Infantile Thoracic Dystrophy. *Radiology*, 91:447–456, 1968.
4. Pirnar, T., and Neuhauser, E. B. D.: Asphyxiating Thoracic Dystrophy of the Newborn. *Am. J. Roentgenol.*, 98:358–364, 1966.

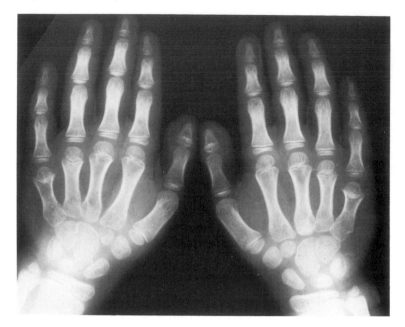

Figure 13–21. Beckwith-Wiedemann syndrome. Six year old female. There is slightly advanced maturation, which is common in this condition. Shortening of the fifth metacarpal was seen only in one patient in this series of Lee. (From Lee, S. A.: *Radiol. Clin. North Am.,* 10:261–276, 1972.)

BECKWITH-WIEDEMANN SYNDROME (EXOMPHALOS-MACROGLOSSIA-GIGANTISM SYNDROME, EMG SYNDROME, SYNDROME OF HYPERPLASTIC FETAL VISCEROMEGALY)

This syndrome consists of macroglossia, omphalocele, gigantism, visceromegaly and neonatal hypoglycemia. The infants are large at birth. They grow slowly initially but then have a very rapid growth spurt. They may be mentally deficient. Their large tongue may interfere with feeding during infancy and may affect their speech in later childhood. Occasionally there is evidence of polycythemia. Most cases are sporadic but autosomal recessive inheritance is suspected because of the occurrence of this disorder in siblings.

RADIOLOGIC FINDINGS IN THE HAND. Hand findings are not particularly characteristic. Cone-shaped epiphyses with shortening of the fifth metacarpals have been reported by Lee (Fig. 13–21).[2] Skeletal maturation is advanced, with the carpals more mature than the phalanges, contrary to the findings in cerebral giantism.[3]

OTHER RADIOLOGIC FINDINGS. These include hemihypertrophy, failure of tubulation of the proximal humerus, flared metaphyses, constricted diaphyses in the lower legs, microcephaly, prognathism, cervical ribs and enlargement of various organs including the liver, kidney and heart. Omphalocele and intestinal malrotation may be

seen. There is often mild breaking of the lumbar vertebrae.

REFERENCES

1. Beckwith, J. B.: Macroglossia, Omphalocele, Adrenal Cytomegaly, Gigantism, and Hyperplastic Visceromegaly. *Birth Defects, Original Article Series,* 5:188–196, 1969.
2. Lee, F. A.: Radiology of the Beckwith-Wiedemann Syndrome. *Radiol. Clin. North Am.,* 10:261–276, 1972.
3. Wiedemann, H.-R.: Exomphalos-Makroglossie-Giantismus-Syndrom, Berardinelli-Seip-Syndrom-eine vergleichende Betrachtung unter ausgewählten Aspekten. *Z. Kinderheik.,* 115:193–207, 1973.
4. McNamara, T. O., Gooding, C. A., Kaplan, S. L., and Clark, R. E.: Exomphalos-Macroglossia-Gigantism (Visceromegaly) Syndrome. *Am. J. Roentgenol.,* 114:264–267, 1972.

BIEMOND SYNDROME I

This syndrome consists of nystagmus and cerebellar ataxia associated with shortening of the fourth metacarpal. According to McKusick, no other families with this syndrome have yet been reported.

REFERENCES

1. Biemond, A.: Brachydactylie, Nystagmus en Cerebellaire Ataxie Als Familiaire Syndroom. *Ned. Tijdschr. Geneeskd.* 78:1423–1431, 1934.
2. McKusick, V. A.: *Mendelian Inheritance in Man. Catalogs of Autosomal Dominant, Autosomal Recessive, and X-Linked Phenotypes,* 3rd Ed. The Johns Hopkins Press, Baltimore, 1971.

BIEMOND SYNDROME II

This condition resembles the Laurence-Moon-Biedl-Bardet syndrome. The findings include coloboma of the iris, mental retardation, obesity, hypogenitalism and postaxial polydactyly. Inherent is an irregular autosomal dominant. The cases described by Grebe[3] and by Blumel and Kniker[2] probably represent the same disease.

RADIOLOGIC FINDINGS IN THE HAND. Postaxial polydactyly is seen.

REFERENCES

1. Biemond, A.: Het Syndroom van Laurence-Biedl en een aanverwant, nieuw Syndroom. *Ned. Tijdschr. Geneeskd.,* 78:1801–1814, 1934.
2. Blumel, J., and Kniker, W. T.: Laurence-Moon-Bardet-Biedl Syndrome. Review of the Literature and a Report of Five Cases Including a Family Group with Three Affected Males. *Tex. Rep. Biol. Med.,* 17:391–410, 1959.
3. Grebe, H.: Contribution au Diagnostic Différentiel du Syndrome de Bardet-Biedl. *J. Genet. Hum.,* 2:127–144, 1953.

BLACKFAN-DIAMOND ANEMIA (CONGENITAL HYPOPLASTIC ANEMIA)

In this rare congenital entity there is subnormal erythropoiesis that causes a profound anemia but no alteration in white cells or platelets.

RADIOLOGIC FINDINGS IN THE HAND. Very little has been written about the hand changes in this entity. Diamond[2] stated that 8 of 30 cases had evidence of triphalangeal thumbs while two had double thumbs. There may also be secondary findings owing to illness of the patient and the repeated transfusions. The children are often retarded in growth and maturation and there may be evidence of osteoporosis.

OTHER RADIOLOGIC FINDINGS. Signs secondary to severe illness may be present.

REFERENCES

1. Aase, J. M., and Smith, D. W.: Congenital Anemia and Triphalangeal Thumbs: A New Syndrome. *J. Pediatr.,* 74:471–474, 1969.
2. Diamond, L. K.: Congenital Hypoplastic Anemia. Oral presentation, Conference on the Clinical Delineation of Birth Defects. Baltimore, 1971.
3. Diamond, L. K., Allen, D. M., and Magill, F. B.: Congenital (Erythroid) Hypoplastic Anemia. *Am. J. Dis. Child.,* 102:403–415, 1961.

CEREBRAL GIANTISM

Cerebral giantism is probably a disorder of the hypothalamus. It was originally described by Sotos et al.[3] It is characterized by accelerated growth rate, nonprogressive

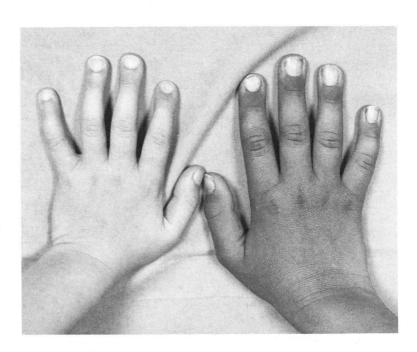

Figure 13–22. Cerebral giantism. The hand of the affected patient is on the right and is considerably larger than the control hand of a child in the 50th percentile for his age. (5 years, 10 months) The soft tissues are markedly thickened. (From Poznanski, A. K., and Stephenson, J. M.: *Radiology,* 88:446–456, 1967.)

mental retardation and characteristic facial appearance. There is a prominence of the mandible, high-arched palate, prominent forehead and supraorbital ridges. The hands and feet are unusually large (Fig. 13–22). The patients are two to three standard deviations above the mean for age but attain a normal adult size. The condition is usually sporadic.

RADIOLOGIC FINDINGS IN THE HAND. There is overall advancement in size and maturation of the hand. Maturation and size are proportionally advanced, so that at maturity the individuals are normal in size. The maturation is dysharmonic, with the phalanges being significantly more advanced than the carpals in all cases.[1,2] The scaphoid is delayed in many of these patients (Fig. 13–23).[1]

OTHER RADIOLOGIC FINDINGS. These include dilatation of the cerebral ventricles, an increased incidence of septum pellucidum cysts, anterior fontanelle bones and minor other radiologic findings.

REFERENCES

1. Poznanski, A. K., Garn, S. M., Kuhns, L. R., and Sandusky, S. T.: Dysharmonic Maturation of the Hand in the Congenital Malformation Syndromes. *Am. J. Phys. Anthropol.*, 35:417–432, 1971.
2. Poznanski, A. K., and Stephenson, J. M.: Radiographic Findings in Hypothalamic Acceleration of Growth Associated with Cerebral Atrophy and Mental Retardation (Cerebral Gigantism). *Radiology*, 88:446–456, 1967.
3. Sotos, J. F., Dodge, P. R., Muirhead, D., Crawford, J. D., and Talbot, N. B.: Cerebral Gigantism in Childhood. A Syndrome of Excessively Rapid Growth with Acromegalic Features and a Nonprogressive Neurologic Disorder. *N. Eng. J. Med.*, 271: 109–116, 1964.

CEREBRO-HEPATO-RENAL SYNDROME (CHRS, ZELLWEGER SYNDROME)

This is a severe, usually fatal congenital abnormality involving multiple systems. The infants are severely hypotonic and may be clinically confused with Down syndrome patients. They have a characteristic facial appearance. Pathologic findings include multiple small cortical renal cysts, liver fibrosis, lissencephaly and evidence of excessive iron storage. The condition is inherited as an autosomal recessive.

RADIOLOGIC FINDINGS IN THE HAND. These are mainly the changes of contractures. Camptodactyly of the fifth fingers is particularly common (Fig. 13–24).

OTHER RADIOLOGIC FINDINGS. The most striking finding is calcification, which is usually in the patellae and is similar to that seen in chondrodysplasia punctata. It is frequently associated with a deformity of the feet. Dilatation of the cerebral ventricles may also be seen.

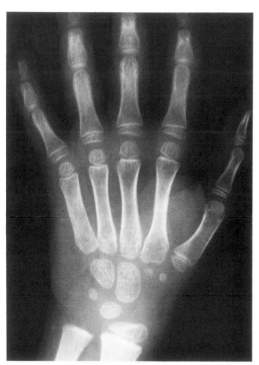

Figure 13–23. Cerebral giantism. Disproportion in phalangeal and carpal ossification. In this 5.3 year old male, the overall maturation is advanced, but there is relative advancement of the phalanges as compared to the carpals. Phalangeal maturation is between eight and nine years, while the carpals are nearer to seven, although there is considerable intercarpal variation. Note the marked delay in scaphoid ossification, which is common in these children. (From Poznanski, A. K., et al.: *Am. J. Phys. Anthropol.*, 35:417–432, 1971.)

REFERENCES

1. Bowen, P., Lee, C. S. N., Zellweger, H., and Lindenberg, R.: A Familial Syndrome of Multiple Congenital Defects. *Johns Hopkins Med. J.*, 114:402–414, 1964.
2. Opitz, J. M., ZuRhein, G. M., Vitale, L., Sha-

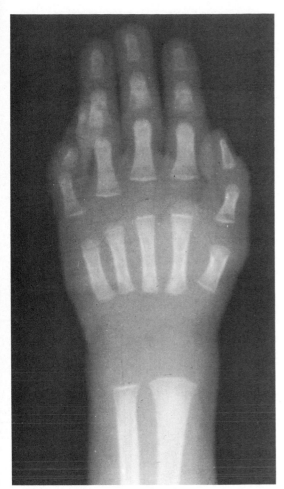

Figure 13-24. Cerebro-hepato-renal syndrome. Newborn infant. There is camptodactyly of the fifth finger. The hand is otherwise unremarkable. There are some nonspecific lucencies in the metaphyses.

hidi, N. T., Howe, J. J., Chou, S. M., Shanklin, D. R., Sybers, H. D., Dood, A. R., and Gerritsen, T.: The Zellweger Syndrome (Cerebro-Hepato-Renal Syndrome). *Birth Defects, Original Article Series*, 5:144–160, 1969.
3. Poznanski, A. K., Nosanchuk, J. S., Baublis, J., and Holt, J. F.: The Cerebro-Hepato-Renal Syndrome (CHRS) (Zellweger's Syndrome). *Am. J. Roentgenol.*, 109:313–322, 1970.

CHONDRODYSPLASIA PUNCTATA (CHONDRODYSTROPHIA CALCIFICANS CONGENITA, STIPPLED EPIPHYSES)

This is a heterogeneous group of conditions associated with calcification in the region of the epiphyses. Spranger et al.[5, 6] considered two main forms of this condition: the Conradi-Hünermann form, which is inherited as an autosomal dominant, and the rhizomelic form, which is inherited as an autosomal recessive. Dwarfism is more severe in the rhizomelic form. Skin changes and cataracts may be seen in both forms. Caffey reported similar findings due to *Listeria monocytogenes* bacteremia.[1]

RADIOLOGIC FINDINGS IN THE HAND. The hallmark of this condition is stippled calcification in the region of the epiphyses. In the hand the bones most commonly affected are the carpals (Figs. 13–25 and 13–26). In the Conradi-Hünermann type there is eventually hypoplasia of the carpus with an appearance similar to an epiphyseal dys-

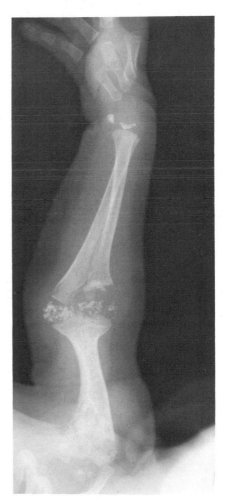

Figure 13-25. Chondrodysplasia punctata (rhizomelic type). There is marked shortening of the humerus. Calcifications are seen in the epiphyseal ends of all the bones.

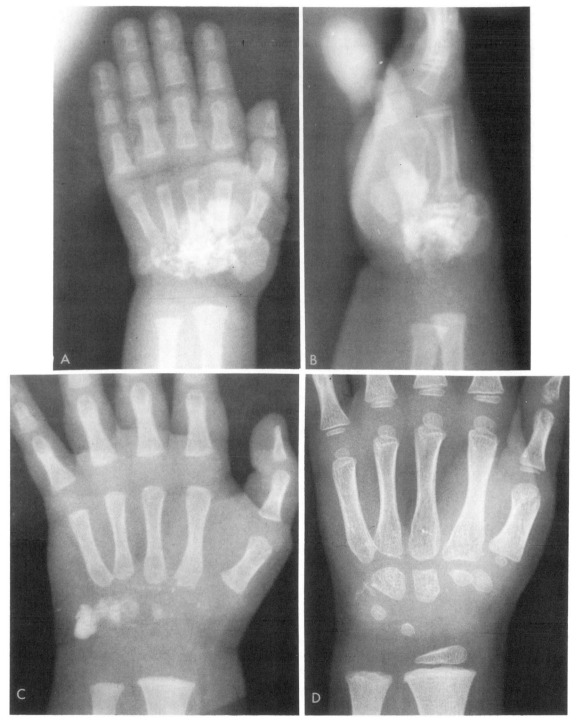

Figure 13–26. Chondrodysplasia punctata (probable Conradi-Hünermann type). *A* and *B*, Antero-posterior and lateral films taken in 1967 shortly after birth. There is extensive calcification outside of the usual distribution of the carpus.

C, Film in 1969. Much of the calcification has now disappeared.

D, Film in 1971. Most of the calcification has now disappeared. The carpal epiphyses are irregular and small with an appearance suggestive of an epiphyseal dysplasia. This case somewhat resembles the cases of postsepticemia calcification that have been described by Caffey.

plasia (Fig. 13–26).[4, 5, 6] In the rhizomelic form calcifications are also seen. The first metacarpal may be short. Other minor anomalies of the hand have also been described. Calcification may be outside the region of the carpal bones, particularly in the cases due to infection.[1]

OTHER RADIOLOGIC FINDINGS. The Conradi-Hünermann type has spondyloepiphyseal localization of the calcifications with deformities. Frequently there may be asymmetry in these findings. The metaphyses are normal. There are deformities of the vertebral bodies with early scoliosis.

The rhizomelic form is characterized by symmetrical severe shortening of the femur and humerus, pronounced metaphyseal ossification problems, coronal clefts in the vertebral bodies and trapeziform dysplasia at the upper ilium.

REFERENCES

1. Caffey, J.: *Pediatric X-Ray Diagnosis*, 6th Ed. Year Book Medical Publishers, Chicago, 1972, Vol. 2.
2. Josephson, B. M., and Oriatti, M. D.: Chondrodystrophia Calcificans Congenita. Report of a Case and Review of the Literature. *Pediatrics*, 28:425–435, 1961.
3. Melnick, J. C.: Chondrodystrophia Calcificans Congenita. *Am. J. Dis. Child.*, 110:218–225, 1965.
4. Silverman, F. N.: Discussion on the Relation Between Stippled Epiphyses and the Multiplex Form of Epiphyseal Dysplasia. *Birth Defects, Original Article Series*, 5: 68–70, 1969.
5. Spranger, J. W., Bidder, U., and Voelz, C.: Chondrodysplasia punctata (Chondrodystrophia calcificans) II. Der rhizomele typ. *Fortschr. Geb. Roentgenstr. Nuklearmed.*, 114:327–335, 1971.
6. Spranger, J. W., Bidder, U., and Voelz, C.: Chondrodysplasia punctata (Chondrodystrophia calcificans) Typ Conradi-Hünermann. *Fortschr. Geb. Roentgenstr. Nuklearmed.*, 113:717–727, 1970.
7. Spranger, J. W., Opitz, J. M., and Bidder, U.: Heterogeneity of Chondrodysplasia Punctata. *Humangenetik*, 11:190–212, 1971.

CHONDROECTODERMAL DYSPLASIA (ELLIS–VAN CREVELD SYNDROME)

This is a well-defined short-limbed dwarfism which is associated with polydactyly and dysplastic fingernails. The limb shortening is more marked in the distal portions of the extremities. Congenital heart disease is seen in 60 per cent of cases, the most common lesion being a single atrium, or a large atrial defect. Other findings include knock-knees and abnormality of the hair and teeth. There is a short upper lip bound by a frenulum. The inheritance pattern is autosomal recessive.

RADIOLOGIC FINDINGS IN THE HAND. There is shortening of all of the hand bones, which is most severe distally and least marked proximally (Fig. 13–27). The distal phalanges may be simply very thin linear shadows of bone, considerably thinner and shorter than the other phalanges. There is also significant shortening of the middle phalanges. Prominent cone-shaped epiphyses may be seen, particularly in the middle phalanges (Fig. 13–28). Epiphyseal centers may ossify late, and in the distal phalanges they often may not be visible. Postaxial polydactyly is common and may vary from a normal-appearing finger to one

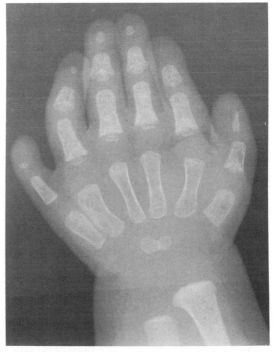

Figure 13–27. Chondroectodermal dysplasia (Ellis-van Creveld syndrome). One year old female. There is postaxial polydactyly. The distal phalanges are markedly hypoplastic: the second is barely perceptible and the sixth is not apparent. Cone-shaped epiphyses are seen in the proximal and middle phalanges. The middle phalanges are particularly short. There is early fusion of the capitate and hamate.

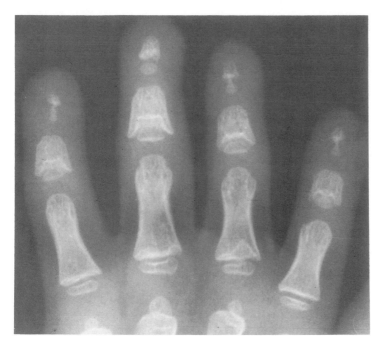

Figure 13-28. Chondroectodermal dysplasia (Ellis–van Creveld syndrome). Cone epiphyses of various types are seen. The elongated cones in the distal phalanges are characteristic of chondroectodermal dysplasia. The middle phalangeal cones are very deep and square shaped. The middle and distal phalanges are particularly shortened. (Courtesy Dr. John Dorst and Dr. Victor McKusick, Johns Hopkins University, Baltimore, Maryland.)

with very small phalanges. The fifth and sixth metacarpals may be fused.

Duplication of the carpal bones is common, with additional carpals in the distal row (Fig. 13–29). This may appear as an elongated hamate or a bone between the hamate and the capitate, or there may simply be a very wide capitate. Although capitate-hamate fusion has been described as a typical finding (Fig. 13–27), it is not a necessary part of the syndrome and many patients fail to show this.

OTHER RADIOLOGIC FINDINGS. Marked shortening of the extremities is often evident. The pelvis has an abnormal configuration, with broad iliac wings. Knock-knee

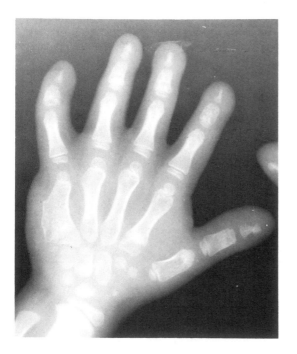

Figure 13-29. Chondroectodermal dysplasia. (Ellis–van Creveld syndrome). There are accessory carpals in the distal row. Instead of the usual four carpals, six are noted. There is widening of the fifth metacarpal, which is evidence of a previously removed accessory digit. Epiphyseal changes in the distal and middle phalanges are noted. (Courtesy Dr. Don Babbitt, Milwaukee, Wisconsin.)

deformity is common. Polydactyly in the feet is less common than in the hands. Often there is a deformity of the epiphyseal cartilages at the proximal ends of the tibiae, the proximal ends of the ulnae, and the distal ends of the radii.

REFERENCES

1. Caffey, J.: Chondroectodermal Dysplasia (Ellis–Van Creveld Disease). Report of Three Cases. *Am. J. Roentgenol.*, 68:875–886, 1952.
2. Ellis, R. W. B., and van Creveld, S.: A Syndrome Characterized by Ectodermal Dysplasia, Polydactyly, Chondro-Dysplasia and Congenital Morbus Cordis. Report of Three Cases. *Arch. Dis. Child.*, 15:65–84, 1940.
3. McKusick, V. A., Egeland, J. A., Eldridge, R., and Krusen, D. E.: Dwarfism in the Amish. I. The Ellis–van Creveld Syndrome. *Johns Hopkins Med. J.*, 115:306–336, 1964.

CHRISTIAN BRACHYDACTYLY SYNDROME (DOMINANT PREAXIAL BRACHYDACTYLY)

This syndrome of mental retardation, with brachydactyly, hallux varus and abducted thumbs, was inherited as an autosomal dominant.

RADIOLOGIC FINDINGS IN THE HAND. The first metacarpals were broad and short and the thumb was deviated radially. The distal phalanx of the thumb was broad and short. Ratios of the first metacarpal and the first distal phalanx as compared to the second metacarpal were significantly below normal limits. The other metacarpals showed evidence of cortical thickening. The middle and distal phalanges of the other fingers were relatively wide, but were more normal on the ulnar than on the radial side of the hand. There was some irregularity of the articular surface of the trapezium.

OTHER RADIOLOGIC FINDINGS. The great toe was grossly abnormal and deviated medially. The first metatarsal was broad and short, and the other metatarsals were unremarkable.

REFERENCE

1. Christian, J. C., Cho, K. S., Franken, E. A., and Thompson, B. H.: Dominant Preaxial Brachydactyly with Hallux Varus and Thumb Abduction. *Am. J. Hum. Genet.*, 24:694–701, 1972.

CLEIDOCRANIAL DYSPLASIA (CLEIDOCRANIAL DYSOSTOSIS, MARIE-SAINTON SYNDROME, MUTATIONAL DYSOSTOSIS)

The chief clinical manifestations of this condition relate to absence of the clavicle, which permits marked anterior shoulder movement. The head is usually brachycephalic with a prominent forehead, a small face and persistence of the anterior fontanelles. Multiple tooth abnormalities are seen. The stature of the patients may be subnormal. The condition is inherited as an autosomal dominant with a wide variability of expression.

RADIOLOGIC FINDINGS IN THE HAND. The distal phalanges are hypoplastic in many cases (Fig. 13–30). This has been seen both in the literature and in our own cases

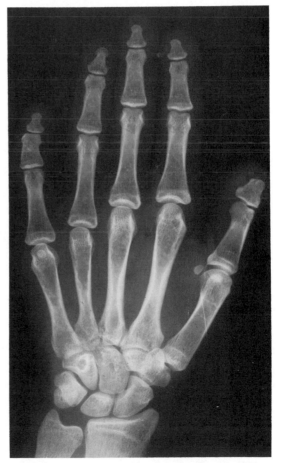

Figure 13–30. Cleidocranial dysplasia. Adult. There is shortening of the distal phalanges and there is minimal clinodactyly of the fifth finger. The second metacarpal is relatively long.

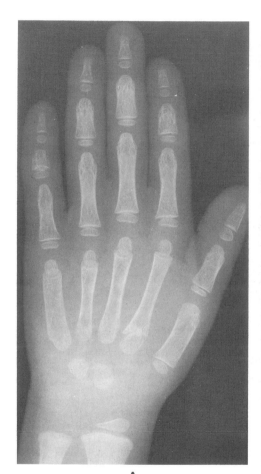
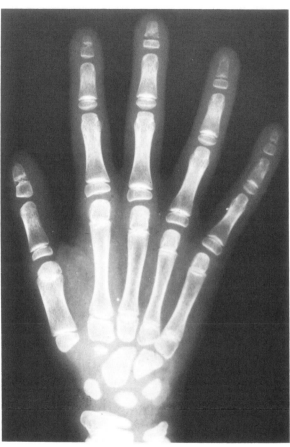

A **B**

Figure 13–31. Cleidocranial dysplasia. *A*, Minimal findings in four year old child. There is minimal thickening of the distal phalangeal epiphyses. There is minimal notching of the distal ends of the middle phalanges and at the bases of the metacarpals. There is a well defined pseudoepiphysis in the second metacarpal.

B, Severe changes in 10 year old girl. Thick epiphyses are much more obvious. There are distinct pseudoepiphyses of all the metacarpals. (Figure *B* courtesy Dr. F. N. Silverman, Cincinnati, Ohio.)

and is evident on pattern profile analysis. The shortening of the distal phalanges is particularly marked in adults. However, the distal phalanges are not reduced in all patients. No characteristic reductions of any other phalanges are apparent from the pattern profiles. Occasionally the second metacarpal is somewhat enlarged compared to the other bones. The literature on the condition is somewhat confusing, since some cases of pycnodysostosis have been included in early reports. The phalangeal epiphyses, particularly in the distal phalanges, may appear somewhat thickened (Fig. 13–31) and there may be some prominent pseudoepiphyses. This latter finding may be of little significance when it occurs in the second metacarpal, where it is a common normal variant. Cone epiphyses may sometimes be seen.

OTHER RADIOLOGIC FINDINGS. An important finding is a defect in the clavicle. This defect may involve only a small portion of the clavicle. In 10 per cent of the cases the clavicles may be completely absent. The skull shows evidence of poor ossification with multiple wormian bones and persistence of fontanelles. There is poor ossification in the pelvis with a wide gap at the symphysis pubis, and there is marked delay in tooth maturation. Multiple other minor congenital defects may also be seen.

REFERENCES

1. Cole, W. R., and Levin, S.: Cleidocranial Dysostosis. Br. J. Radiol., 24:549–555, 1951.
2. Jackson, W. P. U.: Osteo-dental dysplasia (Cleido-cranial Dysostosis). The "Arnold Head." Acta Med. Scand., 139:292–307, 1951.
3. Kalliala, E., and Taskinen, P. J.: Cleidocranial Dysostosis. Report of Six Typical Cases and One Atypical Case. Oral Surg., 15:808–822, 1962.
4. Soule, A. B., Jr.: Mutational Dysostosis (Cleidocranial Dysostosis). J. Bone Joint Surg., 28:81–102, 1946.
5. Srivastava, K. K., Pai, R. A., Kolbhandarai, M. P., and Kant, K.: Cleidocranial Dysostosis. A Clinical and Cytological Study. Clin. Genet., 2:104–110, 1971.

CLOVERLEAF SKULL (KLEEBLATTSCHÄDEL DEFORMITY SYNDROME)

In this bizarre anomaly the skull bulges laterally and superiorly, giving it a cloverleaf appearance. It is often associated with short-limbed dwarfism and is usually fatal at birth or shortly thereafter.

RADIOLOGIC FINDINGS IN THE HAND. These have not been well documented in the literature. There may be syndactyly similar to that seen in the acrocephalosyndactyly syndromes.[5] There may also be broadening of the thumbs. Shortening of the digits is common when associated with short-limbed dwarfism and flexion contractures with inability to extend the fingers have also been noted.

OTHER RADIOLOGIC FINDINGS. The gross skull deformity is probably the most dramatic. However, shortening of other bones may be seen; in some cases there is a picture similar to that of thanatophoric dwarfism. Synostosis of all of the bones about the elbow is also commonly present.

REFERENCES

1. Angle, C. R., McIntire, M. S., and Moore, R. C.: Cloverleaf Skull: Kleeblattschädel-Deformity Syndrome. Amer. J. Dis. Child., 114:198–202, 1967.
2. Bloomfield, J. A.: Cloverleaf Skull and Thanatophoric Dwarfism. Australas. Radiol., 14:420–434, 1970.
3. Comings, D. E.: The Kleeblattschädel Syndrome – A Grotesque Form of Hydrocephalus. J. Pediatr., 67:126–129, 1965.
4. Holtermüller, K., and Wiedemann, H.-R.: Kleeblattschädel-Syndrom. Med. Monatsschr., 14:439–446, 1960.
5. Rosenbaum, K. N., and Weisskopf, B.: Kleeblattschädel Syndrome J. Ky. Med. Assoc., 69:594–597, 1971.

COCKAYNE SYNDROME

This ill-defined syndrome of microcephalic dwarfism is associated with mental retardation and retinal pigmentation. The initial growth is normal but then halts in early childhood.

RADIOLOGIC FINDINGS IN THE HAND. The radiographic findings in the hand are often not particularly specific. Land and Nogrady[2] reported a broad, triangular carpus with short metacarpals and phalanges, squaring and peculiar notching. Dense epiphyses are common in the distal phalanges (Fig. 13–32). There is also some evidence of osteoporosis. Bone age may be retarded, normal or advanced. Riggs and Seibert[3] felt that the bone age was advanced only in the older patients.

OTHER RADIOLOGIC FINDINGS. Other radiographic manifestations include microcephaly, kyphosis, posterior tapering of

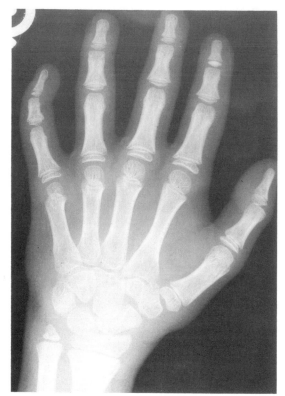

Figure 13–32. Cockayne syndrome. 12³⁄₄ year old boy. Note the ivory epiphysis in the distal phalanx of the index finger. There is clinodactyly of the fifth finger. The maturation of the phalanges is retarded, while the carpals are near normal.

thoracic vertebral bodies, pelvic abnormalities and osteoporosis. There may be evidence of intracranial calcification.

REFERENCES

1. Alton, D. J., McDonald, P., and Reilly, B. J.: Cockayne's Syndrome. *Radiology,* 102: 403–406, 1972.
2. Land, V. J., and Nogrady, M. B.: Cockayne's Syndrome. *J. Can. Assoc. Radiol.,* 20:194–203, 1969.
3. Riggs, W., and Seibert, J.: Cockayne's Syndrome. *Am. J. Roentgenol.,* 116:623–633, 1972.

COFFIN–SIRIS SYNDROME

Coffin and Siris[1] reported three small, severely retarded girls who lacked nails on their fifth fingers and lateral toes. The children were mentally retarded, had severe retardation of postnatal growth and lax joints, and two of the patients had thick features and sparse scalp hair.

RADIOLOGIC FINDINGS IN THE HAND. There is diminution in size of the distal phalanges, most marked in the fifth finger, which may have only two phalanges. The remainder of the hand is usually unremarkable. The bone age was retarded in all cases.

Similar hand findings may be seen in mothers receiving antiepileptic medication (Fig. 9–3C). One such case was included with the Coffin–Siris syndrome in the report of Weiswasser et al.[3]

Short distal phalanges and hypoplastic nails on the toes were noted in the syndrome reported by Senior.[2] In this condition there was also associated shortening of the fifth middle phalanx. It is not clear whether Senior syndrome is simply a mild variant of the Coffin–Siris syndrome. A similar appearance is seen in the Zimmermann–Laband syndrome. Also, similar bony changes without nail abnormalities may occur (Fig. 9–30).

OTHER RADIOLOGIC FINDINGS. There was smallness of the patella. Elbow dislocation, coxa valga and short sternum were also seen.

REFERENCES

1. Coffin, G. S., and Siris, E.: Mental Retardation with Absent Fifth Fingernail and Terminal Phalanx. *Am. J. Dis. Child.,* 119:433–439, 1970.
2. Senior, G.: Impaired Growth and Onychodysplasia. Short Children with Tiny Toenails. *Am. J. Dis. Child.,* 122:7–9, 1971.
3. Weisswasser, W. H., Hall, B. D., Delavan, G. W., and Smith, D. W.: Coffin–Siris Syndrome. *Am. J. Dis. Child.,* 125:838–840, 1973.

COFFIN-SIRIS-WEGIENKA SYNDROME

This condition includes smallness of stature; large, soft hands; pectus carinatum; lax ligaments; and a peculiar facies, particularly prominent frontal bossing, hypertelorism, downward slant of the eyes, prognathism and low-set ears.

RADIOLOGIC FINDINGS IN THE HAND. The soft tissue tapering of the hand from proximal to distal is seen on the roentgenograms. The distal phalanges are somewhat unusual, with a drumstick-like appearance due to overconstriction just beneath the tufts. Procopis and Turner[2] reported children with similar findings.[2]

OTHER RADIOLOGIC FINDINGS. There is hypoplasia of the mastoids, the maxillae, and the zygomatica. Sternal abnormality and thoracolumbar kyphosis are also seen.

REFERENCES

1. Coffin, G. S., Siris, E., and Wegienka, L. C.: Mental Retardation with Osteocartilaginous Anomalies. *Am. J. Dis. Child.*, 112:205–213, 1966.
2. Procopis, P. G., and Turner, B.: Mental Retardation, Abnormal Fingers, and Skeletal Anomalies: Coffin's Syndrome. *Am. J. Dis. Child.*, 124:258–261, 1972.

CRANIOFACIAL DYSOSTOSIS (CROUZON DISEASE)

This is a disorder of bilateral exophthalmos, external strabismus, beak nose, relative mandibular prognathism and a drooping lower lid.

RADIOLOGIC FINDINGS IN THE HAND. Most cases do not have hand involvement. In some cases hand changes similar to that of Apert syndrome have been noted.[1] It is difficult to be certain whether these cases should be placed in the category of Crouzon or of Apert syndrome, since the facial appearance of the two is very similar. They should probably be included in the group acrocephalosyndactyly type II (p. 260). Garcin et al.[2] have reported ectrodactyly in association with Crouzon disease.

REFERENCES

1. Dodge, H. W., Jr., Wood, M. W., and Kennedy, R. L. J.: Craniofacial Dysostosis: Crouzon's Disease. *Pediatrics*, 23:98–106, 1959.
2. Garcin, R., Thurel, R., and Rudaux, P.: Sur un Cas Isole de Dysostose Cranio-Faciale (Maladie de Crouzon), avec Ectrodactylie. *Bull. et Mém. de la Soc. Med. des Hop.*, 3rd series, no. 29, pp. 1458–1466, 1932.
3. Gorlin, R. J., and Pindborg, J. J.: *Syndromes of the Head and Neck.* McGraw-Hill Book Company, New York, 1964.

CRANIOMETAPHYSEAL DYSPLASIA (METAPHYSEAL DYSPLASIA, PYLE DISEASE)

There is some disagreement about whether craniometaphyseal dysplasia and metaphyseal dysplasia are separate disorders. The differentiation is based mainly on the degree of cranial involvement, so that we shall consider them together in this section.

This is a disorder associated with a failure of resorption of spongiosa, which produces lack of modeling of bones and enlargement of the cranial bones. This in turn can lead to cranial nerve impingement with blindness, deafness, nystagmus and paralysis of the facial nerve. The inheritance of this condition is usually autosomal dominant, although recessive forms are also known.[5]

RADIOLOGIC FINDINGS IN THE HAND. The hand findings are similar to those seen in other bones but are milder in their expression. During infancy there may be an area of radiolucency in the ends of the bones (Fig. 13–33). With maturation, the

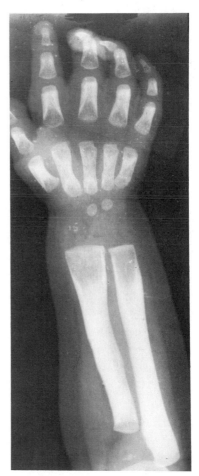

Figure 13–33. Craniometaphyseal dysplasia. Infant. Triangular areas of radiolucency are seen at the proximal ends of the phalanges and to a lesser degree at both ends of the metacarpals. A similar appearance is seen in the distal end of the radius and the ulna. The modeling changes may be relatively mild at this age.

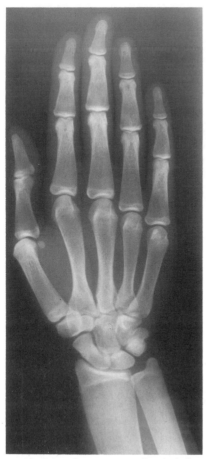

Figure 13–34. Craniometaphyseal dysplasia. 17 year old female. Although definite failure of modeling is seen the distal radius, the findings in the hand are very mild. Some changes are seen in the distal metacarpals, while the phalanges and carpals are relatively uninvolved.

bones become more uniformly ossified and there may be some failure of modeling at the metaphyseal ends, particularly in the metacarpals (Fig. 13–34). Occasionally findings are seen also in the phalanges. The carpals are usually uninvolved.

OTHER RADIOLOGIC FINDINGS. Characteristic Erlenmeyer flask deformity may be seen in the region of the femurs. The findings are similar to those in the hand but are more severe. The skull bones show evidence of increased density.

REFERENCES

1. Carlson, D. H., and Harris, G. B. C.: Craniometaphyseal Dysplasia. A Family with Three Documented Cases. *Radiology,* 103:147–151, 1972.
2. Girdwood, T. G., Gibson, W. J. A., and Mackintosh, T. F.: Craniometaphyseal Dysplasia Congenita—Pyle's Disease in a Young Child. *Br. J. Radiol.,* 42:299–303, 1969.
3. Gorlin, R. J., Spranger, J., and Koszalka, M. F.: Genetic Craniotubular Bone Dysplasias and Hyperostoses. A Critical Analysis. *Birth Defects, Original Article Series,* 5: 79–95, 1969.
4. Holt, J. F.: The Evolution of Cranio-Metaphyseal Dysplasia. *Ann. Radiol.,* 9:209–214, 1965.
5. McKusick, V. A.: *Heritable Disorders of Connective Tissue.* The C. V. Mosby Company, St. Louis, 1972.
6. Rimoin, D. L., Woodruff, S. L., and Holman, B. L.: Craniometaphyseal Dysplasia (Pyle's Disease): Autosomal Dominant Inheritance in a Large Kindred. *Birth Defects, Original Article Series,* 5:96–104, 1969.
7. Walker, N.: Pyle's Disease or Cranio-Metaphyseal Dysplasia. *Ann. Radiol.,* 9:197–207, 1966.

CRYPTODONTIC BRACHYMETACARPALIA

This was a syndrome of short straight clavicles, multiple impacted teeth and hand abnormalities similar to those seen in pseudohypoparathyroidism. No abnormalities in serum calcium or phosphorus were noted, nor were there any other clinical signs of pseudohypoparathyroidism. The inheritance was autosomal dominant.

RADIOLOGIC FINDINGS IN THE HAND. There was shortening of the fourth and fifth metacarpals. Most patients had a short distal phalanx of the thumb, resulting in a small thumb. The roentgen appearance of the hands was similar to that seen in the patient illustrated in Figure 9–14.

OTHER RADIOLOGIC FINDINGS. Shortening of the third and fourth metatarsals was noted. The clavicles were straighter and shorter than normal. The teeth were impacted.

REFERENCE

1. Gorlin, R. J., and Sedano, H. O.: Cryptodontic Brachymetacarpalia. *Birth Defects, Original Article Series,* 7:200–203, 1971.

CRYPTOPHTHALMOS SYNDROME

In this condition the eyeball is hidden by a flap of skin. Severe limb changes are present in the cryptophthalmos syndrome, with marked syndactyly, and a decreased number of digits. Ear deformities are commonly associated with this abnormality. Cleft lip and cleft palate are occasionally present. Laryngeal abnormality may be seen. Males often have mild or severe hypospadias or cryptorchidism. Females may have enlargement of the clitoris and labia.

REFERENCES

1. Holmes, L. B. Moser, H. W., Halldorsson, S., Mack, C., Pant, S. S., and Matzilevich, B.: *Mental Retardation. An Atlas of Diseases with Associated Physical Abnormalities.* The Macmillan Company, New York, 1972.
2. Ide, C. H., and Wollschlaeger, P. B.: Multiple Congenital Abnormalities Associated with Cryptophthalmia. *Arch. Ophthalmol.,* 81: 638–644, 1969.

DE LANGE SYNDROME (BRACHMANN–DE LANGE SYNDROME, CORNELIA DE LANGE SYNDROME, TYPUS DEGENERATIVUS AMSTELODAMENSIS)

This condition is associated with mental retardation, growth failure, microbrachycephaly, micrognathia, small nose with anteverted nostrils, characteristic downturned upper lip, low-pitched growling cry, eyebrows meeting in the middle (synophrys), curly eyelashes and hirsutism. The thumb usually has a proximal insertion and there is frequently a simian crease in the hand (Fig. 13–35B). Syndactyly between the second and third toes is common. A large number of miscellaneous anomalies may occasionally be present. This disorder has a wide spectrum of changes, ranging

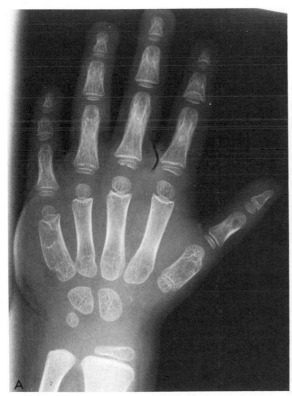
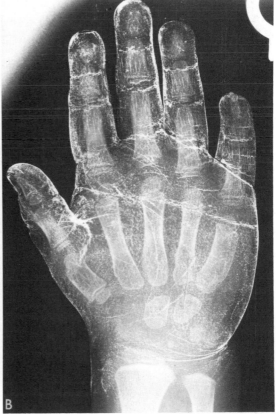

Figure 13–35. de Lange syndrome. *A,* Mild hypoplasia of the thumb and fifth finger. The first metacarpal is hypoplastic, as is the middle phalanx of the fifth finger.

B, Radiodermatography on the opposite hand. Note the simian crease, which is a common finding in this condition.

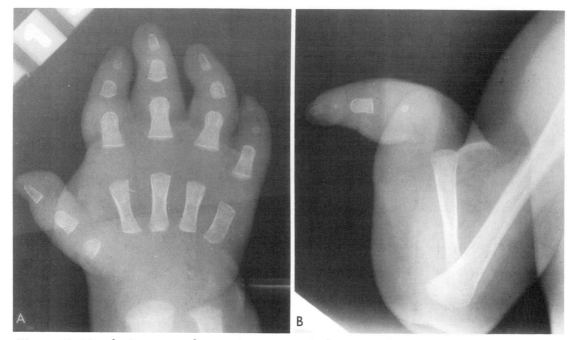

Figure 13–36. de Lange syndrome. Asymmetric findings. *A,* The right hand is typical of the Cornelia de Lange syndrome with a short first metacarpal which is almost a round nodule. There is also marked shortening of the fifth finger, with a very short middle phalanx.

B, Opposite hand of the same patient with the same magnification. There is only one digit. Although this finding is not uncommon in the Cornelia de Lange syndrome, it may occur as an isolated finding.

from very mild to very severe. Patients appear retarded in growth and development at birth and usually fail to thrive. Various chromosomal aberrations have been found in patients with this syndrome, but they are not consistent. The genetic pattern is unknown. Occasional familial cases have been described.

RADIOLOGIC FINDINGS IN THE HAND. In this condition the most characteristic finding is hypoplasia of both the radial and ulnar sides of the hand (Figs. 13–35 and 13–36). The thumb is either very short or completely absent. The most significantly shortened portion of the thumb is the metacarpal, which may be simply a small nodule

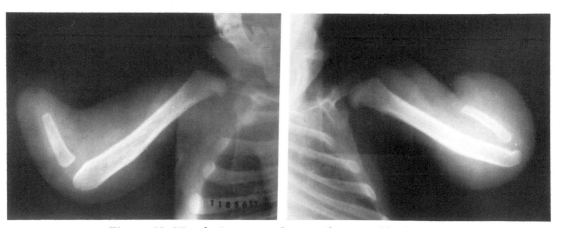

Figure 13–37. de Lange syndrome. Absence of both hands.

(Fig. 13–36A). There may also be some shortening of the distal phalanx of the thumb. The proximal phalanx is usually unremarkable. The hypoplasia of the fifth digit can range from absence of the fifth ray to hypoplasia of its parts. Clinodactyly of the fifth finger is seen in 88 per cent of cases.[7] Other digital abnormalities are variable and include absence of hands (Fig. 13–37) and monodactyly (Fig. 13–36B). Severe hand defects were present in 32 per cent of cases studied by Silver.[7] Skeletal maturation is retarded. McArthur and Edwards[5] reported a case with carpal fusion, but this is not a common manifestation. Lee[3] in 1968 described a de Lange dwarf with Kirner deformity.

OTHER RADIOLOGIC FINDINGS. A large number of other abnormalities may be present, including absence of any of the upper extremity bones. Foot deformity may be present. Rib anomalies, small skull and miscellaneous other abnormalities are well summarized by both Kurlander and De-Meyer,[2] and Lee.[3]

REFERENCES

1. Berg, J. M., McCreary, B. D., Ridler, M. A. C., and Smith, G. F.: The De Lange Syndrome. Pergamon Press, New York, 1970.
2. Kurlander, G. J., and DeMeyer, W.: Roentgenology of the Brachmann-De Lange Syndrome. *Radiology,* 88:101–110, 1967.
3. Lee, F. A.: Generalized Overconstruction of Long Bones and Unilateral Kirner's Deformity in a de Lange Dwarf. *Am. J. Dis. Child.,* 116:599–603, 1968.
4. Lee, F. A., and Kenny, F. M.: Skeletal Changes in the Cornelia de Lange Syndrome. *Am. J. Roentgenol.,* 100:27–39, 1967.
5. McArthur, R. G., and Edwards, J. H.: de Lange Syndrome: Report of 20 Cases. *Can. Med. Assoc. J.,* 96:1185–1198, 1967.
6. Pelc, S., Bollaert, A., and Cremer, N.: A propos du typus degenerativus amstelodamensis. Etude radiologique et pneumo-encéphalographique. *Ann. Radiol.,* 12:903–914, 1969.
7. Silver, H. K.: The de Lange Syndrome. Typus Amstelodamensis. *Am. J. Dis. Child.,* 108: 523–529, 1964.

DIAPHYSEAL DYSPLASIA (ENGELMANN-CAMURATI DISEASE)

This is a rare disorder of bone. The patient is usually underweight and has an un-

usual wide-based gait. The patient appears straight-legged with spindle-shaped limbs, poor musculature and normal mentation. Inheritance is autosomal dominant with marked variability in expression.

RADIOLOGIC FINDINGS IN THE HAND. The hand is infrequently affected in this disorder (Fig. 13–38). It was affected in 16 per cent of cases in the world literature as studied by Benabderrahmane et al.[1] The radiographic findings include increased density of the midshafts of the metacarpals and phalanges and apparent thickening of the cortex (Fig. 13–39). The involvement may be symmetric or asymmetric. In several

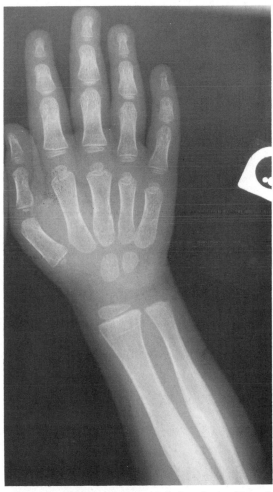

Figure 13–38. Diaphyseal dysplasia (Engelmann-Camurati disease). The patient had extensive skeletal involvement of most of the long bones of the skeleton and even of the spine, but the hands are relatively unaffected. Widening of the diaphysis of the radius and ulna is seen.

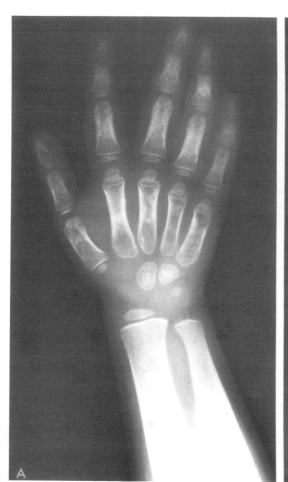

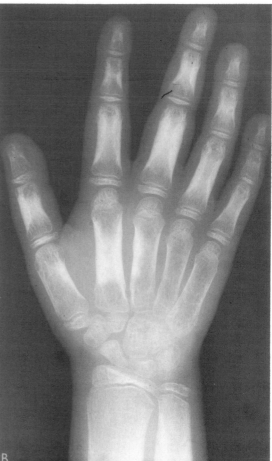

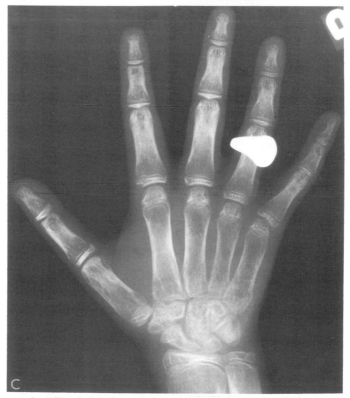

Figure 13-39. *See opposite page for legend.*

of the published cases the radial side of the hand appears more involved than the ulnar. An interesting finding in Mottram and Hill's[3] case was the relative progression, which was then followed by regression (Fig. 13–39).

OTHER RADIOLOGIC FINDINGS. The classic radiographic findings include a fusiform widening of the diaphysis of the long bones. The skull is usually affected and any of the bones can be involved. Occasional cases of spine involvement have also been seen.

REFERENCES

1. Benabderrahmane, M., Siegenthaler, P., Uhlmann, C., and Wettstein, P.: Le syndrome de Camurati-Engelmann. A propos d'un Cas et Revue de la Littérature. *Schweiz. Med. Wochenschr.*, 99:1204–1212, 1969.
2. Lennon, E. A., Schechter, M. M., and Hornabrook, R. W.: Engelmann's Disease. Report of a Case with a Review of the Literature. *J. Bone Joint Surg.*, 43B:273–284, 1961.
3. Mottram, M. E., and Hill, H. A.: Diaphyseal Dysplasia. Report of a Case. *Am. J. Roentgenol.*, 95:162–167, 1965.
4. Sparkes, R. S., and Graham, C. B.: Camurati-Engelmann Disease. Genetics and Clinical Manifestations with a Review of the Literature. *J. Med. Genet.*, 9:73–85, 1972.

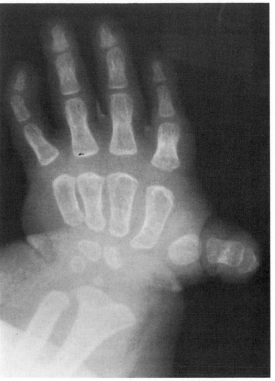

Figure 13–40. Diastrophic dwarfism. Infant with typical "hitchhiker's thumb." The first metacarpal is short and round but of normal width. There is some shortening of all of the digits.

DIASTROPHIC DWARFISM

Diastrophic dwarfism means bent or twisted dwarfism. The condition refers to a form of short-limbed dwarfism, which can be differentiated from achondroplasia by the presence of clubfoot deformity and scoliosis. Deformity of the pinnae of the ears is seen in 82 per cent of cases.[1] Cleft palate may be seen. Intelligence is usually normal. The condition is inherited as an autosomal recessive trait. The patients may live to late adult life.

RADIOLOGIC FINDINGS IN THE HAND. Characteristically, the hand bones are very small. The thumb points away from the hand in a hitchhiker's attitude (Fig. 13–40). The first metacarpal is very small and may be simply a round or oval ossicle. Epiphyseal abnormalities are common; occasionally, vertical clefts are also noted in the phalanges (Fig. 13–41).

The carpals are also abnormal; they may be precocious in appearance. Extra carpals are common particularly in the distal row.

Figure 13–39. Diaphyseal dysplasia (Engelmann-Camurati disease). *A*, Age 4. There are minimal findings in the hand with some sclerosis of the diaphyses.

B, Age 12½ years. Diaphyseal thickening has progressed. The radial side is more involved than the ulnar, with the most marked findings seen in the second metacarpal.

C, Age 18. There has been considerable diminution of the diaphyseal sclerosis since the previous study.

(Films courtesy Dr. M. E. Mottram, San Francisco, California. Figure *B* reproduced courtesy *Am. J. Roentgenol.*, 95:162–167, 1965.)

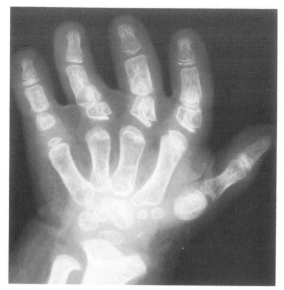

Figure 13–41. Diastrophic dwarfism. Four year old girl. The short oval first metacarpal is again seen. Bizarre epiphyses are seen in the proximal phalanges. Additional carpals are seen in the distal row.

The capitate may be transverse in position. In older individuals with this condition, the joints become very narrow (Fig. 13–42).[3] The carpal angle is often increased (Fig. 13–43).

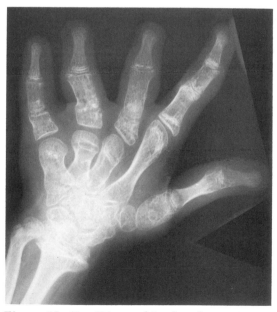

Figure 13–42. Diastrophic dwarfism. 12 year old sister of patient in Figure 13–41. There is irregular shortening of the digits. The intercarpal joints are narrowed.

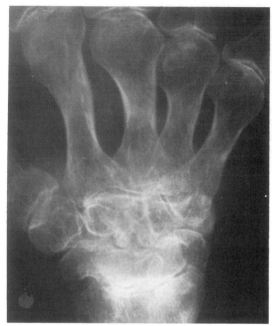

Figure 13–43. Diastrophic dwarfism. Elderly male. There is marked narrowing of the intercarpal joints with increase in the carpal angle. (From Poznanski, A. K. et al.: *Am. J. Roentgenol.,* 112: 443–459, 1971.)

OTHER RADIOLOGIC FINDINGS. Clubfoot deformity and scoliosis are the hallmarks of this disease, although many of the other long bones are also abnormal. Generally the epiphyses are flat and irregular.

REFERENCES

1. Langer, L. O., Jr.: Diastrophic Dwarfism in Early Infancy. *Am. J. Roentgenol.,* 93: 399–404, 1965.
2. Maroteaux, P.: Etude Radiologique De Trois Nouvelles Affections Osseuses Constitutionnelles. *Ann. Radiol.,* 5:551–563, 1962.
3. Poznanski, A. K., and Holt, J. F.: The Carpals in Congenital Malformation Syndromes. *Am. J. Roentgenol.,* 112:443–459, 1971.
4. Stover, C. N., Hayes, J. T., and Holt, J. F.: Diastrophic Dwarfism. *Am. J. Roentgenol.,* 89:914–922, 1963.
5. Taybi, H.: Diastrophic Dwarfism. *Radiology,* 80:1–10, 1963.

DYGGVE-MELCHIOR-CLAUSEN SYNDROME (MORQUIO-ULLRICH DISEASE)

This form of short-limbed dwarfism is inherited as an autosomal recessive trait. The condition is differentiated from Morquio disease by the absence of corneal clouding, dental enamel abnormality, proximal metacarpal pointing, hypoplasia of the vertebral bodies and excretion of keratan sulfate in the urine.

RADIOLOGIC FINDINGS IN THE HAND. The findings in the hand are considerably milder than those in Morquio or Hurler syndrome. There is no pointing of the proximal metacarpals. The main findings are small carpals.

OTHER RADIOLOGIC FINDINGS. The most characteristic finding, according to Kaufman et al.[2] is a lacy appearance of the iliac crest. There is evidence of platyspondyly and pelvic abnormality, and miscellaneous other findings.

DYSCHONDROSTEOSIS (LERI-WEILL SYNDROME)

Dyschondrosteosis is an autosomal dominant condition which is associated with a Madelung-type deformity of the wrist and moderate dwarfism. Most patients are females and most average below five feet in height. Dyschondrosteosis may simply be a part of the wide spectrum of mesomelic dwarfism, the extreme of which is the Langer type (p. 329).[5]

RADIOLOGIC FINDINGS IN THE HAND. A Madelung-type deformity is present, with a decrease in the carpal angle (Fig. 13–44). The phalanges of the hand may be short.

OTHER RADIOLOGIC FINDINGS. There may be a short radius and ulna with deformity, and short tibias and fibulas.

REFERENCES

1. Dyggve, H. V., Melchior, J. C., and Clausen, J.: Morquio-Ullrich's Disease. An Inborn Error of Metabolism? *Arch. Dis. Child.*, 37:525–534, 1962.
2. Kaufman, R. L., Rimoin, D. L., and McAlister, W. H.: The Dyggve-Melchior-Clausen Syndrome. *Birth Defects, Original Article Series*, 7:144–149, 1971.

REFERENCES

1. Berdon, W. E., Grossman, H., and Baker, D. H.: Dyschondrosteose (Léri-Weill Syndrome): Congenital Short Forearms, Madelung-Type Wrist Deformities, and Moderate Dwarfism. *Radiology*, 85:677–681, 1965.
2. Felman, A. H., and Kirkpatrick, J. A., Jr.: Dyschondrosteose, Mesomelic Dwarfism of

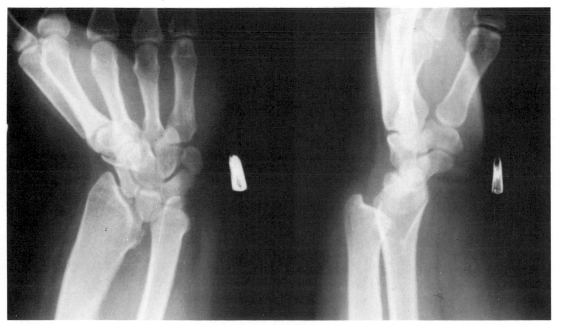

Figure 13–44. Dyschondrosteosis. A Madelung-like deformity of the wrist is seen, with a deep cup formed by the proximal carpals. The ulna is displaced posteriorly. The rest of the hand is unremarkable.

Leri and Weill. *Am. J. Dis. Child.*, 120: 329–331, 1970.
3. Kozłowski, K., and Zychowicz, C.: Dyschondrosteosis. *Acta Radiol.*, 11:459–465, 1971.
4. Langer, L. O., Jr.: Dyschondrosteosis, A Hereditable Bone Dysplasia with Characteristic Roentgenographic Features. *Am. J. Roentgenol.*, 95:178–188, 1965.
5. Silverman, F. N.: Mesomelic Dwarfism. *Progr. Pediat. Radiol.*, 4:546–562, 1973. (*Intrinsic Diseases of Bones*, edited by H. J. Kaufmann, Karger, Basel.)

DYSOSTEOSCLEROSIS

This disorder, named by Spranger et al.[3], is characterized by osteosclerosis and platyspondyly. The limbs are short as compared to the trunk, though the trunk may be deformed. Paralysis of the optic, facial or abducens nerve may be seen early in life. Some degree of spasticity has been noted. Inheritance is probably autosomal recessive.

RADIOLOGIC FINDINGS IN THE HAND. The most striking findings are bands of sclerosis adjacent to the metaphyses of the tubular bones of the hand. There is radiolucency beneath these. There is some failure of modeling, which is less marked in the metacarpals and phalanges than in the distal radius and ulna.

OTHER RADIOLOGIC FINDINGS. Similar sclerotic changes are seen in other bones of the body. One of the important characteristics of this condition is platyspondyly with wide intervertebral spaces. There may be some bowing of the long bones. The base of the skull is thickened.

REFERENCES

1. Gorlin, R. J., Spranger, J., and Koszalka, M. F.: Genetic Craniotubular Bone Dysplasias and Hyperostoses. A Critical Analysis. *Birth Defects, Original Article Series*, 5: 79–95, 1969.
2. Roy, C. Maroteaux, P., Kremp, L., Courtecuisse, V., and Alagille, D.: Un Nouveau Syndrome Osseux Avec Anomalies Cutanees et Troubles Neurologiques. *Arch. Fr. Pediatr.*, 25:393–905, 1968.
3. Spranger, J., Rohwedder, H.-J., and Wiedemann, H.-R.: Die Dysosteosklerose—eine Sonderform der generalisierten Osteosklerose. *Fortschr. Geb. Roentgenstr. Nuklearmed.*, 109:504–512, 1968.

DYSPLASIA EPIPHYSEALIS HEMIMELICA

This is a rare developmental disorder with asymmetrical cartilaginous overgrowth that usually affects the lower extremities. Fairbank[1] reported one case in which the carpus was involved, but this appears to be extremely rare.

REFERENCES

1. Fairbank, T. J.: Dysplasia Epiphysialis Hemimelica (Tarso-epiphysial Aclasis). *J. Bone Joint Surg.*, 38B:237–257, 1956.
2. Kettelkamp, D. B., Campbell, C. J., and Bonfiglio, M.: Dysplasia Epiphysealis Hemimelica: A Report of Fifteen Cases and a Review of the Literature. *J. Bone Joint Surg.*, 48A:746–766, 1966.

ECTODERMAL DYSPLASIA

This is a broad term that includes a number of syndromes. In this section we will exclude certain other syndromes that have ectodermal dysplasia, particularly the Ellis-van Creveld and Rothmund syndrome, which are listed separately. In addition to these two, there are eight different types listed by Smith.[5] Reed et al.[1] classify the hereditary ectodermal dysplasias into six forms, one of which is the Rothmund-Thomson syndrome. The clinical findings depend on the specific form of ectodermal dysplasia and include tooth abnormalities, sparse and thin hair, dystrophy of the nails and abnormality of the sweat glands. The inheritance may be autosomal recessive or dominant, or X-linked recessive, depending on the form.[1]

RADIOLOGIC FINDINGS IN THE HAND. In most of these conditions no radiologic manifestations are seen in the hand. However, in several forms there has been association of cleft hand and missing digits.[3, 4] Hypoplastic thumbs have been seen in one family described by Rosselli and Gulienetti.[3] Although most cases with anhidrotic dysplasia do not show hand abnormalities, these have occasionally been present.[4]

REFERENCES

1. Reed, W. B., Lopez, D. A., and Landing, B.: Clinical Spectrum of Anhidrotic Ectodermal Dysplasia. *Arch. Derm.*, 102:134–143, 1970.

2. Robinson, G. C., Wildervanck, L. S., and Chiang, T. P.: Ectrodactyly, Ectodermal Dysplasia, and Cleft Lip-Palate Syndrome. Its Association with Conductive Hearing Loss. *J. Pediatr.*, 82: 107–109, 1973.
3. Rosselli, D., and Gulienetti, R.: Ectodermal Dysplasia. *Br. J. Plast. Surg.*, 14:190–204, 1961.
4. Rüdiger, R. A., Haase, W., and Passarge, E.: Association of Ectrodactyly, Ectodermal Dysplasia, and Cleft Lip-Palate. *Am. J. Dis. Child.*, 120:160–163, 1970.
5. Smith, D. W.: *Recognizable Patterns of Human Malformation.* W. B. Saunders Company, Philadelphia, 1970.

ENCHONDROMATOSIS (OLLIER DISEASE, DYSCHONDROPLASIA)

This is a syndrome of multiple enchondromas which can appear clinically as multiple swellings of different extremities. There may be severe alterations in length of

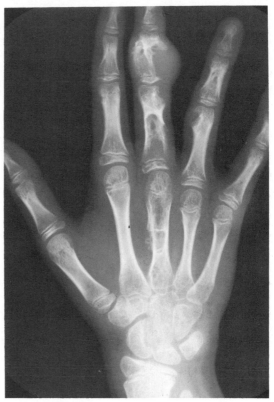

Figure 13–46. Enchondromatosis (Ollier disease). Multiple bizarre lesions are seen within the bones, particularly in the third and fourth digits. There is some soft tissue swelling in the distal portion of the middle finger.

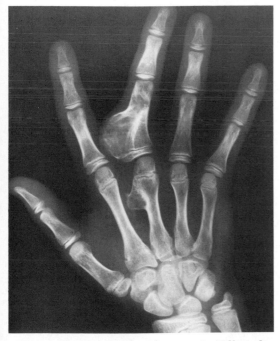

Figure 13–45. Enchondromatosis (Ollier disease). 13 year old male. There are eccentric echondromas on the third proximal phalanx and the third metacarpal. The proximal phalangeal lesion causes deviation of the digit toward the ulnar side. The lesion in the metacarpal could be confused with an exostosis.

the bones. The severity of the disease is variable, ranging from an occasional enchondroma to marked disfiguring changes. According to McKusick,[3] no genetic basis for this disorder has been established, since no familial cases have been noted.

RADIOLOGIC FINDINGS IN THE HAND. The enchondromas in the hand may appear as cartilaginous tumors similar to the isolated variety discussed in Chapter 15. They can range from single expansile radiolucencies within the bone to eccentric lesions which may be difficult to differentiate from exostoses (Fig. 13–45). Occasionally they appear more diffuse, producing bizarre irregular central bone changes (Fig. 13–46). The severity of the disease varies considerably, ranging from minor changes involving only a few bones to extensive changes involving most of the hand (Fig. 13–47). Le-

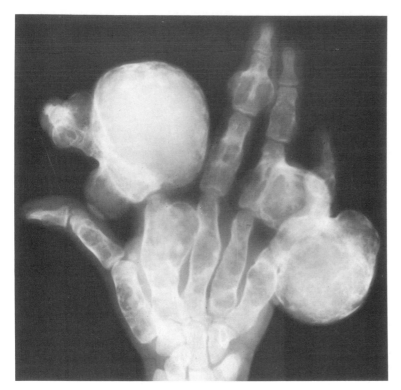

Figure 13–47. Enchondromatosis (Ollier disease). There are marked changes with large tumors involving most of the fingers, particularly the index and the fifth. There is some soft tissue calcification within the tumors. There is gross deformity of the fingers resulting from these large tumors. (Courtesy Dr. E. S. Huckins, Bay City, Michigan.)

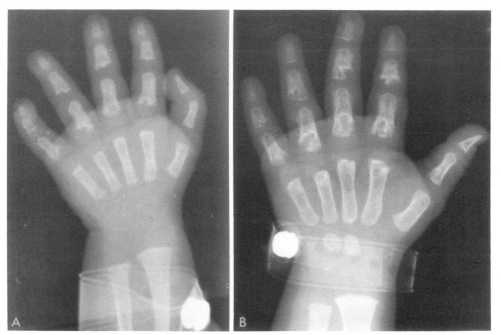

Figure 13–48. Enchondromatosis (Maffucci syndrome). This child also had associated hemangiomas, but the radiologic findings are the same as would be seen in Ollier disease in the infant age group. In *A*, very minimal findings are noted in the neonatal period; there are small punched-out lesions that may be difficult to diagnose. On a follow-up film (*B*) the lesions become more typical in appearance, involving multiple bones. (Courtesy Dr. D. Babitt, Milwaukee, Wisconsin.)

sions are usually asymmetric, affecting one part of the body more than another. When the enchondromas are located near an epiphysis, they can severely affect the growth of a bone, causing deviation of the digits and failure of growth with resultant brachydactyly. In infancy the enchondromas are very subtle (Fig. 13–48), appearing as small lucent defects. With time, they become more typical in appearance. In later life the growth of the enchondromas may spontaneously arrest.[2]

OTHER RADIOLOGIC FINDINGS. There is often evidence of enchondromas elsewhere in other bones, often in a unilateral distribution. The effects on the other bones are similar to those in the hand.

REFERENCES

1. Farriaux, J.-P., Renard, V., Samaille, G., Cordier, R., and L'Hermine, C.: La Dyschondroplasie. Étude d'une Observation suivie de l'Âge de 18 Mois à 7 Ans et Demi. Presse Med., 76: 1240–1243, 1968.
2. Mainzer, F., Minagi, H., and Steinbach, H. L.: The Variable Manifestations of Multiple Enchondromatosis. Radiology, 99:377–388, 1971.
3. McKusick, V. A.: Heritable Disorders of Connective Tissue. The C. V. Mosby Company, St. Louis, 1972.
4. Rubin, P.: Dynamic Classification of Bone Dysplasias. Year Book Medical Publishers, Inc., Chicago, 1964.

ENCHONDROMATOSIS WITH HEMANGIOMA (MAFFUCCI SYNDROME)

This is the association of cavernous hemangioma and enchondromatosis. In many ways it is similar to Ollier disease. All cases of this condition are sporadic and the genetic pattern is not known. Occasionally brain tumors, ovarian teratomas, and sarcomas may be associated with the syndrome.[3]

RADIOLOGIC FINDINGS IN THE HAND. The appearance is that of multiple enchondromas, which can be quite large and can involve many of the hand bones. When large they can affect the growth of the bone, causing distortion in shape and length of these bones. They also may predispose the bone to fracture. In early infancy the enchondromas are less apparent and become

evident as the child grows (Fig. 13–48). In some cases a number of phleboliths can be seen in the associated hemangiomas. On arteriography, multiple arteriovenous malformations may be noted.[4]

OTHER RADIOLOGIC FINDINGS. Enchondromas may be found in other portions of the body, including the long bones and the mandible.

REFERENCES

1. Anderson, I. F.: Maffucci's Syndrome. Report of a Case with a Review of the Literature. S. Afr. Med. J., 39:1066–1070, 1965.
2. Andren, L., Dymling, J. F., Elner, A., and Hogeman, K. E.: Maffucci's Syndrome. Report of 4 Cases. Acta Chir. Scand., 126:397–405, 1963.
3. Banna, M., and Parwani, G. S.: Multiple Sarcomas in Maffucci's Syndrome. Br. J. Radiol., 42: 304–307, 1969.
4. Howard, F. M., and Lee, R. E., Jr.: The Hand in Maffucci Syndrome. Arch. Surg., 103:752–756, 1971.

ENDOSTEAL HYPEROSTOSIS (VAN BUCHEM DISEASE, HYPEROSTOSIS CORTICALIS GENERALISATA)

This is a systemic condition of the skeleton with overgrowth of the skull and mandible. The hyperostosis involves many bones and can cause compression of cranial nerves as they pass through the base of the skull, particularly the facial nerve (in 12 of 15 patients studied by van Buchem). Choked discs also have been seen. Bones are not painful and do not appear to be prone to fracture. The chin becomes widened and thickened beginning in the early teens.

RADIOLOGIC FINDINGS IN THE HAND. There is marked hyperostosis and thickening of the tubular bones of the hand (Fig. 13–49).[1] The metacarpals are most significantly affected, while the carpals are apparently spared. The thickening is mainly confined to the diaphysis, with the ends of the bones appearing relatively clear. In some cases in the literature the findings in the hand are relatively mild.

OTHER RADIOLOGIC FINDINGS. Similar radiologic changes are seen in other bones of the body. The skull and mandible are particularly affected.

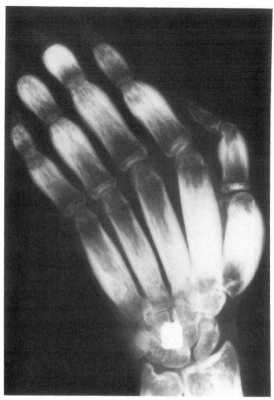

Figure 13–49. Endosteal hyperostosis (van Buchem disease). There is marked increase in the density of the shafts of the bones with considerable thickening. (Courtesy Dr. R. J. Fosmoe and Dr. R. C. Hildreth. From *Radiology*, 90:771–774, 1968.)

REFERENCES

1. Fosmoe, R. J., Holm, R. S., and Hildreth, R. C.: Van Buchem's Disease (Hyperostosis Corticalis Generalisata Familiaris). A Case Report. *Radiology*, 90:771–774, 1968.
2. van Buchem, F. S. P.: Hyperostosis Corticalis Generalisata. Eight New Cases. *Acta Med. Scand.*, 189:257–267, 1971.
3. van Buchem, F. S. P.: The Pathogenesis of Hyperostosis Corticalis Generalisata and Calcitonin. *Proc. K. Ned. Akad. Wet (Biol. Med.)*, 73:243–253, 1970.

EPIDERMOLYSIS BULLOSA

Epidermolysis bullosa is a chronic skin disorder which is due to poor adherence of the epidermis to the dermis, resulting in formation of vesicles, bullae and ulcers. It may be inherited as either a dominant or a recessive. The recessive form is the most severe. Hand deformities are common, with claw-hand or closed-fist configuration.

RADIOLOGIC FINDINGS IN THE HAND. There are flexion contractures of the metacarpophalangeal and interphalangeal joints (Fig. 13–50). Marked webbing occurs between the fingers. There can be trophic changes distally, with pointing of the distal phalanges of the fingers which may resemble scleroderma. The distal tip changes are most likely caused by decreased blood supply.

OTHER RADIOLOGIC FINDINGS. Other findings include esophageal strictures, skeletal demineralization and overconstriction of the long bones.

REFERENCES

1. Becker, M. H., and Swinyard, C. A.: Epidermolysis Bullosa Dystrophica in Children. Radiologic Manifestations. *Radiology*, 90:124–128, 1968.
2. Brinn, L. B., and Khilnani, M. T.: Epidermolysis Bullosa with Characteristic Hand Deformities. *Radiology*, 89:272–274, 1967.
3. Horner, R. L., Wiedel, J. D., and Bralliar, F.: Involvement of the Hand in Epidermolysis Bullosa. *J. Bone Joint Surg.*, 53A:1347–1356, 1971.

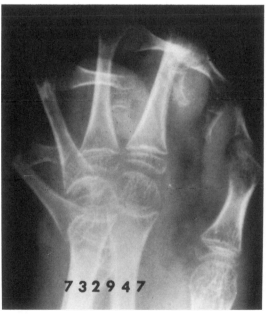

Figure 13–50. Epidermolysis bullosa. There is marked demineralization of the bones of the hand, which are severely contracted. The distal phalanges are pointed and shortened; this is best seen in the thumb.

EPIPHYSEAL DYSPLASIA (MULTIPLE EPIPHYSEAL DYSPLASIA, DYSPLASIA EPIPHYSEALIS MULTIPLEX, FAIRBANK DISEASE)

The term "multiple epiphyseal dysplasia" usually refers to the Fairbank form of the disease, though various authors have used the term for different conditions. The term probably includes a group of diseases rather than a single entity. The main finding in these conditions is an abnormality of the epiphyses that results in shortness of stature which is usually not severe. Clinical manifestations may also include evidence of arthritis, particularly in the hips. There is some overlap between this disease and other abnormalities that involve the epiphyses, in particular chondrodysplasia punctata. Silverman[7] has noted a case of chondrodysplasia punctata which with time appeared as an epiphyseal dysplasia. Most reported cases are inherited as an autosomal dominant,[5] although some cases of recessive inheritance have also been described.[4]

RADIOLOGIC FINDINGS IN THE HAND. A wide spectrum of abnormalities may be seen in the hand, depending on the type of epiphyseal dysplasia. In many cases the hands are much less involved than are the hips or the knees.

In some forms the carpals are irregular and fuzzy in their outline and they may sometimes be fragmented (Fig. 13–51). The capitate is most frequently affected. Carpal maturation, in particular that of the capitate, is often markedly delayed. Alterations in the carpal angle have been noted.[6] Usually there is an increase in the carpal angle (Figs. 13–52 to 13–54), although even this is variable. In the family reported by Juberg and Holt,[4] most individuals had an increased carpal angle, while in some the carpal angle was smaller than normal.

The epiphyseal abnormalities also vary with the type of epiphyseal dysplasia. The epiphyses may be irregular and fragmented (Fig. 13–51). They may have some increase in sclerosis, sometimes mimicking dense epiphyses. In some patients with epiphyseal dysplasia the epiphyses may be very late in appearing (Fig. 13–54). The epiphyses often appear thinner than usual.

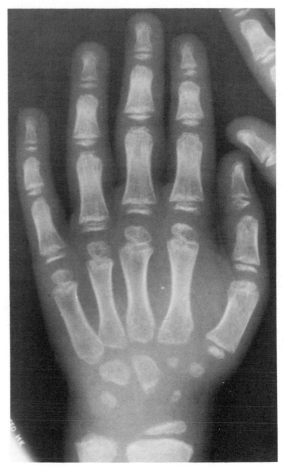

Figure 13–51. Epiphyseal dysplasia. There is irregularity of the outline of the carpal bones as well as of the phalangeal epiphyses. Pseudoepiphyses are noted at the distal end of the proximal phalanges. The bones of the hands are not markedly altered in size.

The dense sclerotic epiphyses reach their most marked form in Thiemann disease, which is discussed separately in this chapter.

Various bone length alterations also may be seen. The bones may be relatively normal in length in some patients (Figs. 13–51 and 13–53), while in others severe brachydactyly may be noted (Fig. 13–55). This was particularly noticeable in the cases reported by Juberg and Holt,[4] some of which had shortening of the fourth and other metacarpals as adults. This may be related to early

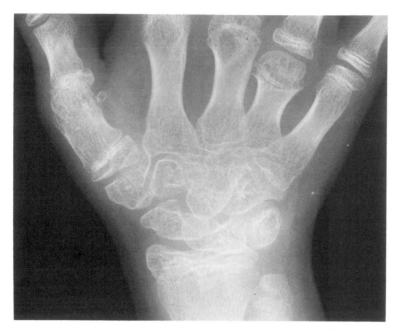

Figure 13–52. Epiphyseal dysplasia. Nine year old female. There is a marked increase in the carpal angle. The proximal carpals are almost lined up in a straight row. The carpals are somewhat small. There is shortening of the fourth metacarpal with an abnormal epiphysis. The first metacarpal is also shortened. This is a member of the family reported by Juberg and Holt.

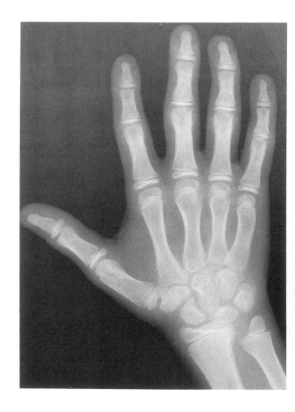

Figure 13–53. Epiphyseal dysplasia. 11 year old male. The hand changes are relatively minimal. There is only some flattening of the epiphyses of the middle phalanges and perhaps also some of the metacarpal heads. Elsewhere in the skeleton the patient had more typical findings, including a cleft in the patella. His brother was also affected.

closure or absence of epiphyses (Fig. 13–54). The pattern of alteration of bone length in those conditions does not seem to be characteristic.

OTHER RADIOLOGIC FINDINGS. Most epiphyses are affected. The most marked changes occur in the hips, and these may mimic Perthes disease. A common finding is a coronal cleft in the patella.

Multiple epiphyseal dysplasia must be differentiated from other conditions with epiphyseal involvement, particularly diastrophic dwarfism, pseudoachondroplastic dysplasia, spondyloepiphyseal dysplasia and spondylometaphyseal dysplasia. A useful differentiating factor is that in multiple epiphyseal dysplasia the spine is not significantly involved.

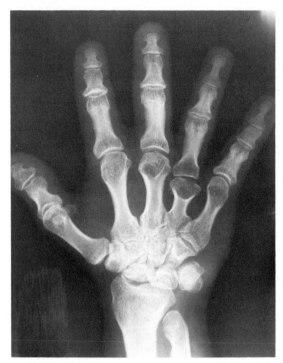

Figure 13–55. Epiphyseal dysplasia. This patient is related to the patient described in Figure 13–52. The carpal angle is flattened and there is marked shortening of some of the metacarpals.

REFERENCES

1. Fairbank, T.: Dysplasia Epiphysialis Multiplex. *Br. J. Surg.*, 134:225–232, 1947.
2. Hulvey, J. T., and Keats, T.: Multiple Epiphyseal Dysplasia. A Contribution to the Problem of Spinal Involvement. *Am. J. Roentgenol.*, 106: 170–177, 1969.
3. Jacobs, P.: Multiple Epiphyseal Dysplasia. *Progr. Pediatr. Radiol.*, 4:309–324, 1973. (*Intrinsic Diseases of Bones*, edited by H. J. Kaufmann, Karger, Basel.)
4. Juberg, R. C., and Holt, J. F.: Inheritance of Multiple Epiphyseal Dysplasia, Tarda. *Am. J. Hum. Genet.*, 20:549–563, 1968.
5. Kozlowski, K., and Lipska, E.: Hereditary Dysplasia Epiphysealis Multiplex. *Clin. Radiol.*, 18:330–336, 1967.
6. Poznanski, A. K., and Holt, J. F.: The Carpals in Congenital Malformation Syndromes. *Am. J. Roentgenol.*, 112:443–459, 1971.
7. Silverman, F. N.: Dysplasies Épiphysaires: Entité Protéiforme. *Ann. Radiol.*, 4:833–867, 1961.

FARBER DISEASE (LIPOGRANULOMATOSIS)

This is an inborn error of lipid metabolism which manifests itself with develop-

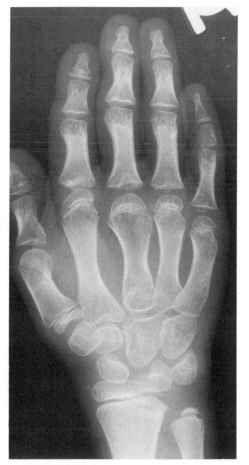

Figure 13–54. Epiphyseal dysplasia. Eight year old male. There is marked delay in onset of ossification of the epiphyses of the phalanges. The carpals appear relatively normal.

ment of tender, swollen joints particularly in the hands. The condition is fatal, usually within two years. It is probably inherited as an autosomal recessive.

RADIOLOGIC FINDINGS IN THE HAND. These have been poorly defined. They consist of soft tissue swelling in periarticular areas, contractures and, occasionally, destructive changes in bone.

REFERENCES

1. Farber, S., Cohen, J., and Uzman, L. L.: Lipogranulomatosis. A New Lipo-Glyco-Protein "Storage" Disease. *Mt. Sinai J. Med. N.Y.*, 24:816–837, 1957.
2. Schanche, A. F., Bierman, S. M., Sopher, R. L., and O'Loughlin, B. J.: Disseminated Lipogranulomatosis: Early Roentgenographic Changes. *Radiology*, 82:675–678, 1964.
3. Zetterström, R.: Disseminated Lipogranulomatosis (Farber's Disease). *Acta Paediatr.*, 47:501–510, 1958.

FIBROUS DYSPLASIA (JAFFE-LICHTENSTEIN DISEASE, WITH SEXUAL PRECOCITY–THE McCUNE-ALBRIGHT SYNDROME)

This condition of unknown cause is included in this chapter because it has been considered with the bone dysplasias in the European classification. Pathologically it is a fibrous replacement of portions of the medullary cavities. It may be monostotic or polyostotic. Most cases can be traced back to childhood (131 of 148 cases studied by Pritchard).[5] Clinical symptoms may be due to bone expansion and consequent soft tissue thickening, or due to fracture, which occurs in about 40 per cent of cases.[3] Bowing of the bones may also be seen. The polyostotic form is often associated with café au lait spots. Sexual precocity is seen in 20 per cent of cases[3] and occurs almost entirely in females. Other endocrine dysfunctions may also be seen in these patients, particularly hyperthyroidism[6] and Cushing disease.[1]

RADIOLOGIC FINDINGS IN THE HAND. The characteristic appearance is that of a widened medullary space which often may have a ground-glass appearance (Fig. 13–56). The bone involvement may be spotty,

sparing some fingers while affecting others. Another manifestation is areas of radiolucency which may appear as punched-out lesions (Fig. 13–56). Any of the bones of the hand may be involved, including the carpals. When associated with precocious puberty there is advancement of skeletal maturation (Fig. 13–57). Fibrous dysplasia has also been seen in association with myositis ossificans progressiva[4] and its consequent radiologic changes (Fig. 13–106).

OTHER RADIOLOGIC FINDINGS. The findings in the remainder of the skeleton are similar to those in the hand. Skull changes may mimic Paget disease, and fractures and pseudoarthroses may be seen with this condition.

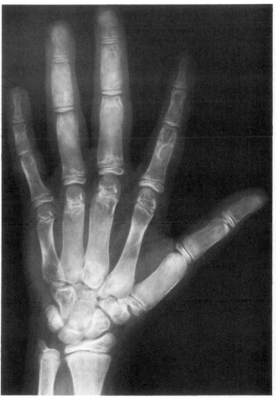

Figure 13–56. Fibrous dysplasia. 12 year old boy who had multiple fractures and café au lait spots. There is expansion and swelling of several of the metacarpals and phalanges, particularly in the third and fourth fingers. The bones involved have a ground-glass appearance. Some lucent defects are seen, particularly in the region of the index finger and in the scaphoid. This boy had no evidence of sexual precocity.

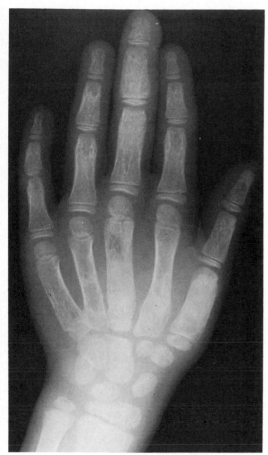

Myositis Ossificans Progressiva. *Am. J. Dis. Child.*, 124:120–122, 1972.
5. Pritchard, J. E.: Fibrous Dysplasia of the Bones. *Am. J. Med. Sci.*, 222:313–332, 1951.
6. Zangeneh, F., Lulejian, G. A., and Steiner, M. M.: McCune-Albright Syndrome with Hyperthyroidism. *Am. J. Dis. Child.*, 111:644–648, 1966.

Figure 13–57. Fibrous dysplasia (McCune-Albright syndrome). This five year old girl had precocious puberty. She had only a few café au lait spots. Radiograph of the hand shows typical changes of fibrous dysplasia, with widening of several of the bones and a ground-glass appearance. Occasional focal areas of radiolucency are seen, particularly in the third metacarpal. The bone age is markedly advanced, which is consistent with the precocious puberty. The typical changes of fibrous dysplasia were also seen elsewhere in her body.

FOCAL DERMAL HYPOPLASIA (GOLTZ SYNDROME)

This is a syndrome of dermal hypoplasia, with linear areas of dermal hypoplasia associated with altered pigmentation. There may be telangiectasia and lipomatous nodules in areas of skin atrophy. The nails are dystrophic and hypoplastic. There is also hypoplasia of the teeth. Eye abnormalities may be present. The condition is almost entirely limited to females; the reported male cases have been rare.

RADIOLOGIC FINDINGS IN THE HAND. The most common finding is syndactyly, which may occur between various digits but which is most frequent between the third and fourth fingers. Although the cutaneous form is more common, syndactyly may involve the bones. In occasional cases polydactyly may be present, although this is more common in the feet than in the hands. Cleft hand or absence of digits may also occur, and these manifestations may be variable. Clinodactyly and camptodactyly are also common.

OTHER RADIOLOGIC FINDINGS. Other skeletal abnormalities are nonspecific. Walbaum et al.[4] reviewed the literature and found cases of scoliosis, microcephaly, spina bifida, genu valgum and hip abnormalities.

REFERENCES

1. Aarskog, D., and Tveteraas, E.: McCune-Albright's Syndrome Following Adrenalectomy for Cushing's Syndrome in Infancy. *J. Pediatr.*, 73:89–96, 1968.
2. Aegerter, E., and Kirkpatrick, J. A., Jr.: *Orthopedic Diseases. Physiology · Pathology · Radiology*, 2nd Ed. W. B. Saunders Company, Philadelphia, 1964.
3. Edeiken, J., and Hodes, P. J.: *Roentgen Diagnosis of Diseases of Bone.* The Williams & Wilkins Co., Baltimore, 1967.
4. Frame, B., Azad, N., Reynolds, W. A., and Saeed, S. M.: Polyostotic Fibrous Dysplasia and

REFERENCES

1. Ginsburg, L. D., Sedano, H. O., and Gorlin, R. J.: Focal Dermal Hypoplasia Syndrome. *Am. J. Roentgenol.*, 110:561–571, 1970.
2. Goltz, R. W., Henderson, R. R., Hitch, J. M., and Ott, J. E.: Focal Dermal Hypoplasia Syndrome. A Review of the Literature and Report of Two Cases. *Arch. Derm.*, 101:1–11, 1970.
3. Gorlin, R. J., Meskin, L. H., Peterson, W. C., Jr., and Goltz, R. W.: Focal Dermal Hypoplasia Syndrome. *Acta Derm. Venereol.*, 43:421–440, 1963.
4. Walbaum, R., Samaille, G., and Dehaene, P.: Syndrome de Goltz Chez un Garcon. *Pediatrie*, 25:911–920, 1970.

FRONTODIGITAL SYNDROME

This was a rare autosomal dominant syndrome of frontal bossing, prominent bony sagittal ridge, syndactyly of the hands and feet and broad thumbs. The appearance was similar to that in some of the acrocephalosyndactyly syndromes; however, there was a good prognosis for mental and physical development.

RADIOLOGIC FINDINGS IN THE HAND. There may be postaxial polydactyly, broadening of the thumb and syndactyly.

OTHER RADIOLOGIC FINDINGS. There was absence of cranial synostosis and a relatively normal-appearing skull, and preaxial polydactyly of the feet.

REFERENCE

1. Marshall, R. E., and Smith, D. W.: Frontodigital Syndrome: A Dominantly Inherited Disorder with Normal Intelligence. *J. Pediatr.*, 77:129–133, 1970.

FRONTOMETAPHYSEAL DYSPLASIA

This condition is characterized by pronounced overgrowth of the supraorbital ridges, agenesis of the frontal sinuses, underdevelopment of the mandible, metaphyseal splaying of the tubular bones, flaring of the iliac bones, conductive deafness and hirsutism.

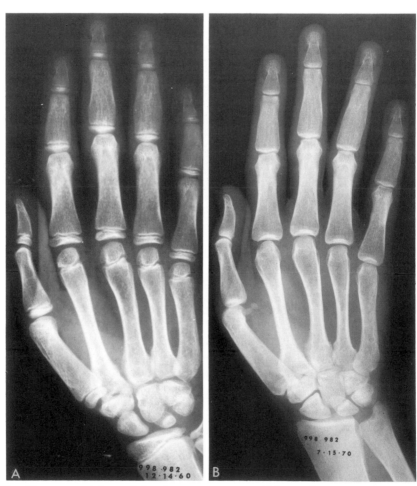

Figure 13–58. Frontometaphyseal dysplasia. *A*, 11 year old boy. There is elongation and failure of modeling of the metacarpals and phalanges. The middle phalanges in particular are wide and long. The carpal angle is elevated. The lunate is somewhat retarded in onset of ossification. (From Holt, J. F., et al.: *Radiol. Clin. North Am.*, 10:225–243, 1972.)

B, Age 21. The carpals remain small and the bones are slender. The failure of modeling of the middle phalanges is again noted.

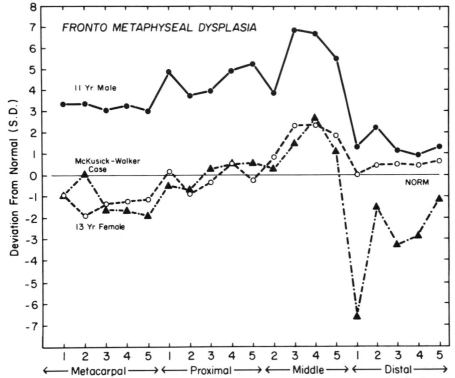

Figure 13–59. Frontometaphyseal dysplasia. Pattern profile. There is a relative elongation of the middle and proximal phalanges as compared to the distals. There is a fair degree of similarity between the cases of Holt et al. and that described by McKusick and Walker.

RADIOLOGIC FINDINGS IN THE HAND. There is lack of modeling in the elongated metacarpals and phalanges. In particular, there is widening of the middle phalanges. The carpal angle is increased. Some of the carpals are hypoplastic (Fig. 13–58).

Pattern profile analysis shows that the middle phalanges of the third, fourth and fifth fingers are relatively longer than the distal and proximal phalanges. There is also relative elongation of the first proximal phalanx (Fig. 13–59).

OTHER RADIOLOGIC FINDINGS. These include a Nazi-helmet configuration of the cranial vault, internal hyperostosis, perisutural sclerosis, supraorbital exostosis, absent frontal sinuses, arched superior border of the maxillary sinuses, defective dentition, antegonial notching of the mandible, thoracic scoliosis, irregular vertebral contours, coat-hanger deformity of the lower ribs, accentuated iliac flare, protrusio acetabuli, coxa valga and lack of modeling in the elongated metatarsals and phalanges.

REFERENCES

1. Danks, D. M., Mayne, V., Hall, R. K., and McKinnon, M. C.: Frontometaphyseal Dysplasia. *Am. J. Dis. Child.*, 123:254–258, 1972.
2. Gorlin, R. J., and Cohen, M. M.: Frontometaphyseal Dysplasia. A New Syndrome. *Am. J. Dis. Child.*, 118:487–494, 1969.
3. Holt, J. F., Thompson, G. R., and Arenberg, I. K.: Frontometaphyseal Dysplasia. *Radiol. Clin. North Am.*, 10:225–243, 1972.

GM₁ GANGLIOSIDOSIS, TYPE 1 (NEUROVISCERAL STORAGE DISEASE, NEUROVISCERAL LIPIDOSIS, INFANTILE GENERALIZED GANGLIOSIDOSIS, PSEUDO-HURLER)

This is another Hurler-like condition which occurs early in infancy and may be very similar to mucolipidosis II (I-cell) disease. Affected children usually die at about two years of age. There is decreased motion at the joints; about one-half of the children may have cherry red macular spots.[3] The basic defect is a deficiency of beta galactosidase activity and accumulation of GM₁ ganglioside in the cells. The condition is inherited as an autosomal recessive.

RADIOLOGIC FINDINGS IN THE HAND. These are very similar to those seen in I-cell disease except that they are probably more severe and occur somewhat earlier. There is lack of tubulation of the bones of the hands, particularly the metacarpals; the bony cortex of the metacarpals is thin owing to the severe osteoporosis that is commonly present. There is pointing of the proximal ends of the metacarpals.

OTHER RADIOLOGIC FINDINGS. There are other Hurler-like changes, including beaking of the spine. A distinctive feature of this disease is periosteal cloaking, which is seen in many of the long bones.

REFERENCES

1. Grossman, H., and Danes, B. S.: Neurovisceral Storage Disease. Roentgenographic Features and Mode of Inheritance. *Am. J. Roentgenol.*, 103:149–153, 1968.
2. O'Brien, J. S.: G_{M1} Gangliosidoses. *In* Stanbury, J. B., Wyngaarden, J. B., and Fredrickson, D. S.: *The Metabolic Basis of Inherited Disease*, 3rd Ed. McGraw-Hill Book Company, New York, 1972.
3. Spranger, J. W., Langer, L., and Wiedemann, H.-R.: *Bone Dysplasias: An Atlas of Constitutional Disorders of Skeletal Development*. W. B. Saunders Company, Philadelphia, 1974.

HAND-FOOT-UTERUS SYNDROME

This is a congenital disorder characterized by small feet with short great toes and by abnormal hands with hypoplasia of the thumb. It is transmitted as an autosomal dominant with full penetrance and variable expression. Varying degrees of duplication of the female genital tract have been noted.

RADIOLOGIC FINDINGS IN THE HAND. The thumb is markedly shortened due to a short first metacarpal which is normal in diameter. The metacarpal 2 to metacarpal 1 ratio was more than two standard deviations above normal in 12 of 16 cases. The short metacarpals have a pseudoepiphysis in almost all affected children (Fig. 13–60). The distal phalanx of the thumb is pointed, lacking its normal tuft, but is usually of normal size. Most of the patients have a short middle phalanx and clinodactyly of the fifth finger (Figs. 13–60 and 13–61). A pseudoepiphysis of the middle phalanx of the fifth finger is common. Fusion of the scaphoid and trapezium is common in adults (Fig. 13–61) but is usually not apparent in children. An os centrale is frequently present. Dysharmonic maturation of the carpals may be seen.

OTHER RADIOLOGIC FINDINGS. The feet are small with a short great toe due to shortening of the first metatarsal. The distal phalanx of the great toe is pointed. A pseudoepiphysis of the proximal phalanx is frequently present. There is fusion of the middle and distal phalanges of many of the toes. Tarsal fusions are common, involving particularly the cuneiforms. The calcaneus is short and the navicular is abnormal in configuration.

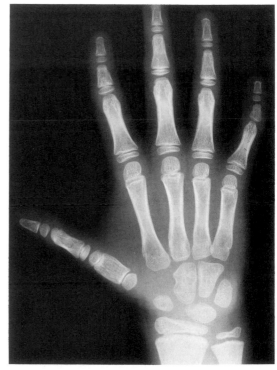

Figure 13–60. Hand-foot-uterus syndrome. 11 year old boy. There is shortening of the middle phalanx of the fifth finger with slight clinodactyly. The trapezium and trapezoid are markedly retarded in onset ossification. The first metacarpal is short with a prominent pseudoepiphysis. There is a cone epiphysis at the middle phalanx of the index finger, which is also shortened. (From Poznanski, A. K., et al.: *Radiology*, 95:129–134, 1970.)

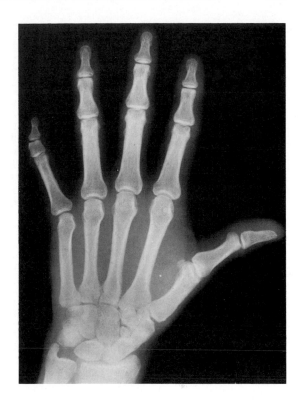

Figure 13-61. Hand-foot-uterus syndrome. Adult male. There is fusion of the trapezium and scaphoid, and an os centrale is also seen. There is shortening of the middle phalanx of the fifth finger with some clinodactyly. The thumb is short. (From Poznanski, A. K., and Holt J. F.: *Am. J. Roentgenol.*, 112:443–459, 1971.)

REFERENCES

1. Poznanski, A. K., Garn, S. M., and Holt, J. F.: The Thumb in the Congenital Malformation Syndromes. *Radiology,* 100:115–129, 1971.
2. Poznanski, A. K., Stern, A. M., and Gall, J. C., Jr.: Radiographic Findings in the Hand-Foot-Uterus Syndrome (HFUS). *Radiology,* 95:129–134, 1970.
3. Stern, A. M., Gall, J. C., Jr., Perry, B. L., Stimson, C. W., Weitkamp, L. R., and Poznanski, A. K.: The Hand-Foot-Uterus Syndrome. A New Hereditary Disorder Characterized by Hand and Foot Dysplasia, Dermatoglyphic Abnormalities, and Partial Duplication of the Female Genital Tract. *J. Pediatr.,* 77:109–116, 1970.

HOLT-ORAM SYNDROME AND OTHER CARDIOMELIC SYNDROMES

The Holt-Oram syndrome consists of characteristic upper limb abnormalities associated with congenital heart disease. The limb deformities are bilateral but not necessarily symmetric, and are variable in severity within families. Clinically they range from phocomelia to abnormal thumbs and in some cases are only detectable radiologically. The cardiac lesions are variable and include mainly atrial and ventricular defects. However, pulmonary hypertension and rhythmic disturbances are common. The condition is inherited as an autosomal dominant.

RADIOLOGIC FINDINGS IN THE HAND. The carpal findings are probably the most characteristic, with some abnormality of the scaphoid being present in almost all cases (Fig. 13–62). Extra carpals are quite common and may include a single os centrale or several carpals in the middle carpal row. Some patients have three carpals along the radial side. Carpal fusions are occasionally seen, and there may be evidence of narrowing of the intercarpal joints.

The thumb is almost always abnormal. The changes can vary from absence of the thumb to a finger-like triphalangeal thumb (Figs. 13–63 and 13–64). When the thumb is enlarged, it is usually curved. The defect in the thumb may include absence of the metacarpal or of the phalanges. Cases in the same family may have a triphalangeal thumb, an absent thumb, or even phocomelia (Fig. 13–64).

The middle phalanges of the fifth fingers

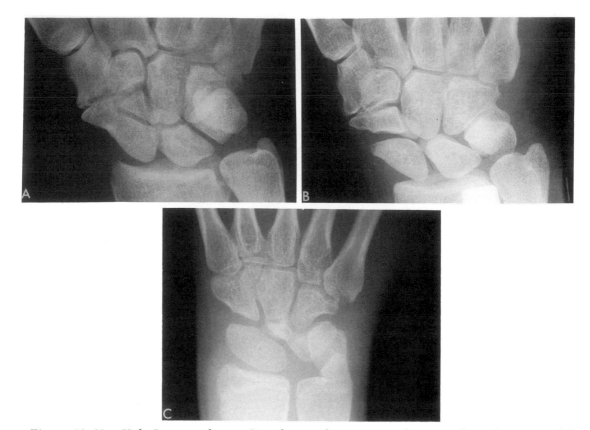

Figure 13–62. Holt-Oram syndrome. Carpal anomalies. *A,* Typical os centrale in the center of the wrist. The trapezium-scaphoid joint is irregular and narrow, and the trapezium is somewhat longer than normal.

B, Rare accessory bone along the radial aspect; it extends into the region of the usual os centrale. There is narrowing of the joint between this bone and the trapezium.

C. Lunate-scaphoid fusion. An os centrale is also present. There is also fusion of the trapezium and trapezoid. (From Poznanski, A. K., et al.: *Radiology,* 94:45, 1970.)

are short and there is usually associated clinodactyly. Pattern profile analysis is most often characteristic, with increased length of the metacarpals and reduction of all of the middle phalanges (Fig. 13–65). The most marked findings are the increase in the length of the first metacarpal and the shortening of the fifth middle phalanx. When the ratios of the thumb bones and the second metacarpal are considered, the most discriminatory bone length is that of metacarpal 1 to distal 1.[5]

OTHER RADIOLOGIC FINDINGS. Various other upper extremity abnormalities occur. The lower extremities are not involved. The shoulders are usually abnormal with outwardly rotated scapulas. In young infants the clavicles are curved, short and angulated laterally. In older individuals the clavicles are thick and often have prominent coracoid processes which may

articulate with the coracoid process of the scapula. There is an increased incidence of accessory ossicles about the shoulder, and prominent deltoid ridges of the humerus. Frequently the medial epicondyles of the humeri project medially and posteriorly, and occasionally abnormalities of the humeral head may be present. The radial head is deformed but the radius is rarely absent.

Other Cardiomelic Syndromes

There are a number of other syndromes in which the hand and heart may be affected.[7, 8] A common disorder, termed ventriculoradial dysplasia, includes unilateral absence of the radius associated with congenital heart disease, usually a ventricular defect (Fig. 13–66). This entity is probably

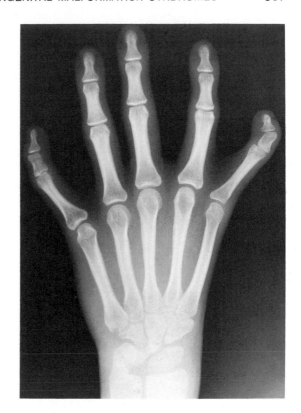

Figure 13–63. Holt-Oram syndrome. Triphalangeal thumb. The first metacarpal is slender. The thumb is triphalangeal with deviation of the thumb toward the ulnar side. There is cliniodactyly of the fifth finger with a short middle phalanx. An accessory carpal is also present.

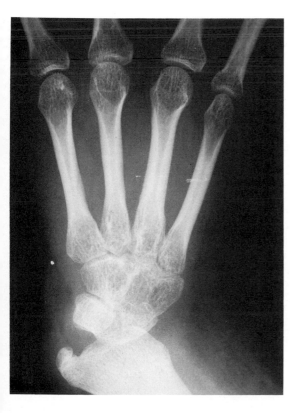

Figure 13–64. Holt-Oram syndrome. Absence of the thumb and phocomelia. Adult male. This was the father of a family with the Holt-Oram syndrome. His daughters had typical triphalangeal thumbs. There is evidence of massive carpal fusion. (From Poznanski, A. K., et al.: *Radiol. Clin. North Am.* 9:435–458, 1971.)

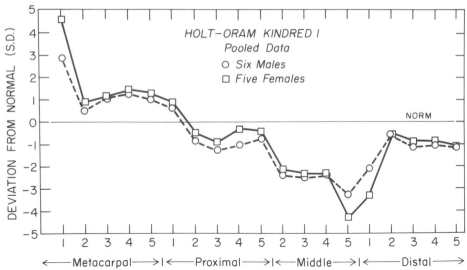

Figure 13–65. Holt-Oram syndrome. Pattern profiles. Mean patterns from our first family. Note the elongation of the metacarpals as well as other similarities between the males and females. The middle phalanx of the fifth finger appears short. The pattern would be somewhat different in the families that have short thumbs rather than elongated thumbs.

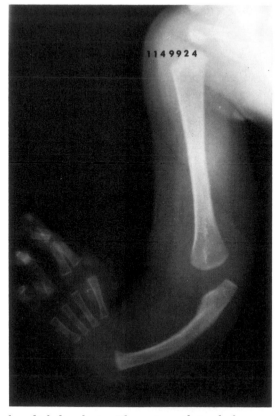

Figure 13–66. Ventriculoradial dysplasia. There is unilateral absence of the radius with a hypoplastic thumb. This is probably different from the Holt-Oram syndrome. The patient had a ventricular septal defect. (From Poznanski, A. K., et al.: *Radiol. Clin. North Am.,* 9:435–458, 1971.)

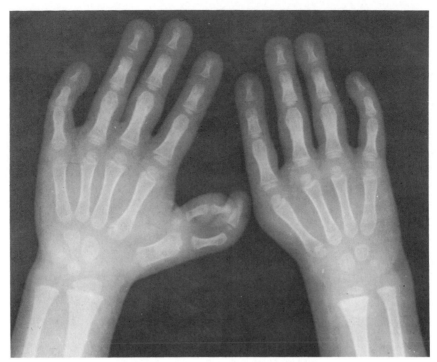

Figure 13–67. Cardiomelic syndrome. Unusual type. This child had a ventricular septal defect and patent ductus arteriosus. The thumb is absent on one side, and there is a double thumb on the other side. Although the radiologic findings are compatible with the Holt-Oram syndrome, the patient also had some abnormalities in the lower extremities, including dislocated patellas, which suggest that this may be a different condition.

different from the Holt-Oram syndrome. Further discussion on the association of radial defects and congenital heart disease can be found in Chapter 9.

A number of other ill-defined syndromes may also be associated with abnormalities of the heart and hand (Fig. 13–67). In some of these the abnormalities do not affect the upper extremities and should probably not be included in the term "Holt-Oram."

REFERENCES

1. Gall, J. C., Jr., Stern, A. M., Cohen, M. M., Adams, M. S., and Davidson, R. T.: Holt-Oram Syndrome: Clinical and Genetic Study of a Large Family. *Am. J. Hum. Genet.*, 18:187–200, 1966.
2. Harris, L. C., and Osborne, W. P.: Congenital Absence or Hypoplasia of the Radius with Ventricular Septal Defect: Ventriculo-Radial Dysplasia. *J. Pediatr.*, 68:265–272, 1966.
3. Holmes, L. B.: Congenital Heart Disease and Upper Extremity Deformities. A Report of Two Families. *N. Engl. J. Med.*, 272:437–444, 1965.
4. Lewis, K. B., Bruce, R. A., Baum, D., and Motulsky, A. G.: The Upper Limb-Cardiovascular Syndrome. An Autosomal Dominant Genetic Effect on Embryogenesis. *J.A.M.A.*, 193:1080–1086, 1965.
5. Poznanski, A. K., Gall, J. C., Jr., and Stern, A. M.: Skeletal Manifestations of the Holt-Oram Syndrome. *Radiology*, 94:45–53, 1970.
6. Poznanski, A. K., Garn, S. M., Gall, J. C., Jr., and Stern, A. M.: Objective Evaluation of the Hand in the Holt-Oram Syndrome. *Birth Defects, Original Article Series*, 8:125–131, 1972.
7. Poznanski, A. K., Stern, A. M., and Gall, J. C., Jr.: Skeletal Anomalies in Genetically Determined Congenital Heart Disease. *Radiol. Clin. North Am.*, 9:435–458, 1971.
8. Poznanski, A. K., Stern, A., and Gall, J.: The Upper Limb Cardiovascular Syndrome. Letter to the Editor. *Am. J. Dis. Child.*, 125:622, 1973.

HOMOCYSTINURIA

This is an inborn error of metabolism. The basic abnormality is a deficiency of the enzyme cystathionine synthetase, which catalyzes the condensation of homocystine and serine to form cystathionine. In affected individuals homocystine appears in the urine. The ocular, skeletal and vascular changes in homocystinuria

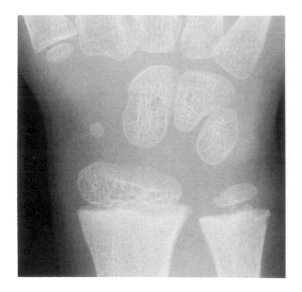

Figure 13–68. Homocystinuria. There is a marked delay of the lunate, trapezium and trapezoid. Metaphyseal spicules are seen in the ulna. (From Poznanski, A. K., et al.: *Am. J. Phys. Anthropol.*, 35:417–432, 1971.)

are similar to those seen in Marfan syndrome. Osteoporosis or thrombosis, however, is a distinguishing feature of homocystinuria, and some of the patients with homocystinuria are mentally retarded. It is inherited as an autosomal recessive trait.

RADIOLOGIC FINDINGS IN THE HAND. Most of the findings occur only in children. Holt and Allen[2] reported the presence of focal calcifications and spicules in the radial and ulnar metaphyses (Fig. 13–68). The carpal bones may be abnormal. Dysharmonic maturation is common and gives the appearance of relative enlargement of the capitate and hamate and relative hypoplasia of the lunate (Fig. 13–68). Although narrowing between the carpal joints has been reported, this finding does not occur in most patients. Overall skeletal maturation may be delayed or normal. In both adults and children there may be evidence of arachnodactyly. Osteoporosis is common.

OTHER RADIOLOGIC FINDINGS. The most commonly present findings include osteoporosis, which is marked in the spine. Scoliosis is also common. Sternal abnormalities are seen in a small percentage of cases. Arterial abnormalities are common and include thromboses and emboli.

REFERENCES

1. Brenton, D. P., Dow, C. J., James, J. I. P., Hay, R. L., Wynne-Davies, R.: Homocystinuria and Marfan's Syndrome. A Comparison. *J. Bone Joint Surg.*, 54B:277–298, 1972.
2. Holt, J. F., and Allen, R. J.: Radiologic Signs in the Primary Aminoacidurias. *Ann. Radiol.*, 10:317–321, 1967.
3. Morreels, C. L., Jr., Fletcher, B. D., Weilbaecher, R. G., and Dorst, J. P.: The Roentgenographic Features of Homocystinuria. *Radiology*, 90: 1150–1158, 1968.
4. Poznanski, A. K., Garn, S. M., Kuhns, L. R., and Sandusky, S. T.: Dysharmonic Maturation of the Hand in the Congenital Malformation Syndromes. *Am. J. Phys. Anthropol.*, 35:417–432, 1971.
5. Schedewie, H., Willich, E., Gröbe, H., Schmidt, H., and Müller, K. M.: Skeletal Findings in Homocystinuria. A Collaborative Study. *Pediatr. Radiol.*, 1:12–23, 1973.

HYPERCALCEMIA – INFANTILE (HYPERCALCEMIA– SUPRAVALVULAR AORTIC STENOSIS SYNDROME)

Affected children have a characteristic facial appearance and associated supravalvular aortic stenosis and peripheral pulmonary stenosis. They are usually mentally retarded and of short stature. Abnormalities of the teeth are common. Familial cases have been reported, particularly in association with supravalvular aortic stenosis.

RADIOLOGIC FINDINGS IN THE HAND. There may be a generalized osteosclerosis or there may be associated bands of increased density in the tubular bones of the hand, but these are less marked than in

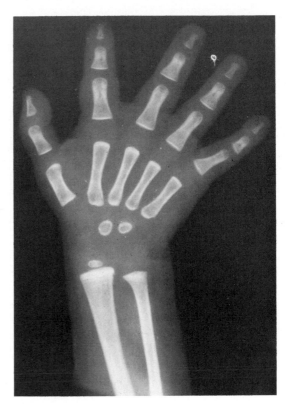

Figure 13-69. Hypercalcemia. Infantile. Ten month old infant. There is some increase in the density of the cortex of the metacarpals. The ends of the bones also appear dense and no soft tissue calcification is seen. (Courtesy Dr. F. Silverman, Cincinnati, Ohio.)

the long bones (Fig. 13–69). Soft tissue calcification and vascular calcification may sometimes be seen.

OTHER RADIOLOGIC FINDINGS. Abnormally formed teeth and mandibles may be seen. Absence of some of the teeth, particularly the lateral incisors and second premolars of the maxilla, is common. There is generalized osteosclerosis and increased density in other bones. Cranial suture synostosis may be noted.

REFERENCES

1. Beuren, A. J.: Supravalvular Aortic Stenosis: A Complex Syndrome With and Without Mental Retardation. *Birth Defects, Original Article Series,* 8:45–56, 1972.
2. Friedman, W. F.: Vitamin D and the Supravalvular Aortic Stenosis Syndrome. *Advances in Teratology,* 3:85–96, 1968.
3. Ottesen, O. E., Antia, A. U., and Rowe, R. D.: Peripheral Vascular Anomalies Associated with the Supravalvular Aortic Stenosis Syndrome. *Radiology,* 86:430–435,443, 1966.
4. Shiers, J. A., Neuhauser, E. B. D., and Bowman, J. R.: Idiopathic Hypercalcemia. *Am. J. Roentgenol.,* 78:19–29, 1957.
5. Singleton, E. B.: The Radiographic Features of Severe Idiopathic Hypercalcemia of Infancy. *Radiology,* 68:721–726, 1957.

HYPOCHONDROPLASIA

This form of dwarfism is similar to achondroplasia but has much milder clinical and radiologic manifestations. The clinical findings include disproportionately short limbs as compared to the trunk, but the face does not show the depressed nasal bridge and frontal bossing seen in achondroplasia. Distinction from other forms of dwarfism may be made radiologically. Inheritance of the condition is autosomal dominant.

RADIOLOGIC FINDINGS IN THE HAND. The hand is small with short tubular bones, but no inherent abnormality is seen (Figs. 13–70 and 13–71). In the infant the hand does not appear to have the trident configuration seen in achondroplasia. Also, there is usually no cupping of the metaphyses. The hand findings are not particularly characteristic. In contradistinction to

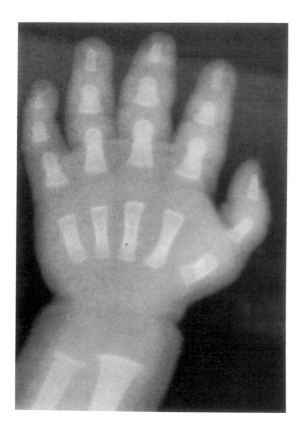

Figure 13–70. Hypochondroplasia. Infant. Mild shortening of the tubular bones. The appearance may be difficult to distinguish from achondroplasia or even from normal. (Courtesy Dr. William McAlister, St. Louis, Missouri.)

Figure 13–71. Hypochondroplasia. Adult. Father of infant in Figure 13–70. Again, mild shortening of the hand bones is seen. (Courtesy Dr. William McAlister, St. Louis, Missouri.)

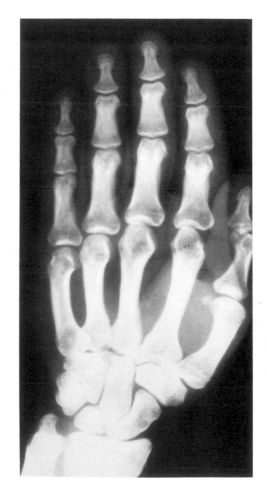

achondroplasia, little alteration in pattern profile is evident.

OTHER RADIOLOGIC FINDINGS. Probably the most positive finding is lack of normal widening of the interpediculate distance from L1 to L5; this is similar to that seen in achondroplasia. The spinal canal is also decreased in anteroposterior diameter, but the changes are considerably milder than those in achondroplasia and no neurologic findings have been described in hypochondroplasia. The skull has a normal configuration. The tubular bones are comparatively short, giving them a relatively wide appearance.

REFERENCES

1. Beals, R. K.: Hypochondroplasia. A Report of Five Kindreds. *J. Bone Joint Surg.*, 51A:728–736, 1969.
2. Kozlowski, K.: Hypochondroplasia. *Progr. Pediatr. Radiol.*, 4:238–249, 1973. (*Intrinsic Diseases of Bones*, edited by H. J. Kaufmann, Karger, Basel.)
3. Walker, B. A., Murdoch, J. L., McKusick, V. A., Langer, L. O., and Beals, R. K.: Hypochondroplasia. *Am. J. Dis. Child.*, 122:95–104, 1971.

HYPOPHOSPHATASIA

This inherited metabolic abnormality is characterized by low serum and tissue alkaline phosphatase and the presence of excess phosphoethanolamine in the urine. The changes vary significantly in severity, ranging from a fatal form with almost no bone, to very mild changes seen mainly in adult life. Most cases are inherited as an autosomal recessive, although a few families with autosomal dominant transmission have been reported.[5]

RADIOLOGIC FINDINGS IN THE HAND. The basic radiologic finding is that of rickets. However, because of the variations in severity, the roentgen appearance may be very different in the severe forms as compared to the mild. In the very severe cases the infant may be born with essentially no bones in the hand (Fig. 13–72). The few bones that are present appear deeply cupped (Fig. 13–73). In the intermediate cases there may be changes which are similar to those of rickets, occasionally with some evidence of healing (Fig. 13–74). In older individuals the rachitic changes

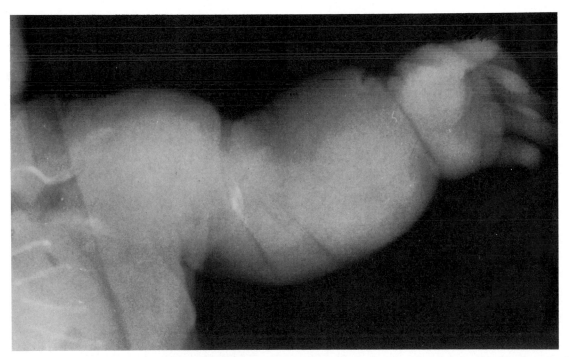

Figure 13–72. Hypophosphatasia. Severe. This infant died shortly after birth. His brother had well-documented hypophosphatasia. There are no bones visible in the hand at all, and only a small amount of bone is seen in the remainder of the arm. This is case 1 reported by Macpherson, R. I., et al.: *J. Can. Assoc. Radiol.*, 23:16–26, 1972. (Courtesy Dr. R. Macpherson, Winnipeg, Canada; and Dr. S. Houston, Saskatoon, Canada.)

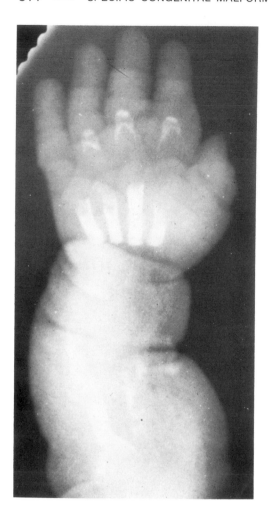

Figure 13-73. Hypophosphatasia. Severe. This case is somewhat less severe than that shown in Figure 13-72. However, there is no ossification in many of the hand bones. The remaining hand bones show deep cups at their ends. (Courtesy Dr. William McAlister, St. Louis, Missouri.)

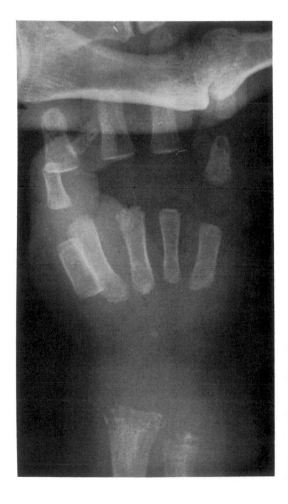

Figure 13-74. Hypophosphatasia. More moderate findings. Three and one half year old male. Changes suggestive of healing rickets are seen in the distal radius and at the ends of the metacarpals. This is case 6 reported by Macpherson, R. I., et al.: *J. Can. Assoc. Radiol.*, 23:16-26, 1972. (Courtesy Dr. S. Houston, Saskatoon, Canada, and Dr. R. Macpherson, Winnipeg, Canada.)

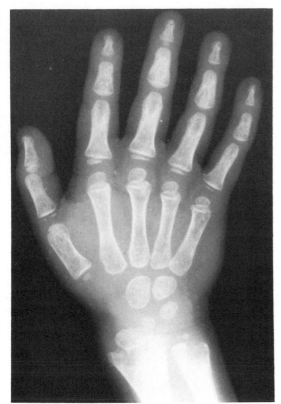

Figure 13-75. Hypophosphatasia. Deep cups are seen in the radial and ulna metaphyses, but the hands are relatively normal. This is a common manifestation in this condition, with the hand being relatively less involved than the remainder of the skeleton.

are mainly in the radius and ulna and the hand is usually spared (Fig. 13-75). The rachitic changes in this condition are somewhat exaggerated compared to other forms of rickets, and the cups in the metaphyses appear deeper and more sharply defined.

OTHER RADIOLOGIC FINDINGS. Metaphyseal defects are present in various areas of the body. Fractures and premature synostosis of the cranial sutures may be seen. In the severe newborn forms there is a lack of bone in almost the entire skeleton.

REFERENCES

1. Currarino, G.: Hypophosphatasia. *Progr. Pediatr. Radiol.*, 4:469–494, 1973. (*Intrinsic Diseases of Bones*, edited by H. J. Kaufmann, Karger, Basel.)

2. Currarino, G., Neuhauser, E. B. D., Reyersbach, G. C., and Sobel, E. H.: Hypophosphatasia. *Am. J. Roentgenol.*, 78:392–419, 1957.
3. Jardon, O. M., Burney, D. W., and Fink, R. L.: Hypophosphatasia in an Adult. *J. Bone Joint Surg.*, 52A:1477–1484, 1970.
4. Macpherson, R. I., Kroeker, M., and Houston, C. S.: Hypophosphatasia. *J. Can. Assoc. Radiol.*, 23: 16–26, 1972.
5. Silverman, J. L.: Apparent Dominant Inheritance of Hypophosphatasia. *Arch. Int. Med.*, 110: 191–198, 1962.

INSENSITIVITY TO PAIN— CONGENITAL (CONGENITAL INDIFFERENCE TO PAIN, CONGENITAL ANALGIA)

Lack of response to pain stimuli may be caused by a number of syndromes, including the condition of congenital indifference to pain as well as familial dysautonomia, congenital sensory neuropathy, hereditary sensory radicular neuropathy, familial sensory neuropathy with anhidrosis, acquired sensory neuropathy (toxic and infectious) and syringomyelia. The condition of indifference to pain has its onset at birth, and the patient has a normal physiologic pain reaction, sense perception, temperature perception, axon reflexes, nerve conduction, motor strength, sensory nerves, skin biopsy, brain and intelligence. The sensory loss distribution is universal. Inheritance of the congenital insensitivity to pain syndrome is autosomal recessive; some of the other conditions may have dominant or recessive inheritance. The differential diagnosis between these conditions is well described in Tachdjian.[6]

RADIOLOGIC FINDINGS IN THE HAND. Children will occasionally bite their hands, causing partial amputations (Fig. 13–76). New lesions in the hands are less common as the patients get older, since they become more cognizant of the need to be more careful not to inflict injury upon themselves. The changes in the hand include erosion of the tufts, amputations and areas of osteomyelitis. Similar changes may be seen in the Lesch-Nyhan syndrome and in the other causes of insensitivity listed above.

OTHER RADIOLOGIC FINDINGS. These include multiple fractures, and the condition may sometimes have to be differentiated from the battered child syndrome. Arthropathy of various joints, dislocations and osteomyelitis may be seen. Areas of

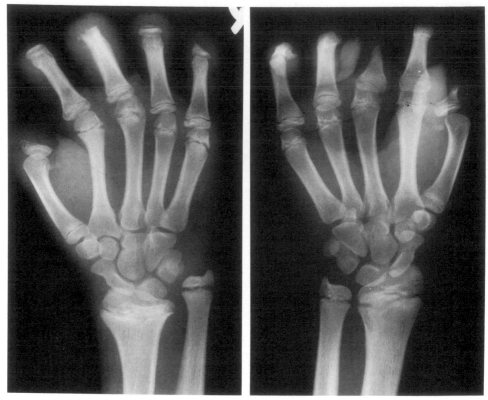

Figure 13–76. Insensitivity to pain. Congenital. There is absence of the terminal portions of the digits bilaterally. Some of the digits have a pointed distal portion. Epiphyseal damage is seen in the radius on the left illustration. (Courtesy Dr. M. Ozonoff, Newington, Connecticut.)

aseptic necrosis, particularly in weight-bearing portions of the skeleton, may be noted.

REFERENCES

1. Gwinn, J. L., and Barnes, G. R., Jr.: Radiological Case of the Month. *Am. J. Dis. Child.,* 112: 583–584, 1966.
2. MacEwen, G. D., and Floyd, G. C.: Congenital Insensitivity to Pain and Its Orthopedic Implications. *Clin. Orthop.,* 68:100–107, 1970.
3. McKusick, V. A.: *Mendelian Inheritance in Man. Catalogs of Autosomal Dominant, Autosomal Recessive, and X-Linked Phenotypes,* 3rd Ed. The Johns Hopkins Press, Baltimore, 1971.
4. Siegelman, S. S., Heimann, W. G., and Manin, M. C.: Congenital Indifference to Pain. *Am. J. Roentgenol.,* 97:242–247, 1966.
5. Silverman, F. N., and Gilden, J. J.: Congenital Insensitivity to Pain: A Neurologic Syndrome with Bizarre Skeletal Lesions. *Radiology,* 72: 176–190, 1959.
6. Tachdjian, M. O.: *Pediatric Orthopedics.* W. B. Saunders Company, Philadelphia, 1972, Vols. I and II.

JUBERG-HAYWARD SYNDROME

This is a syndrome of a cleft lip–cleft palate, microcephaly and hypoplastic thumbs in a family reported by Juberg and Hayward.[1] One member of this family was later shown to have congenital heart disease. Inheritance is autosomal recessive.

RADIOLOGIC FINDINGS IN THE HAND. The thumb is hypoplastic, with a particularly slender, short first metacarpal which may be missing its proximal epiphysis (Fig. 13–77); as is often the case in this situation, a distal pseudoepiphysis may be present. The metacarpal is slender. The radial carpals, particularly the scaphoid and trapezium, may be delayed or absent. An additional phalanx was seen in one of the patients in the original family.[2] The ap-

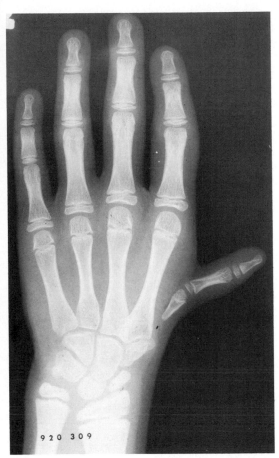

Figure 13-77. Juberg-Hayward syndrome. There is hypoplasia of the thumb, particularly involving the first metacarpal, which has an epiphysis at the distal rather than the proximal end. There is hypoplasia of the radial carpals as well.

pearance of the hand is not particularly characteristic of this condition and may be seen in other radial hypoplasia syndromes with short slender first metacarpals.

OTHER RADIOLOGIC FINDINGS. Microcephaly was present in a number of patients. Syndactyly of the toes was also seen. A horseshoe kidney was present in one patient and signs of congenital heart disease were noted in another.

REFERENCES

1. Juberg, R. C., and Hayward, J. R.: A New Familial Syndrome of Oral, Cranial, and Digital Anomalies. *J. Pediatr.*, 74:755–762, 1969.
2. Poznanski, A. K., Garn, S. M., and Holt, J. F.: The Thumb in the Congenital Malformation Syndromes. *Radiology*, 100:115–129, 1971.

JUVENILE IDIOPATHIC OSTEOPOROSIS (JUVENILE OSTEOPOROSIS)

This condition, described by Dent, is an osteogenesis imperfecta–like syndrome which can be distinguished from osteogenesis imperfecta by the following features, as stated by Dent:[2] (1) Absolute normality clinically and radiologically in the first years of life; (2) fairly constant age of presentation (8 to 12 years); (3) severity in acuteness of the process when it does reveal itself; (4) characteristic radiologic appearance of the bone in the more severe cases; (5) spontaneous healing; (6) absence of family history and of blue sclerae; and (7) normal teeth. The condition appears to heal at puberty although the healing may not be complete and the condition may later develop into senile osteoporosis.

RADIOLOGIC FINDINGS IN THE HAND. These are not particularly typical and are simply manifestations of osteoporosis.

OTHER RADIOLOGIC FINDINGS. There is vertebral collapse due to osteoporosis. Distinction between this disease and osteogenesis imperfecta may be quite difficult. The very slender bones of osteogenesis imperfecta are usually not present in juvenile osteoporosis. However, the tarda form of osteogenesis imperfecta may be difficult to differentiate from juvenile osteoporosis.

REFERENCES

1. Cumming, W. A.: Idiopathic Juvenile Osteoporosis. *J. Can. Assoc. Radiol.*, 21:21–26, 1970.
2. Dent, C. E.: Idiopathic Juvenile Osteoporosis (IJO). *Birth Defects, Original Article Series*, 5:134–139, 1969.
3. Gooding, C. A., and Ball, J. H.: Idiopathic Juvenile Osteoporosis. *Radiology*, 93:1349–1350, 1969.
4. Guibaud, P., Larbre, F., Hermier, M., Frédérich, A., and Meunier, P.: "Ostéoporose Idiopathique" ou Ostéogénèse Imparfaite. *Pediatrie*, 25:553–562, 1970.

KASCHIN-BECK DISEASE

This rare disease was described in Manchuria and Russia. The condition was a form of dwarfism with disproportionately short extremities as compared with the head and trunk. Patients assumed a characteristic posture with the head pulled backwards and the knees slightly bent. There was frequently enlargement and deformity of the joints of the hands and the legs. Associated lordosis, kyphosis or scoliosis was present in some instances.

RADIOLOGIC FINDINGS IN THE HAND. Cone-shaped epiphyses were seen in the phalanges. When they affected the middle phalanges they produced a deformity which was somewhat akin to that seen in the tricho-rhino-phalangeal syndrome. However, the pattern profile of this condition does not seem to match with that seen in the latter. The distal phalanges in Kaschin-Beck disease appear somewhat short. The carpals were delayed in maturation and in severe cases showed considerable irregularity. The appearance in some cases is somewhat suggestive of that seen in Thiemann disease and in the epiphyseal dysplasias.

OTHER RADIOLOGIC FINDINGS. There was underdevelopment and shortening of many of the long bones and there was deformity of the femur.

REFERENCE

1. Takamori, T.: *Kaschin-Beck's Disease (Dysostosis Enchondralis Endemica).* Professor Tokio Takamori Foundation, Gifu, Japan, 1968.

KEUTEL SYNDROME

This condition included peripheral pulmonary stenoses without cardiac abnormalities, neural hearing loss and widespread abnormal cartilage calcifications. It is inherited as an autosomal recessive.

RADIOLOGIC FINDINGS IN THE HAND. There was shortening of the distal phalanges of many of the fingers. The short phalanges appeared somewhat broad. Abnormal epiphyses were noted in these phalanges and may have been the cause of the shortening.

OTHER RADIOLOGIC FINDINGS. There was calcification in the cartilage of the ears, larynx, trachea and nose.

REFERENCE

1. Keutel, J., Jörgensen, G., and Gabriel, P.: A New Autosomal Recessive Syndrome: Peripheral Pulmonary Stenoses, Brachytelephalangism, Neural Hearing Loss and Abnormal Cartilage Calcifications/Ossification. *Birth Defects, Original Article Series,* 8:60–68, 1972.

KLIPPEL-TRENAUNAY-WEBER SYNDROME (PARKES WEBER SYNDROME, ANGIO-OSTEOHYPERTROPHIC SYNDROME, OSTEOHYPERTROPHIC–VARICOSE NEVUS SYNDROME)

This syndrome of hypertrophy of skeletal and soft tissues usually affects one extremity or one side. It is associated with angiomas, nevi, varices and sometimes lipomas. There is scant evidence that there is a genetic tendency in this condition.

RADIOLOGIC FINDINGS IN THE HAND. The hand findings are mainly those of soft tissue and osseous enlargement of the involved digit, which makes it longer and wider than normal (Fig. 13–78). Usually only several digits are involved rather than the entire hand. Syndactyly has been reported.[2] Most often only one hand is involved.

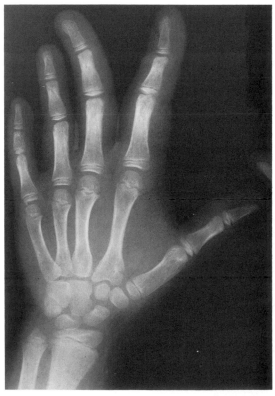

Figure 13–78. Klippel-Trenaunay-Weber syndrome. 11½ year old boy. There is enlargement of the thumb and of the second and third digits, along with some curvature of these digits. Both the bones and soft tissues are enlarged. This patient had multiple capillary hemangiomas and a large lipoma on the abdominal wall.

OTHER RADIOLOGIC FINDINGS. Similar involvement may be seen in the foot. The veins in the involved area may be enlarged, and arteriovenous fistulas may be seen. Psoriasis has also been associated with this condition, as have lipomas in various portions of the body.

REFERENCES

1. Brooksaler, F.: The Angioosteohypertrophy Syndrome. Klippel-Trenaunay-Weber Syndrome. Am. J. Dis. Child., 112:161–164, 1966.
2. Fainsinger, M. H., and Harris, L. C.: Generalised Lipomatosis Involving Bone. Report of a Case. Br. J. Radiol., 23:274–278, 1950.
3. Kuffer, F. R., Starzynski, T. E., Girolami, A., Murphy, L., and Grabstald, H.: Klippel-Trenaunay Syndrome, Visceral Angiomatosis and Thrombocytopenia. J. Pediatr. Surg., 3: 65–72, 1968.
4. McCarthy, D. M., Dorr, C. A., and Mackintosh, C. E.: Unilateral Localised Gigantism of the Extremities with Lipomatosis, Arthropathy and Psoriasis. J. Bone Joint Surg., 51B:348–353, 1969.
5. Mullins, J. F., Naylor, D., and Redetski, J.: The Klippel-Trenaunay-Weber Syndrome. Naevus Vasculosus Osteohypertrophicus. Arch. Dermatol., 86:202–206, 1962.
6. Schönenberg, H., and Redemann, M.: Klippel-Trénaunay-Weber-Syndrom. Klin. Pädiat., 184: 449–460, 1972.

KNIEST DWARFISM

This form of dwarfism is associated with prominent eyes and a depressed nasal bridge. There is a restriction of joint mobility and, according to Spranger,[3] cleft palate is seen in 50 per cent of cases. The patients walk in a crouched position. Inheritance is autosomal dominant and X-linked.

RADIOLOGIC FINDINGS IN THE HAND. The tubular bones of the hand are somewhat short with broad metaphyses that may somewhat mimic the changes seen in metatropic dwarfism. The epiphyses, however, appear large. There may also be early carpal ossification.

OTHER RADIOLOGIC FINDINGS. Platyspondyly with anterior wedging is common. The pelvis has a fairly characteristic configuration, with a broad femoral neck and a very late appearance of the femoral ossification center. Both metaphyseal and epiphyseal changes may be present in the long bones. The acetabula have a somewhat bubbly appearance.

REFERENCES

1. Bailey, J. A.: Disproportionate Short Stature. Diagnosis and Management. W. B. Saunders Company, Philadelphia, 1973.
2. Kniest, W.: Zur Abgrenzung der Dysostosis enchondralis von der Chondrodystrophie. Z. Kinderheilkd., 70:633–640, 1952.
3. Spranger, J. W., Langer, L., and Wiedemann, H.-R.: Bone Dysplasias: An Atlas of Constitutional Disorders of Skeletal Development. W. B. Saunders Company, Philadelphia, 1974.

LARSEN SYNDROME

This is a poorly defined syndrome, with the most common finding being bilateral anterior dislocation of the knees. It is usually associated with bilateral dislocations of the hip, equinovarus and equinovalgus of the feet, dislocation of the elbows and a characteristic facial configuration. The eyes are widely spaced, and there is a prominent forehead; depression of the nasal bridge produces a flattened facial appearance. Associated abnormalities include deformities of the soft palate, or a cleft palate or uvula. Both dominant and recessive forms of inheritance have been seen.

RADIOLOGIC FINDINGS IN THE HAND. The digits are somewhat broad, particularly in their distal portions (Fig. 13–79). Shortening of various digits may be seen. The metacarpals are most frequently affected.[2, 4] Pattern profile analysis of cases in the literature and those of Spranger[5] are somewhat similar to the pattern profile analysis of the oto-palato-digital syndrome (Fig. 13–81). Multiple carpal bones may be seen in older individuals, and these are scattered in a rather random fashion (Fig. 13–79). These carpals do not resemble normal carpal bones. Not all patients with Larsen syndrome have these carpal abnormalities[4] (Fig. 13–80),[4] even though the tubular bones may show the typical alterations in length (Fig. 13–81).

OTHER RADIOLOGIC FINDINGS. The most characteristic finding is a double ossification center of the calcaneus, which is seen along the posterior portion and which eventually fuses with the calcaneus. Multiple and abnormal tarsal bones are also present. Dislocations of the knee and pseudoacetabula at birth from congenital dislocation in utero are also seen. Shortening of the metatarsals may be noted.

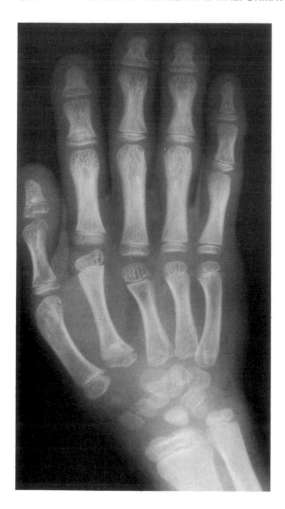

Figure 13–79. Larsen syndrome. There is short-ening of several of the metacarpals and phalanges. The fingers appear broad. This is particularly no-ticeable in the distal phalanges. The carpals are bizarre in configuration, having the appearance of being simply thrown together. Specific carpal bones cannot be identified. (Courtesy Dr. G. Currarino, Dallas, Texas.)

Figure 13–80. Larsen syndrome. These roentgen findings are somewhat atypical. There is some shortening of the digits, which is better seen in the pattern profile of Figure 13–81. No extra carpals are seen. Considerable bony de-mineralization is present.

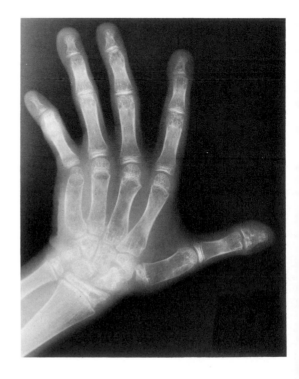

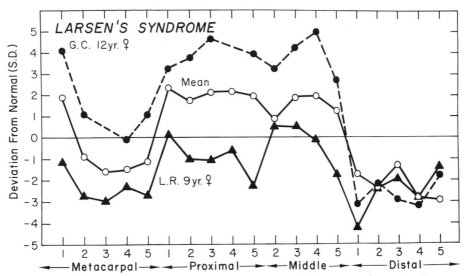

Figure 13–81. Larsen syndrome. Pattern profiles. Plots of the case of Dr. G. Currarino (G. C.) shown in Figure 13–79, and our own case (L.R.) shown in Figure 13–80, compared to the mean from cases including our own as well as those of Dr. J. Spranger, Kiel, Germany.

REFERENCES

1. Harris, R., and Cullen, C. H.: Autosomal Dominant Inheritance in Larsen's Syndrome. *Clin. Genet.*, 2:87–90, 1971.
2. Larsen, L. J., Schottstaedt, E. R., and Bost, F. C.: Multiple Congenital Dislocations Associated with Characteristic Facial Abnormality. *J. Pediatr.*, 37:574–581, 1950.
3. Latta, R. J., Graham, C. B., Aase, J., Scham, S. M., and Smith, D. W.: Larsen's Syndrome: A Skeletal Dysplasia with Multiple Joint Dislocations and Unusual Facies. *J. Pediatr.*, 78:291–298, 1971.
4. Silverman, F. N.: Larsen's Syndrome: Congenital Dislocation of the Knees and Other Joints, Distinctive Facies, and, Frequently, Cleft Palate. *Ann. Radiol.*, 15:297–328, 1972.
5. Spranger, J.: Personal communication.
6. Steel, H. H., and Kohl, E. J.: Multiple Congenital Dislocations Associated with Other Skeletal Anomalies (Larsen's Syndrome) in Three Siblings. *J. Bone Joint Surg.*, 54A:75–82, 1972.

LAURENCE-MOON-BIEDL-BARDET SYNDROME

This syndrome consists of obesity, retinitis pigmentosa, polydactyly and hypogonadism. Mental retardation is common. It is inherited as an autosomal recessive and is more common in males than in females. This syndrome must be differentiated from Carpenter syndrome.[4] However, in the latter condition the facial appearance is abnormal and there is also acrocephaly; also, in Carpenter syndrome the patients do not have retinal degeneration. The syndrome should also be differentiated from Biedmond II syndrome.[2, 5] In the latter, besides preaxial polydactyly, obesity and hypogenitalism, there are also colobomas of the iris.

RADIOLOGIC FINDINGS IN THE HAND. The most common finding, postaxial polydactyly, may not be seen in all patients, although the majority do have it.[2, 3, 4] The polydactyly may be asymmetrical. According to Temtamy[4] there may be shortening of metacarpals and distal phalanges and of the middle phalanx of the fifth finger. Syndactyly may be seen, although it is not certain whether the reported cases of syndactyly were really patients with Laurence-Moon-Biedl-Bardet syndrome or whether they represented other cases of Carpenter syndrome.

REFERENCES

1. Bell, J.: The Laurence-Moon Syndrome, *In* Penrose, L. S. (Ed.): The *Treasury of Human Inheritance*. Volume V, *On Hereditary Digital Anomalies*, Cambridge University Press, Cambridge, England, 1958.
2. Klein, D., and Ammann, F.: The Syndrome of Laurence-Moon-Bardet-Biedl and Allied Diseases in Switzerland. Clinical, Genetic and Epidemiological Studies. *J. Neurol. Sci.*, 9:479–513, 1969.

3. Seringe, P., Allaneau, C., Fores, C., and Guimbaud, P.: Le Syndrome de Bardet-Biedl et ses Troubles Endocriniens. *Ann. Endocrinol.*, 30:641–657, 1969.
4. Temtamy, S. A.: Carpenter's Syndrome: Acrocephalopolysyndactyly. An Autosomal Recessive Syndrome. *J. Pediatr.*, 69:111–120, 1966.
5. Temtamy, S. A.: Genetic Factors in Hand Malformations. Thesis. The Johns Hopkins University, 1966.

LENTIGINES SYNDROME (LEOPARD SYNDROME)

This is a disorder consisting of short stature, multiple lentigines, electrocardiographic changes, ocular hypertelorism, deafness, genital anomalies and a cardiac lesion which is usually valvular pulmonary stenosis. It has a dominant mode of inheritance.

RADIOLOGIC FINDINGS IN THE HAND. In many cases the findings are negligible; however, a family described by Forney et al.[1] had many similarities to the lentigines syndrome and had associated carpal and tarsal fusions.

OTHER RADIOLOGIC FINDINGS. Cervical spine fusions and tarsal fusions have been seen in Forney's patients, and minimal cervical spinal fusion has been seen in our cases of the lentigines syndrome.

REFERENCES

1. Forney, W. R., Robinson, S. J., and Pascoe, D. J.: Congenital Heart Disease, Deafness, and Skeletal Malformations: A New Syndrome? *J. Pediatr.*, 68:14–26, 1966.
2. Gorlin, R. J., Anderson, R. C., and Blaw, M.: Multiple Lentigines Syndrome. *Am. J. Dis. Child.*, 117:652–662, 1969.
3. Poznanski, A. K., Stern, A. M., and Gall, J. C., Jr.: Skeletal Anomalies in Genetically Determined Congenital Heart Disease. *Radiol. Clin. North Am.*, 9:435–458, 1971.

LENZ MICROPHTHALMIA SYNDROME

This is an X-linked syndrome of microphthalmia or anophthalmia, with or without microcephaly, which may be associated with abnormalities in the vertebral column, the clavicles and the extremities. Renal aplasia, dental abnormalities, hypospadias and cryptorchidism have also been seen. The patients may be mentally retarded.[1]

RADIOLOGIC FINDINGS IN THE HAND. These are variable and include camptodactyly and clinodactyly of the fifth finger. Cutaneous syndactyly may also be seen.

REFERENCES

1. Hermann, J., and Opitz, J. M.: The Lenz Microphthalmia Syndrome. *Birth Defects, Original Article Series*, 5:138–143, 1969.
2. Hoefnagel, D., Keenan, M. E., and Allen, F. H., Jr.: Heredofamilial Bilateral Anophthalmia. *Arch. Ophthalmol.*, 69:760–764, 1963.
3. Lenz, W.: Recessiv-geschlechtsgebundene Mikrophthalmie mit multiplen Missbildungen. *Z. Kinderheilkd.*, 77:384–390, 1955.

LÉRI PLEONOSTEOSIS

This somewhat ill-defined syndrome consists of shortness of stature; mongoloid

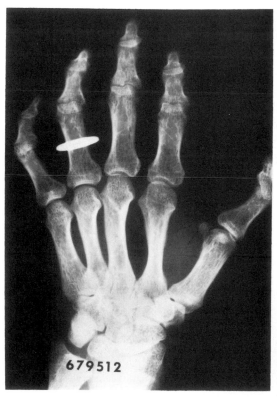

Figure 13–82. Léri pleonosteosis. The bones are coarse and thick and have undergone contracture in this affected adult. The patient is a member of the family reported by Rukavina et al.

facies; short, spade-like hands; broad thumbs held in valgus position; genu recurvatum; flexion contractures of the digits, hands and feet; cubitus valgus; and limitation of motion of the joints. There may be a mongoloid slant to the palpebral fissures. Inheritance is autosomal dominant with full penetrance.

RADIOLOGIC FINDINGS IN THE HAND. There is thickening of the various bones of the hand as well as some contractures (Fig. 13–82).

REFERENCES

1. Léri, A.: Dystrophie Osseuse Generalisee, Congenitale et Hereditaire: La Pléonostéose Familiale. *Presse Med.*, 30:13–16, 1922.
2. Léri, A.: Sur La Pléonostéose Familiale (2), (Presentation de Pieces et de Radiographies). *Bull. et Memories de la Societe Med. des Hosp. de Paris*, 48:216–220, 1924.
3. Rukavina, J. G., Falls, H. F., Holt, J. F., and Block, W. D.: Léri's Pleonosteosis. *J. Bone Joint Surg.*, 41A:397–408, 1959.
4. Watson-Jones, R.: Léri's Pleonosteosis, Carpal Tunnel Compression of the Median Nerves and Morton's Metatarsalgia. *J. Bone Joint Surg.*, 31B:560–571, 1949.

LESCH-NYHAN SYNDROME (CONGENITAL HYPERURICOSURIA)

This is an X-linked recessive syndrome consisting of choreoathetosis, mental retardation, motor dysfunction, self-mutilation and hyperuricemia. The condition is due to an enzyme defect and can be diagnosed by the inability of affected individuals to incorporate hypoxanthine into their cells.

RADIOLOGIC FINDINGS IN THE HAND. These changes are the result of self-mutilation, with destructive changes seen mainly in the distal phalanges (Fig. 13–83). There is usually delayed skeletal maturation. The appearance of the changes in the hand is similar to that seen in congenital indifference to pain.

OTHER RADIOLOGIC FINDINGS. Bilateral coxa valga and subluxation of the hips may be seen. Some cases have been reported with cerebral atrophy. Tophaceous gout may occur.

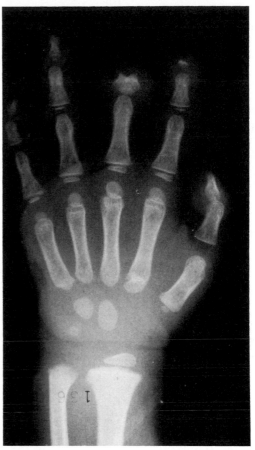

Figure 13–83. Lesch-Nyhan syndrome (congenital hyperuricosuria). There is loss of the tips of the index and middle fingers. There is some widening of the middle phalanx of the third finger as well. These are acquired changes due to trauma and infection. (Courtesy Dr. Melvin Becker. From Becker, M., and Wallin, J.: *Radiol. Clin. North Am.*, 6:239–243, 1968.)

REFERENCES

1. Becker, M. H., and Wallin, J. K.: Congenital Hyperuricosuria. Associated Radiologic Features. *Radiol. Clin. North Am.*, 6:239–243, 1968.
2. Nyhan, W. L., Oliver, W. J., and Lesch, M.: A Familial Disorder of Uric Acid Metabolism and Central Nervous System Function II. *J. Pediatr.*, 67:257–263, 1965.

LIEBENBERG SYNDROME

This association of elbow and wrist abnormalities was described in five generations of a South African family. The fingers were short with small, grooved nails. The condition was inherited as an autosomal dominant.

RADIOLOGIC FINDINGS IN THE HAND. The triquetrum was large and abnormal in configuration. It was fused to the pisiform in some patients. Other carpals, particularly the hamate, were also abnormal in configuration. Brachydactyly involving mainly the distal phalanges was seen.

OTHER RADIOLOGIC FINDINGS. There was underdevelopment of the humeral condyles, and deformity of the radial head and olecranon.

REFERENCE

1. Liebenberg, F.: A Pedigree with Unusual Anomalies of the Elbows, Wrists and Hands in Five Generations. S. Afr. Med. J., 47:745–748, 1973.

LIPODYSTROPHY—CONGENITAL, TOTAL

This is a condition associated with absence of body adipose tissue. The other clinical findings include hepatomegaly, hyperlipemia, an insulin-resistant diabetes, accelerated growth and maturation, hyperpigmentation and muscular overdevelopment. The cause of this condition is unknown but it may be related to an abnormality of the diencephalon. There is some resemblance between this condition and the diencephalic syndrome of infancy in that in both there is loss of fat, although no tumors are seen in congenital lipodystrophy. There is also a similarity between congenital lipodystrophy and cerebral gigantism, since in both of these conditions some individuals have a large size and advanced skeletal maturation. However, none of the other findings of cerebral gigantism is seen in lipodystrophy. Brunzell et al. reported an unusual family with lipodystrophy associated with congenital angiomatosis. These patients had multiple lucent defects throughout the hand bones and the remainder of the skeleton.

RADIOLOGIC FINDINGS IN THE HAND. The main abnormalities in the hand are those of advanced skeletal maturation. For example, the patient of Wesenberg et al.[3] had a bone age of 12 at age eight. There is also loss of the normal fat lines, which can be seen in the extremities but in the hand

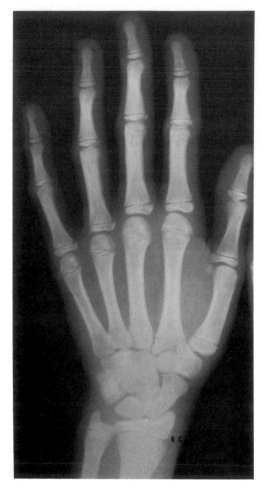

Figure 13–84. Lipodystrophy. Note lack of subcutaneous fat. The bone age is only slightly advanced in this 10 year old female. (Courtesy Dr. John Gwinn, Los Angeles, California.)

are better noted in the region of the wrist (Fig. 13–84).

OTHER RADIOLOGIC FINDINGS. Some cases have been described with dilatation of the third ventricle with or without concomitant enlargement of the lateral ventricles. Since a similar syndrome can be due to tumor, pneumoencephalography may sometimes reveal the primary cause of the disorder.

REFERENCES

1. Brunzell, J. D., Shankle, S. W., and Bethune, J. E.: Congenital Generalized Lipodystrophy Ac-

companied by Cystic Angiomatosis. *Ann. Int. Med.*, 69:501–516, 1968.

2. Seip, M., and Trygstad, O.: Generalized Lipodystrophy. *Arch. Dis. Child.*, 38:447–453, 1963.

3. Wesenberg, R. L., Gwinn, J. L., and Barnes, G. R., Jr.: The Roentgenographic Findings in Total Lipodystrophy. *Am. J. Roentgenol.*, 103:154–164, 1968.

MANDIBULOACRAL DYSPLASIA

This was a condition associated with mandibular hypoplasia, mild cranial dysplasia, hypoplasia of the clavicles, stiff joints and cutaneous atrophy. The inheritance was not known.

RADIOLOGIC FINDINGS IN THE HAND. There was acroosteolysis of the phalangeal tufts. The erosion was nonspecific in appearance. Since there was tuft erosion as well as absence of the clavicles, this condition somewhat resembles pycnodysostosis. However, no osteosclerosis was seen in mandibuloacral dysplasia.

OTHER RADIOLOGIC FINDINGS. Widening of the cranial sutures, wormian bones, small mandible, hypoplasia of the clavicles, lumbar scoliosis and coxa valga were seen.

REFERENCE

1. Young, L. W., Radebaugh, J. F., Rubin, P., Sensenbrenner, J. A., Fiorelli, G., and McKusick, V. A.: New Syndrome Manifested by Mandibular Hypoplasia, Acroosteolysis, Stiff Joints and Cutaneous Atrophy (Mandibuloacral Dysplasia) in Two Unrelated Boys. *Birth Defects, Original Article Series*, 7:291–297, 1971.

MANDIBULOFACIAL DYSOSTOSIS (TREACHER COLLINS SYNDROME)

This is a syndrome of hypoplasia of the face. The patients have a down-turned palpebral fissure, abnormalities of the lower lid, malar hypoplasia, mandibular hypoplasia and abnormally formed ears. There may be a projection of scalp hair onto the lateral cheek.

RADIOLOGIC FINDINGS IN THE HAND. Many patients show no abnormality in the hand; however, a number of assorted anomalies have been seen, including aplasia of the thumb, polydactyly and cleft hand. The appearance of the hand is not specific in this disorder.

OTHER RADIOLOGIC FINDINGS. Abnormality of the mastoids, mandible, ears and face may be seen.

REFERENCES

1. Franceschetti, A., and Klein, D.: The Mandibulo-Facial Dysostosis. A New Hereditary Syndrome. With 85 Figures. *Acta Ophthalmol.*, 27: 143–224, 1949.

2. Gorlin, R. J., and Pindborg, J. J.: *Syndromes of the Head and Neck.* McGraw-Hill Book Company, New York, 1964.

3. Stovin, J. J., Lyon, J. A., Jr., and Clemmens, R. L.: Mandibulofacial Dysostosis. *Radiology*, 74: 225–231, 1960.

MARFAN'S SYNDROME

This syndrome of arachnodactyly and hyperextensibility is associated with lens subluxation, aortic dilatation and other forms of congenital heart disease. Patients have a tendency to be tall. They may have pectus excavatum or pectus carinatum.

RADIOLOGIC FINDINGS IN THE HAND. Arachnodactyly is well seen clinically but is often difficult to document radiologically (Figs. 13–85 and 13–86). Steinberg[4] described the sign of the long thumb, which when clasped projects beyond the ulnar margin of the hand, but this is a clinical rather than a radiologic sign (Fig. 13–87). Sinclair[3] described a metacarpal index, which was the ratio of the length to width at midshaft of metacarpals one to four (see Chapter 2). In the normal group this index varied from 5.4 to 7.9, while in the Marfan group it ranged from 8.4 to 10.4. Parish[2] measured ratios of bone lengths to bone widths in the hand bones, and in some cases of Marfan syndrome he found a relative slenderness of the proximal phalanges as well as metacarpals. Pattern-profile analysis failed to reveal any characteristic pattern for this disorder. Clinodactyly may occasionally occur in Marfan syndrome.[1]

OTHER RADIOLOGIC FINDINGS. Other findings include disproportion and elongation of the lower limbs, proximal position of the patella, and long thin feet with prominent elongation of the first metatarsal and great toe. Sometimes there is severe flat-foot deformity; other deformities have also been described. Dislocation of various joints may be seen. Kyphoscoliosis is common and may be severe. Usually it is idio-

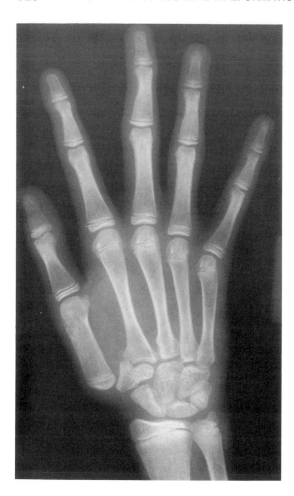

Figure 13–85. Marfan syndrome. There are long slender fingers, with dislocation of the thumb. (Courtesy Dr. L. Desautels, Calgary, Alberta, Canada.)

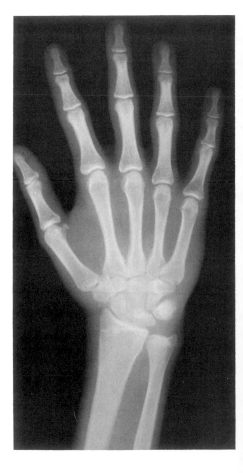

Figure 13–86. Marfan syndrome. Note the slightly slender bones, which are difficult to appreciate on simple observation. The slenderness ratios, using Parish's normal standards, were significantly abnormal.

3. Sinclair, R. J. G., Kitchin, A. H., and Turner, R. W. D.: The Marfan Syndrome. *Q. J. Med.,* 53:19–46, 1960.
4. Steinberg, I.: A Simple Screening Test for the Marfan Syndrome. *Am. J. Roentgenol.,* 97:118–124, 1966.
5. Wilner, H. I., and Finby, N.: Skeletal Manifestations in the Marfan Syndrome. *J.A.M.A.,* 187: 490–495, 1964.

MARSHALL SYNDROME

Marshall et al.[1] described a syndrome characterized by unusual facial features, failure to thrive and marked acceleration of osseous maturation. Facial abnormalities included coarse eyebrows, shallow orbits and an underdeveloped upturned nose. Patients had severe motor and mental retardation.

RADIOLOGIC FINDINGS IN THE HAND. There was markedly advanced skeletal maturation. At age 16 months, one of their patients had a maturation of at least six years. The hands were otherwise unremarkable except perhaps for some slenderness of the distal phalanges.

OTHER RADIOLOGIC FINDINGS. The orbits were rather shallow.

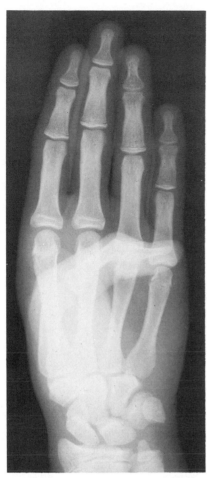

Figure 13–87. Marfan syndrome. There is a questionably positive Steinberg sign with the thumb across the hand—the edge of the thumb normally does not go beyond the margin of the hand. In this patient, the finding is borderline.

pathic and evident after 10 to 12 years of age. Skull findings are variable, ranging from dolichocephaly to brachycephaly. Sternal deformities have been seen, varying from pectus excavatum to pectus carinatum.

REFERENCES

1. McKusick, V. A.: *Heritable Disorders of Connective Tissue,* 4th Ed. The C. V. Mosby Company, St. Louis, 1972.
2. Parish, J. G.: Skeletal Hand Charts in Inherited Connective Tissue Disease. *J. Med. Genet.,* 4:227–238, 1967.

REFERENCE

1. Marshall, R. E., Graham, C. B., Scott, C. R., and Smith, D. W.: Syndrome of Accelerated Skeletal Maturation and Relative Failure to Thrive: A Newly Recognized Clinical Growth Disorder *J. Pediatr.,* 78:95–101, 1971.

MECKEL SYNDROME (DYSENCEPHALIA SPLANCHNOCYSTICA)

The features of this syndrome are occipital encephalocele, cleft lip and cleft palate, polydactyly and polycystic kidneys. There may be associated microcephaly, short-limbed dwarfism and a variety of other anomalies. The appearance may be somewhat reminiscent of trisomy 13 but the karyotype is normal.

RADIOLOGIC FINDINGS IN THE HAND. The main hand finding is evidence of polydactyly of the postaxial type. Syndactyly may also be seen.

REFERENCES

1. Fitch, N., and Pinsky, L.: The Meckel Syndrome with Limited Expression in Relatives. *Clin. Genet.,* 4:33–37, 1973.
2. Hsia, Y. E., Bratu, M., and Herbordt, A.: Genetics of the Meckel Syndrome (Dysencephalia Splanchnocystica). *Pediatrics,* 48:237–247, 1971.
3. Mecke, S., and Passarge, E.: Encephalocele, Polycystic Kidneys, and Polydactyly as an Autosomal Recessive Trait Simulating Certain Other Disorders: The Meckel Syndrome. *Ann. Genet.,* 14:97–103, 1971.

MELORHEOSTOSIS

This is a hyperostosis of bone which resembles melting wax dripping down one side of a candle. The clinical symptoms are usually pain, stiffness and limitation of motion. Contractures may be seen and the skin over the lesions may be tense. No hereditary factors are known.

RADIOLOGIC FINDINGS IN THE HAND. There are increased areas of radiopacity which follow the long axis of some of the hand bones. Usually only a few of the hand bones are involved, but the disease process appears to extend from the forearm to the carpal bones, into the metacarpals, and then to the phalanges, as though a line were drawn across these bones (Fig. 13–88). The finding may be very minimal in infancy, but the disease is rapidly progressive in childhood and is best seen in adults. The cortical thickening may encroach on the medullary canal of the bones.

OTHER RADIOLOGIC FINDINGS. Distribution of the disease may be monostotic, polyostotic or monomelic, with an appearance similar to that seen in the hand. The lower extremities are involved much more often than the upper extremities.

REFERENCES

1. Campbell, C. J., Papademetriou, T., and Bonfiglio, M.: Melorheostosis. *J. Bone Joint Surg.,* 50A: 1281–1304, 1968.

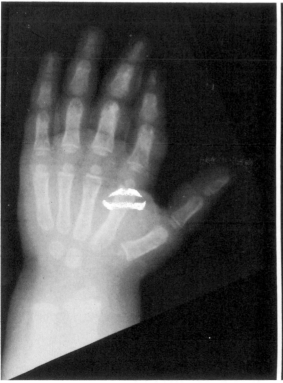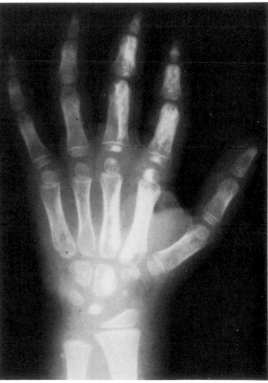

Figure 13–88. Melorheostosis. Ages two years and six years. The earlier film shows relatively little sclerosis, while on the later film definite sclerotic changes are seen along the index and middle fingers. In addition, the capitate is crossed by a line of sclerosis. (Courtesy Dr. C. J. Campbell, Albany, New York. From Campbell, C. J., et al.: *J. Bone Joint Surg.,* 50A:1281–1304, 1968.)

2. Morris, J. M., Samilson, R. L., and Corley, C. L.: Melorheostosis. *J. Bone Joint Surg.*, 45A:1191–1206, 1963.

MENKES SYNDROME (KINKY HAIR SYNDROME)

This is a condition of failure to thrive, cerebral degeneration, kinky hair, hypothermia and convulsions. Pathologically, gliosis and cystic degeneration of the brain are seen, probably due to obliteration of cerebral arteries in association with fragmentation of the elastic layer. Similar arterial changes are evident in the rest of the body. The syndrome is due to a defect in copper absorption from the gut and has an X-linked pattern of inheritance.

RADIOLOGIC FINDINGS IN THE HAND. These are minimal. The main findings are in the wrist, with flaring of the distal radius and ulna and small spurs, which may somewhat resemble rickets. The findings may be similar to other causes of copper deficiency (see Chapter 21). Arterial changes in the hand can also be expected, since most of the arteries of the body are involved.

OTHER RADIOLOGIC FINDINGS. Flaring of the ends of most of the bones may be seen with some spurring. Arteriographic changes are dramatic, with corkscrew vessels seen in the brain and most other regions. Many of the vessels may be obstructed. Persistent wormian bones may be seen in the skull.

REFERENCES

1. Danks, D. M., Campbell, P. E., Stevens, B. J., Mayne, V., and Cartwright, E.: Menkes's Kinky Hair Syndrome. An Inherited Defect in Copper Absorption with Widespread Effects. *Pediatrics*, 50:188–201, 1972.
2. Wesenberg, R. L., Gwinn, J. L., and Barnes, G. R., Jr.: Radiological Findings in the Kinky-Hair Syndrome. *Radiology*, 92:500–506, 1969.

MESOMELIC DWARFISM—TYPE LANGER (MESOMELIC DWARFISM OF THE HYPOPLASTIC ULNA, FIBULA, MANDIBLE TYPE)

This is a form of short-limbed dwarfism evident from birth and associated with mesomelic shortening, i.e., the middle segment of the extremity is short. This includes the forearm and the shank. The affected individuals have normal intelligence.

Silverman[2] postulated a relationship between this condition and dyschondrosteosis. He reported a mother with typical manifestations of dyschondrosteosis and two of her children who had a typical Langer-type of mesomelic dwarfism. Inheritance in Langer's cases was believed to be autosomal recessive, while in Silverman's family as well as in dyschondrosteosis it is dominant.

RADIOLOGIC FINDINGS IN THE HAND. The fingers appear normal on casual inspection, although abnormal pattern profiles may be seen. The proximal carpals form a decreased carpal angle (Fig. 13–89). This is probably related to the cup formed by the radius and ulna. The appearance is similar to that seen in dyschondrosteosis, but the radial and ulnar shortening is much more severe in Langer disease.

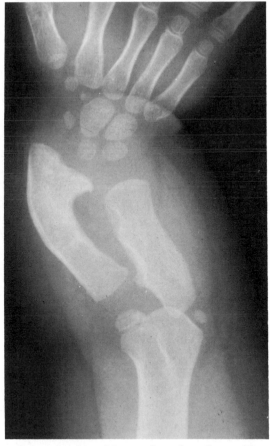

Figure 13–89. Mesomelic dwarfism. Type Langer. In this condition the radius and ulna are particularly short and bowed. The hand was relatively normal except for a decrease in carpal angle. (Courtesy Dr. David Corbett, Detroit, Michigan.)

OTHER RADIOLOGIC FINDINGS. There is marked shortening of the fibula, radius and ulna. To a lesser degree the humerus and femur are also shortened. The mandible is hypoplastic.

REFERENCES

1. Langer, L. O., Jr.: Mesomelic Dwarfism of the Hypoplastic Ulna, Fibula, Mandible Type. *Radiology*, 89:654–660, 1967.
2. Silverman, F. N.: Mesomelic Dwarfism. *Progr. Pediatr. Radiol.*, 4:546–562, 1973. (*Intrinsic Diseases of Bones*, edited by H. J. Kaufmann, Karger, Basel.)

METAPHYSEAL CHONDRODYSPLASIA—TYPE JANSEN

This is a rare form of dwarfism associated clinically with severe anterior bowing of the legs which produces an unusual mon-

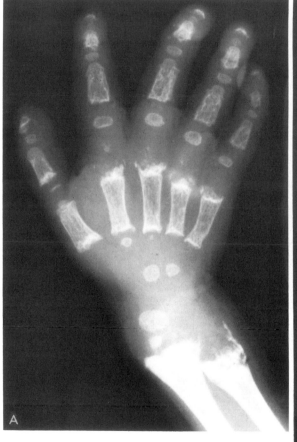
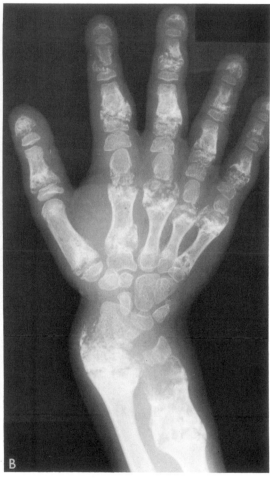

Figure 13–90. Metaphyseal chondrodysplasia. Type Jansen. *A*, Two and one half year old child. There is cupping of the ends of the bones with slight irregular calcification in the cupped ends. There is marked widening of the epiphyseal plate, which is best seen in the proximal phalanges, where the epiphyses are widely separated from the rest of the shaft. The changes are similar to those of rickets. The distal phalanges are very poorly ossified, the nonepiphyseal ends appearing as crescents of bone. The epiphyses are relatively uninvolved.

B, Follow up at age 13½years. There is now marked irregularity at the ends of the bones. The previously unossified area now contains amorphous calcification, in some cases with a cystic-like pattern. The epiphyses appear somewhat thicker than usual but do not contain this abnormal calcification. The fingers are somewhat short. (This is the patient reported by Holt, J. F., and Poznanski, A. K.: *Seminars in Roentgenology*, 8:166–167, 1973, by permission.)

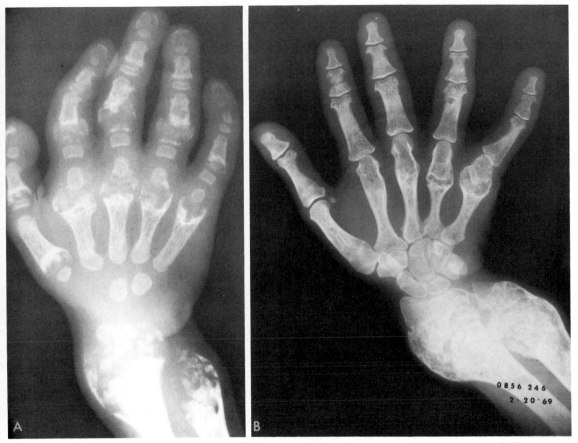

Figure 13–91. Metaphyseal chondrodysplasia. Type Jansen. *A*, There is irregular calcification in the metaphyses, which appear swollen and thickened. Crescent-shaped distal phalanges are again seen.

B, Follow-up film. There is now marked healing of the previously described changes. Some of the bones appear relatively normal. There is still a defect in the middle of the middle phalanx of the index finger. The phalanges are relatively shortened. (This is the patient reported by Gram, P. B., et al.: *J. Bone-Joint Surg.*, 41A:951–959, 1959.)

key-like squatting stance. The dwarfism is pronounced. There is swelling of the wrists, knees and other joints, and a prominent rosary may be seen in the costochondral region. The facial configuration is fairly typical, with hypertelorism, exophthalmos and a receding chin. Most patients have evidence of hypercalcemia. The condition is inherited as an autosomal dominent.

RADIOLOGIC FINDINGS IN THE HAND. At birth there is fraying of the metaphysis and some scalloping in this region (Fig. 13–90 A). As the patient gets older there is bizarre ossification in the metaphyseal region, with foci of calcification that may ap-

pear cyst-like (Fig. 13–90 B). The epiphyses in the hand appear somewhat broad but have a normal architecture. The distal phalanges appear as a broad line, deeply scalloped along their epiphyseal border (Fig. 13–91 A). There is delay in bone maturation. With maturity, much of the irregularity of the metaphyseal calcification disappears and the bones regain a more normal appearance (Fig. 13–91 B).

OTHER RADIOLOGIC FINDINGS. Findings similar to those of the hand are seen in the other bones with prominent areas of calcification. The bowing is most marked in the lower extremities and can be very dramatic.

REFERENCES

1. De Haas, W. H. D., De Boer, W., and Griffioen, F.: Metaphysial Dysostosis. A Late Follow-up of the First Reported Case. *J. Bone Joint Surg.*, 51B:290–299, 1969.
2. Gram, P. B., Fleming, J. L., Frame, B., and Fine, G.: Metaphyseal Chondrodysplasia of Jansen. *J. Bone Joint Surg.*, 41A:951–959, 1959.
3. Holt, J. F., and Poznanski, A. K.: Metaphyseal Chondrodysplasia—Type Jansen. *Seminars in Roentgenology*, 8:166–167, 1973.
4. Ozonoff, M. B.: Metaphyseal Dysostosis of Jansen. *Radiology*, 93:1047–1050, 1969.

METAPHYSEAL CHONDRODYSPLASIA (METAPHYSEAL DYSOSTOSIS)— OTHER TYPES

There are various other types of metaphyseal chondrodysplasia, including the Peña, the Schmidt, the Spahr and the McKusick forms. This is a rather broad group of disorders characterized by dwarfism and rachitic-like changes of the metaphyses of the long bones. The Jansen type, which was separately described, has the most severe

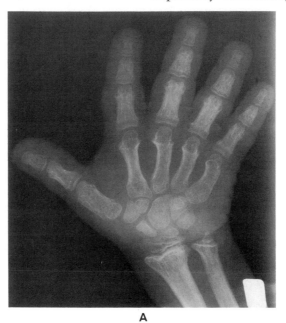

A

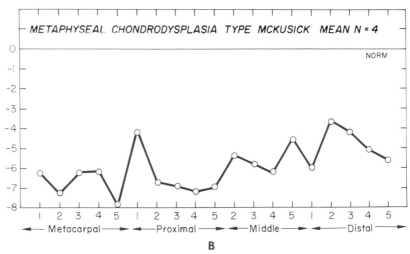

B

Figure 13–92. *A*, Metaphyseal chondrodysplasia. Type McKusick. (Hair-cartilage hypoplasia.) There is decrease in size of the hand bones. The metaphyses are slightly irregular, but the findings are otherwise not diagnostic.

B, Pattern profile. The hand bones are very small. The metacarpals are six to eight standard deviations below the mean.

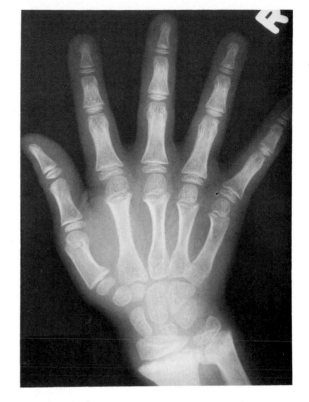

Figure 13–93. Metaphyseal chondrodysplasia. Type Schmidt. The radius and ulna show some irregularity, but the hand bones are unremarkable.

radiographic findings. In the McKusick type there is associated hair-cartilage hypoplasia. Some forms have been described in association with spine changes and have been termed spondylometaphyseal dysplasia. Some forms have been associated with pancreatic insufficiency and chronic neutropenia.[1, 5]

The genetic pattern of the various types differs. The Schmidt type is an autosomal dominant, while the hair-cartilage hypoplasia is an autosomal recessive.

RADIOLOGIC FINDINGS IN THE HAND. The radiologic changes in these disorders affect both the metaphyses and the length of the hand bones.

The radiologic findings in cartilage–hair hypoplasia were evaluated by Ray and Dorst.[3] They found that the hand is disproportionately small in this disease, with all of the metacarpals, phalanges and carpal bones markedly diminished in size (Fig. 13–92). A characteristic pattern profile is shown in Figure 13–92*B*. The metaphyses of the phalanges are mildly cupped, with the epiphyses fitting into the cups, giving them a cone-shaped configuration. The distal phalanges are not only short but also very slender, particularly during infancy; they widen somewhat at their bases during preadolescence. The middle phalanges have a narrow distal end to match the distal phalanges, and eventually they develop a bullet-shaped configuration. Similar findings are seen in the proximal phalanges. This bullet-shape disappears when adulthood is reached. The carpal bones are somewhat irregular in size, and the entire carpus appears small. There may be an increase in carpal angle in some patients.[3]

In the Schmidt type of metaphyseal chondrodysplasia, the shortening of the hand bones is relatively mild (Fig. 13–93), and in some cases the metaphysis of the radius may be within normal limits.

In the Peña type, irregular defects in ossification are seen which extend significantly into the metaphyseal shafts of the metacarpals and phalanges.[5]

In adult patients, in both the hair–cartilage and Schmidt forms of metaphyseal chondrodysplasia, the radiographic findings may be nondiagnostic. There may simply be evidence of shortening.

OTHER RADIOLOGIC FINDINGS. There are metaphyseal changes in the other bones, probably most marked about the knees. Dwarfism is variable in these different types of metaphyseal chondrodysplasia.

REFERENCES

1. Giedion, A., Prader, A., Hadorn, B., Shmerling, D. H., and Auricchio, S.: Metaphysäre Dysostose und angeborene Pankreasinsuffizienz. *Fortschr. Geb. Roentgenstr. Nuklearmed.*, 108: 51–57, 1968.
2. McKusick, V. A., Eldridge, R., Hostetler, J. A., Ruangwit, U., and Egeland, J. A.: Dwarfism in the Amish. II. Cartilage-Hair Hypoplasia. Johns Hopkins Med. J., 116:285–326, 1965.
3. Ray, H. C., and Dorst, J. P.: Cartilage-Hair-Hypoplasia. *Progr. Pediatr. Radiol.*, Vol. 4, 1973. (*Intrinsic Diseases of Bones*, edited by H. J. Kaufmann, Karger, Basel.)
4. Rimoin, D. L., and McAlister, W. H.: Metaphyseal Dysostosis, Conductive Hearing Loss and Mental Retardation: A Recessively Inherited Syndrome. *Birth Defects, Original Article Series,* 7:116–122, 1971.
5. Sutcliffe, J., and Stanley, P.: Metaphyseal Chondrodysplasias. *Progr. Pediatr. Radiol.*, 4:250–269, 1973. (*Intrinsic Diseases of Bones*, edited by H. J. Kaufmann, Karger, Basel.)
6. Taybi, H., Mitchell, A. D., and Friedman, G. D.: Metaphyseal Dysostosis and the Associated Syndrome of Pancreatic Insufficiency and Blood Disorders. *Radiology*, 93:563–571, 1969.
7. Wiedemann, H.-R., Spranger, J., and Kosenow, W.: Knorpel-Haar-Hypoplasie. *Arch. Kinderheilkd.*, 176:74–85, 1967.

METATROPIC DWARFISM

This is a form of dwarfism described by Maroteaux, Spranger and Wiedemann in 1966.[4] It somewhat resembles achondroplasia at birth, since it is associated with disproportionately short limbs. Later, as the spine changes become more severe with flattening and scoliosis, it clinically appears more like Morquio disease. The joints may appear prominent and stiff. There may be a small caudal appendage or tail present in some of these patients. The condition is probably inherited as an autosomal recessive.

RADIOLOGIC FINDINGS IN THE HAND. In the infant the hands have a fairly characteristic appearance. The proximal phalanges seem to have an hourglass configuration (Fig. 13–94). The indentation in the middle phalanges is partially related to the relatively bulbous ends of these bones. To some degree the same configuration may be seen in other bones of the hand. The bones of the hand are short and in the older individual there is evidence of metaphyseal and epiphyseal abnormality. The carpal bones are irregular in contour (Fig. 13–95 *B*). Maturation is markedly delayed in this condition (Fig. 13–95).

OTHER RADIOLOGIC FINDINGS. At birth there is overmodeling, with prominent bulbous ends of the long bones. The pelvis has a fairly characteristic appearance. There is markedly decreased height of the vertebral bodies but little change in appearance of the pedicles. Kyphoscoliosis may be seen. As the child grows, the height of the intervertebral spaces decreases, kyphoscoliosis progresses and platyspondyly persists.

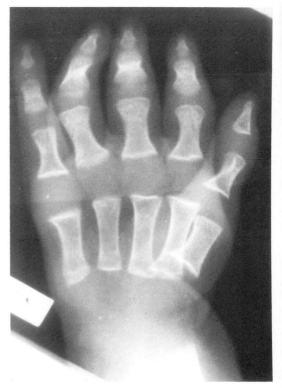

Figure 13–94. Metatropic dwarfism. Infant. The hand has a characteristic configuration, with an hourglass appearance most marked in the middle phalanges.

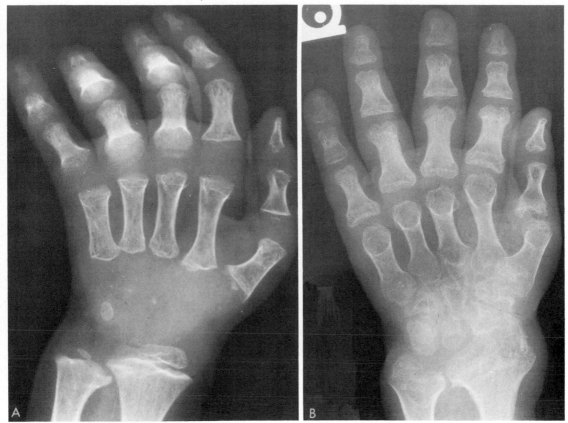

Figure 13-95. Metatropic dwarfism. *A,* 3 9/12 female. Again, the hourglass configuration of the middle phalanges makes the film diagnostic of this condition. A similar appearance is seen in other bones of the hand. There is evidence of shortening of the hand bones and there is marked delay in maturation. The carpal bones are barely perceptible.

B, Age 14 years. There is still some hourglass deformity of the bones of the hands, which have now matured somewhat. Brachydactyly is quite evident.

REFERENCES

1. Bailey, J. A., II, Dorst, J. P., and Saunderson, R. W., Jr.: Metatropic Dwarfism, Recognized Retrospectively from the Roentgenographic Features. *Birth Defects, Original Article Series,* 5:376–381, 1969.
2. Jenkins, P., Smith, M. B., and McKinnell, J. S.: Metatropic Dwarfism. *Br. J. Radiol.,* 43:561–565, 1970.
3. Maroteaux, P.: Spondyloepiphyseal Dysplasias and Metatropic Dwarfism. *Birth Defects, Original Article Series,* 5:35–44, 1969.
4. Maroteaux, P., Spranger, J., and Wiedemann, H.-R.: Der metatropische Zwergwuchs. *Arch Kinderheilkd.,* 173:211–226, 1966.
5. Tucker, A. S., and Iannacone, G.: Differential Diagnosis of Metatropic Dwarfism. *Ann. Radiol.,* 14:361–363, 1970.

MÖBIUS SYNDROME (CONGENITAL FACIAL DIPLEGIA)

This is a syndrome of congenital paralysis of the cranial nerves, particularly the sixth and seventh. The patients have a mask-like face at birth, their eyes do not close and their mouth remains open. The paralysis may be asymmetric and other cranial nerves may be affected. Ear anomalies are sometimes seen. The patients may be mentally retarded. Inheritance is not certain but may be autosomal dominant.

RADIOLOGIC FINDINGS IN THE HAND. A variety of hand defects can be seen, the most common of which is syndactyly. Some

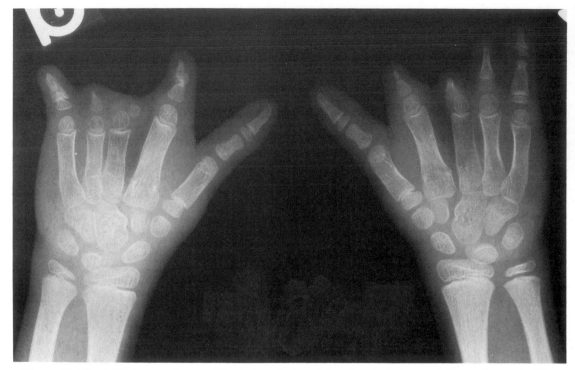

Figure 13–96. Möbius syndrome. There is aplasia of the distal phalanges bilaterally, with bizarre remnants of the phalanges.

patients have associated absence of digits, polydactyly, brachydactyly and various disordered positions of the fingers (Fig. 13–96).

OTHER RADIOLOGIC FINDINGS. Clubfoot is a common abnormality and may be either unilateral or bilateral. Miscellaneous other abnormalities, such as congenital dislocation of the hip, have been seen. Absence of the pectoral muscle has also been noted.

REFERENCES

1. Dalloz, J.-C., and Nocton, F.: Le Syndrome de Moebius. A propos de Deux Observations Nouvelles. *Arch. Fr. Pediat.*, 21:1027–1047, 1964.
2. Gorlin, R. J., and Sedano, H.: Moebius Syndrome. *Modern Medicine*, 40:110, 1972.
3. Gorlin, R. J., and Pindborg, J. J.: *Syndromes of the Head and Neck*, McGraw-Hill Book Company, New York, 1964.
4. Hanissian, A. S., Fuste, F., Hayes, W. T., and Duncan, J. M.: Moebius Syndrome in Twins. *Am. J. Dis. Child.*, 120:472, 1970.
5. Holmes, L. B., Moser, H. W., Halldorsson, S., Mac, C., Pant, S. S., and Matzilevich, B.: *Mental Retardation. An Atlas of Diseases with Asso-*
ciated Physical Abnormalities. The Macmillan Company, New York, 1972.

MUCOLIPIDOSIS II (I-CELL DISEASE, LEROY DISEASE)

This is a Hurler-like condition which differs from Hurler syndrome in that its onset is early; it may even be apparent at birth. It is difficult to differentiate from GM_1 gangliosidosis. The clinical findings progress, so that between the sixth and eighteenth month they are very severe. There is no increase in excretion of mucopolysaccharides in the urine. Histologically, the most striking finding is the presence of inclusions in the cells in tissue culture; hence the term I-cell disease. This disease is inherited as an autosomal recessive.

RADIOLOGIC FINDINGS IN THE HAND. The findings are indistinguishable from those of Hurler disease (mucopolysaccharidosis I). The only radiologic distinguishing factor is the relatively greater severity of the findings that are present in Hurler disease. In particular, the proximal ends of the

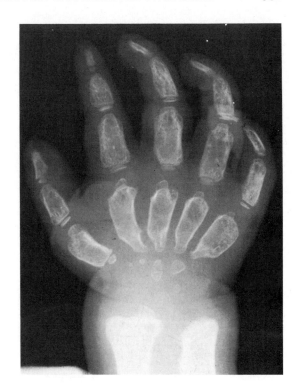

Figure 13–97. Mucolipodosis II (I-cell disease, Leroy disease). There is pointing at the proximal ends of the metacarpals and failure of modeling of the phalanges, which appear as thick in their center portions as in their ends. The carpals are irregular. There is some curvature of the fingers. The appearance of the hand is similar to that seen in Hurler syndrome except that the changes are more severe for the age of the patient.

metacarpals have a pointed appearance. The bones are thickened. Carpal maturation is markedly delayed. There is cupping of the distal radius and ulna (Fig. 13–97).

OTHER RADIOLOGIC FINDINGS. These are the same as those of Hurler disease and GM₁ gangliosidosis.

REFERENCES

1. Leroy, J. G., Spranger, J. W., Feingold, M., Opitz, J. M., and Crocker, A. C.: I-Cell Disease: A Clinical Picture. *J. Pediatr.*, 79:360–365, 1971.
2. Spranger, J. W., and Wiedemann, H.-R.: The Genetic Mucolipidoses. Diagnosis and Differential Diagnosis. *Humangenetik*, 9:113–139, 1970.
3. Taber, P., Gyepes, M. T., Philippart, M., and Ling, S.: Roentgenographic Manifestations of Leroy's I-Cell Disease. *Am. J. Roentgenol.*, 118:213–221, 1973.

MUCOLIPIDOSIS III (PSEUDO-HURLER POLYDYSTROPHY)

This is a condition which clinically resembles Hurler disease, with coarse facies, claw hands and mild corneal opacities. However, there is no excretion of an abnormal amount of mucopolysaccharide in the urine, but there is evidence of increased visceral and mesenchymal storage of acid mucopolysaccharides and glycolipids, which can be demonstrated on tissue culture. Joint stiffness is a prominent feature. There is mild mental retardation later in childhood, and dwarfism is common. The condition is probably inherited as an autosomal recessive trait.

RADIOLOGIC FINDINGS IN THE HAND. The changes in the hand are variable. Some patients have short metacarpals and phalanges while in other patients these bones are relatively normal in length. There is often proximal pointing of the metacarpals with a claw configuration of the hand. However, the diaphyses are never as wide as the metaphyses, as may sometimes be seen in Hurler syndrome.[1] The carpals ossify late and may be small and irregular. The overall appearance of the hand is similar to that seen in Hurler disease but is usually significantly milder (Fig. 13–98).

OTHER RADIOLOGIC FINDINGS. These are similar to those of Hurler disease.

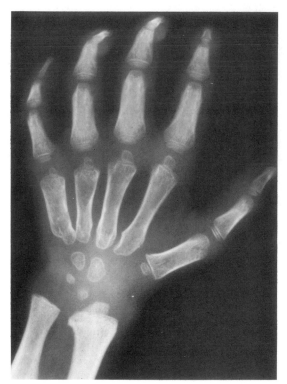

Figure 13–98. Probable mucolipidosis III (pseudo-Hurler polydystrophy). This is a seven year old female with Hurler-like findings but with no abnormal mucopolysacchariduria. There is some pointing of the metacarpals and some modeling errors. The patient had considerable stiffness of the joints. (Tissue culture not yet done.) (Courtesy Dr. R. Allen, Ann Arbor, Michigan.)

REFERENCES

1. Maroteaux, P., and Lamy, M.: La Pseudo-Poly-dystrophie de Hurler. *Presse Med.,* 74:2889–2892, 1966.

2. Melhem, R., Dorst, J. P., Scott, C. I., Jr., and Mc-Kusick, V. A.: Roentgen Findings in Muco-lipidosis III (Pseudo-Hurler Polydystrophy). *Radiology,* 106:153–160, 1973.

MUCOPOLYSACCHARIDOSES (HURLER SYNDROME, HUNTER SYNDROME, SANFILIPPO SYNDROME, MAROTEAUX-LAMY)

There are at least six well-defined syndromes involving mucopolysaccharide abnormality. These six syndromes exhibit mucopolysacchariduria, and their various characteristics are listed in Table 13–1. In these six types the radiologic findings are very similar, except in Morquio syndrome, or type IV, which will be discussed separately.

The Hurler form, or gargoylism, is the most severe and best known and is characterized by clouding of the cornea, severe dwarfism, mental retardation and deafness. The Hunter form is a sex-linked form which occurs only in males and generally appears milder. In the Sanfilippo form, patients have very severe mental defects but relatively mild somatic features. The type V or Scheie form is now felt to be due to the same biochemical defect as the Hurler form and should probably be called type IS.[4] It is characterized by the fact that there is little or no intellectual impairment. In the type VI, or Maroteaux-Lamy form, there are marked osseous and corneal changes which are similar to those in the Hurler syndrome, but there is no intellec-

TABLE 13–1. Mucopolysaccharidoses*

TYPE	I (1H)	II	III	IV	V (1S)	VI
EPONYM	Hurler	Hunter	Sanfilippo	Morquio	Scheie	Maroteaux-Lamy
GARGOYLE-LIKE APPEARANCE	+++†	++	+	−	++	++
TIME OF ONSET	Infancy	1–2 years	4–6 years	1–2 years	Late ?	2–6 years
GROWTH RETARDATION	+++	++	−	+++	+	++
MENTAL RETARDATION	+++	++	+++	−	−	−
CORNEAL OPACITIES	+	−	−	+	+	+
SEVERITY OF BONY CHANGES	+++	++	+	+++ different from others	+	++
OTHER	Die before 10 years	Males only; wide range of severity	Die at puberty	Typical facies	May survive to adulthood	May survive to adulthood

*After Spranger, J. W., et al.: *Helv. Paediatr. Acta,* 25:337–362, 1970; and McKusick, V. A.: *Heritable Disorders of Connective Tissue.* The C. V. Mosby Company, St. Louis, 1972.
†− Indicates mild.
+ Indicates present, mild.
+++ Indicates present, severe.

tual impairment. A newly described type VII, which is due to beta glucuronidase deficiency,[5] is not yet well defined.

There are some differences between these various syndromes in the types of mucopolysaccharide excreted, and biochemical differences are beginning to be defined. Clinically and radiologically the Hurler syndrome resembles I-cell disease (Leroy disease, mucolipidosis II), except that mucolipidosis II has more severe manifestations earlier in infancy than does Hurler disease. Most of these conditions are inherited as an autosomal recessive except Hunter's, which is X-linked.

RADIOLOGIC FINDINGS IN THE HAND. The most severe findings are present in the Hurler form of the syndrome (Fig. 13–

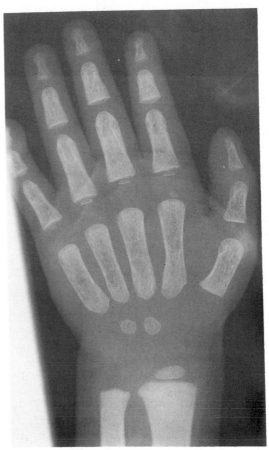

Figure 13–100. Mucopolysaccharidosis III (San Filippo syndrome). 2½ year old. There are minimal changes in the hand bones with perhaps slight pointing of the metacarpals. There is some delay in maturation.

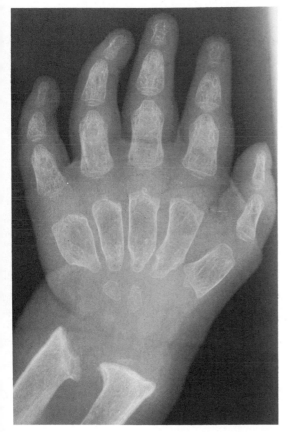

Figure 13–99. Mucopolysaccharidosis I (Hurler disease). 5⁸/₁₀ year old female. There is severe tapering of the proximal ends of the metacarpals, which appear pointed. All the bones of the hand appear broad and irregular. The bony cortex is thinned. There is some pointing of the distal radius and ulna, which are more cupped than normal. There is marked delay in maturation for the patient's stated age. The hand has a somewhat claw-like configuration with curvature of the fingers.

99), and they are progressively milder in the Hunter and milder yet in the Sanfilippo (Fig. 13–100). Severe bony changes are seen in the Maroteaux-Lamy, and less severe changes occur in the Scheie. In all types, the severity in the findings progresses during the course of the disease, so that each of the forms may appear mild or severe, depending on when it is seen. The characteristic findings in all these types are short, poorly modeled metacarpals with tapering of the proximal portions (Fig. 13–99). There is pointing of the radius and ulna with a decreased carpal angle. Flexion contracture occurs in severe cases. Maturation is retarded. Small carpal cysts may be seen in Scheie syndrome.[9]

OTHER RADIOLOGIC FINDINGS. Similar coarsening and thickening of the bones is seen in other portions of the skeleton. There may be enlargement of the sella turcica from subarachnoid cysts. The pelvis may have a characteristic configuration. There is flattening or beaking of some of the vertebral bodies, but this is not as marked as in Morquio syndrome.

REFERENCES

1. Danks, D. M., Campbell, P. E., Cartwright, E., Mayne, V., Taft, L. I., and Wilson, R. G.: The Sanfilippo Syndrome: Clinical, Biochemical, Radiological, Haematological and Pathological Features of Nine Cases. *Aust. Paediatr. J.*, 8:174–186, 1972.
2. Langer, L. O.: The Radiographic Manifestations of the HS-Mucopolysaccharidosis of Sanfilippo. *Ann. Radiol.*, 7:315–325, 1964.
3. Leroy, J. G., and Crocker, A. C.: Clinical Definition of the Hurler-Hunter Phenotypes. *Am. J. Dis. Child.*, 112:518–530, 1966.
4. McKusick, V. A.: *Heritable Disorders of Connective Tissue*. The C. V. Mosby Company, St. Louis, 1972.
5. Sly, W. S., Quinton, B. A., McAlister, W. H., and Rimoin, D. L.: Beta Glucuronidase Deficiency: Report of Clinical, Radiologic, and Biochemical Features of a New Mucopolysaccharidosis. *J. Pediatr.*, 82:249–257, 1973.
6. Spranger, J. W.: The Genetic Mucopolysaccharidoses. *Birth Defects, Original Article Series*, 5:145–156, 1969.
7. Spranger, J. W.: The Systemic Mucopolysaccharidoses. *Ergeb. Inn. Med. Kinderheilkd.*, 32: 165–265, 1972.
8. Spranger, J. W., Koch, F., McKusick, V. A., Natzschika, J., Wiedemann, H.-R., and Zellweger, H.: Mucopolysaccharidosis VI (Maroteaux-Lamy's Disease). *Helv. Paediatr. Acta*, 25: 337–362, 1970.
9. Dorst, J.: Personal communication.

MUCOPOLYSACCHARIDOSIS IV (MORQUIO DISEASE, MORQUIO-BRAILSFORD DISEASE)

This mucopolysaccharidosis differs clinically and chemically from the others. The

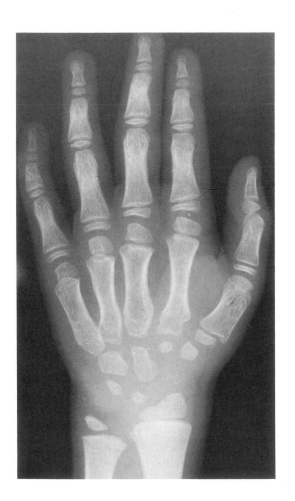

Figure 13–101. Mucopolysaccharidosis IV (Morquio disease). There is some shortening of the metacarpals. The carpals appear small and irregular in contour. The proximal ends of the metacarpals are also somewhat irregular. (Courtesy Dr. William Reynolds, Henry Ford Hospital, Detroit, Michigan.)

clinical findings include a short trunk and a waddling gait which becomes apparent at about two years of age. Keratan sulfate is excreted in the urine. Corneal opacities and dental abnormalities are seen in all patients. The condition is inherited as an autosomal recessive.

RADIOLOGIC FINDINGS IN THE HAND. The hand findings are not in themselves very characteristic of this condition. In the young child there are conical bases of the second through fifth metacarpals. As the child becomes older the carpal bones become somewhat irregular in configuration (Fig. 13–101). There may be marked delay in the ossification of the scaphoid.[1] Modeling of the metacarpals remains unremarkable in these patients. In the older child or adult there may still be a decreased number of ossified carpal bones. The metacarpals in particular are shortened. The hand may be in ulnar deviation because of the shortening of the ulna. In some cases skeletal maturation may be within normal limits.

OTHER RADIOLOGIC FINDINGS. The most characteristic appearance is that of a specific pattern of universal platyspondyly. Abnormalities of the odontoid are also present. In the hip there is often compression of the capital femoral epiphysis with subsequent erosion and disappearance of the femoral neck.

REFERENCES

1. Langer, L. O., Jr., and Carey, L. S.: The Roentgenographic Features of the KS Mucopolysaccharidosis of Morquio (Morquio-Brailsford's Disease). *Am. J. Roentgenol.,* 97:1–20, 1966.
2. McKusick, V. A.: *Heritable Diseases of Connective Tissue.* The C. V. Mosby Company, St. Louis, 1972.
3. Maroteaux, P., Lamy, M., and Foucher, M.: La Maladie de Morquio. Étude Clinique, Radiologique et Biologique. *Presse Med.,* 71:2091–2094, 1963.

MULTIPLE CARTILAGINOUS EXOSTOSES (DIAPHYSEAL ACLASIS, MULTIPLE OSTEOCHONDROMAS, CARTILAGINOUS EXOSTOSES, DEFORMING CHONDROPLASIA)

This bone dysplasia is associated with multiple osteochondromas involving many of the bones. Clinical symptoms are due to pressure of the exostoses or their protrusion through the skin. There may also be pressure on adjacent organs. Inheritance is autosomal dominant.

RADIOLOGIC FINDINGS IN THE HAND. The configuration of the multiple exostoses is similar to that of the isolated ones which are further described in Chapter 15. Generally speaking, the exostoses are much more subtle in the hand than they are in the other bones, and sometimes only their influence on growth may be visualized. They may cause deformity of the growth plate, which may result in curvature (Fig. 13–102) or shortening (Fig. 13–103) of the phalanges or metacarpals. They may appear as bony projections from the bones, generally involving the bones near their ends. The carpals may also occasionally be involved.[3]

OTHER RADIOLOGIC FINDINGS. Exostoses may be seen near the ends of almost any bone. Occasionally they may undergo

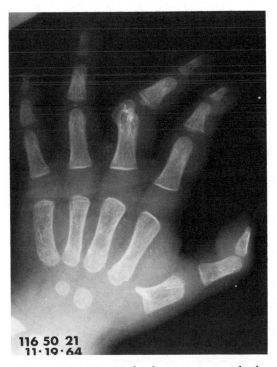

116 50 21
11·19·64

Figure 13–102. Multiple exostoses with clinodactyly. The exostosis in the distal portion of the proximal phalanx of the third finger causes deviation of this digit. There is some shortening of the first metacarpal as well. (From Poznanski, A. K., et al.: *Radiology,* 93:573–582, 1969.)

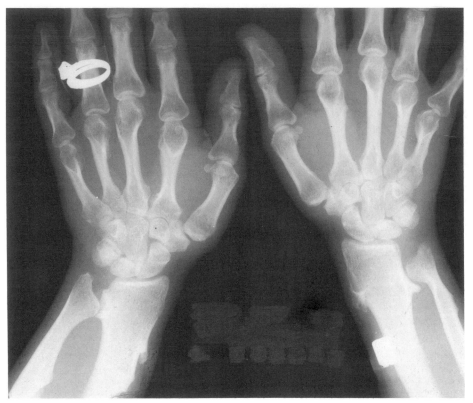

Figure 13–103. Multiple exostoses with bizarre brachydactyly. There is shortening of various bones of the hand. The exostoses are poorly seen except in the radius and ulna.

malignant degeneration. They may sometimes be seen even in the spine, where they can compress the spinal cord.[4] Exostoses may be seen in a number of other conditions, including pseudopseudohyperparathyroidism, as a result of previous irradiation and in myositis ossificans progressiva.

REFERENCES

1. Krooth, R. S., Macklin, M. T., and Hilbish, T. F.: Diaphysial Aclasis (Multiple Exostoses) on Guam. *Am. J. Hum. Genet.,* 13:340–347, 1961.
2. Poznanski, A. K., Pratt, G. B., Manson, G., and Weiss, L.: Clinodactyly, Camptodactyly, Kirner's Deformity, and Other Crooked Fingers. *Radiology,* 93:573–582, 1969.
3. Solomon, ·L.: Hereditary Multiple Exostosis. *J. Bone Joint Surg.,* 45B:292–304, 1963.
4. Vinstein, A. L., and Franken, E. A., Jr.: Hereditary Multiple Exostoses. *Am. J. Roentgenol.,* 112:405–407, 1971.

MULTIPLE FIBROMATOSIS (GENERALIZED HAMARTOMATOSIS, STOUT FIBROMATOSIS)

In this condition, nodules of well-differentiated fibrous tissue are scattered throughout the skeleton, subcutaneous tissues and viscera. In the terminology of Kauffman and Stout,[2] multiple fibromatosis indicates a condition in which the lesions are limited to the subcutaneous tissue, whereas generalized fibromatosis is a widespread condition involving viscera as well as bones. In some individuals the lesions regress spontaneously.

RADIOLOGIC FINDINGS IN THE HAND. The hand is not frequently involved, but when it is, there are small lucent areas within the hand bones (Fig. 13–104) which may expand the shaft.

OTHER RADIOLOGIC FINDINGS. Lucent densities can be seen in a number of bones, including the skull.

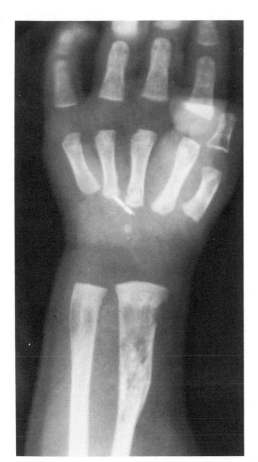

Figure 13–104. Multiple fibromatosis. Well-defined defects are seen in the distal radius and ulna and are similar to those that were seen in the remainder of the skeleton. The hand is minimally involved, with some lucency in the proximal phalanx of the thumb.

REFERENCES

1. Heiple, K. G., Perrin, E., and Aikawa, M.: Congenital Generalized Fibromatosis. A Case Limited to Osseous Lesions. *J. Bone Joint Surg.,* 54A:663–669, 1972.
2. Kauffman, S. L., and Stout, A. P.: Congenital Mesenchymal Tumors. *Cancer,* 18:460–476, 1965.
3. Mackenzie, D. H.: The Fibromatoses: A Clinicopathological Concept. *Br. Med. J.,* 4:277–281, 1972.
4. Morettin, L. B., Mueller, E., and Schreiber, M.: Generalized Hamartomatosis (Congenital Generalized Fibromatosis). *Am. J. Roentgenol.,* 114:722–734, 1972.
5. Schaffzin, E. A., Chung, S. M. K., and Kaye, R.: Congenital Generalized Fibromatosis with Complete Spontaneous Regression. *J. Bone Joint Surg.,* 54A:657–662, 1972.

MYOSITIS OSSIFICANS PROGRESSIVA (FIBRODYSPLASIA OSSIFICANS PROGRESSIVA)

This is a disorder of connective tissue which is characterized by progressive ossification adjacent to striated muscle. The onset is usually in early childhood. The first findings are swelling and pain, mostly around the paravertebral areas, shoulders and arms. Hypoplasia of the great toe and sometimes the thumb is clinically evident from birth, long before the clinical symptoms occur.

RADIOLOGIC FINDINGS IN THE HAND. The thumb is hypoplastic. A review of the literature by Lutwak[2] showed thumb ab-

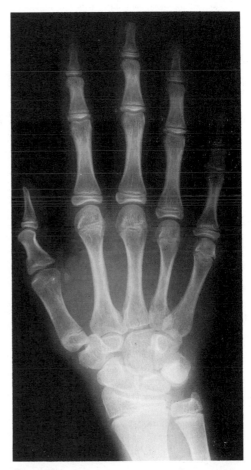

Figure 13–105. Myositis ossificans progressiva. There is a short proximal phalanx of the thumb and there is some shortening of the middle phalanx of the fifth finger. The first metacarpal is relatively unremarkable. More dramatic changes were seen in the feet.

normalities in 87 of 264 cases. The thumb findings are less common than those in the great toe. There is hypoplasia of the proximal phalanx of the thumb (Fig. 13–105). Some cases also show evidence of hypoplasia of the first metacarpal, although no definite shortening was seen in our five cases. A short middle phalanx of the fifth finger is a common finding and was present in all of our cases, as was evident in the pattern profile analysis. Pattern profile analysis also showed some relative shortening of the first proximal phalanx, which may not be visible on clinical inspection. A case of associated myositis ossificans progressiva and fibrous dysplasia was reported by Frame et al. (Fig. 13–106).[1]

OTHER RADIOLOGIC FINDINGS. A short great toe and lateral deviation associated with a hypoplastic proximal phalanx is probably the most classic finding. The areas of ossification in regions of tendons and muscles are seen beginning in the region of the shoulder girdle and the back. Exostoses are common around many of the long bones. Fusion of the cervical spine may be present in some cases.

REFERENCES

1. Frame, B., Azad, N., Reynolds, W. A., and Saeed, S. M.: Polyostotic Fibrous Dysplasia and Myositis Ossificans Progressiva. *Am. J. Dis. Child.*, 124:120–122, 1972.
2. Lutwak, L.: Myositis Ossificans Progressiva. Mineral, Metabolic and Radioactive Calcium Studies of the Effects of Hormones. *Am. J. Med.*, 37:269–293, 1964.
3. Singleton, E. B., and Holt, J. F.: Myositis Ossificans Progressiva. *Radiology*, 62:47–54, 1954.

NEUROFIBROMATOSIS

This is a condition with multiple neurofibromas, café au lait spots and multiple bone lesions. The inheritance pattern is autosomal dominant with high penetrance but with a wide variability in expression.

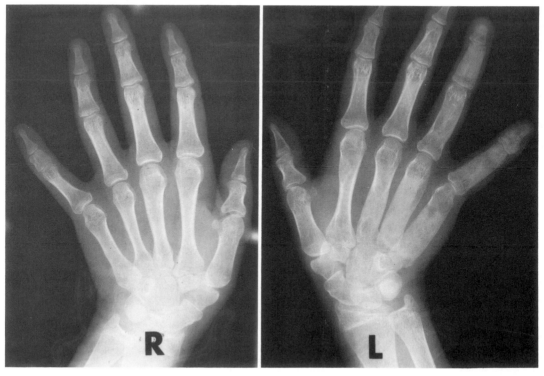

Figure 13–106. Myositis ossificans progressiva associated with fibrous dysplasia. This is a rather unusual combination. The short middle phalanx of the thumb is well seen, as is the short middle phalanx of the fifth finger. However, superimposed on this is marked widening of the metacarpals and phalanges in the left hand (L), which is evidence of polyostotic fibrous dysplasia. (Courtesy Dr. William Reynolds and Dr. B. Frame, Henry Ford Hospital. From *Am. J. Dis. Child.*, 124:120–122, 1972. Copyright 1972, American Medical Association.)

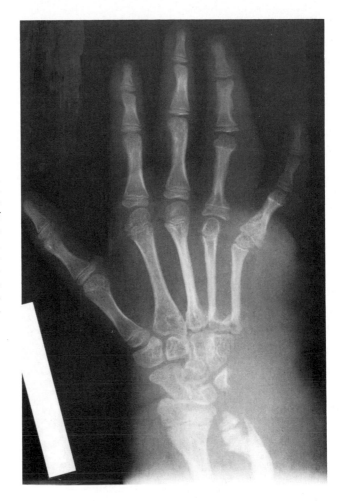

Figure 13-107. Neurofibromatosis. There is hypoplasia of the lateral metacarpals, which are thin and pointed in their proximal portions. There is deformity of the distal ulna and carpus with considerable soft tissue thickening along the lateral aspect of the hand. Unusual cone epiphyses are seen in the fourth and fifth proximal phalanges, and an abnormality of the shaft of the fourth middle phalanx is also noted. There is thickening of the soft tissues about the ring finger.

RADIOLOGIC FINDINGS IN THE HAND. The hand is not commonly involved. A variety of lesions can be seen, including hypoplasia, hyperplasia, thinning of the bones and localized gigantism (Fig. 13–107).

OTHER RADIOLOGIC FINDINGS. Many findings, too numerous to mention, in other bones and in the viscera may also be seen.

REFERENCES

1. Holt, J. F., and Wright, E. M.: The Radiologic Features of Neurofibromatosis. *Radiology,* 51: 647–664, 1948.
2. Meszaros, W. T., Guzzo, F., and Schorsch, H.: Neurofibromatosis. *Am. J. Roentgenol.*, 98:557–569, 1966.
3. Pitt, M. J., Mosher, J. F., and Edeiken, J.: Abnormal Periosteum and Bone in Neurofibromatosis. *Radiology*, 103:143–146, 1972.

NEVOID BASAL CELL CARCINOMA (BASAL CELL NEVUS SYNDROME)

This syndrome of multiple cutaneous nevi that may become multiple basal cell epitheliomas is associated with cysts of the jaw, rib anomalies and, frequently, mental retardation. The facial appearance is characteristic, with a broad nasal root, frontal and temporal bossing and prominent supraorbital ridges. These patients have an increased incidence of medulloblastoma. The condition is transmitted as an autosomal dominant with full penetrance.

RADIOLOGIC FINDINGS IN THE HAND. The most common abnormality is shortening of the fourth metacarpal, or there may be shortening of the third, fourth and fifth metacarpals. The appearance of the hand resembles that seen in pseudohypoparathyroidism, or brachydactyly E. Occasionally other findings are present in the hand, including a short distal phalanx of the

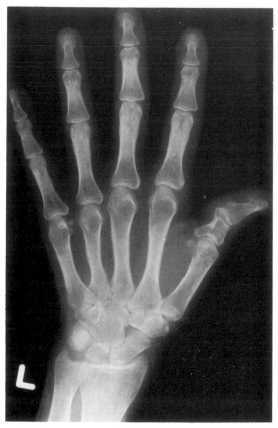

Figure 13–108. Nevoid basal cell carcinoma syndrome. There is shortening of the proximal phalanx of the thumb and minimal shortening of the fourth metacarpal.

thumb,[5] a short proximal phalanx (Fig. 13–108)[4], polydactyly,[2] syndactyly[2] and arachnodactyly.[2]

OTHER RADIOLOGIC FINDINGS. These include spine changes, particularly spina bifida and kyphoscoliosis, and, less commonly, Klippel-Feil deformity and thoracic lack of segmentation. Follicular or dentigerous cysts may be seen, usually in the mandible but occasionally in the maxilla, as can tooth abnormalities. Bifid ribs or synostosis of the ribs is common. Many patients have calcification of the falx cerebri. There may be ectopic calcification, particularly in the region of the pelvis. Hypertelorism is frequently seen. Occasionally polydactyly of the feet may be noted.[3, 4] Calcification of the petroclinoid ligament is common.[2]

REFERENCES

1. Becker, M. H., Kopf, A. W., and Lande, A.: Basal Cell Nevus Syndrome: Its Roentgenologic

Significance. *Am. J. Roentgenol.*, 99:817–825, 1967.
2. Gorlin, R. J., and Sedano, H. O.: The Multiple Nevoid Basal Cell Carcinoma Syndrome Revisited. *Birth Defects, Original Article Series*, 7:140–148, 1971.
3. Gorlin, R. J., Vickers, R. A., Kelln, E., and Williamson, J. J.: The Multiple Basal-Cell Nevi Syndrome. An Analysis of a Syndrome Consisting of Multiple Nevoid Basal-Cell Carcinoma, Jaw Cysts, Skeletal Anomalies, Medulloblastoma, and Hyporesponsiveness to Parathormone. *Cancer*, 18:89–104, 1965.
4. Lausecker, H.: Beitrag zu den Naevo-Epitheliomen. *Arch. Dermat. u. Syph.*, 194:639–662, 1952.
5. Lile, H. A., Rogers, J. F., and Gerald, B.: The Basal Cell Nevus Syndrome. *Am. J. Roentgenol.*, 103:214–217, 1968.
6. McEvoy, B. F., and Gatzek, H.: Multiple Nevoid Basal Cell Carcinoma Syndrome: Radiological Manifestations. *Br. J. Radiol.*, 42:24–28, 1969.

NOONAN SYNDROME (MALE TURNER, TURNER PHENOTYPE)

This is a Turner-like condition with a normal karyotype. As in XO Turner's syndrome, the clinical findings include short stature, web neck, cubitus valgus and prominent ears. There is frequently associated cryptorchidism in males. The condition may be seen in both males and females. There is an increased incidence of cardiovascular anomalies, and pulmonary stenosis is the most common lesion. Many cases are familial although the hereditary pattern is not clear.

RADIOLOGIC FINDINGS IN THE HAND. The hand does not show the short fourth metacarpal and increased carpal angle which are the usual changes of XO Turner's syndrome. The main radiologic finding in the hand is clinodactyly of the fifth finger, which occurred in seven of eight cases studied by Nora and Sinha.[3] Char et al.[1] found widening of the proximal ends of the middle phalanges in 70 per cent of cases and also described modeling errors in the metacarpals. Pattern profile analysis of this condition does not reveal a characteristic pattern. It certainly does not look like that of Turner syndrome, although relatively few cases have been studied so far. The bone age is somewhat retarded.

OTHER RADIOLOGIC FINDINGS. The most typical other finding is pectus carinatum, usually with shortening of the sternum. There is also flattening of the distal femoral and tibial epiphyses. There is an increased incidence of Klippel-Feil anomaly and scoliosis. A number of other miscellaneous abnormalities have also been reported.[1]

REFERENCES

1. Char, F., Rodriquez-Fernandez, H. L., Scott, C. I., Borgaonkar, D. S., Bell, B. B., and Rowe, R. D.: The Noonan Syndrome—A Clinical Study of Forty-Five Cases. *Birth Defects, Original Article Series,* 8:110–118, 1972.
2. Noonan, J. A.: Hypertelorism with Turner Phenotype. A New Syndrome with Associated Congenital Heart Disease. *Am. J. Dis. Child.,* 116:373–380, 1968.
3. Nora, J. J., and Sinha, A. K.: Direct Familial Transmission of the Turner Phenotype. *Am. J. Dis. Child.,* 116:343–350, 1968.
4. Riggs, W., Jr.: Roentgen Findings in Noonan's Syndrome. *Radiology,* 96:393–395, 1970.

OCULO-CEREBRO-RENAL SYNDROME (LOWE SYNDROME)

This condition is characterized by growth retardation, mental deficiency, hypotonia, bilateral congenital cataracts, glaucoma and a renal tubular dysfunction. Biochemical abnormalities include metabolic acidosis and a generalized hyperaminoaciduria.

RADIOLOGIC FINDINGS. These include evidence of both osteoporosis and rickets.

The rickets is relatively sensitive to vitamin D, responding to doses of about 1500 international units.

REFERENCES

1. Abbassi, V., Lowe, C. U., and Calcagno, P. L.: Oculo-Cerebro-Renal Syndrome. A Review. *Am. J. Dis. Child.,* 115:145–168, 1968.
2. Lowe, C. U., Terrey, M., and MacLachlan, E. A.: Organic-Aciduria, Decreased Renal Ammonia Production, Hydrophthalmos, and Mental Retardation. *Am. J. Dis. Child.,* 83:164–184, 1952.

OCULO-DENTO-OSSEOUS DYSPLASIA (OCULO-DENTO-DIGITAL SYNDROME)

This syndrome includes ocular anomalies, such as hypotelorism, microphthalmia and iridic changes; a characteristic facial appearance with slenderness of the nose; severe hypoplasia of the enamel of all of the teeth; and multiple digital abnormalities. Dominant inheritance has been demonstrated in this condition.[3, 5]

RADIOLOGIC FINDINGS IN THE HAND. The most common radiologic findings are camptodactyly and clinodactyly of the fifth finger (Figs. 13–109 and 13–110). Syndac-

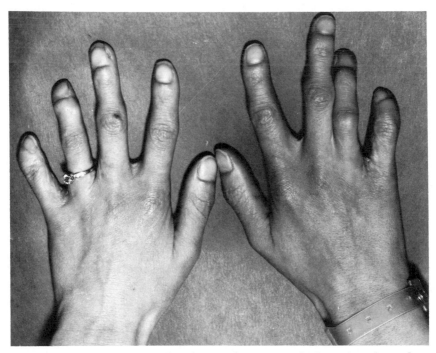

Figure 13–109. Oculo-dento-osseous dysplasia. There is marked syndactyly and camptodactyly together with abbreviation of some of the digits. (Courtesy of Dr. H. S. Sugar, Detroit, Michigan; and Dr. H. Falls, Ann Arbor, Michigan.)

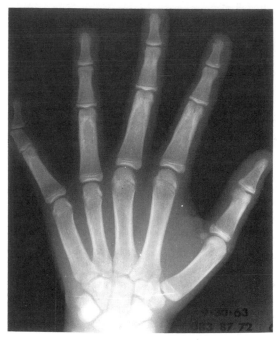

Figure 13–110. Oculo-dento-osseous dysplasia. The patient has only clinodactyly of the fifth finger. (From Poznanski, A. K., et al.: *Radiology*, 93:573–582, 1969.)

tyly between the fourth and fifth fingers is also common. There may be tapering of the digits. Some cases have shown evidence of osteoporosis.

OTHER RADIOLOGIC FINDINGS. The mandible appears quite broad. This is most visible in the submental-vertical view. Foot changes resemble those of the hand. The teeth may show evidence of amelogenesis imperfecta.[3]

REFERENCES

1. Gorlin, R. J., Meskin, L. H., and St. Geme, J. W.: Oculodentodigital dysplasia. *J. Pediat.*, 63: 69–75, 1963.
2. Kurlander, G. J., Lavy, N. W., and Campbell, J. A.: Roentgen Differentiation of the Oculodentodigital Syndrome and the Hallermann-Streiff Syndrome in Infancy. *Radiology*, 86:77–85, 1966.
3. Rajic, D. S., and de Veber, L. L.: Hereditary Oculodentoosseous Dysplasia. *Ann. Radiol.*, 9:224–231, 1965.
4. Reisner, S. H., Kott, E., Bornstein, B., Salinger, H., Kaplan, I., and Gorlin, R. J.: Oculodentodigital Dysplasia. *Am. J. Dis. Child.*, 118:600–607, 1969.

5. Taysi, K., Say, B., Tanju, F., and Gürsu, G.: Oculodentodigital Dysplasia Syndrome. Case Report. *Acta Paediatr. Scand.*, 60:235–238, 1971.

ORO-DIGITO-FACIAL SYNDROME, TYPE I (PAPILLON-LÉAGE AND PSAUME SYNDROME, ORO-FACIO-DIGITAL SYNDROME, OFD I)

This syndrome is characterized by an abnormal frenulum, a cleft tongue and palate, a median cleft of the upper lip, hypoplasia of the ala nasi, digital anomalies and mental retardation. The syndrome is almost never manifested in males. The mode of inheritance is X-linked dominant. The form seen in males is that of the Mohr syndrome (oro-facio-digital syndrome II).[4]

RADIOLOGIC FINDINGS IN THE HAND. The main findings are those of a generalized brachydactyly, mild syndactyly and occasionally polydactyly. There is usually irregular demineralization of the phalanges, giving the digits a mottled appearance. Clinodactyly is common in this condition.

OTHER RADIOLOGIC FINDINGS. The skull has a steep anterior fossa. There is elevation of the cribriform plate and the lesser sphenoid wings. The floor of the posterior fossa also slopes. Clefts may be seen in the alveolar ridge. Polydactyly of the toes is seen in the Mohr form but not in the Papillon-Léage and Psaume type.

REFERENCES

1. Doege, T. C., Thuline, H. C., Priest, J. H., Norby, D. E., and Bryant, J. S.: Studies of a Family with the Oral-Facial-Digital Syndrome. *N. Engl. J. Med.*, 271:1073–1080, 1964.
2. Gorlin, R. J., and Psaume, J.: Orodigitofacial Dysostosis—A New Syndrome. *J. Pediatr.*, 61:520–530, 1962.
3. Papillon-Leage, and Psaume, J.: Une Malformation Héréditaire de la Muqueuse Buccale Brides et Freins Anormaux. *Rev. Stomatol. Chir. Maxillofac.*, 55:209–227, 1954.
4. Rimoin, D. L., and Edgerton, M. T.: Genetic and Clinical Heterogeneity in the Oral-Facial-Digital Syndromes. *J. Pediatr.*, 71:94–102, 1967.

ORO-DIGITO-FACIAL SYNDROME, TYPE II (MOHR SYNDROME, ORO-FACIO-DIGITAL II, OFD II)

This is a condition similar to the oro-digito-facial I syndrome or Papillon-Léage and Psaume syndrome in that it includes a lobate tongue with nodularity, midline cleft lip, broad nasal root and dystopia canthorum, as well as hand abnormalities. It differs from type I in that it may be associated with a hearing defect and polysyndactyly of the toes. The nose in the Mohr form is broad and may have a dimple within it, while in type I alar hypoplasia may be seen. The inheritance of the Mohr type is autosomal recessive and may be seen in males or females (type I is sex-linked).

RADIOLOGIC FINDINGS IN THE HAND. Brachydactyly is common and may affect any of the phalanges. Polydactyly may also be seen in the hand. It is sometimes post-axial.[1] One of Rimoin and Edgerton's cases[2] had some bizarre areas of increased density in the tubular bones of the hand. Syndactyly may be seen.

OTHER RADIOLOGIC FINDINGS. Preaxial polydactyly of the great toes is probably the most important finding in differentiating it from the other form. The great toe may be short with an abnormal first metatarsal.

REFERENCES

1. Gustavson, K.-H., Kreuger, A., and Petersson, P. O.: Syndrome Characterized by Lingual Malformation, Polydactyly, Tachypnea, and Psychomotor Retardation (Mohr Syndrome). *Clin. Genet.*, 2:261–266, 1971.
2. Rimoin, D. L., and Edgerton, M. T.: Genetic and Clinical Heterogeneity in the Oral Facial Digital Syndromes. *J. Pediatr.*, 71:94–102, 1967.

OSTEOECTASIA WITH HYPERPHOSPHATASIA

This rare abnormality of bone is associated with a gross elevation of serum alkaline and acid phosphatase. There is also a massive urinary excretion of hydroxyproline and proline-containing peptides. The patients are dwarfed, have a large head, a saddle nose and an early loss of deciduous teeth. Histologically there is a rapid turnover of bone in these patients. The disorder is probably inherited as an autosomal recessive.

RADIOLOGIC FINDINGS IN THE HAND. There appear to be significant differences between the few patients that have been reported (Figs. 13–111 to 13–114). Generally speaking, there is cortical thickening and

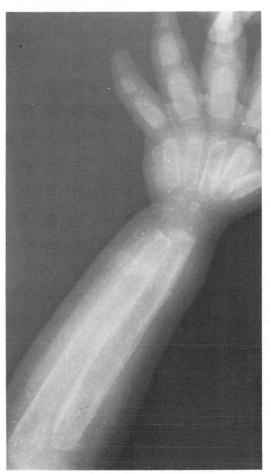

Figure 13–111. Osteoectasia with hyperphosphatasia. There is widening of the radius and ulna and of the various phalanges, particularly the proximals. The metacarpals are less involved. (Courtesy Dr. H. Rosenbaum, Lexington, Kentucky.)

widening of some of the hand bones (Fig. 13–111). This affects the proximal phalanges more than the metacarpals. In some members of a family, however, there may be the appearance of demineralized bone, particularly in the metacarpals (Fig. 13–112). The intercarpal joints may be narrowed.

OTHER RADIOLOGIC FINDINGS. Coarsening of the medullary trabecular pattern, generalized widening of bones and local areas of widening in bones may be seen throughout the skeleton (Fig. 13–113). The cortical thickening appears spotty. The condition somewhat resembles Paget's disease and has been considered to be a juvenile form of this entity. A case has also been reported in association with pseudoxanthoma elasticum.

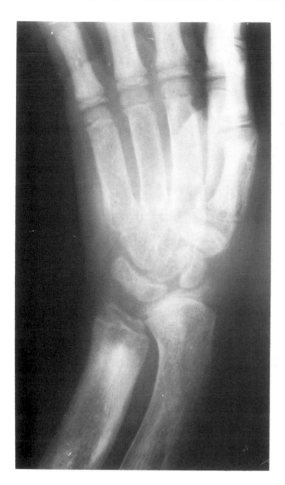

Figure 13–112. Osteoectasia with hyperphosphatasia. Nine year old male. There is thickening of the proximal phalanges with an irregular configuration. The metacarpals are less affected. There is marked involvement of the radius and ulna. (Courtesy Dr. Walter Berdon, New York, New York.)

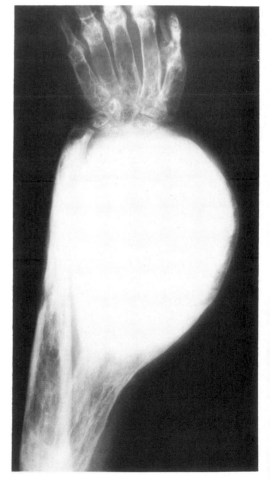

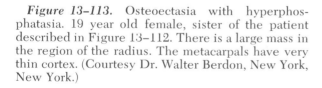

Figure 13–113. Osteoectasia with hyperphosphatasia. 19 year old female, sister of the patient described in Figure 13–112. There is a large mass in the region of the radius. The metacarpals have very thin cortex. (Courtesy Dr. Walter Berdon, New York, New York.)

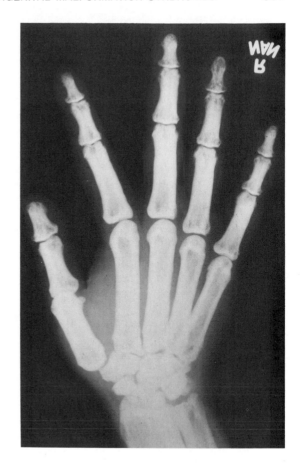

Figure 13–114. Osteoectasia with hyperphosphatasia. Generalized cortical thickening is seen in all the bones. This manifestation is somewhat different from those in other cases illustrated. (Courtesy Dr. William McAlister, St. Louis, Missouri.)

REFERENCES

1. Caffey, J.: Familial Hyperphosphatasemia with Ateliosis and Hypermetabolism of Growing Membranous Bone; Review of the Clinical, Radiographic and Chemical Features. *Bull. Hosp. Joint Dis.*, 33:81–110, 1972.
2. Choremis, C., Yannakos, D., Papadatos, C., and Baroutsou, E.: Osteitis deformans (Paget's Disease) in an 11 Year Old Boy. *Helv. Paediatr. Acta*, 13:185–188, 1958.
3. Eyring, E. J., and Eisenberg, E.: Congenital Hyperphosphatasia. A Clinical, Pathological, and Biochemical Study of Two Cases. *J. Bone Joint Surg.*, 50A:1099–1117, 1968.
4. Mitsudo, S. M.: Chronic Idiopathic Hyperphosphatasia Associated with Pseudoxanthoma Elasticum. *J. Bone Joint Surg.*, 53A:303–314, 1971.
5. Swoboda, W.: Hyperostosis corticalis deformans juvenilis. Ungewöhnliche generalisierte Osteopathie bei zwei Geschwistern. *Helv. Paediatr. Acta*, 13:292–312, 1958.
6. Thompson, R. C., Jr., Gaull, G. E., Horwitz, S. J., and Schenk, R. K.: Hereditary Hyperphosphatasia. Studies of Three Siblings. *Am. J. Med.*, 47:209–219, 1969.

OSTEOGENESIS IMPERFECTA (CONGENITA FORM – VROLIK DISEASE, FRAGILITAS OSSIUM, OSTEOPSATHYROSIS; TARDA FORM – LOBSTEIN DISEASE)

This is a somewhat heterogeneous group of conditions. The congenital form is very severe. The infants have multiple fractures at birth which may be associated with shortening of the limbs, thus mimicking achondroplasia. The skull is soft. In the tarda form the only clinical finding may be the blue sclera. Fractures may occasionally be seen. In the severe cases of the tarda form there may be bowing of the bones and scoliosis. The skin is often translucent. Deafness may occur and there may be some tooth abnormality. The condition is due to a disorder of collagen. The more common tarda form is inherited as an autosomal dominant, while the congenital form is

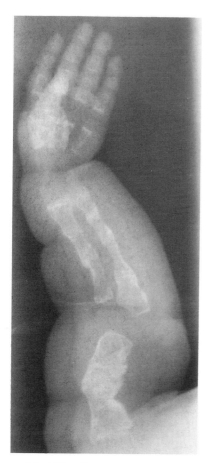

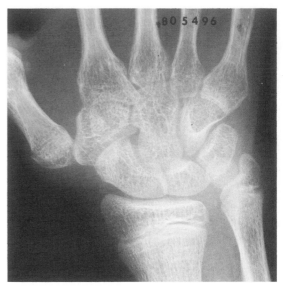

Figure 13–116. Osteogenesis imperfecta. There is coarsening of the osseous trabecular pattern in the bones of the hand. No other abnormality is seen.

Figure 13–115. Osteogenesis imperfecta. Congenita form. Multiple fractures of the forearm are seen with telescoping of the bones, but the hand is relatively spared. Only slight demineralization is seen within the hand.

more commonly associated with recessive inheritance.[3, 4]

RADIOLOGIC FINDINGS IN THE HAND. The appearance of the hand is usually not diagnostic. In the severe juvenile form there may be some bone demineralization, but even when multiple fractures are seen in other bones, the hand bones are usually spared (Fig. 13–115). There may be various manifestations of poor bone formation, including a coarsened trabecular pattern (Fig. 13–116) or slender bones (Fig. 13–117), although in most cases the bones are not as slender in the hand as they are in the remainder of the skeleton. Fractures of the hand may occasionally be seen (Fig. 13–

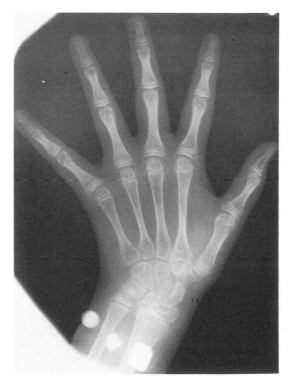

Figure 13–117. Osteogenesis imperfecta. There is thinning of the hand bones, particularly of the metacarpals. This degree of thinning is unusual in most cases of osteogenesis imperfecta, since the hand is rarely involved in this severely.

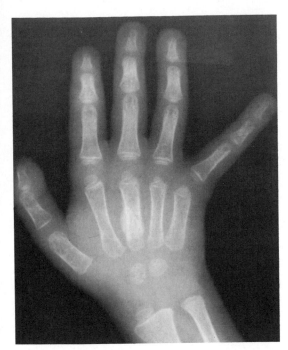

Figure 13–118. Osteogenesis imperfecta with a fracture of third metacarpal. There is good callus formation, which is common in osteogenesis imperfecta. The cortex of the metacarpals appears somewhat thin, but otherwise the bones are unremarkable.

118), but they are uncommon. The fractures heal with good callus formation.

OTHER RADIOLOGIC FINDINGS. In the tarda form very slender bones are often seen, particularly in the lower extremities. Also, there may be platyspondyly, multiple wormian bones in the skull and very poor mineralization in the acute stage. In the congenital form multiple fractures may be noted, with telescoping of the long bones.

REFERENCES

1. Caffey, J.: *Pediatric X-Ray Diagnosis*, 6th Ed. Year Book Medical Publishers, Chicago, 1972, Vol. 2.
2. King, J. D., and Bobechko, W. P.: Osteogenesis Imperfecta. An Orthopaedic Description and Surgical Review. *J. Bone Joint Surg.*, 53B:72–89, 1971.
3. McKusick, V. A.: *Heritable Disorders of Connective Tissue.* The C. V. Mosby Company, St. Louis, 1972.
4. Spranger, J. W., Langer, L., and Wiedemann, H.-R.: *Bone Dysplasias: An Atlas of Constitutional Disorders of Skeletal Development.* W. B. Saunders Company, Philadelphia, 1974.

OSTEO-ONYCHO-DYSOSTOSIS (NAIL-PATELLA SYNDROME, ONYCHO-OSTEO-ARTHRO-DYSPLASIA)

This is a syndrome of patellar absence, hypoplasia of the nails and various other abnormalities. Bony spurs in the posterior portion of the ilium are common, as are elbow abnormalities and other knee abnormalities. Renal signs, particularly proteinuria with or without hematuria, and renal insufficiency, are seen in a significant percentage of the cases and are due to an associated nephropathy.

RADIOLOGIC FINDINGS IN THE HAND. The most common radiologic finding is clinodactyly of the fifth finger, with a short middle phalanx. This is seen more commonly than is represented in the literature.[2] Contrary to many conditions with hypoplastic nails, the distal phalanges are often normal in this entity, as evidenced by pattern profile analysis. A number of other anomalies of the hand have been described, including shortening of the third to fifth metacarpals, but none of these findings appears to be consistent.

OTHER RADIOLOGIC FINDINGS. Absence of the patella and iliac spurs are the common radiographic findings. There are also abnormalities around the elbow, with a hypoplastic head of the radius and capitellum. Clubfoot deformity may sometimes be seen.

REFERENCES

1. de Beaumont, F.: L'Onycho-Ostéodysplasie. *J. Genet. Hum.*, 14:93–131, 1965.
2. Cowell, H. R.: Hereditary Onycho-osteodysplasia. Report of a Kindred with Dysplasia of the Fifth Finger. *Clin. Orthop.*, 76:43–53, 1971.
3. Fauré, C., and Petrel, P.: L'Ostéo-Onycho-Dysplasie Héréditaire. *Ann. Radiol.*, 11:376–388, 1967.
4. McCluskey, K. A.: The Nail-Patella Syndrome: (Hereditary Onycho-Mesodysplasia). *Can. J. Surg.*, 4:192–204, 1961.
5. Mino, R. A., Mino, V. H., and Livingstone, R. G.: Osseous Dysplasia and Dystrophy of the Nails. A Review of the Literature and Report of a Case. *Am. J. Roentgenol.*, 60:633–641, 1948.
6. Preger, L., Miller, E. H., Winfield, J. S., and Choy, S. H.: Hereditary Onycho-Osteo-Arthrodysplasia. *Am. J. Roentgenol.*, 100:546–549, 1967.

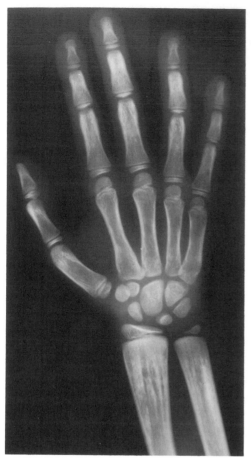

Figure 13–119. Osteopathia striata. Linear streaks of density are seen in the radius and ulna. Attempts at this streaking are seen in some of the metacarpals, particularly the first. The changes are much milder in the hand than they are in the radius.

OSTEOPATHIA STRIATA

This is a rare form of bone dysplasia associated with longitudinal sclerotic streaks in the long bones. McKusick reported a case in association with cataracts and deafness.

RADIOLOGIC FINDINGS IN THE HAND. The streaks are rarely seen in the hand and only a suggestion may be noted (Fig. 13–119).

OTHER RADIOLOGIC FINDINGS. Similar striations may be seen in other bones of the body.

REFERENCES

1. Fairbank, H. A. T.: Osteopathia Striata. *J. Bone Joint Surg.*, 32B:117–125, 1950.

2. McKusick, V. A.: *Heritable Disorders of Connective Tissue.* The C. V. Mosby Company, St. Louis, 1972.

OSTEOPETROSIS (ALBERS-SCHÖNBERG DISEASE, MARBLE BONE DISEASE)

This disease is associated with the persistence of calcified cartilage. Bone resorption and formation are slowed in certain areas.[1] There may be encroachment upon the marrow spaces, which may result in anemia. Enlargement of the bone can cause encroachment upon various cranial nerves, particularly the optic, causing optic atrophy. The bone becomes brittle and susceptible to fracture. The spectrum of clinical manifestations is wide, ranging from the "malignant" form, which manifests itself in infancy with hepatosplenomegaly anemia and early death from infection, to a "benign" form

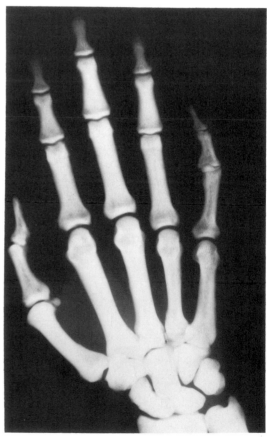

Figure 13–120. Osteopetrosis. The bones are dense and sclerotic. There is a decrease in size of the medullary cavity. Modeling of the bones is unremarkable.

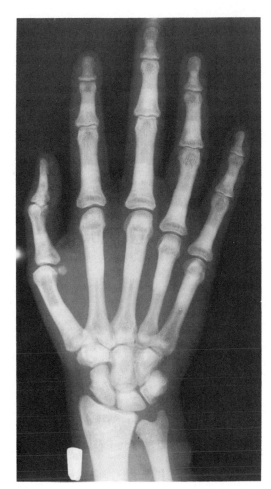

Figure 13-121. Osteopetrosis. Adult. Bands of increased and decreased density are seen within the hand bones. There is some encroachment upon the medullary canal of all of the metacarpals. This is the case studied histologically by Frost, et al.: *Clin. Orthop.*, 65:203–217, 1969.

which is diagnosed accidentally during radiography for some other disorder. The malignant form is usually inherited as an autosomal recessive, while the more benign forms of the disease usually have an autosomal dominant inheritance.

RADIOLOGIC FINDINGS IN THE HAND. There is somewhat less involvement of the hand than of some of the other bones. However, manifestations in the hand are similar to those elsewhere. There are several patterns of involvement which may represent different forms of the disease. There may be dense sclerosis of the bones with lack of normal trabecular structure in some cases (Fig. 13-120). The sclerosis may be evenly distributed throughout the bones (Fig.

13-120) or there may be linear bands of sclerosis and lucency (Fig. 13-121). These bands may give the bones, particularly the carpals, a bone-in-bone appearance (Fig. 13-122). Some bones that appear uniformly dense on conventional radiographs may show considerable internal structure when overexposed films are obtained.[2] These areas of radiolucency are not as pronounced as in dysosteosclerosis. Failure of modeling is more apparent in the long bones than in the hand bones, but may be seen in juvenile cases (Fig. 13-123). Moss and Mainzer[4] reported some cases of terminal tuft erosion in this condition; however, this is an uncommon finding. In most cases the presence of tuft erosion suggests pycnodysostosis rather than osteopetrosis.

OTHER RADIOLOGIC FINDINGS. Dense bone and failure of modeling are seen elsewhere in the skeleton, and the bones are prone to fracture. The lack of platyspondyly

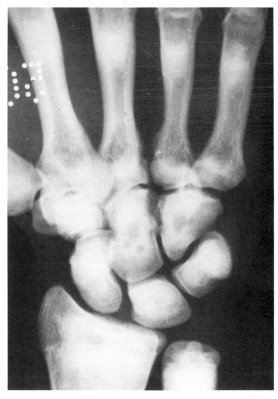

Figure 13-122. Osteopetrosis. Bone-in-bone appearance is seen, owing to areas of sclerosis and lucency. There is some failure of modeling in the metacarpals, and the medullary canal is thinned.

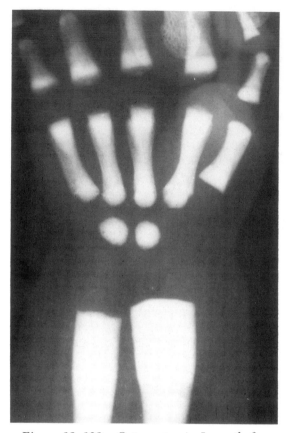

Figure 13–123. Osteopetrosis. Juvenile form. Although there is marked modeling abnormality in the distal radius and ulna, the changes are relatively mild in the bones of the hand. There is increased bone density, with triangular areas of increased density at the ends of the hand bones.

is helpful in differentiating osteopetrosis from dysosteosclerosis.

REFERENCES

1. Frost, H. M., Villanueva, A. R., Jett, S., and Eyring, E.: Tetracycline-based Analysis of Bone Remodelling in Osteopetrosis. *Clin. Orthop.*, 65: 203–217, 1969.
2. Graham, C. B., Rudhe, U., and Eklöf, O.: Osteopetrosis. *Progr. Pediatr. Radiol.* 4:375–402, 1973. (*Intrinsic Diseases of Bones*, edited by H. J. Kaufmann, Karger, Basel.)
3. Johnston, C. C., Jr., Lavy, N., Lord, T., Vellios, F., Merritt, A. D., and Deiss, W. P., Jr.: Osteopetrosis. A Clinical, Genetic, Metabolic, and Morphologic Study of the Dominantly Inherited, Benign Form. *Medicine*, 47:149–167, 1968.
4. Moss, A. A., and Mainzer, F.: Osteopetrosis: An Unusual Cause of Terminal-Tuft Erosion. *Radiology*, 97:631–632, 1970.
5. Yu, J. S., Oates, R. K., Walsh, K. H., and Stuckey, S. J.: Osteopetrosis. *Arch. Dis. Child.*, 46:257–263, 1971.
6. Zetterström, R.: Osteopetrosis (Marble Bone Disease) Clinical and Pathological Review. *Mod. Probl. Pädiatr.*, 3:488–508, 1957.

OTO-PALATO-DIGITAL SYNDROME (OPD SYNDROME, TAYBI SYNDROME)

The term oto-palato-digital syndrome was coined by Dudding, Gorlin and Langer[1] because their patients had deafness, cleft palate and digital anomalies. However, not all of these findings are present in affected individuals. Although initially it was felt that only males were affected, Gall et al.[2] demonstrated that the condition is manifested in females but with much less severe changes than in the males.

The facial configuration in this condition is typical, including a prominent supraorbital ridge, a broad nasal bridge with an appearance suggesting hypertelorism, a flat face and a somewhat antimongoloid slant of the palpebral fissures. Most males have a midline cleft palate, while most females do not have this finding. Deafness is present in some cases but, at least clinically, is not significant. In many other patients deafness may be related to ear infections.

The mode of inheritance is still in doubt. It appears that the inheritance is compatible either with X-linkage with intermediate expression in female heterozygotes, or with autosomal dominant inheritance with sex differences in expression.[4]

RADIOLOGIC FINDINGS IN THE HAND. The roentgen appearance of the hand is fairly characteristic in this condition. The thumbs are small with a broad, short distal phalanx which in boys is associated with a cone-shaped epiphysis (Fig. 13–125). The pseudoepiphysis in the proximal portion of the second metacarpal is prominent in children and in adults remains as a pointed proximal end of this bone. Failure of modeling is evident in most of the bones of the hands but particularly in the metacarpals.

The configuration of the carpals also may be typical of the syndrome, with a transverse capitate, an angulated comma-shaped trapezoid and a double ossification center of the lunate (Fig. 13–126). Accessory ossicles may also be seen. These findings, how-

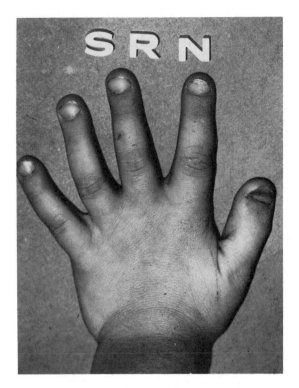

Figure 13-124. Oto-palato-digital syndrome. Typical hand of a patient with this disease. Note the thick fingers and thumb.

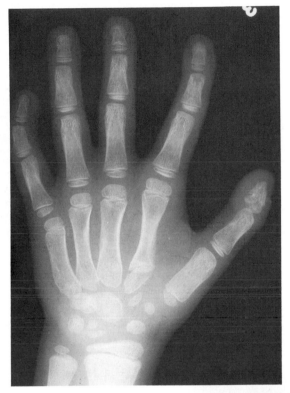

Figure 13-125. Oto-palato-digital syndrome. Typical affected male. The fingers appear somewhat broad. There is some failure of modeling of some of the metacarpals. The thumb appears broad with a prominent cone epiphysis in the distal phalanx. There is a bizarre pseudoepiphysis of the second metacarpal, which is characteristic of this condition. This is associated with an abnormally shaped trapezoid. There is a double ossification center of the lunate, and the capitate appears transverse in position. There is a clinodactyly of the fifth finger. (From Poznanski, A. K., et al.: *Birth Defects, Original Article Series,* in press.)

Figure 13-126. Oto-palato-digital syndrome. Young male. Note the typical transverse capitate and the accessory carpal in the distal row near the hamate. There is also an abnormally shaped trapezoid and a double ossification center of the lunate.

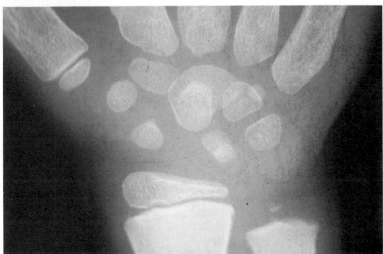

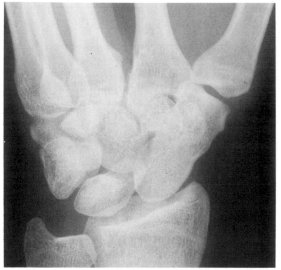

Figure 13–127. Oto-palato-digital syndrome. Adult female. There is trapezium-scaphoid fusion, which is more common in females than in males.

ever, are seen mainly in young males. In adults, trapezium-scaphoid fusion may be noted (Fig. 13–127) and the position of the capitate has a more normal configuration. Additional carpals in the middle or distal row are common during childhood. The mean carpal angle is increased.

Pattern profile analysis shows characteristic alteration in length of the hand bones (Fig. 13–128), and the pattern may

sometimes be similar to that seen in Larsen syndrome. The pattern is more consistent in males than in females.

OTHER RADIOLOGIC FINDINGS. The foot changes are quite striking, with short great toes involving both phalanges, and with multiple tarsal fusions particularly affecting the distal tarsals and the metatarsals. Abnormalities of the fifth metatarsal are common. Changes are also seen in the skull, with prominence of the frontal and occipital areas. Sinusitis and sinus hypoplasia are common, and mastoid disease may be noted. The iliac wings are small and there is flattening of the acetabular angle. Anomalies of the spine may also be noted.

REFERENCES

1. Dudding, B. A., Gorlin, R. J., and Langer, L. O.: The Oto-Palato-Digital Syndrome. A New Symptom-Complex Consisting of Deafness, Dwarfism, Cleft Palate, Characteristic Facies, and a Generalized Bone Dysplasia. *Am. J. Dis. Child.,* 113:214–221, 1967.
2. Gall, J. C., Jr., Stern, A. M., Poznanski, A. K., Garn, S. M., Weinstein, E. D., and Hayward, J. R.: Oto-Palato-Digital Syndrome: Comparison of Clinical and Radiographic Manifestations in Males and Females. *Am. J. Hum. Genet.,* 24: 24–36, 1972.
3. Langer, L. O., Jr.: The Roentgenographic Features of the Oto-Palato-Digital (OPD) Syndrome. *Am. J. Roentgenol.,* 100:63–70, 1967.
4. Poznanski, A. K., Macpherson, R. I., Gorlin, R. J., Garn, S. M., Nagy, J. M., Gall, J. C., Jr., Stern, A. M., and Dijkman, D. J.: The Hand in the

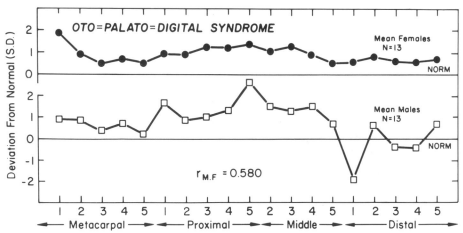

Figure 13–128. Oto-palato-digital syndrome. Pattern profile. There is a significant difference in pattern between males and females. Generally speaking, the females are much more mildly involved. The characteristics of the pattern are a short distal phalanx of the thumb and a relatively long proximal fifth phalanx. The distal phalanges are generally shorter than the other bones.

Oto-Palato-Digital Syndrome. *Ann. Radiol.*, 16:203–209, 1973.
5. Taybi, H.: Generalized Skeletal Dysplasia with Multiple Anomalies. A Note on Pyle's Disease. *Am. J. Roentgenol.*, 88:450–457, 1962.

PACHYDERMOPERIOSTOSIS (IDIOPATHIC HYPERTROPHIC OSTEOARTHROPATHY, FAMILIAL IDIOPATHIC OSTEOARTHROPATHY)

This is a syndrome of unknown cause which is associated with clubbing of the digits; periosteal new bone formation, particularly over the distal ends of the long bones; coarsening of the facial features; and furrowing of the scalp, known as cutis verticis gyrata. The condition is inherited as an autosomal dominant with marked variability in expression.[5]

The syndrome may be incomplete, in that thickening of the skin or pachyderma is missing.[1]

RADIOLOGIC FINDINGS IN THE HAND. Soft tissue clubbing may be seen. There is thickening of the bones of the hand (Fig. 13–129). Occasional periosteal elevation may be seen. The terminal phalanges sometimes show atrophic changes. Arteriography reveals sluggish arterial flow with marked vascular stasis and tortuosity of the vessels to the hand. Joint narrowing may be evident.

OTHER RADIOLOGIC FINDINGS. Periosteal changes are seen in other bones, including the feet. The manifestations of the disease are identical to those seen in hypertrophic osteoarthropathy. In the milder forms, such as the one described by Harbison and Nice,[4] the disease may be confused with acromegaly. A case of pachydermoperiostosis with Marfanoid features has also been reported.[2]

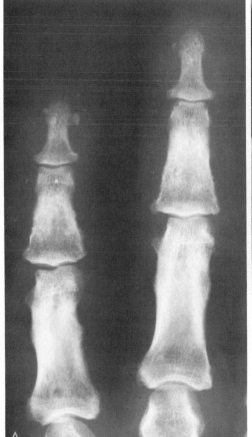
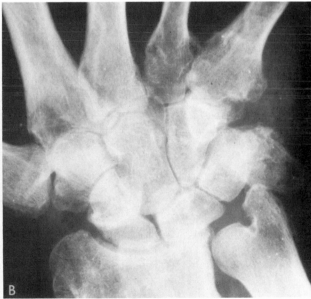

Figure 13–129. Pachydermoperiostosis. *A*, There is thickening of the bones of the fingers with irregularity of the cortical margins. The proximal and middle phalanges are most involved. This patient had the characteristic furrows in his forehead and the typical osseous changes in other bones as well.

B, Carpal abnormalities are seen. The pisiform is particularly irregular in contour. The distal radius and ulna also appear thickened.

REFERENCES

1. Currarino, G., Tierney, R. C., Giesel, R. G., and Weihl, C.: Familial Idiopathic Osteoarthropathy. *Am. J. Roentgenol.*, 85:633–644, 1961.
2. De Deuxchaisnes, C. N., Huaux, J. P., Vandooren-Deflorenne, R., and Lachapelle, J. M.: Pachydermoperiostose, Cryptorchidie et Aspect Marfanoide. *Arch. Belg. Dermatol. Syphiligr.*, 23: 121–135, 1967.
3. Gougeon, J., and Labram, C.: Hippocratisme Digital Idiopathique Avec Periostose Engainante Respectant Les Extrémités: Forme Incomplete de Pachydermo-Périostose. *Rev. Rhum. Mal. Osteoartic.*, 36:333–338, 1969.
4. Harbison, J. B., and Nice, C. M.: Familial Pachydermoperiostosis Presenting as an Acromegaly-Like Syndrome. *Am. J. Roentgenol.*, 112:532–536, 1971.
5. Rimoin, D. L.: Pachydermoperiostosis (Idiopathic Clubbing and Periostosis). Genetic and Physiologic Considerations. *N. Engl. J. Med.*, 272: 923–931, 1965.
6. Touraine, A., Solente, G., and Golé, L.: Un Syndrome Ostéodermopathique: La Pachydermie Plicaturée avec Pachypériostose des Extrémités. *Presse Med.*, 43:1820–1824, 1935.

PANCYTOPENIA-DYSMELIA SYNDROME (FANCONI ANEMIA)

This congenital anemia with pancytopenia is associated with pigmentation of the skin and multiple congenital abnormalities. Symptoms develop at about 5 to 10 years of age and include bleeding and recurrent infection. The marrow is hypoplastic. Most of the patients are of small stature and have hypoplastic genitalia; cryptorchidism is common. The condition is transmitted as an autosomal recessive and is more common in males than in females.

RADIOLOGIC FINDINGS IN THE HAND. The most characteristic changes are those in the thumb. These were seen in 34 of

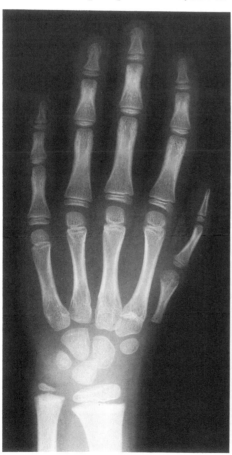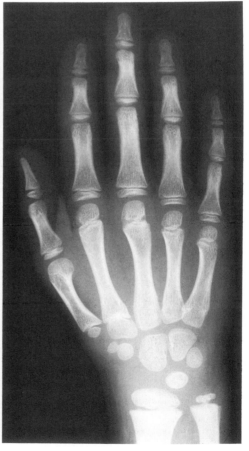

Figure 13–130. Pancytopenia-dysmelia syndrome (Fanconi anemia). There is asymmetry in the appearance of the thumb bilaterally. The left hand is more severely involved, with absence of the normal epiphysis of the first metacarpal and a pseudoepiphysis along its distal end. There is hypoplasia of the radial row of carpals, particularly the scaphoid. (From Poznanski, A. K., et al.: *Radiology*, 100:115, 1971.)

44 cases reviewed by Minagi and Steinbach.[2] Hypoplasia of the phalanges of the thumb (Fig. 13–130) was seen in 12 of their cases, while absent thumbs occurred in 15. Supernumerary thumbs are occasionally seen (Fig. 13–131). Generally speaking, the first metacarpal is more slender than usual, but its length is variable. The metacarpal 2 to metacarpal 1 ratio, both in our cases and in those of the literature, varied from a marked increase to more than two standard deviations below normal.[3] With hypoplasia of the metacarpal, the usual proximal epiphysis is often absent and only a distal pseudoepiphysis is seen. The distal phalanx of the thumb is short in most cases, even though the metacarpal may be normal. Frequently the changes in the hand are asymmetrical. Associated with the thumb hypoplasia there is often hypoplasia of the scaphoid, particularly in the developing child; however, the scaphoid may become normal in older life. Occasionally the thumb is completely absent, and this is often associated with an absent radius. Clinodactyly of the fifth finger is a common finding.

OTHER RADIOLOGIC FINDINGS. A variety of other congenital anomalies may be seen with this disorder. These include congenital hip dislocation, webbing of the toes, flat feet and Klippel-Feil deformity. Other isolated anomalies have also been noted. Renal abnormalities are common, being seen in more than one-quarter of the cases.[2]

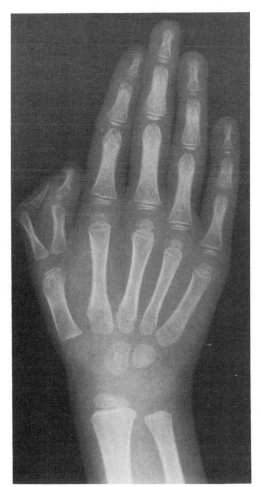

Figure 13–131. Pancytopenia-dysmelia syndrome (Fanconi anemia). Double thumb in a boy with this condition. This is a less common manifestation.

REFERENCES

1. Juhl, J. J., Wesenberg, R. L., and Gwinn, J. L.: Roentgenographic Findings in Fanconi's Anemia. *Radiology*, 89:646–653, 1967.
2. Minagi, H., and Steinbach, H. L.: Roentgen Appearance of Anomalies Associated with Hypoplastic Anemias of Childhood: Fanconi's Anemia and Congenital Hypoplastic Anemia (Erythrogenesis Imperfecta). *Am. J. Roentgenol.*, 97:100–109, 1966.
3. Poznanski, A. K., Garn, S. M., and Holt, J. F.: The Thumb in the Congenital Malformation Syndromes. *Radiology*, 100:115–129, 1971.
4. Poznanski, A. K., and Holt, J. F.: The Carpals in Congenital Malformation Syndromes. *Am. J. Roentgenol.*, 112:443–459, 1971.

PARASTREMMATIC DWARFISM

This is a rare form of dwarfism, identified by Langer et al.[1] The name comes from the Greek term *parastremma*, meaning distorted limb. Abnormality was seen in the first year, with scoliosis giving the patient the appearance of a twisted dwarf. There was asymmetry of the legs, and the arms appeared relatively long as compared to the legs. The mode of inheritance was probably dominant.

RADIOLOGIC FINDINGS IN THE HAND. The hands were short and stubby with shortening of the metacarpals and phalanges. The carpal angle was decreased owing to an angulation of the distal radius and ulna. There was irregularity of the carpal bones and of the epiphyses and metaphyses. The radiologic appearance suggested a metaphyseal and epiphyseal dysplasia.

OTHER RADIOLOGIC FINDINGS. Scoliosis was severe. During childhood there was a lacy ossification in the pelvis, particularly around the iliac wings, which may be characteristic of this disorder. Flakes of calcification were seen in areas of endochondral ossification and may somewhat mimic those seen in Jansen's type of metaphyseal chondrodysplasia. The differential diagnosis of this condition includes Morquio disease, diastrophic dwarfism and Jansen disease.

REFERENCE

1. Langer, L. O., Petersen, D., and Spranger, J.: An Unusual Bone Dysplasia: Parastremmatic Dwarfism. *Am. J. Roentgenol.*, 110:550–560, 1970.

PECTORAL APLASIA–DYSDACTYLY SYNDROME (POLAND SYNDROME, PECTORAL MUSCLE ABSENCE AND SYNDACTYLY SYNDROME)

This syndrome includes unilateral absence of the sternocostal portion of the pectoralis major muscle in association with hypoplasia and syndactyly of the ipsilateral hand. The condition is sporadic and affected individuals are usually otherwise normal. Seventy-eight per cent of cases occur in males, and 75 per cent of cases occur on the right side.[3] Absence of the nipples occurs in 10 per cent.[3] There is a high incidence of attempted abortion early in pregnancy in mothers of patients with this condition.[1]

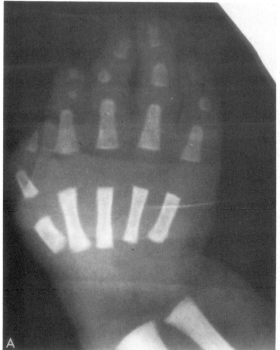 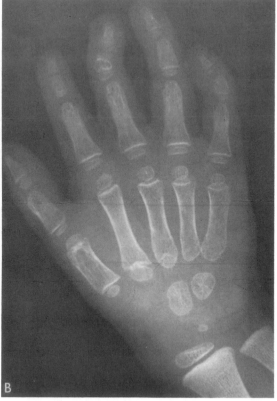

Figure 13–132. Pectoral aplasia-dysdactyly syndrome (Poland syndrome). *A,* One day old infant with characteristic findings of hypoplasia of the middle phalanges, some syndactyly and clinodactyly. The findings were unilateral. The radiologic diagnosis of Poland syndrome was suggested but could not be confirmed since pectoral muscle evaluation is difficult in the neonate.

B, Same patient at 3¹⁰/₁₂ years of age. At this time the pectoral muscle deficiency was obvious clinically. Abnormal epiphyses are seen in some of the middle phalanges. The hypoplasia of the middle phalanges has persisted and the curvature has become somewhat more severe.

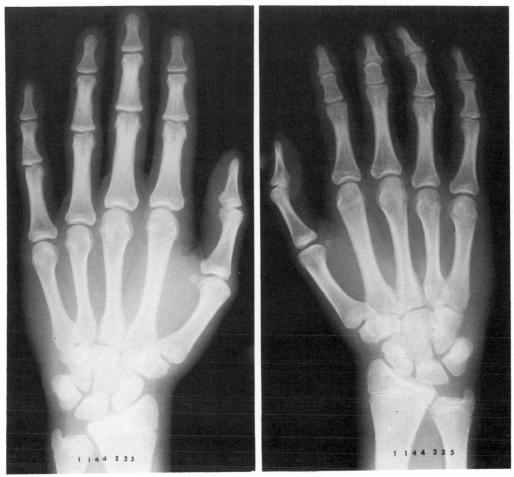

Figure 13-133. Pectoral aplasia–dysdactyly syndrome (Poland syndrome). This boy was admitted for evaluation of an unrelated abnormality. The unilateral hypoplasia of the middle phalanges and of some of the distal phalanges is characteristic of this condition. As is more common, the patient was male and the involvement was on the right side.

RADIOLOGIC FINDINGS IN THE HAND. Various patterns of syndactyly may be seen, involving only two of the digits or the whole hand. Associated with the syndactyly is considerable hypoplasia of the digits. The middle phalanges are most severely affected (Figs. 13-132 and 13-133). Other phalanges may be hypoplastic as well, particularly the distals (Fig. 13-134).

The presence of unilateral syndactyly and short middle phalanges in an otherwise normal-appearing infant should suggest the diagnosis of Poland syndrome. Often during infancy, as in the case illustrated in Figure 13-132, the hand deformity is evident at birth but the partial pectoral muscle abnormality may be missed until later in life.[4] The hand in brachydactyly A-1 may be similar to that seen in Poland syndrome. However, the findings in the former are bilateral, which easily differentiates it from Poland syndrome. Carpenter syndrome is also associated with short middle phalanges and a small hand, but it also is bilateral, and its other clinical manifestations easily differentiate it from Poland syndrome.

OTHER RADIOLOGIC FINDINGS. Hypoplasia of the forearm and of the arm may occur in some cases, as may some abnormalities about the elbow. The chest may appear more lucent because of the lack of pectoral muscles, and rib anomalies have been noted in a few cases.

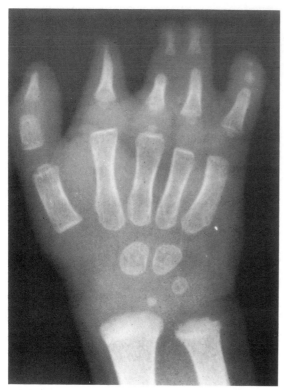

Figure 13-134. Pectoral aplasia-dysdactyly syndrome (Poland syndrome). Severe unilateral hand change was associated with absence of the pectoral muscle. This finding is more severe than usual.

REFERENCES

1. David, T. J.: Nature and Etiology of the Poland Anomaly. *N. Engl. J. Med.*, 287:487–489, 1972.
2. Février, J.-C.: Agénésie du Pectoral Associée à une Malformation Congénitale de la Main: Syndactylie et Ectrodactylie. *Ann. Chir. Plast.*, 14:335–340, 1969.
3. Mace, J. W., Kaplan, J. M., Schanberger, J. E., and Gotlin, R. W.: Poland's Syndrome. Report of Seven Cases and Review of the Literature. *Clin. Pediatr.*, 11:98–102, 1972.
4. Pearl, M., Chow, T. F., and Friedman, E.: Poland's Syndrome. *Radiology*, 101:619–623, 1971.
5. Stein, H. L.: Roentgen Diagnosis of Congenital Absence of Pectoralis Muscles. *Radiology*, 83: 63–66, 1964.

POPLITEAL-PTERYGIUM SYNDROME (POPLITEAL WEB SYNDROME)

This is a syndrome of multiple anomalies, including cleft lip and palate, pits of the lower lip, digital and genital anomalies and popliteal webbing. Toenail dysplasia is another common finding. Various modes of inheritance have been described. The recessive form is more severe than the dominant form.[1]

RADIOLOGIC FINDINGS IN THE HAND. These include syndactyly, symphalangism, absent phalanges or digits, and curved fingers.

OTHER RADIOLOGIC FINDINGS. Foot deformity, abnormality of the pelvis, vertebral anomalies and scoliosis have been seen in this condition.

REFERENCES

1. Bartsocas, C. S., and Papas, C. V.: Popliteal Pterygium Syndrome: Evidence for a Severe Autosomal Recessive Form. *J. Med. Genet.*, 9:222–226, 1972.
2. Gorlin, R. J., Sedano, H. O., and Cervenka, J.: Popliteal Pterygium Syndrome. A Syndrome Comprising Cleft Lip-Palate, Popliteal and Intercrural Pterygia, Digital and Genital Anomalies. *Pediatrics*, 41:503–509, 1968.
3. Hecht, F., and Jarvinen, J. M.: Heritable Dysmorphic Syndrome with Normal Intelligence. *J. Pediatr.*, 70:927–935, 1967.
4. Klein, D.: Cas Observé. Un Curieux Syndrome Héréditaire: Chéilo-Palatoschizis avec Fistules de la Lèvre Inferieure Associe à une Syndactylie, une Onychodysplasie Particulière, un Ptérygion Poplité Unilatéral et des Pieds Varus Équins. *J. Genet. Hum.*, 11:65–71, 1962.

PORPHYRIA – CONGENITAL

This rare defect of porphyrin metabolism was clinically associated with severe photosensitivity, hemolytic anemia and splenomegaly. The solar sensitivity resulted in erythema, which was followed by bullous formation that could eventually have become infected. There was subsequent loss of some of the soft tissues. The condition was inherited as a Mendelian recessive.

RADIOLOGIC FINDINGS IN THE HAND. There was loss of the soft tissues at the ends of the fingers with subsequent loss of the tufts of the distal phalanges or even larger portions of these bones. Soft tissue calcification was seen. The radiologic findings were not particularly characteristic and may be seen in a number of conditions.

OTHER RADIOLOGIC FINDINGS. Bone changes similar to those of the anemias may be noted. There may be some lucencies in the skull.

REFERENCE

1. Small, P., and Dickson, R.: The Radiological Features of Congenital Porphyria. *Br. J. Radiol.*, 43:732–734, 1970.

PRADER-WILLI SYNDROME

This syndrome consists of neonatal hypotonia, sexual infantilism, obesity and mental retardation.

RADIOLOGIC FINDINGS IN THE HAND. The hands are characteristically small, although this has been a somewhat subjective evaluation. The bony cortex is thin and there may be overtubulation. Clinodactyly is occasionally seen. Bone age may be delayed or normal.

OTHER RADIOLOGIC FINDINGS. These include small sella turcica, coxa valga, scoliosis and fatty infiltration of muscle. There may be asymmetry in length of the long bones.

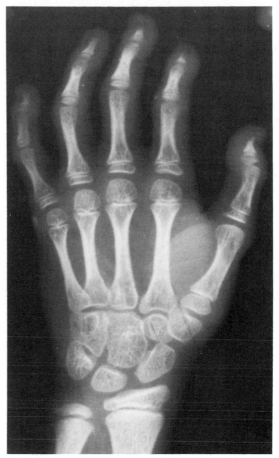

Figure 13-135. Progeria. There is some erosion at the tips of the distal phalanges, particularly on the radial aspect of the hand. The bones appear overtubulated. The appearance of acroosteolysis is not specific for this condition. (Courtesy Dr. M. Ozonoff, Newington, Connecticut.)

REFERENCES

1. Hall, B. D., and Smith, D. W.: Prader-Willi Syndrome. A Resumé of 32 Cases Including an Instance of Affected First Cousins, One of Whom is of Normal Stature and Intelligence. *J. Pediatr.*, 81:286–293, 1972.
2. Landwirth, J., Schwartz, A. H., and Grunt, J. A.: Prader-Willi Syndrome *Am. J. Dis. Child.*, 116:211–217, 1968.
3. Pearson, K. D., Steinbach, H. L., and Bier, D. M.: Roentgenographic Manifestations of the Prader-Willi Syndrome. *Radiology*, 100:369–377, 1971.
4. Zellweger, H., and Schneider, H. J.: Syndrome of Hypotonia-Hypomentia-Hypogonadism-Obesity (HHHO) or Prader-Willi Syndrome. *Am. J. Dis. Child.*, 115:588–598, 1968.

PROGERIA (HUTCHINSON-GILFORD SYNDROME)

These patients exhibit a scleroderma-like skin, midfacial cyanosis and a sculptured nasal tip. The changes begin early in infancy, with deficient growth in the first year of life. The appearance is somewhat like that of aging but is differentiated from other conditions with premature aging. Alopecia is common. Degenerative processes occur early and include arteriosclerosis.

RADIOLOGIC FINDINGS IN THE HAND. There is a progressive osteolysis of the distal phalanges (Fig. 13–135). The pattern of acroosteolysis is similar to that seen in many other conditions. The hand appears somewhat demineralized. The bone age is retarded.

OTHER RADIOLOGIC FINDINGS. Acroosteolysis is also seen in the feet. There is loss of subcutaneous fat. The facial bones are hypoplastic. The cranial sutures are open, with persistent fontanelles. The clavicles are thin and short and may be affected by progressive osteolysis. Coxa valga deformity may be seen.

REFERENCES

1. DeBusk, F. L.: The Hutchinson-Gilford Progeria Syndrome. *J. Pediatr.*, 80:697–724, 1972.
2. Margolin, F. R., and Steinbach, H. L.: Progeria. Hutchinson-Gilford Syndrome. *Am. J. Roentgenol.*, 103:173–178, 1968.
3. Ozonoff, M. B., and Clemett, A. R.: Progressive Osteolysis in Progeria. *Am. J. Roentgenol.*, 100:75–79, 1967.
4. Reichel, W., Bailey, J. A., II, Zigel, S., Garcia-Bunuel, R., and Knox, G.: Radiologic Findings in Progeria. *J. Am. Geriatr. Soc.*, 19:657–674, 1971.

PSEUDOACHONDROPLASTIC DYSPLASIA (PSEUDOACHONDROPLASTIC SPONDYLOEPIPHYSEAL DYSPLASIA)

This form of short-limb dwarfism clinically resembles achondroplasia but is not evident at birth. The facial appearance of these patients is normal. Because of the spine involvement, it is somewhat related to spondyloepiphyseal dysplasia. According to Hall and Dorst,[2] four different forms of this entity are described. There is a Koz-lowski dominant and recessive form, and there is a Maroteaux-Lamy dominant and recessive form. The Kozlowski types are milder than those of Maroteaux and Lamy.

RADIOLOGIC FINDINGS IN THE HAND. The hand changes in all of the various forms include shortening of the metacarpals and phalanges (Figs. 13–136 and 13–137). In some patients there is irregularity of the epiphyses, the distal radius and ulna and occasionally the phalanges and metacarpals. Ossification of the carpals is late. The appearance of the hand is similar to that seen in other epiphyseal dysplasias. As in many of the bone dysplasias, when seen in the adult the findings in the hand may not be diagnostic.

OTHER RADIOLOGIC FINDINGS. There is shortening of all of the limbs, and a relatively large trunk. The definite changes are not evident until later in infancy or childhood. Vertebral changes are seen, with some flattening and tongue-like projection anteriorly. The height of the vertebrae may vary from normal to flat, depending on the severity and type. Various epiphyses throughout the skeleton may be irregular in configuration and delayed in formation.

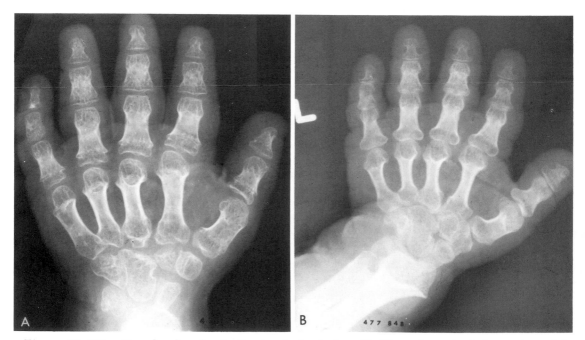

Figure 13–136. Pseudoachondroplastic dysplasia. *A,* Age 13. There is marked shortening of the bones of the hand. There is some irregularity of the epiphyses. The carpal angle appears decreased. *B,* Age 39. Short digits are difficult to differentiate from other causes of small hand.

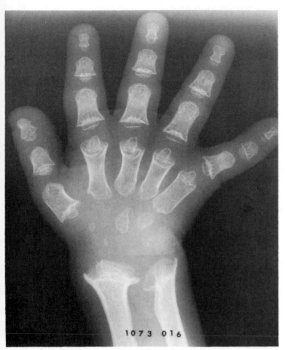

Figure 13–137. Pseudoachondroplastic dysplasia. 24 month old child of the patient described in Figure 13–136. There is marked shortening of the bones of the hand. The epiphyses are somewhat wide. All of the bones are short. The carpal bones are irregular in outline, as are the distal radius and ulna.

REFERENCES

1. Ford, N., Silverman, F. N., and Kozlowski, K.: Spondylo-Epiphyseal Dysplasia (Pseudoachondroplastic Type). *Am. J. Roentgenol.,* 86:462–472, 1961.
2. Hall, J. G., and Dorst, J. P.: Pseudoachondroplastic SED, Recessive Maroteaux-Lamy Type. *Birth Defects, Original Article Series,* 5:254–259, 1969.
3. Hall, J. G., and Grossman, M.: Pseudoachondroplastic SED: Recessive Kozlowski Type. *Birth Defects, Original Article Series,* 5:247–249, 1969.
4. Lindseth, R. E., Danigelis, J. A., Murray, D. G., and Wray, J. B.: Spondylo-Epiphyseal Dysplasia (Pseudoachondroplastic Type). *Am. J. Dis. Child.,* 113:721–726, 1967.
5. Maloney, F. P.: Four Types of Pseudoachondroplastic Spondyloepiphyseal Dysplasia (SED). Dominant Kozlowski Type in Father and Three Children. *Birth Defects, Original Article Series,* 5:242–246, 1969.
6. Maroteaux, P., and Lamy, M.: Les Formes Pseudo-Achondroplasiques Des Dysplasies Spondylo-Epiphysaires. *Presse Med.,* 67:383–386, 1959.
7. Wadia, R.: Pseudoachondroplastic Spondyloepi-

physeal Dysplasia: Dominant Maroteaux-Lamy Type in Three Generations of Whom Three Affected Persons are Described Here. *Birth Defects, Original Article Series,* 5:250–253, 1969.

PSEUDOTHALIDOMIDE SYNDROME (SC SYNDROME)

This is a syndrome of reduction defects in the limbs, flexion contractures of various joints and other abnormalities, including capillary hemangioma of the face, forehead and ears; hypoplasia of the cartilages of the ear and nose; micrognathia, cloudy cornea and lenses; intrauterine growth retardation; growth failure; and possibly mental retardation. It is inherited as an autosomal recessive.

RADIOLOGIC FINDINGS IN THE HAND. Various hand abnormalities were seen in the few cases that have been reported. In most of them the thumb is absent and there is also some hypoplasia of the fifth digit. In some there is fusion of the fourth and fifth metacarpals. Clinodactyly of the second and fifth digits is common.

OTHER RADIOLOGIC FINDINGS. Multiple shortenings in the lower extremities are also noted, with absence of bones and hypoplasia or bowing of some of the bones; clubfoot deformities were seen in some patients. Humeroradial synostosis may also occur.

REFERENCES

1. Hall, B. D., and Greenberg, M. H.: Hypomelia-Hypotrichosis-Facial Hemangioma Syndrome. (Pseudothalidomide, SC Syndrome, SO Phocomelia Syndrome). *Am. J. Dis. Child.,* 123:602–604, 1972.
2. Herrmann, J., Feingold, M., Tuffli, G. A., and Opitz, J. M.: A Familial Dysmorphogenetic Syndrome of Limb Deformities, Characteristic Facial Appearance and Associated Anomalies: The "Pseudothalidomide" or "SC-Syndrome." *Birth Defects, Original Article Series,* 5:81–89, 1969.

PSEUDOXANTHOMA ELASTICUM (PXE)

This is a hereditary disorder characterized by degenerative changes in elastic tissues. It involves multiple systems. The condition is named after the xanthoma-like skin lesions that are seen, usually about the neck. Symptoms may include gastrointestinal hemorrhage and loss of visual acuity. The condition is inherited, probably as an autosomal recessive.

RADIOLOGIC FINDINGS IN THE HAND. A variety of changes may be seen, including soft tissue calcification which may be within the skin or periarticular in its location.[3] Calcification may also be seen in arteries. There may be evidence of an erosion of the tufts of the fingers, which may be related to arterial occlusion.[1]

OTHER RADIOLOGIC FINDINGS. Other soft tissue calcification, vascular calcification and occlusions can be demonstrated. There may be a cardiac abnormality with dilatation of the aorta. Angioid streaks of the optic fundus may be seen.

REFERENCES

1. James, A. E., Jr., Eaton, S. B., Blazek, J. V., Donner, M. W., and Reeves, R. J.: Roentgen Findings in Pseudoxanthoma Elasticum (PXE). *Am. J. Roentgenol.*, 106:642–647, 1969.
2. McKusick, V. A.: *Heritable Disorders of Connective Tissue.* The C. V. Mosby Company, St. Louis, 1972.
3. Najjar, S. S., Farah, F. S., Kurban, A. K., Melhem, R. E., and Khatchadourian, A. K.: Tumoral Calcinosis and Pseudoxanthoma Elasticum. *J. Pediatr.*, 72:243–247, 1968.

PYCNODYSOSTOSIS (PYKNODYSOSTOSIS)

This is a syndrome of short stature, increased bone density, a relatively large head with open fontanelles and sutures and an increased tendency to fracture. Tooth abnormalities are common. Deciduous teeth may persist into adulthood. Sometimes a double row of teeth may be seen. Patients are occasionally mentally retarded. The disorder is inherited as an autosomal recessive.

RADIOLOGIC FINDINGS IN THE HAND. There is osteolysis of the tips of the distal phalanges of the hand. This may vary from minimal loss of tuft to severe loss of most of the phalanx (Figs. 13–138 and 13–139). On occasion several small fragments may be seen in place of the tuft. The changes are more severe with advancing age. The thumb is occasionally involved (Fig. 13–139). The bones generally are very dense and radiopaque. Various bone shortenings may occur from previous fractures.

OTHER RADIOLOGIC FINDINGS. Dense bones are seen throughout the skeleton, and there is an increased tendency for transverse fractures. The skull shows delayed closure of the sutures and an increased number of wormian bones. The mandible has an obtuse angle. In occasional cases there may be loss of the acromial end of the clavicle. Because of the radiographic

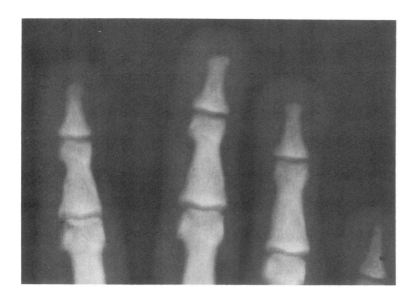

Figure 13–138. Pycnodysostosis. There is some erosion of the distal portions of the tufts. There is increased bone density. These are minimal findings of pycnodysostosis. (Courtesy Dr. John Dorst, Johns Hopkins Hospital, Baltimore, Maryland.)

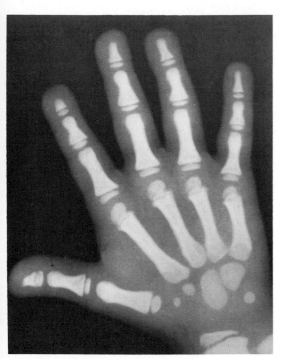

Figure 13-139. Pycnodysostosis. More severe changes. There is more destruction of the tufts than in the case shown in Figure 13-138. (Courtesy Dr. Charles Bream, University of North Carolina, Chapel Hill, North Carolina.)

findings, pycnodysostosis must be differentiated from cleidocranial dysostosis, osteopetrosis and various forms of acroosteolysis.

REFERENCES

1. Elmore, S. M.: Pycnodysostosis: A Review. *J. Bone Joint Surg.*, 49A:153–161, 1967.
2. Maroteaux, P., and Lamy, M.: La Pycnodysostose. *Presse Med.*, 70:999–1002, 1962.
3. Sedano, H. D., Gorlin, R. J., and Anderson, V. E.: Pycnodysostosis. *Am. J. Dis. Child.*, 116:70–77, 1968.
4. Shiraishi, S.: Pycnodysostosis. *Acta Orthop. Scand.*, 42:227–243, 1971.

ROTHMUND SYNDROME (ROTHMUND-THOMSON SYNDROME)

This is a syndrome of congenital poikiloderma associated with congenital cataracts. Tooth abnormalities are common, as is short stature. The condition is inherited as an autosomal recessive.

RADIOLOGIC FINDINGS IN THE HAND. These mainly include phalangeal tuft resorption. Soft tissue calcification may also be evident. The findings in the hand may be similar to those of Werner syndrome.

REFERENCES

1. Maurer, R. M., and Langford, O. L.: Rothmund's Syndrome. A Cause of Resorption of Phalangeal Tufts and Dystrophic Calcification. *Radiology*, 89:706–708, 1967.
2. Silver, H. K.: Rothmund-Thomson Syndrome: An Oculocutaneous Disorder. *Am. J. Dis. Child.*, 111:182–190, 1966.
3. Taylor, W. B.: Rothmund's Syndrome—Thomson's Syndrome. Congenital Poikiloderma With or Without Juvenile Cataracts. A Review of the Literature, Report of a Case, and Discussion of the Relationship of the Two Syndromes. *Arch. Dermatol.*, 75:236–244, 1957.
4. Thannhauser, S. J.: Werner's Syndrome (Progeria of the Adult) and Rothmund's Syndrome: Two Types of Closely Related Heredofamilial Atrophic Dermatoses with Juvenile Cataracts and Endocrine Features: A Critical Study with Five New Cases. *Ann. Int. Med.*, 23:559–626, 1945.
5. Thomson, M. S.: An Hitherto Undescribed Familial Disease. *Br. J. Dermatol. Syph.*, 35:455–462, 1923.

RUBINSTEIN-TAYBI SYNDROME (BROAD THUMBS SYNDROME)

This is a syndrome of mental retardation associated with broad thumbs and great toes. The patients are of short stature and have a small skull. There is a characteristic facies with a beaked or straight nose. They have an antimongoloid slant of the palpebral fissures, high-arched palate and, in males, incomplete or delayed descent of testes. Most cases are sporadic.

RADIOLOGIC FINDINGS IN THE HAND. The most typical findings in the hand are those affecting the thumb, which is broad and usually deviates radially. The distal phalanx of the thumb is short in the severely affected cases, but in mild cases it appears normal in length. The first proximal phalanx, however, is markedly abnormal and in the extreme cases has a comma or triangular shape which accounts for the radial curvature of the thumb. (Fig. 13–140). This triangular configuration was encountered in 35 of the 91 cases reviewed by Rubinstein.[1] The other distal phalanges may also be broad. Rubinstein reported them widened

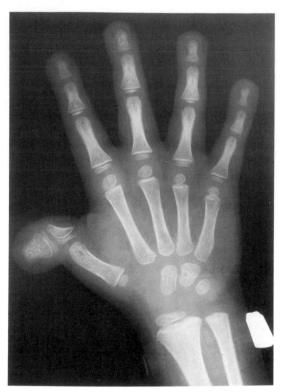

Figure 13–140. Rubinstein-Taybi syndrome. Two year old male with a broad thumb. There is a bizarre proximal phalanx of the thumb, which is characteristic of this condition. The distal phalanx of the thumb appears broad.

in 63 of 114 cases. Twenty-nine of his patients had clinodactyly of the fifth finger.

OTHER RADIOLOGIC FINDINGS. There is often angulation deformity in the foot, with an abnormal proximal phalanx of the first metatarsal, which may be duplicated. Pelvic anomalies are occasionally seen, with flat acetabular angles and flaring of the ilia. Vertebral anomalies, including spina bifida, kyphosis, lordosis and scoliosis, were seen in a number of patients. Sternum or rib anomalies were also present.

REFERENCES

1. Rubinstein, J. H.: The Broad Thumbs Syndrome— Progress Report 1968. *Birth Defects, Original Article Series*, 5:25–41, 1969.
2. Rubinstein, J. H., and Taybi, H.: Broad Thumbs and Toes and Facial Abnormalities. A Possible Mental Retardation Syndrome. *Am. J. Dis. Child.*, 105:588–608, 1963.
3. Taybi, H., and Rubinstein, J. H.: Broad Thumbs and Toes, and Unusual Facial Features. A Probable Mental Retardation Syndrome. *Am. J. Roentgenol.*, 93:362–366, 1965.

RÜDIGER SYNDROME

This was a condition of shortened extremities, coarse facial features, abnormally thick palms and soles, lack of cartilage formation in the ears, cleft soft palate, hydronephrosis, failure of development of motor control, and early death. It was probably inherited as an autosomal recessive.

RADIOLOGIC FINDINGS IN THE HAND. The fingers and toes were small, and there was hypoplasia of the middle and distal phalanges. The nails were also very small. The syndrome was similar radiologically to that in the Coffin-Siris syndrome and to hypoplasia of the distal phalanges associated with maternal use of anticonvulsants during pregnancy (page 158).

OTHER RADIOLOGIC FINDINGS. Hydronephrosis was seen.

REFERENCE

1. Rüdiger, R. A., Schmidt, W., Loose, D. A., and Passarge, E.: Severe Developmental Failure with Coarse Facial Features, Distal Limb Hypoplasia, Thickened Palmar Creases, Bifid Uvula, and Ureteral Stenosis: A Previously Unidentified Familial Disorder with Lethal Outcome. *J. Pediatr.*, 79:977–981, 1971.

RUVALCABA SYNDROME

Ruvalcaba et al. described two siblings with an unusual syndrome consisting of mental retardation, short stature, microcephaly, peculiar facies, a narrow thoracic cage with pectus carinatum, hypoplastic genitalia, hypoplastic skin lesions, and skeletal deformities. The mode of inheritance is undetermined.

RADIOLOGIC FINDINGS IN THE HAND. There was marked shortening of the third to fifth metacarpals with broadening of the distal ends, which was associated with early fusion of the epiphyses. The distal phalanges were described as short, although this was not visible on the published radiographs. One of the patients had triquetrum-lunate fusion. The bone age was relatively normal and was not as significantly depressed as the height age.

OTHER RADIOLOGIC FINDINGS. Shortening of the lateral metatarsals was seen. Scheuermann-like changes were noted in the spine.

REFERENCE

1. Ruvalcaba, R. H. A., Reichert, A., and Smith, D. W.: A New Familial Syndrome with Osseous Dys-

plasia and Mental Deficiency. *J. Pediatr.*, 79: 450–455, 1971.

SALDINO-NOONAN SYNDROME (SHORT-RIB POLYSYNDACTYLY, SALDINO-NOONAN TYPE)

This severe form of dwarfism is usually fatal at birth. Infants have a hydropic appearance with a very small chest and usually die from cardiopulmonary problems. Multiple anomalies of the heart, lungs and genital tract and anal atresia may be seen. The limbs are all extremely short. The condition is inherited as an autosomal recessive trait.

RADIOLOGIC FINDINGS IN THE HAND. Postaxial polydactyly with six or seven fingers may be seen. The fingers are extremely short with absent nails. On radiography only a small amount of calcification is seen within the hands.

OTHER RADIOLOGIC FINDINGS. There is polydactyly of the feet. Coronal clefts are present in the spine. The long bones have an unusually short form with somewhat pointed ends, which differentiates them from thanatophoric dwarfism. The bizarre short extremities also differentiate this condition from Jeune asphyxiating thoracic dystrophy. The ribs are extremely short horizontally. The condition is somewhat different from a form of dwarfism described by Majewski et al., which is associated with cleft lip and smooth ends of the tubular bones.

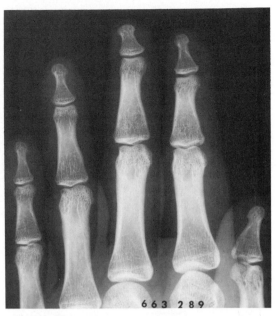

Figure 13–141. Scalp defect syndrome. There is hypoplasia of the distal phalanges. Much more severe changes were present in the feet. The patient had focal areas of scalp hypoplasia.

REFERENCES

1. Majewski, F., Pfeiffer, R. A., Lenz, W., Müller, R., Feil, G., and Seiler, R.: Polysyndaktylie, verkürzte Gliedmassen und Genitalfehlbildungene: Kennzeichen eines selbständigen Syndroms? Z. *Kinderheilk.*, 111:118–138, 1971.
2. Saldino, R. M., and Noonan, C. D.: Severe Thoracic Dystrophy with Striking Micromelia, Abnormal Osseous Development, Including the Spine, and Multiple Visceral Anomalies. *Am. J. Roentgenol.*, 114:257–263, 1972.
3. Spranger, J. W., Langer, L., and Wiedemann, H.-R.: *Bone Dysplasias: An Atlas of Constitutional Disorders of Skeletal Development.* W. B. Saunders Company, Philadelphia, 1974.

SCALP DEFECTS AND HAND ANOMALIES

It is not clear whether this represents a definite syndrome or simply an association of anomalies. A number of cases in the literature have familial focal defects of the scalp which are sometimes associated with hand and foot abnormalities. Since siblings have been affected, inheritance may be autosomal recessive.

RADIOLOGIC FINDINGS IN THE HAND. Various combinations of brachydactyly and syndactyly may be noted. In our own cases the hypoplasia of the digits was much more marked in the feet; in the hands (Fig. 13–141) there was only minimal hypoplasia of the distal phalanges. There appears to be considerable variation in the appearance of the hand changes.

REFERENCES

1. Kahn, E. A., and Olmedo, L.: Congenital Defect of the Scalp. With a Note on the Closure of Large Scalp Defects in General. *Plast. Reconstr. Surg.*, 6:435–440, 1950.
2. Liepman, M.: Familial Aplasia Cutis Congenita with Skeletal and Other Anomalies: Case Reports, in press.
3. Lynch, P. J., and Kahn, E. A.: Congenital Defects of the Scalp. A Surgical Approach to Aplasia Cutis Congenita. *J. Neurosurg.*, 33:198–202, 1970.

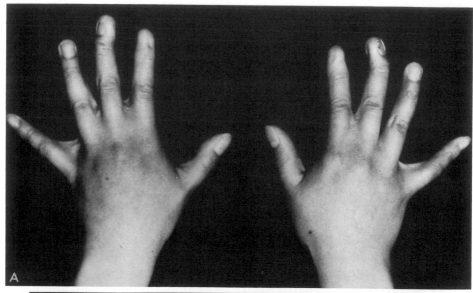

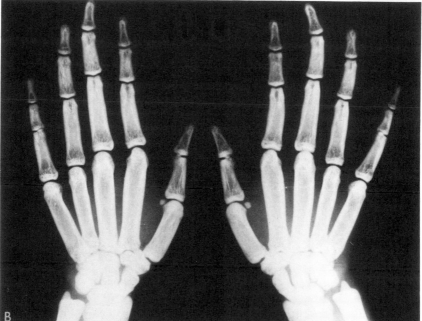

Figure 13–142. Sclerosteosis. *A,* There is cutaneous syndactyly.
B, Thickening of the cortex of the bones with failure of modeling is noted. There is some deviation of the third and ring fingers radially. (Courtesy Dr. Y. Sugiura, Nagoya, Japan.)

SCLEROSTEOSIS

This is a disorder characterized by hyperostosis of the calvarium, mandible, clavicles and pelvis; the hyperostosis is probably different from that observed in van Buchem disease.[1] The appearance of patients is characterized by a steep high forehead, hypertelorism and a broad flat nasal roof. Deafness may occur early. The condition was previously included in some reports of osteopetrosis.

RADIOLOGIC FINDINGS IN THE HAND. The most characteristic findings in the hand are syndactyly associated with increased bone density (Fig. 13–142). There is failure of tubulation of the bones of the hand, which appear wide. Another finding in a number of these cases is the radial deviation of the index or other fingers (Fig. 13–142 B). There is often an associated decrease in size of the middle phalanx of the index finger, which may be triangular in shape.

OTHER RADIOLOGIC FINDINGS. Increased bone density and failure of modeling may be seen in many of the tubular bones. The calvarium is thickened and the optic canal is narrowed. The body of the mandible is considerably thickened.

REFERENCES

1. Gorlin, R. J., Spranger, J., and Koszalka, M. F.: Genetic Craniotubular Bone Dysplasias and Hyperostoses—A Critical Analysis. *Birth Defects, Original Article Series,* 5:79–95, 1969.
2. Higinbotham, N. L., and Alexander, S. F.: Osteopetrosis. Four Cases in One Family. *Am. J. Surg.,* 54:444–454, 1941.
3. Truswell, A. S.: Osteopetrosis with Syndactyly. A Morphological Variant of Albers-Schönberg's Disease. *J. Bone Joint Surg.,* 40B:208–218, 1958.

SECKEL DWARFS (BIRD-HEADED DWARFS, VIRCHOW-SECKEL DWARFS)

This form of dwarfism is so-called because of a "bird-headed" appearance of the face which, however, is not unique to the Seckel form of dwarfism. There is evidence of intrauterine retardations, hypoplasia of the facial bones, low-set ears and microcephalic head. The dwarfism is proportional. Inheritance may well be autosomal recessive.

RADIOLOGIC FINDINGS IN THE HAND. There was evidence of dysharmonic maturation with marked delay in appearance of the lunate bone in Seckel's original cases. Clinodactyly of the second and fifth fingers may be seen. Absence of the thumb has also been reported.[3]

OTHER RADIOLOGIC FINDINGS. Radiologic findings elsewhere are not particularly characteristic of the syndrome.

REFERENCES

1. Harper, R. G., Orti, E., and Baker, R. K.: Bird-Headed Dwarfs (Seckel's Syndrome). A Familial Pattern of Developmental, Dental, Skeletal, Genital and Central Nervous System Anomalies. *J. Pediatr.,* 70:799–804, 1967.
2. Holmes, L. B., Moser, H. W., Halldorsson, S., Mack, C., Pant, S. S., and Matzilevich, B.: *Mental Retardation. An Atlas of Diseases with Associated Physical Abnormalities.* The Macmillan Company, New York, 1972.
3. McKusick, V. A., Mahloudji, M., Abbott, M. H., Lindenberg, R., and Kepas, D.: Seckel's Bird-Headed Dwarfism. *N. Engl. J. Med.,* 277:279–286, 1967.
4. Seckel, H.: *Bird-Headed Dwarfs.* Charles C Thomas, Publisher, Springfield, Illinois, 1960.

SILVER SYNDROME (RUSSELL-SILVER DWARF)

This form of dwarfism is evident from birth. There is usually associated asymmetry. The patients have a triangular face with down-turned corners of the mouth. Occasionally there may be café au lait spots, and in some of the patients there is altered sexual maturation. Some patients are mentally deficient.

RADIOLOGIC FINDINGS IN THE HAND. Clinodactyly of the fifth finger with radial deviation is seen in almost all cases. When this is associated with asymmetry in size, which is often evident in the hand films, the diagnosis of Silver syndrome can be suggested (Fig. 13–143). The bone age is retarded except when there is associated sexual precocity. There is often asymmetry in skeletal maturation, with the larger hand being more mature than the smaller. Another abnormality occasionally seen in Silver syndrome is Kirner deformity.

OTHER RADIOLOGIC FINDINGS. Hemihypertrophy and asymmetry are seen in other portions of the body, and other sites

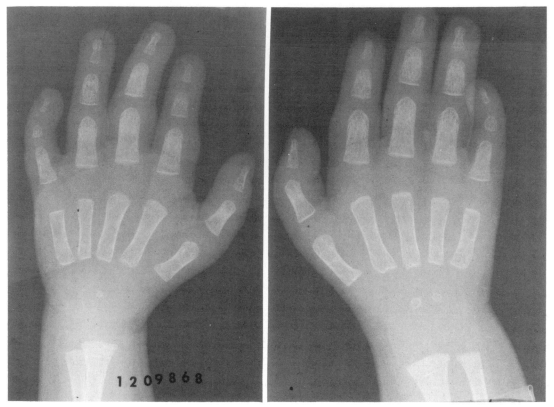

Figure 13-143. Silver syndrome. One year old boy. There is clinodactyly of the fifth finger bilaterally, with short middle phalanges. The right hand is larger than the left and the right carpals are more advanced in maturation than those of the left. The overall maturation, however, is retarded. (From Poznanski, A. K., and Holt, J. F.: *Seminars in Roentgenology*, April, 1973, by permission.)

of asymmetry of maturation may also be evident.

REFERENCES

1. Moseley, J. E., Moloshok, R. E., and Freiberger, R. H.: The Silver Syndrome: Congenital Asymmetry, Short Stature and Variations in Sexual Development. Roentgen Features. *Am. J. Roentgenol.*, 97:74–81, 1966.
2. Poznanski, A. K., Garn, S. M., Kuhns, L. R., and Sandusky, S. T.: Dysharmonic Maturation of the Hand in the Congenital Malformation Syndromes. *Am. J. Phys. Anthropol.*, 35:417–432, 1971.
3. Silver, H. K.: Asymmetry, Short Stature, and Variations in Sexual Development. *Am. J. Dis. Child.*, 107:495–515, 1964.

SMITH-LEMLI-OPITZ SYNDROME

This is a congenital syndrome consisting of anteverted nostrils, which may be associated with ptosis of the eyelid, syndactyly of the second and third toes, hypospadias and cryptorchidism in the male.

RADIOLOGIC FINDINGS IN THE HAND. Hand manifestations are not particularly characteristic. Different minor anomalies have been seen in a number of hands. Fine et al.[2] demonstrated the presence of cutaneous syndactyly in the hand and hypoplastic, low-set thumbs. Short fingers and rudimentary polydactyly have also been seen.

OTHER RADIOLOGIC FINDINGS. Syndactyly is more evident in the feet. Other foot deformities have also been noted. Congenital heart disease may be seen in 20 per cent of cases.[3]

REFERENCES

1. Dallaire, L.: Syndrome of Retardation with Urogenital and Skeletal Anomalies (Smith-Lemli-

Opitz Syndrome): Clinical Features and Mode of Inheritance. *J. Med. Genet.*, 6:113–120, 1969.
2. Fine, R. N., Gwinn, J. L., and Young, E. F.: Smith-Lemli-Opitz Syndrome. Radiologic and Postmortem Findings. *Am. J. Dis. Child.*, 115: 483–488, 1968.
3. Robinson, C. D., Perry, L. W., Barlee, A., and Mella, G. W.: Smith-Lemli-Opitz Syndrome with Cardiovascular Abnormality. *Pediatrics*, 47:844–847, 1971.

SPHEROPHAKIA BRACHYMORPHIA (MARCHESANI SYNDROME, WEILL-MARCHESANI SYNDROME, CONGENITAL MESODERMAL DYSMORPHODYSTROPHY)

This condition occurs in association with a small spherical lens, short stature and brachydactyly. There is usually myopia and glaucoma. Cardiac anomalies are occasionally seen.

RADIOLOGIC FINDINGS IN THE HAND. These include very mild brachydactyly, which is nonspecific. Measurements are not available. There is retardation of skeletal maturation.

OTHER RADIOLOGIC FINDINGS. There are occasional tooth malformations. The skull is broad with shallow orbits.

REFERENCES

1. Feinberg, S. B.: Congenital Mesodermal Dysmor-pho-Dystrophy. *Radiology*, 74:218–224, 1960.
2. Sellem, C., Rosenberg, D., Chatelain, R., Picaud, S., and Monnet, P.: Syndrome De Weill-Marchesani. *Pediatrie*,25:771–775, 1970.
3. Zabriskie, J., and Reisman, M.: Marchesani Syndrome. *J. Pediat.*, 52:158–169, 1958.

SPONDYLOEPIPHYSEAL DYSPLASIA CONGENITA

This is a hereditary form of disproportionate dwarfism which is evident at birth. The main characteristics are a short trunk and neck with a normal head. Myopia with retinal detachment is an important complication. Some flattening of the face may also be seen. The disease is differentiated from Morquio disease by its roentgen features, lack of corneal clouding and keratosulfaturia, as well as by a different mode of inheritance. The inheritance of spondyloepiphyseal dysplasia is autosomal dominant, although it is somewhat more common in males than in females.

RADIOLOGIC FINDINGS IN THE HAND. Only minimal changes are present in the hand and may not be manifested until later in life. The tubular bones in the hand are unremarkable, although Spranger has occasionally noted shortening. Pseudoepiphyses are common. The carpals, particularly the proximal row, are retarded (Fig. 13–144). The epiphyses of the phalanges may be flattened and may appear somewhat sclerotic. The involvement of the proximal and middle phalanges differentiates it from normal ivory epiphyses.

OTHER RADIOLOGIC FINDINGS. These are too numerous to discuss in detail. The main ones include flattening of the verte-

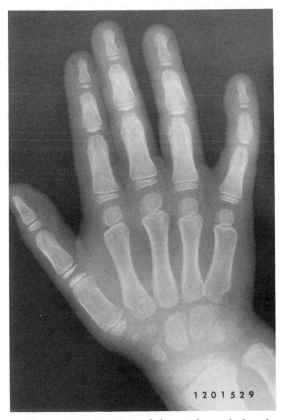

Figure 13–144. Spondyloepiphyseal dysplasia congenita. The hand changes are minimal, but there is some flattening of the epiphyses and retarded maturation of the proximal row of carpal bones. The skeletal findings in the remainder of the skeleton were much more severe. The patient's brother was also affected.

bral bodies, odontoid hypoplasia and pelvic abnormality with coxa vara.

REFERENCES

1. Kozlowski, K., Bittel-Dobrzynska, N., and Budzynska, A.: Spondylo-Epiphyseal Dysplasia Congenita. *Ann. Radiol.*, 11:367–375, 1967.
2. Spranger, J. W., and Langer, L. O., Jr.: Spondyloepiphyseal Dysplasia Congenita. *Radiology*, 94:313–322, 1970.

SPONDYLOMETAPHYSEAL DYSPLASIA (KOZLOWSKI)

This form of dwarfism becomes manifest in early childhood. It affects the vertebral

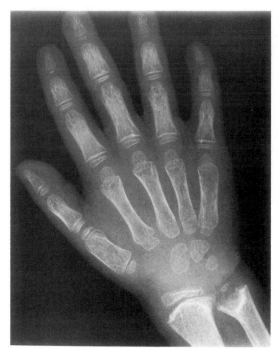

Figure 13–146. Spondylometaphyseal-epiphyseal dysplasia. Both epiphyseal and metaphyseal changes were seen in the skeleton. In the hand, mainly the metaphyseal component is seen in the radius and ulna.

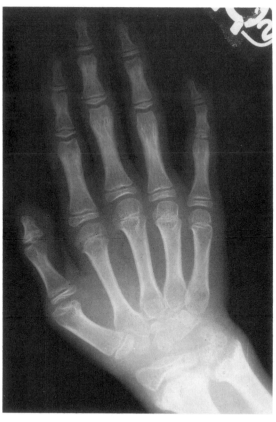

Figure 13–145. Spondylometaphyseal dysplasia. There are metaphyseal irregularities in the radius and ulna. The carpals are markedly hypoplastic, particularly in the proximal row. The fingers are relatively uninvolved. The distal phalanx of the thumb appears somewhat short. (Courtesy Dr. William Reynolds, Henry Ford Hospital, Detroit, Michigan.)

column. There are associated metaphyseal changes which predominantly involve the long bones. These patients differ from those with Morquio disease in that they have no visceral abnormality, corneal clouding, deafness or abnormal mucopolysaccharides.

RADIOLOGIC FINDINGS IN THE HAND. The manifestations in the phalanges are less marked than those in the carpals. The carpals are markedly retarded in onset, particularly those in the proximal row (Fig. 13–145), and in some reported cases were not present when phalangeal ossification centers were well developed. The carpals may be irregular in outline. Some cases which have both epiphyseal and metaphyseal components have been termed spondylo-metaphyseal-epiphyseal dysplasia (Fig. 13–146).[1]

OTHER RADIOLOGIC FINDINGS. There is marked platyspondyly involving the entire spine. The principal metaphyseal changes are in the proximal skeleton and result in coxa vara with shortening of the neck of the femur.

REFERENCES

1. Kozlowski, K., Filipiak-Miastkowska, I., Narebska, E., Nowicki, S., and Chylinska, H.: Dysplasia spondylometa-epiphysaria Congenita und Dysplasia spondyloepiphysaria congenita mit Brachymetakarpie und -metatarsie. Ein Beitrag zur Differentialdiagnose der Dysplasia spondyloepiphysaria congenita. *Fortschr. Geb. Roentgenstr. Nuklearmed.*, 114:824–832, 1971.
2. Kozlowski, K., Maroteaux, P., and Spranger, J.: La Dysostose Spondylo-Metaphysaire. *Presse Med.*, 75:2769–2774, 1967.
3. Michel, J., Grenier, B., Castaing, J., Augier, J. L., and Desbuquois, G.: Deux Cas Familiaux de Dysplasie Spondylo-Metaphysaire. *Ann. Radiol.*, 13:251–254, 1969.
4. Piffaretti, P. G., Delgado, H., and Nussle, D.: La Dysostose Spondylo-Metaphysaire de Kozlowski, Maroteaux et Spranger. *Ann. Radiol.*, 13:405–417, 1970.
5. Refior, H. J.: Zur spondylo-metaphysären Dysostose (Typ Kozlowski-Maroteaux-Spranger). *Arch. Orthop. Unfallchir.*, 66:334–346, 1969.
6. Riggs, W., Jr., and Summitt, R. L.: Spondylometaphyseal Dysplasia (Kozlowski). Report of Affected Mother and Son. *Radiology*, 101:375–381, 1971.

THANATOPHORIC DWARFISM

This fatal form of bone dysplasia has in the past been confused with achondroplasia. The cartilage growth in this condition is markedly irregular, in contradistinction to the regular cartilage seen in achondroplasia.[6] The clinical appearance is that of a short-limbed form of dwarfism with a narrow chest. The infants are usually either stillborn or die a few days after birth. The condition may be clinically difficult to differentiate from achondrogenesis.

RADIOLOGIC FINDINGS IN THE HAND. The hand bones are extremely short and cupped. Some of the phalangeal bones may be shorter in length than in width (Fig. 13–147). The bones of the hand are considerably shorter than those in homozygous achondroplasia, which can somewhat mimic this condition.[4] The appearance of the hand may be similar to that seen in achondrogenesis. The shortening is usually more marked than that seen in metatropic dwarfism.

OTHER RADIOLOGIC FINDINGS. There is marked platyspondyly involving the vertebral bodies. The ossification of the vertebrae is greater than in achondrogenesis, and the trunk is not decreased in size. This helps differentiate the two conditions. All of the long bones are short and cupped,

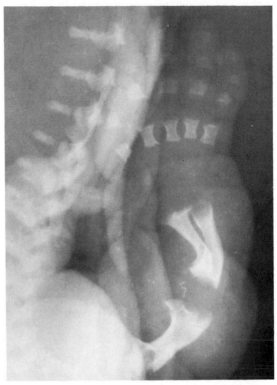

Figure 13–147. Thanatophoric dwarfism. Note the marked shortening of the hand bones, with some cupping at the ends of each of the bones. The hand partially overlies the vertebral spine, where the markedly flattened vertebral bodies are seen. The humerus, radius and ulna are short and bent.

and there is marked bowing of the femora and humeri.

REFERENCES

1. Giedion, A.: Thanatophoric Dwarfism. *Helv. Paediatr. Acta*, 2:175–183, 1968.
2. Kaufman, R. L., Rimoin, D. L., McAlister, W. H., and Kissane, J. M.: Thanatophoric Dwarfism. *Am. J. Dis. Child.*, 120:53–57, 1970.
3. Keats, T. E., Riddervold, H. O., and Michaelis, L. L.: Thanatophoric Dwarfism. *Am. J. Roentgenol.*, 108:473–480, 1970.
4. Langer, L. O., Jr., Spranger, J. W., Greinacher, I., and Herdman, R. C.: Thanatophoric Dwarfism. A Condition Confused with Achondroplasia in the Neonate, with Brief Comments on Achondrogenesis and Homozygous Achondroplasia. *Radiology*, 92:285–294, 303, 1969.
5. Maroteaux, P., Lamy, M., and Robert J.-M.: Le Nanisme Thanatophore. *Presse Med.*, 75:2519–2524, 1967.
6. O'Malley, B. P., Parker, R., Saphyakhajon, P., and Qizilbash, A. H.: Thanatophoric Dwarfism. *J. Can. Assoc. Radiol.*, 23:62–68, 1972.

THIEMANN DISEASE (EPIPHYSEAL ACRODYSPLASIA—THIEMANN, OSTEOCHONDROPATHY OF THE FINGERS)

This somewhat poorly defined condition has been described mainly in the German literature and was originally identified by Thiemann. The main symptoms are swelling about the fingers. The condition occurs mainly in males, usually in their late teens. Dominant inheritance has been seen, or the condition may be related to trauma. There is some similarity between this entity and epiphyseal dysplasia.

RADIOLOGIC FINDINGS IN THE HAND. The characteristic appearance is that of an irregularity to the epiphyses of the fingers, involving particularly the middle fingers. The epiphyses appear sclerotic and fragmented (Fig. 13–148) and may project outward with a moustache-like configuration.[2] There is some similarity between these changes and those of an epiphyseal dysplasia. Similar findings may also be seen in Kaschin-Beck disease.

OTHER RADIOLOGIC FINDINGS. These are not well defined. When Thiemann disease is associated with epiphyseal dysplasia, there may be flattening of epiphyses in other areas of the body.

REFERENCES

1. Dessecker, C.: Zur Epiphyseonekrose der Mittelphalangen beider Hände. *Deutsche Zeitschrift fur Chirurgie*, 229:327–336, 1930.

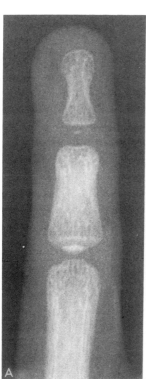
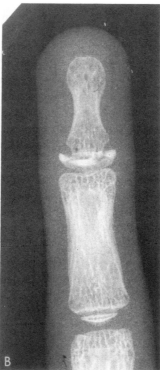
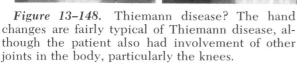

Figure 13–148. Thiemann disease? The hand changes are fairly typical of Thiemann disease, although the patient also had involvement of other joints in the body, particularly the knees.

A, Age 5½ years. Normal appearance.

B, Age 10½ years. There is a sclerotic, fragmented epiphysis, which is wider than the base of the phalanx. This appearance is fairly typical of Thiemann disease.

C, Entire hand of the same patient at 10½ years of age. There is some flattening of other epiphyses as well, and the carpal bones are diminished in size. This patient could easily be considered to have a form of epiphyseal dysplasia rather than Thiemann disease.

2. Giedion, A.: Acrodysplasias, Cone Epiphyses, Peripheral Dysostosis, Thiemann's Disease and Acrodysostosis. *Prog. Pediatr. Radiol.*, 4:325–345, 1973.
3. Poschel, M.: Juvenile Osteo-Chondro-Nekrosen. Anhang: Coxa Vara Congenita und Protrusio Acetabuli Coxae. *In:* Diethelm, L. (Ed.): *Handbuch der Medizinischen Radiologie.* Springer-Verlag, Berlin, 1971, Teil 4.
4. Reinberg, S. A., and Graziansky, W. P.: Multiple Osteochondropathy of the Phalanges of the Fingers. *Am. J. Roentgenol.*, 34:617–628, 1935.
5. Thiemann, H.: Juvenile Epiphysenstörungen. *Fortschr. Roentgen.*, 14:79–87, 1909.

THROMBOCYTOPENIA–RADIAL APLASIA SYNDROME (THROMBOCYTOPENIA–RADIAL HYPOPLASIA SYNDROME, THROMBOCYTOPENIA–ABSENT RADIUS SYNDROME, TAR SYNDROME, THROMBOCYTOPENIA–PHOCOMELIA SYNDROME)

This is an association of hypomegakaryocytic thrombocytopenia with bilateral absence of the radius. The hematologic findings occur at birth or during infancy and usually decrease after one year if the patient survives. Bone marrow examination reveals a decreased number of, or abnormal, megakaryocytes. Elevation of the leukocyte count or leukemoid reactions are seen in a significant number of cases, particularly in infants. Anemia may be the result of hemorrhage. The condition is differentiated both clinically and radiologically from Fanconi's anemia, in which a pancytopenia occurs and in which symptoms appear later.

RADIOLOGIC FINDINGS IN THE HAND. The hand findings are characteristic of this condition. A five-fingered hand in association with absent radius appears to occur mainly in this condition (Fig. 13–149). Other causes of absent radius or phocomelia, such as those associated with thalidomide embryopathy, Fanconi's anemia or the Holt-Oram syndrome, are usually associated with an absent thumb. The most extensive review of the radiographic findings was made by Hall et al.[2] They reported limited extension of the hand in 21 of 30 cases, club hand in six cases, hypoplastic or fused phalanges in 17, finger syndactyly in nine, carpal hypoplasia or fusion in five and radial deviation in 16. Clinodactyly of the fifth finger is

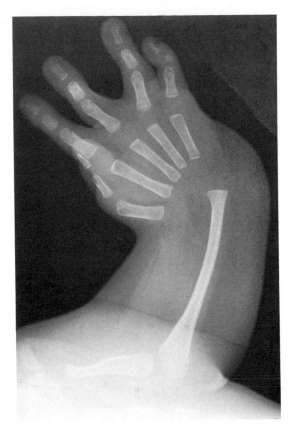

Figure 13–149. Thrombocytopenia–radial aplasia syndrome. There is absence of the radius and hypoplasia of the humerus. The hand has five digits. The thumb is reasonably well formed and the middle phalanx of the fifth finger is short with associated clinodactyly.

a common finding, with absence or marked hypoplasia of the middle phalanx (Figs. 13–149 and 13–150). The ulna is short, malformed and frequently absent. There is also hypoplasia about the shoulder. In some cases there may be severe phocomelia with the hand attached to the shoulder area (Fig. 13–150).

OTHER RADIOLOGIC FINDINGS. Although the hand and upper extremity findings are the most characteristic, changes are also seen in other bones. In our two cases there was absence of the distal femoral ossification centers at birth, even though infants were term and tooth maturation indicated a normal length of gestation. The feet are frequently abnormal with an overriding fifth toe, calcaneus valgus, club foot or other foot deformity. Coxa valga abnormalities about the knee are also seen.

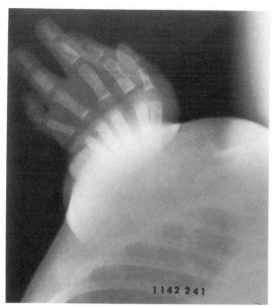

Figure 13–150. Thrombocytopenia-radial aplasia syndrome. There is phocomelia, with the hand attached to the shoulder region. The thumb is relatively uninvolved. There is curvature of the fingers, particularly clinodactyly of the fifth with a short middle phalanx.

REFERENCES

1. Dignan, P. St. J., Mauer, A. M., and Frantz, C.: Phocomelia with Congenital Hypoplastic Thrombocytopenia and Myeloid Leukemoid Reactions. *J. Pediatr.*, 70:561–573, 1967.
2. Hall, J. G., Levin, J., Kuhn, J. P., Ottenheimer, E. J., van Berkum, K. A. P., and McKusick, V. A.: Thrombocytopenia with Absent Radius (TAR). *Medicine*, 48:411–439, 1969.

TRICHO-RHINO-PHALANGEAL SYNDROME (GIEDION SYNDROME, ACRODYSPLASIA)

This syndrome is characterized by a bulbous nose, hypoplasia or slow growth of the hair and, sometimes, short stature. The patients are occasionally mentally retarded. Hypoglycemia may be evident. In most cases the condition is inherited as a Mendelian dominant, although a few cases of recessive transmission have been noted.[4]

RADIOLOGIC FINDINGS IN THE HAND. The hand radiographs are pathognomonic. Cone-shaped epiphyses of the Giedion type 12 are seen particularly in the middle phalanges (Figs. 13–151 to 13–153). The cen-

tral portion of these cones is often fused with the remainder of the shaft. In adults, stigmata of the previous cones may be seen by splaying of the distal end of the bone (Fig. 13–153). Ivory epiphyses are common in the distal phalanges, and their distribution is similar to that seen in normal individuals. Various degrees of brachydactyly may be seen. This is best delineated on pattern profile analysis (Fig. 13–154), which shows that the middle phalanges are most commonly shortened but the metacarpals may also be involved. There may be curvature of the fingers owing to the abnormal epiphyses, which usually becomes manifest after age 10. There is considerable variation in the severity of the hand findings.

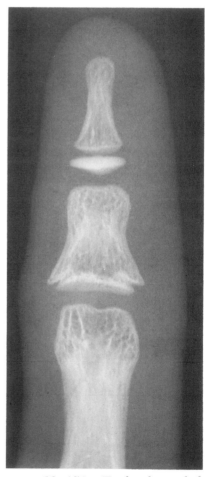

Figure 13–151. Tricho-rhino-phalangeal syndrome. Finger of a 10 year old female with this disease. The ivory epiphysis in the distal phalanx is typically seen in this condition; as is the splaying of the middle phalanx with the broad cone fused to the phalanx (Giedion type 12 cone).

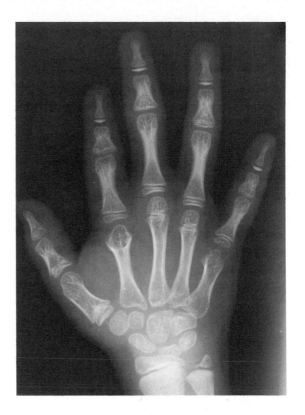

Figure 13–152. Tricho-rhino-phalangeal syndrome. This is the entire hand of the patient shown in Figure 13–151. Multiple ivory epiphyses are seen. Also, there are multiple cones involving even the thumb and brachydactyly involving the second and fifth metacarpals with abnormal epiphyses of these metacarpal heads.

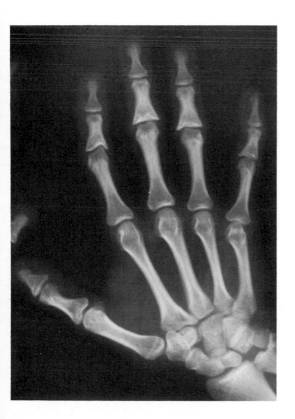

Figure 13–153. Tricho-rhino-phalangeal syndrome. Adult male. Note the splaying of the middle phalanges, which are signs that cone epiphyses were previously present at this site.

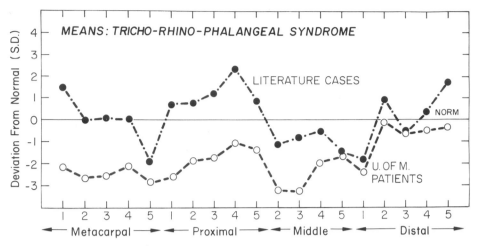

Figure 13–154. Tricho-rhino-phalangeal syndrome. Pattern profile analysis including both our patients (U. of M. patients) and those from the literature. Note that the most marked shortening is in the middle phalanges, while the distal and proximal phalanges are relatively long. Note also the relatively common shortening of the fifth metacarpal and of the first distal phalanx.

OTHER RADIOLOGIC FINDINGS. Changes similar to those in the hand may also be seen in the feet. Legg-Perthes changes in the hips may occasionally be seen. Exostoses are sometimes associated with this condition, but probably this represents a different syndrome (so-called Langer-Giedion syndrome).

REFERENCES

1. Fontaine, G., Maroteaux, P., Farriaux, J.-P., Richard, J., and Roelens, B.: Le Syndrome Trichio-Rhino-Phalangien. *Arch. Fr. Pediatr.*, 27:635–647, 1970.
2. Giedion, A.: Cone-Shaped Epiphyses of the Hands and Their Diagnostic Value. The Tricho-Rhino-Phalangeal Syndrome. *Ann. Radiol.*, 10:322–329, 1967.
3. Giedion, A.: Das tricho-rhino-phalangeale Syndrom. *Helv. Paediatr. Acta*, 5:475–482, 1966.
4. Giedion, A., Burdea, M., Fruchter, Z., Meloni, T., and Trosc, V.: Autosomal-Dominant Transmission of the Tricho-Rhino-Phalangeal Syndrome. Report of 4 Unrelated Families, Review of 60 cases. *Helv. Paediat. Acta*, 28:249–259, 1973.
5. Gorlin, R. J., Cohen, M. M., Jr., and Wolfson, J.: Tricho-Rhino-Phalangeal Syndrome. *Am. J. Dis. Child.*, 118:595–599, 1969.
6. Poznanski, A. K., Schmickel, R. D., and Harper, H. A.: Tricho-Rhino-Phalangeal Syndrome. *Birth Defects, Original Article Series*, in press.

TUBEROUS SCLEROSIS

This is a congenital malformation syndrome with associated adenoma sebaceum, tuber-like neurologic proliferations in the cerebral cortex and a multitude of other lesions. There is usually mental retardation. The skin lesions are not seen in all of the patients. Recent evidence suggests these patients have abnormal endocrine function of the pituitary, adrenal and thyroid glands, as well as abnormalities in the glucose tolerance test.[3] Tuberous sclerosis is probably inherited as an autosomal dominant.

RADIOLOGIC FINDINGS IN THE HAND. In Holt and Dickerson's classic series,[1] 66 per cent of their 30 cases with radiographs of the hands and feet had changes in these areas. The changes included cyst-like foci in the phalanges (Figs. 13–155 and 13–156) and a distinct periosteal reaction in the metacarpals (Fig. 13–158). The periosteal reaction is less marked in the metacarpals than in the metatarsals. There are also areas of sclerosis in bone adjacent to the areas of lucency. The total pattern is very characteristic for this lesion. The lesions in the hand increase with age (Fig. 13–157), and are more marked in older than in younger individuals.

OTHER RADIOLOGIC FINDINGS. Calcifications in the skull, dense lesions through-

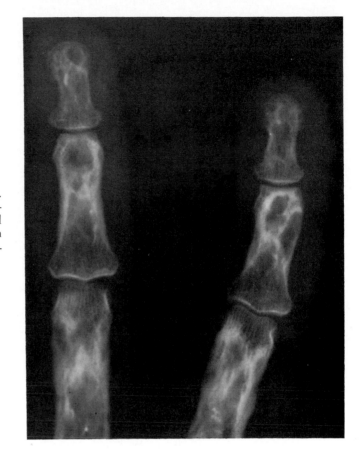

Figure 13–155. Tuberous sclerosis. Typical digital changes of tuberous sclerosis with punched-out lesions as well as areas of increased sclerosis. (From Holt, J. F., and Dickerson, W. W.: *Radiology*, 58:1–8, 1952.)

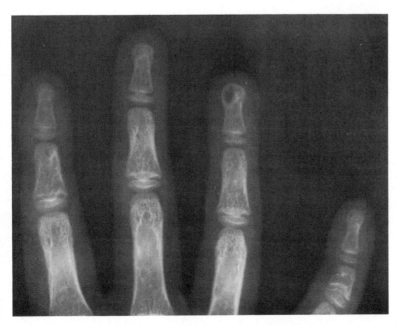

Figure 13–156. Tuberous sclerosis in a young child. There is a lucent defect in the distal phalanx of the ring finger.

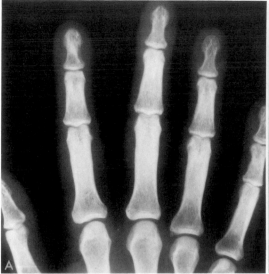 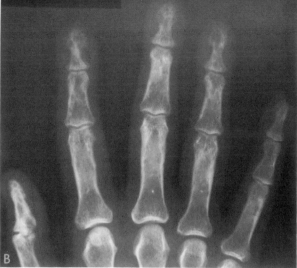

Figure 13–157. Tuberous sclerosis progressing with time over a 12-year period in a young adult. *A,* On the initial film, only minimal sclerotic changes can be seen in the distal phalanx of the index finger, and minor lucencies can be seen in the other distal phalanges.

B, Twelve years later, however, the changes are much more extensive. The areas of lucencies have become larger and better defined. (From Holt, J. F., and Dickerson, W. W.: *Radiology,* 58:1–8, 1952.)

out the remainder of the skeleton, renal masses, renal cystic disease, abnormality of the cerebral ventricles, pulmonary manifestations and cardiac tumors are also found.

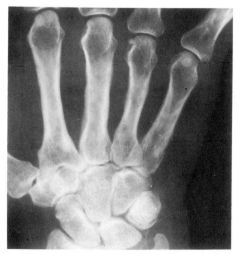

Figure 13–158. Tuberous sclerosis. Irregular cortical margins in the metacarpals are less common in the hand than in the foot. (From Holt, J. F., and Dickerson, W. W.: *Radiology,* 58:1–8, 1952.)

REFERENCES

1. Holt, J. F., and Dickerson, W. W.: The Osseous Lesions of Tuberous Sclerosis. *Radiology,* 58: 1–8, 1952.
2. Lagos, J. C., and Gomez, M. R.: Tuberous Sclerosis: Reappraisal of a Clinical Entity. *Mayo Clin. Proc.,* 42:26–49, 1967.
3. Sareen, C. K., Ruvalcaba, H. A., Scotvoid, M. J., Mahoney, C. P., and Kelley, V. C.: Tuberous Sclerosis. Clinical, Endocrine, and Metabolic Studies. *Am. J. Dis. Child.,* 123:34–39, 1972.

TUBULAR STENOSIS (KENNY-CAFFEY SYNDROME, MEDULLARY STENOSIS SYNDROME)

This is a syndrome of medullary stenosis associated with hypocalcemic tetany. The condition is associated with dwarfism and retardation of skeletal maturation.

RADIOLOGIC FINDINGS IN THE HAND. There is marked narrowing of the medullary canals of the hand bones. This condition is similar to that seen in the so-called normal medullary stenosis (Fig. 13–159), which may also be associated with short stature but which is without any of the

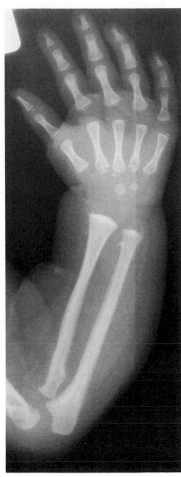

Figure 13-159. Tubular stenosis with hypocalcemia. There is increased modeling of the tubular bones of the hand. This is particularly marked in the metacarpals and in the proximal phalanges. This is the same patient reported by Frech, R. S., and McAlister, W. H.: *Radiology*, 91:457–461, 1968. (Courtesy Dr. William McAlister, St. Louis, Missouri.)

biochemical changes. The medullary stenosis is most noticeable in the metacarpals; the first and fifth are the least affected. The medullary canals of the proximal phalanges are more stenosed than those of the distal phalanges. The carpal bones appear uninvolved.

OTHER RADIOLOGIC FINDINGS. Similar overstenosis is seen in the other bones, which have some flaring of the metaphyses. In the skull there is lack of differentiation of the diploic space and of the outer and inner table. The anterior fontanelle may be large.

REFERENCES

1. Caffey, J.: Congenital Stenosis of Medullary Spaces in Tubular Bones and Calvaria in Two Proportionate Dwarfs—Mother and Son; Coupled with Transitory Hypocalcemic Tetany. *Am. J. Roentgenol.*, 100:1–11, 1967.
2. Frech, R. S., and McAlister, W. H.: Medullary Stenosis of the Tubular Bones Associated with Hypocalcemic Convulsions and Short Stature. *Radiology*, 91:457–461, 1968.
3. Garn, S. M., Davila, G. H., and Rohmann, C. G.: Population Frequencies and Altered Remodeling Mechanisms in Normal Medullary Stenosis. *Am. J. Phys. Anthropol.*, 29:425–428, 1968.
4. Kenny, F. M., and Linarelli, L.: Dwarfism and Cortical Thickening of Tubular Bones. *Am. J. Dis. Child.*, 111:201–208, 1966.

UNILATERAL ECTROMELIA–ICHTHYOSIS SYNDROME

This condition consists of an erythematous skin disorder which is sharply demarcated to one side of the midline. The condition usually does not involve the entire side; the face is usually spared. There is hypoplasia of the extremities on the affected side. The condition is probably inherited as an autosomal recessive.

RADIOLOGIC FINDINGS IN THE HAND. The phalanges may be absent or hypoplastic, or monodactyly may be seen.

OTHER RADIOLOGIC FINDINGS. There is hypoplasia of all the bones in the upper and lower extremities. Congenital heart disease may sometimes be present.

REFERENCES

1. Cullen, S. I., Harris, D. E., Carter, C. H., and Reed, W. B.: Congenital Unilateral Ichthyosiform Erythroderma. *Arch. Derm.*, 99:724–729, 1969.
2. Rossman, R. E., Shapiro, E. M., and Freeman, R. G.: Unilateral Ichthyosiform Erythroderma. *Arch. Derm.*, 88:567–571, 1963.
3. Shear, C. S., Nyhan, W. L., Frost, P., and Weinstein, G. D.: Syndrome of Unilateral Ectromelia, Psoriasis and Central Nervous System Anomalies. *Birth Defects, Original Article Series*, 7:197–203, 1971.

WERNER SYNDROME

This syndrome includes shortened stature, premature graying of the hair, premature baldness, scleropoikiloderma, trophic ulcers of the legs, juvenile cataracts, hypogonadism, tendency to diabetes, calcification of blood vessels, osteoporosis and metastatic calcifications. It tends to occur in siblings. Most of the changes occur in patients in their 20s and 30s. It must be differentiated from progeria, in which cataracts, hyperkeratosis, skin ulcers and diabetes are usually not found. It must also be differentiated from Rothmund syndrome, in which premature graying, shortness of stature, atrophy of the extremity, osteoporosis, diabetes and arteriosclerosis are not present. The condition is inherited as an autosomal recessive.

RADIOLOGIC FINDINGS IN THE HAND. Osteoporosis is a common radiographic finding, which is, of course, nonspecific. According to Epstein et al.,[1] it occurs in about half the patients. Soft tissue calcification is observed in about one-third of the patients; a significant portion occurs in the tendons around the hand. Vascular calcification may also be noted within the hands.

OTHER RADIOLOGIC FINDINGS. These include degenerative changes elsewhere and significant osteoporosis, as well as calcification both in soft tissue and in blood vessels.

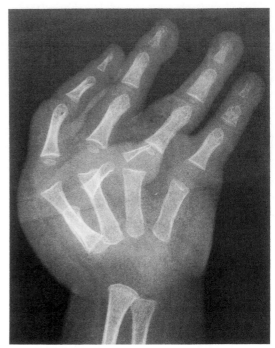

Figure 13–160. Whistling face syndrome (Freeman-Sheldon syndrome). 15 month old female. There is marked deviation of the thumb, which is in a clasp overlying the hand. There is also deviation of the remaining digits. Marked dysharmonic maturation is noted, with that of the phalangeal epiphyses considerably ahead of that of the carpals.

REFERENCES

1. Epstein, C. J., Martin, G. M., Schultz, A. L., and Motulsky, A. G.: Werner's Syndrome. A Review of Its Symptomatology, Natural History, Pathologic Features, Genetics and Relationship to the Natural Aging Process. *Medicine*, 45:177–221, 1966.
2. Jacobson, H. G., Rifkin, H., and Zucker-Franklin, D.: Werner's Syndrome: A Clinical-Roentgen Entity. *Radiology*, 74:373–385, 1960.
3. Rosen, R. S., Cimini, R., and Coblentz, D.: Werner's Syndrome. *Br. J. Radiol.*, 43:193–198, 1970.
4. Thannhauser, S. J.: Werner's Syndrome (Progeria of the Adult) and Rothmund's Syndrome: Two Types of Closely Related Heredofamilial Atrophic Dermatoses with Juvenile Cataracts and Endocrine Features: A Critical Study with Five New Cases. *Ann. Int. Med.*, 23:559–626, 1945.

WHISTLING FACE SYNDROME (FREEMAN-SHELDON SYNDROME, CRANIO-CARPO-TARSAL DYSPLASIA)

This is a syndrome with a typical facial configuration suggesting the appearance of whistling. The affected individuals have a somewhat puckered mouth with a dimple in the region of the chin. The face is flat and the nose is small. The condition is associated with delayed growth. It is inherited as an autosomal dominant but most cases are sporadic.

RADIOLOGIC FINDINGS IN THE HAND. Usually no osseous abnormalities are seen. There is flexion contracture of the thumb, which may be severe (Fig. 13–160). There is ulnar deviation of the digits. Miscellaneous other minor anomalies have been described, but few roentgenograms are available in the literature. We have seen markedly dysharmonic maturation in one patient.

OTHER RADIOLOGIC FINDINGS. Talipes equinovarus is the most common and consistent abnormality. Miscellaneous other findings include pectus deformity, hypoplasia of the mandible and abnormalities of the angle of the jaw.

REFERENCES

1. Rintala, A. E.: Freeman-Sheldon's Syndrome, Cranio-Carpo-Tarsal Dystrophy. Case Report. *Acta Paediat. Scand.*, 57:553–556, 1968.
2. Walbaum, R., Lejeune, M., Poupard, B., Lacheretz, M., and Fontaine, G.: Le Syndrome de Freeman-Sheldon (Syndrome du Siffleur). *Ann. Pediat.*, 20:357–364, 1973.
3. Weinstein, S., and Gorlin, R. J.: Cranio-Carpo-Tarsal Dysplasia or the Whistling Face Syndrome. *Am. J. Dis. Child.*, 117:427–435, 1969.

ZIMMERMANN-LABAND SYNDROME

This is a condition of gingival fibromatosis; absence or dysplasia of the nails; clubbed-tree, frog-like fingers and toes, hyperextensibility of the metacarpophalangeal joints; soft bulky cartilage in nose and ears, producing a bulbous, soft nose and thick, floppy ears; and hepatosplenomegaly.

RADIOLOGIC FINDINGS IN THE HAND.
The main radiologic finding is that of hypoplasia of the distal phalanges, sometimes in association with hypoplastic nails. The appearance resembles that in the Coffin-Siris syndrome.

OTHER RADIOLOGIC FINDINGS. Tuft hypoplasia in the toes is similar to that seen in the fingers.

REFERENCES

1. Jacoby, N. M., Ripman, H. A., and Munden, J. M.: Partial Anonychia (Recessive) with Hypertrophy of the Gums and Multiple Abnormalities of the Osseous System. Report of a Case. *Guy's Hosp. Rep.*, 90:34–40, 1940–1941.
2. Laband, P. F., Habib, G., and Humphreys, G. S.: Hereditary Gingival Fibromatosis. Report of an Affected Family with Associated Splenomegaly and Skeletal and Soft-Tissue Abnormalities. *Oral Surg.*, 17:339–351, 1964.
3. Witkop, C. J.: Heterogeneity in Gingival Fibromatosis. *Birth Defects*, Original Article Series, 7: 210–221, 1971.

Part IV

ACQUIRED DISEASES

Chapter 14

INFECTIONS OF THE HAND

PYOGENIC INFECTION
  Pyogenic Osteomyelitis
  **Neutrophil Dysfunction Syndrome (Chronic
      Granulomatous Disease of Childhood,
      Quie Syndrome)**
  Pyogenic Infectious Arthritis
  Gas Gangrene of the Hand
TUBERCULOSIS OF THE HAND AND WRIST
  Tuberculosis of the Wrist
  Tuberculous Dactylitis
OTHER MYCOBACTERIA
  Leprosy (Hansen Disease)

FUNGAL INFECTIONS
  Actinomycosis of Bone
  Blastomycosis
  Coccidioidomycosis
  Sporotrichosis
  Mycetoma
  Histoplasma duboisii **Dactylitis**
OTHER INFECTIONS AND INFESTATIONS
  Syphilis
  Yaws
  Smallpox (Osteomyelitis Variolosa)
  Other Viruses
  Seal Finger (Blubber Finger)
  Parasitic Infestations of the Hand

There are a number of important infectious conditions of the hand. Many of these involve only the various fascial planes, tendon sheaths, and other soft tissues; and bones are not involved. In this chapter, however, we will consider primarily infections of bone, since these are more commonly associated with significant radiologic findings.

Various pyogenic organisms can cause infections in the hand, as can tuberculosis and leprosy. Spirochetal diseases, including syphilis and yaws, are very uncommon in North America, but in other portions of the world they cause significant pathologic changes in the hand. Similarly, a number of fungi have been shown to involve the hand, as have some viral infections.

PYOGENIC INFECTION

Pyogenic Osteomyelitis

Pyogenic osteomyelitis of the hand is most often associated with some local predisposing factors. External wounds may predispose to infection. This is exemplified by infection associated with compound fractures (Fig. 14–1), lacerations, puncture wounds and human bites. Patients with burn damage to hand (Fig. 14–2) are also

prone to osteomyelitis of the underlying bone, as are individuals with loss of sensation, such as may be seen in congenital insensitivity to pain or in the neurologic deficit due to syringomyelia (Fig. 14–3).

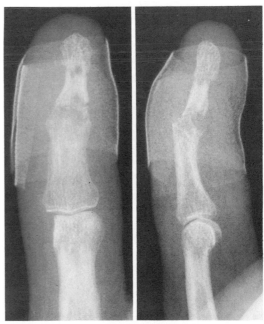

Figure 14–1. Osteomyelitis. There is destruction of the distal interphalangeal joint and the adjacent borders of the phalanges. There is some sclerosis in the distal phalanx suggesting dead bone. There is demineralization of the middle phalanx. (Courtesy Dr. W. Reynolds, Henry Ford Hospital, Detroit, Michigan.)

391

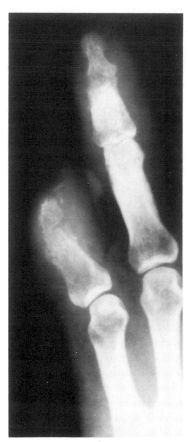

Figure 14-2. Osteomyelitis following a burn. This patient suffered extensive burns to his hand, involving most of the hand surface, and developed an infection with coagulase-positive *Staphylococcus aureus*. There is destruction of the distal portion of the fifth finger with considerable bony demineralization. There is also some bony destruction around the distal interphalangeal joint of the fourth finger. (Courtesy Dr. W. Martel, Ann Arbor, Michigan.)

Osteomyelitis of the distal phalanx may be a complication of a felon.[7, 8] In this condition the pulp space in the digit fills and becomes severely distended due to the infection. The pressure will block the blood supply to the distal portion of the finger, and there may be death of bone with subsequent osseous infection. In the child the damage occurs mainly to the diaphysis, and the epiphysis is usually spared.[2]

Human bites[1, 5] are particularly hazardous. They involve various soft tissue planes but may also be associated with injury to the bones and joints of the hand. In the 50 cases reported by Farmer and Mann,[5] 50 per cent developed complications: 16 per cent developed osteomyelitis and 12 per cent de-

veloped septic arthritis. A variety of organisms may be found in a human bite wound. Most cases associated with complications contained coagulase-positive *Staphylococcus aureus*.[5] This organism is responsible for most hand infections.

Another predisposing cause of pyogenic osteomyelitis of the hand is sickle cell disease. Children with sickle cell disease appear to be more prone to salmonella osteomyelitis, which may both radiologically and clinically be difficult to distinguish from the hand-foot syndrome of sickle cell disease (Chapter 18) (Fig. 14-4).

The relative rarity of primary hematologic osteomyelitis affecting the hand is illustrated in the series of Winters and Cahen,[9] in which none of the 66 cases of acute hema-

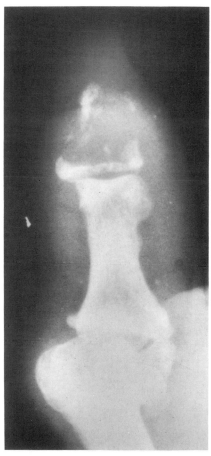

Figure 14-3. Osteomyelitis in a patient with syringomyelia. In the distal phalanx of the thumb, the patient developed a focus of infection which quickly destroyed most of the phalanx. There is considerable soft tissue swelling. (Courtesy Dr. R. Rapp, Veterans Administration Hospital, Ann Arbor, Michigan.)

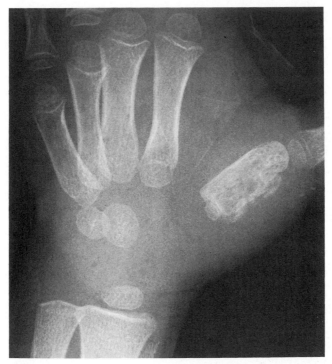

A

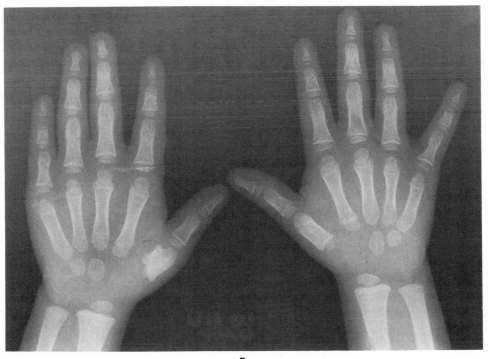

B

Figure 14–4. Osteomyelitis and sickle cell disease. This patient developed swelling of the thumb. Initially only soft tissue swelling was seen. Subsequently some bony destruction was present.

A, The differential diagnosis was between infarction as part of sickle cell hand-foot syndrome, and osteomyelitis. Salmonella was cultured from the blood and was recovered from the lesion at biopsy.

B, Follow-up films show resultant shortening of the first metacarpal.

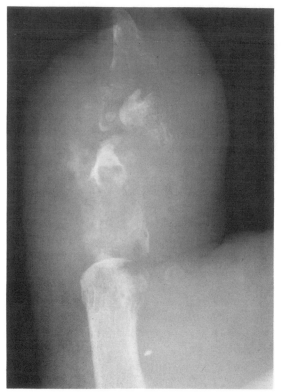

Figure 14–5. Osteomyelitis with sequestrum. This patient had an infection in the thumb for two months. There is tremendous destruction of the middle and distal phalanges, with some foci of sclerotic bone, which is the sequestrum.

togenous osteomyelitis had hand involvement.

The radiologic findings of osteomyelitis of the hand are similar to those of osteomyelitis elsewhere in the body. The first signs are changes in the soft tissues. These include edema of the fat with obliteration of the lucent planes between the muscles, which may be seen in the wrist. This sign is of less value in the fingers, where the normal fat planes are less well defined. Soft tissue swelling, however, can be more readily visualized in this region. The amount of bone destruction visible on the radiographs is usually considerably less than the bone destruction that is actually present,[3] and the bones usually appear normal until about 10 days after the onset of symptoms.

The first osseous sign is periosteal new bone formation or, occasionally, destructive foci. In later phases the destructive foci can be remarkably large and there may be some sequestrum formation (Fig. 14–5). Because

of the new bone formation, during healing the bones in the hand may appear considerably larger than originally.

REFERENCES

1. Boyce, F. F.: Human Bites. An Analysis of 90 (Chiefly Delayed and Late) Cases from Charity Hospital of Louisiana at New Orleans. *South. Med. J.*, 35:631–638, 1942.
2. Boyes, J. H.: *Bunnell's Surgery of the Hand*, 5th Ed., J. B. Lippincott Co., Philadelphia, 1970.
3. Capitanio, M. A., and Kirkpatrick, J. A.: Early Roentgen Observations in Acute Osteomyelitis. *Am. J. Roentgenol.*, 108:488–496, 1970.
4. Constant, E., Green, R. L., and Wagner, D. K.: Salmonella Osteomyelitis of Both Hands and the Hand-Foot Syndrome. *Arch. Surg.*, 102: 148–151, 1971.
5. Farmer, C. B., and Mann, R. J.: Human Bite Infections of the Hand. *South. Med. J.*, 59:515–518, 1966.
6. Gray, E. D., and Patton, J. T.: Periostitis and Osteomyelitis. *In*: Shanks, S. C., and Kerley, P. (Eds.): *A Textbook of X-Ray Diagnosis*, 4th Ed. H. K. Lewis & Co., London, 1971, Vol. 6, Part 5, Sect. 1, Chap. 22, pp. 265–292.
7. Koch, S. L.: Osteomyelitis of the Bones of the Hand. *Surg., Gynec. Obstet.*, 64:1–8, 1937.
8. Macey, H. B.: Paronychia and Bone Felon. *Am. J. Surg.*, 50:553–557, 1940.
9. Winters, J. L., and Cahen, I.: Acute Hematogenous Osteomyelitis. A Review of Sixty-Six Cases. *J. Bone Joint Surg.*, 42A:691–704, 1960.

Neutrophil Dysfunction Syndrome (Chronic Granulomatous Disease of Childhood, Quie Syndrome)

The occurrence of what is apparently hematogenous osteomyelitis of the bones of the hand without predisposing local factors should suggest the possibility of the neutrophil dysfunction syndrome (chronic granulomatous disease of childhood), particularly when several bones are involved (Fig. 14–6). This disease is usually transmitted as an X-linked recessive trait and affects male children. A similar syndrome may more rarely occur in females.

This is usually a fatal disorder. The common presenting signs and symptoms are granulomatous and eczematoid skin lesions, adenitis, repeated pneumonia and osteomyelitis affecting most commonly the small bones of the hands and feet. The radiologic appearance of the osteomyelitis is not particularly characteristic (Figs. 14–6 and 14–7).

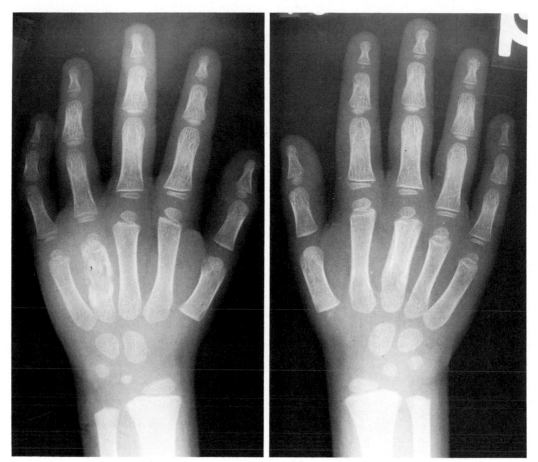

Figure 14-6. Neutrophil dysfunction syndrome in a boy with repeated pulmonary infections. There is a destructive process in the fourth left metacarpal involving most of the bone. Also, considerable bony sclerosis and some bone expansion are evident. There is some periosteal cloaking of the third right metacarpal.

The presence of several areas of osteomyelitis in the hands strongly suggests the diagnosis of neutrophil dysfunction syndrome or the so-called granulomatous disease of childhood. The infectious agent was *Serratia marcescens*.

Figure 14-7. Neutrophil dysfunction syndrome. There is marked expansion of the fourth metacarpal owing to infection with *Serratia marcescens*. The wide expansion of bone is common in this disorder.

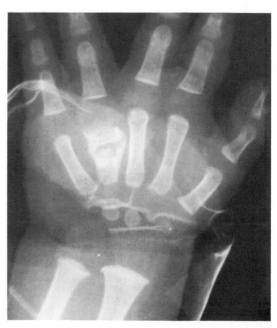

The neutrophils from patients affected with this disease are able to ingest bacteria, but they fail to kill certain types because of a lack of an oxidative enzyme.[5] The most important organisms that cannot be killed include *Staphylococcus aureus*, *Serratia marcescens* and other bacteria which produce catalase.

REFERENCES

1. Bannatyne, R. M., Skowron, P. N., and Weber, J. L.: Job's Syndrome—A Variant of Chronic Granulomatous Disease. Report of a Case. *J. Pediatr.*, 75:236–242, 1969.
2. Gold, R. H., Douglas, S. D., Preger, L., Steinbach, H. L., and Fudenberg, H. H.: Roentgenographic Features of the Neutrophil Dysfunction Syndromes. *Radiology*, 92:1045–1054, 1969.
3. Johnston, R. B., Jr., and Baehner, R. L.: Chronic Granulomatous Disease: Correlation Between Pathogenesis and Clinical Findings. *Pediatrics*, 48:730–739, 1971.
4. Sutcliffe, J.: Chronic Granulomatous Disease. *Ann. Radiol.*, 13:305–310, 1970.
5. Wolfson, J. J., Kane, W. J., Laxdal, S. D., Good, R. A., and Quie, P. G.: Bone Findings in Chronic Granulomatous Disease of Childhood. A Genetic Abnormality of Leukocyte Function. *J. Bone Joint Surg.*, 51A:1573–1583, 1969.

Pyogenic Infectious Arthritis

Pyogenic arthritis may occur from the same forms of trauma that result in osteomyelitis. Felons may involve the distal joints. Radial and ulnar bursal infection can spread to the wrist joint. Hematogenous spread is less common.

The radiologic findings include narrowing of the joint spaces due to damaged cartilage, and an associated demineralization with eventual bone destruction. Osteomyelitis may also occur. The same organisms that cause osteomyelitis may involve the joints of the hand. These include primarily staphylococcus; the specific organisms usually cannot be distinguished by radiologic signs. Brucellosis represents a rare form of infection of the wrist. Of the 36 cases of bone brucellosis studied by Kelly et al.[2] only one involved the phalanx. Arct,[1] in a study of 250 patients with brucellosis of bone, saw four cases which involved the carpal bones. The appearance was not particularly specific, with marked local demineralization. The hand involve-

ment was seen only in cases of long duration in which there was evidence of bone disease in other areas of the body. The lesion can be confused with that of rheumatoid arthritis.

REFERENCES

1. Arct, W. A.: Brucelozowe Uszkodzenia Nadgarstka. *Wiad. Lek.*, 23:1831–1834, 1970.
2. Kelly, P. J., Martin, W. J., Schirger, A., and Weed, L. A.: Brucellosis of the Bones and Joints. Experience with Thirty-six Patients. *J.A.M.A.*, 174:347–353, 1960.

Gas Gangrene of the Hand

Gas gangrene can be caused by a variety of bacteria, but most commonly various species of clostridia are involved. This is a serious complication which may be rapidly fatal, even when it involves only the hand. According to MacLennan,[2] there are three types of clostridial contamination: simple contamination, anaerobic cellulitis and anaerobic myonecrosis (gas gangrene). Clostridial cellulitis is usually a nonfatal gas infection which spreads along fascial planes without involving the healthy muscle. Anaerobic myonecrosis is a more fulminating infection characterized by necrosis of normal muscle and damage by the trauma. Radiologically, gas occurs in muscle bundles and dissects between the muscle fibers.

Sometimes gas in soft tissues may be present without evidence of infection, as was shown in several cases by Filler et al.[1] and by Rubenstein et al.[3] In this situation, gas may enter the soft tissues simply by way of a laceration.

REFERENCES

1. Filler, R. M., Griscom, N. T., and Pappas, A.: Post-Traumatic Crepitation Falsely Suggesting Gas Gangrene. *New Eng. J. Med.*, 278:758–761, 1968.
2. MacLennan, J. D.: The Histotoxic Clostridial Infections of Man. *Bacteriol. Rev.*, 26:177–275, 1962.
3. Rubenstein, A. D., Tabershaw, I. R., and Daniels, J.: Pseudo-Gas Gangrene of the Hand. *J.A.M.A.*, 129:659–662, 1945.
4. Wills, M. R., and Reece, M. W.: Non-Clostridial Gas Infections in Diabetes Mellitus. *Br. Med. J.*, 2:566–568, 1960.

TUBERCULOSIS OF THE HAND AND WRIST

Although formerly a relatively common lesion, tuberculosis of the hand and wrist is now rarely seen in North America. It is, however, still common in Africa[1] and Asia.[3]

Hand and wrist tuberculosis makes up a relatively small portion of all bone tuberculosis. In 290 lesions studied in adult patients at the Glen Lake Sanatorium,[4] one per cent were in the wrist and 2.2 per cent were in the hand. Similarly, in the study of 2000 cases of bone tuberculosis in Hong Kong studied by Hodgson and Smith,[3] 0.7 per cent were in the wrist. In 200 adults with skeletal tuberculosis examined by Feldman et al.,[2] 10 occurred in the hand distal to the wrist. Generally speaking, tuberculous dactylitis is more frequent in children, while wrist tuberculosis is more common in adults. However, both conditions can be seen in all age groups. Of 95 tuberculous cases in the wrist and hand examined by Robins,[8] there were 17 cases of dactylitis. Of these, nine were in children.

Tuberculosis of the Wrist

There is some relationship between tuberculous synovitis — the so-called com-

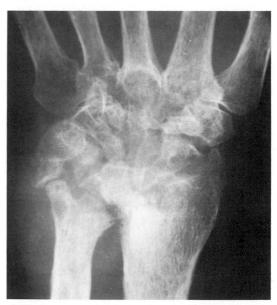

Figure 14–8. Tuberculosis of a wrist. A 73 year old male presented with a painless swelling. There is extensive demineralization, loss of bony margins and destruction of articular surfaces of the carpals. The whole carpus is diminished in size. There are also scattered radiolucencies in the radius and ulna.

pound palmar ganglion — and cases of wrist tuberculosis. In 29 patients with "compound palmar ganglia" of the hand due to tuberculosis seen by Pimm and Waugh,[6] six developed infection of the wrist. On the

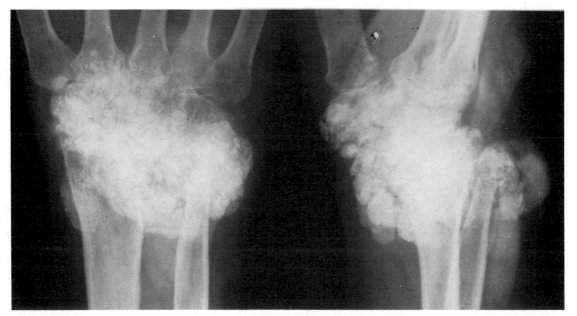

Figure 14–9. Tuberculosis of the wrist from tuberculous synovitis. Extensive soft tissue calcification about the wrist partially obscures the destructive process in the carpus. The radius and ulna are separated from each other and the ulna is displaced dorsally. This is a late phase of tuberculosis.

other hand, other authors suggest that wrist involvement is usually not associated with synovitis.[3]

The first radiologic sign of tuberculosis in the wrist may be simply a soft tissue swelling. Osteoporosis usually follows and corresponds to synovial involvement. After several months there may be early bone destruction which results in an appearance, as described by Hodgson and Smith, "like nibbling of cheese." Usually all of carpals are affected since the intercarpal joints communicate with each other. This is followed by narrowing of the joint spaces (Fig. 14–8). Once bone involvement in the wrist has occurred, the findings are usually permanent. The healing phase is associated with some recalcification, and in some instances there may be secondary new bone formation and fusion of the carpals. If the lesion is secondarily infected, the new bone formation can be excessive. Calcification in the lesion (Fig. 14–9), particularly in abscesses, may also be seen in the healing phase. In the early stages, tuberculosis of the wrist may be confused with rheumatoid arthritis. However, unlike rheumatoid arthritis, the wrist involvement in tuberculosis is usually monarticular.

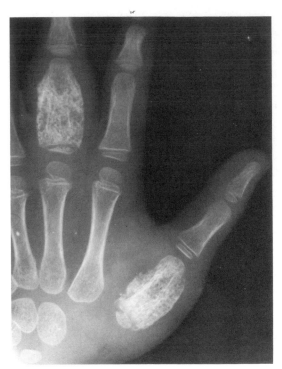

Figure 14–11. Tuberculosis with exuberant periosteal reaction. This is a juvenile form of tuberculosis. The involved bones are markedly expanded. The shadow of the old bone is seen within this exuberant bone production. The epiphyses are relatively uninvolved. (Courtesy Dr. H. H. Brueckner, Canton, Ohio.)

Tuberculous Dactylitis

Tuberculous dactylitis is more frequent in children than in adults. Tuberculous dactylitis has, however, also been described in adults.[2] It may be multiple, particularly during childhood. The radiographic findings in the adult dactylitis may be different from those in the childhood dactylitis. According to Feldman et al.,[2] pathologic fractures are more common in adults than in children. Fistula formation, sequestrum formation, expansion of bone (spina ventosa), involvement of multiple bones and positive chest roentgenograms are more common in children than in adults.

Soft tissue swelling is usually the first finding and can be quite extensive. It may be the sole finding for a long time. Periosteal elevation can be seen in both children and adults (Fig. 14–10). This may be minor, or it may be very exuberant (Fig. 14–11), particularly when associated with a destructive lesion. Expansion of bone

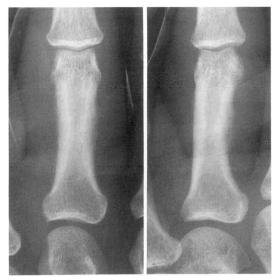

Figure 14–10. Tuberculosis, postinjury. There is minimal periosteal elevation along both sides of the proximal phalanx. There is considerable soft tissue swelling. No definite destruction is seen. Aspiration of the lesion revealed tuberculous bacilli both on smear and guinea pig inoculation. (Courtesy Dr. W. Reynolds, Henry Ford Hospital, Detroit, Michigan.)

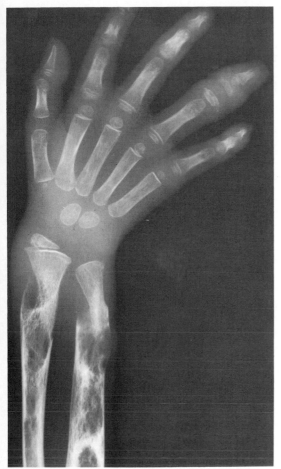

Figure 14–12. Tuberculosis with cystic lesions. There is an extensive destructive process in the fourth middle phalanx and in the radius and ulna.

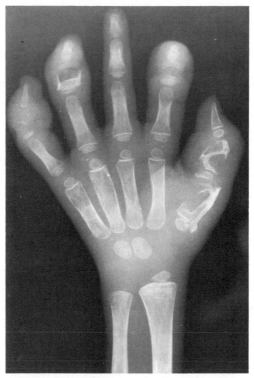

Figure 14–13. Spina ventosa from tuberculosis. Multiple cyst-like lesions are evident in many of the bones. There is some expansion of the metacarpals, with radiolucency within them. There is considerable soft tissue swelling. (Film is lightly retouched.) (Courtesy Dr. H. Brueckner, Canton, Ohio.)

with a cystic-like lesion is particularly common in childhood and has been termed spina ventosa (Figs. 14–12 and 14–13). There may be dense stippling of bone within the lucent areas. The destructive foci are usually diaphyseal but may occasionally involve the epiphysis. Sequestrum formation is uncommon and sometimes is associated with small sinus tracts through which bony fragments may be extruded.[2] Epiphyseal involvement may result in disruption of normal growth and brachydactyly.

Occasionally, instead of focal lesions there may be a more permeative type of involvement, with demineralization which may be associated with pathologic fracture. These areas may be more similar to those seen in pyogenic osteomyelitis. Small localized lesions can also occur but are less common.[2]

For some reason, the prognosis for normal function in the cystic form, particularly in children, is usually better than in some of the other forms.[3]

The differential diagnosis of tuberculosis of the hand or wrist includes a number of entities, depending on the manifestations. Pyogenic infections, brucellosis and various fungal infections such as coccidioidomycosis may be confused with tuberculosis. Other mycobacteria can cause bone lesions similar to tuberculosis. Some of the cystic lesions in bone can be confused with bone tumor. The early tuberculous changes in the wrist may give the impression of rheumatoid arthritis.

REFERENCES

1. Cremin, B. J., Fisher, R. M., and Levinsohn, M. W.: Multiple Bone Tuberculosis in the Young. *Br. J. Radiol.*, 43:638–645, 1970.
2. Feldman, F., Auerbach, R., and Johnston, A.:

Tuberculous Dactylitis in the Adult. *Am. J. Roentgenol.* 112:460–479, 1971.

3. Hodgson, A. R., and Smith, T. K.: Tuberculosis of the Wrist. With a Note on "Chemotherapy." *Clin. Orthop.*, 83:73–83, 1972.
4. LaFond, E. M.: An Analysis of Adult Skeletal Tuberculosis. *J. Bone Joint Surg.*, 40A:346–364, 1958.
5. Nathanson, L., and Cohen, W.: A Statistical and Roentgen Analysis of Two Hundred Cases of Bone and Joint Tuberculosis. *Radiology*, 36: 550–567, 1941.
6. Pimm, L. H., and Waugh, W.: Tuberculous Tenosynovitis. *J. Bone Joint Surg.*, 39B:91–101, 1957.
7. Poppel, M. H., Lawrence, L. R., Jacobson, H. G., and Stein, J.: Skeletal Tuberculosis. A Roentgenographic Survey with Reconsideration of Diagnostic Criteria. *Am. J. Roentgenol.*, 70: 936–963, 1953.
8. Robins, R. H. C.: Tuberculosis of the Wrist and Hand. *Br. J. Surg.*, 54:211–218, 1967.
9. Sanchis-Olmos, V.: *Skeletal Tuberculosis.* The Williams & Wilkins Co., Baltimore, 1948.

OTHER MYCOBACTERIA

A variety of other mycobacteria besides *Mycobacterium tuberculosis* infect bone.

These comprise a number of species, including photochromogens, scotochromogens, nonchromogens and rapid growers.[4] An atypical mycobacterial osteomyelitis has been reported by Dalinka and Hemming[2] in a patient with acute lymphoblastic leukemia. *Mycobacterium marinum*, a rapidly growing photochromogen that infects cold-blooded animals, can also infect man. The infection is carried either from the bite of an infected animal or, more commonly, through skin abrasion or laceration.[4,6]

These organisms can produce focal bone lesions which are usually well defined and often have a sclerotic margin. They are frequently multiple, involving many bones of the body, including the hands and feet. They can produce a variety of other lesions, such as expansile processes or periosteal reaction (Fig. 14–14) or destructive joint lesions. Their appearance is not specific: they may resemble tuberculosis or other inflammatory diseases, or they may be confused with rheumatoid arthritis or gout.[6]

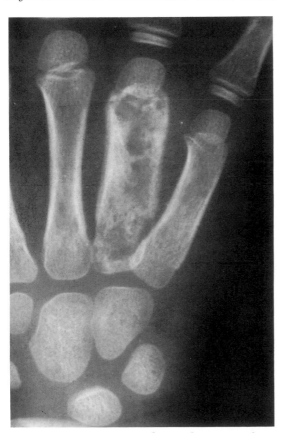

Figure 14–14. Atypical mycobacteria. There is a destructive lesion in the fourth metacarpal with evidence of bony expansion. (Courtesy Dr. I. Krieger. Reproduced with permission from *J. Pediatr.*, 65:340–349, 1964.)

REFERENCES

1. Cortez, L. M., and Pankey, G. A.: *Mycobacterium marinum* Infections of the Hand. Report of Three Cases and Review of the Literature. *J. Bone Joint Surg.*, 55A:363–370, 1973.
2. Dalinka, M. K., and Hemming, V. G.: Atypical Mycobacterial Osteomyelitis. Report of a Case Associated with Acute Lymphoblastic Leukemia. *J. Can. Assoc. Radiol.*, 22:173–175, 1971.
3. Danigelis, J. A., and Long, R. E.: Anonymous Mycobacterial Osteomyelitis. A Case Report of a Six-Year-Old Child. *Radiology*, 93:353–354 and 1084, 1969.
4. Heitzman, E. R., Bornhurst, R. A., and Russell, J. P.: Disease Due to Anonymous Mycobacteria. Potential for Specific Diagnosis. *Am. J. Roentgenol.*, 103:533–539, 1968.
5. Krieger, I., Hahne, O. H., and Whitten, C. F.: Atypical Mycobacteria as a Probable Cause of Chronic Bone Disease. A Report of two Cases. *J. Pediatr.*, 65:340–349, 1964.
6. Williams, C. S., and Riordan, D. C.: *Mycobacterium marinum* (Atypical Acid-Fast Bacillus) Infections of the Hand. A Report of Six Cases. *J. Bone Joint Surg.*, 55A:1042–1050, 1953.
7. Yakovac, W. C., Baker, R., Sweigert, C., and Hope, J. W.: Fatal Disseminated Osteomyelitis Due to an Anonymous Mycobacterium. *J. Pediatr.*, 59:909–914, 1961.

Leprosy (Hansen Disease)

Leprosy, although relatively rare in the United States, is present in the southern states of Texas, Louisiana and Florida. It has also been seen in California, Hawaii and New York City.[2] It is much more common in Africa, Asia and South America.

The disease is caused by *Mycobacterium leprae*, which appears to have a predilection for the cooler areas of the body;[2] thus, skin, nasal mucous membrane and the peripheral nerves of the extremities are involved. There may be some arterial involvement as well, which may be the cause of some of the roentgen findings.[1] This disorder may be seen in both adults and children. According to Newman et al.,[5] one-third of new cases occurred prior to age 15. It is twice as common in males as in females.

Radiologic changes are of two basic types. They may be specific, due to infection by *M. leprae*, or they may be secondary to trauma and infection in a denervated hand.

Specific bone lesions in leprosy are uncommon. They occur in 3 to 5 per cent of cases among hospitalized patients.[7] The initial radiographic findings are those of soft tissue swelling, sometimes associated with demineralization and with increased prominence of the vascular foramina. Destructive lesions in bone may be seen, and these appear to occur mainly in the ends of the bones, particularly the proximal and middle phalanges (Fig. 14–15). There may be a honeycomb or cystic appearance to the bone, and the bone may be prone to fracture. The destructive process in bone may lead to deviation of the digits, which may become permanent. Periostitis is sometimes seen.

Secondary changes may be due to trauma, or to infection in a denervated hand. A claw configuration of the hand is common, as is osteoporosis. Many of the radiologic changes may be similar to those seen in other neurotrophic conditions, such as congenital insensitivity to pain and syringomyelia. One of the classic features is absorption of the fingers, which have a "licked candystick" appearance; progression results in a fingerless hand (Fig. 14–16). This manifestation does not occur if the fingers are not used for grasping. Charcot-like joints may be seen about the wrist secondary to

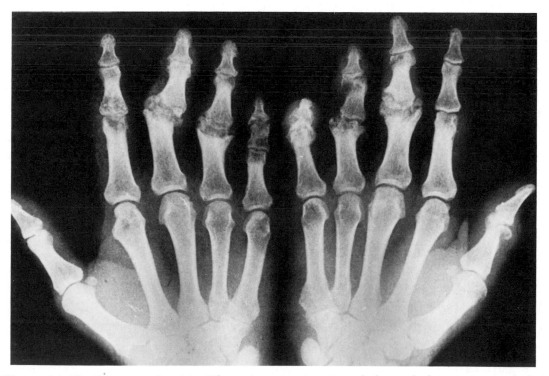

Figure 14–15. Leprosy. Osteitis. There is extensive interphalangeal destruction with bony erosions. There is considerable lucency in the fifth middle phalanx on the right. (Courtesy Dr. C. Enna. Reproduced with permission of *Radiology*, 100:295–306, 1971.)

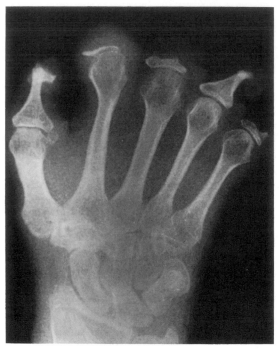

Figure 14–16. Leprosy. Neurotrophic changes. There is marked absorption of the fingers due to a denervated hand. These are the results of trauma and infection. (Courtesy Dr. C. Enna. Reproduced with permission from *Radiology*, 100:295–306, 1971.)

the neuropathy, and evidence of osteomyelitis and fractures may be noted. A rare finding in leprosy is nerve calcification.[8]

Arteriography has been performed in patients with leprosy.[1,7] In one case, Cave et al.[1] showed evidence of obstruction of the external collateral artery of the second and fourth fingers, and of the internal collateral artery of the fifth finger in a patient who had no definite bone involvement. It may be that the arterial changes in this disease are related to the resorption and other findings that occur. Whether these bone changes are due to specific arteritis or are themselves on the basis of neurotrophic change is not clear. Patterson[6] showed defects in the vascular end loops associated with bone absorption, as well as delays in venous emptying and evidence of venous shunting. In the presence of local, nonspecific infections, there may be dilatation of the vessels.

REFERENCES

1. Cave, L., Fustec, R., and Basset, A.: Radiologie de la Lepre. *Ann. Radiol.*, 8:61–76, 1965.

2. Enna, C. D., Jacobson, R. R., and Rausch, R. O.: Bone Changes in Leprosy: A Correlation of Clinical and Radiographic Features. *Radiology*, 100:295–306, 1971.
3. Esguerra-Gomez, G., and Acosta, E.: Bone and Joint Lesions in Leprosy. A Radiologic Study. *Radiology*, 50:619–638, 1948.
4. Faget, G. H.: Bone Changes in Leprosy: A Clinical and Roentgenologic Study of 505 Cases. *Radiology*, 42:1–13, 1944.
5. Newman, H., Casey, B., DuBois, J. J., and Gallaher, T.: Roentgen Features of Leprosy in Children. *Am. J. Roentgenol.*, 114:402–410, 1972.
6. Patterson, D. E.: Radiological Bone Changes and Angiographic Findings in Leprosy with Special Reference to the Pathogenesis of 'Atrophic' Conditions of the Digits. *J. Faculty of Radiol.*, 7:35–56, 1955.
7. Patterson, D. E.: Bone Changes in Leprosy. Their Incidence, Progress, Prevention and Arrest. *Int. J. Lepr.*, 29:393–422, 1961.
8. Trapnell, D. H.: Case reports. Calcification of Nerves in Leprosy. *Br. J. Radiol.*, 38:796–797, 1965.

FUNGAL INFECTIONS

The fungi causing hand infections include coccidioidomycosis, sporotrichosis, blastomycosis, actinomycosis, *Histoplasma duboisii* and mycetoma. These various infections may not have a very specific appearance (except perhaps for the mycetomas). They occur in different parts of the world and have a different degree of predilection for the bones of the hand.

Actinomycosis of Bone

Actinomycosis usually originates from the oral cavity and rarely involves the hand bones except through a bite from an affected individual.[2] Since actinomycosis may occur in the mouth without evidence of disease, the individual who causes the bite is not necessarily apparently affected. The reported cases of involvement in the hand have been summarized by Mendelsohn.[2] The radiologic appearance is that of a destructive lesion and appears nonspecific.

REFERENCES

1. Kanavel, A. R.: *Infections of the Hand. A Guide to the Surgical Treatment of Acute and Chronic Suppurative Processes in the Fingers, Hand and Forearm.* Lea and Febiger, Philadelphia, 1939.
2. Mendelsohn, B. G.: Actinomycosis of a Metacarpal Bone. Report of a Case. *J. Bone Joint Surg.*, 47B:739–742, 1965.

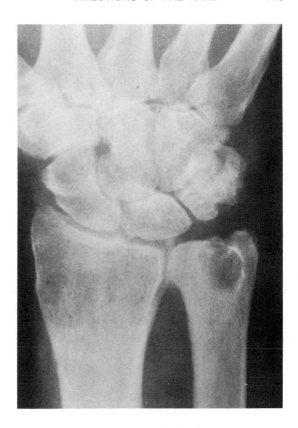

Figure 14-17. Blastomycosis. Destructive changes in the carpals and distal ulna are evident. (From Gehweiler, J., et al., Observations on the Roentgen Patterns in Blastomycosis of Bone. *American Journal of Roentgenology, Radium Therapy and Nuclear Medicine*, 108: 497–510, 1970. Courtesy Charles C Thomas, Publisher, Springfield, Illinois.)

Blastomycosis

Blastomycosis, or North American blastomycosis, is caused by infection directly from the soil which contains the fungus *Blastomyces dermatitidis.* In the United States it is found most commonly along the Ohio Valley, the Mississippi Valley and in the Middle Atlantic States, although it has been seen in other parts of the United States and in the remainder of the world.

The disease appears in two forms: a primary cutaneous form which has no significant radiologic manifestation, and a pulmonary, systemic or disseminated form which is associated with bone involvement. According to various series, 23 to 50 per cent of patients with blastomycosis develop skeletal involvement.[2] The hand is an uncommon site of bone involvement. In a series of 67 cases with 197 lesions, reviewed by Colonna and Gucker,[1] there were 10 cases with lesions in the carpus, 5 with lesions in the metacarpals and 3 with lesions in the phalanges. In the series of Gehweiler et al.,[2] a similar incidence

was found, with 5.6 per cent of the lesions in the carpus and 2.2 per cent in the metacarpals.

The radiologic appearance of the disease is variable. In the carpal bones there may be sharply defined cystic-like areas with sclerotic margins and with little joint involvement (Fig. 14–17). Multiple carpal bones may be involved. Occasionally a diffuse destructive process may be seen with less well-defined margins. In the tubular bones the destruction may be well defined or diffuse, mimicking osteomyelitis or tumor.[3]

REFERENCES

1. Colonna, P. C., and Gucker, T.: Blastomycosis of the Skeletal System. A Summary of Sixty-Seven Recorded Cases and a Case Report. *J. Bone Joint Surg.*, 26:322–328, 1944.
2. Gehweiler, J. A., Capp, M. P., and Chick, E. W.: Observations on the Roentgen Patterns in Blastomycosis of Bone. A Review of Cases from the Blastomycosis Cooperative Study of the Veterans Administration and Duke University

Medical Center. *Am. J. Roentgenol.*, 108: 497–510, 1970.
3. Gelman, M. I., and Everts, C. S.: Blastomycotic Dactylitis. *Radiology*, 107:331–332, 1973.

Coccidioidomycosis

This is a disorder caused by the fungus *Coccidioides immitis.* The disseminated form of the disease is relatively uncommon, but when it does occur, approximately 20 per cent of patients have osseous lesions.[1] The fungus is endemic to the southwestern United States and also to Central and South America. The hands are uncommonly involved. One patient of 14 reported by Dalinka et al.[1] had involvement of a phalanx. The lesions in the hands and feet have poorly defined borders and have the appearance of an inflammatory process with soft tissue swelling, destruction of bone and periosteal reaction (Fig. 14–18). The appearance is not particularly specific.

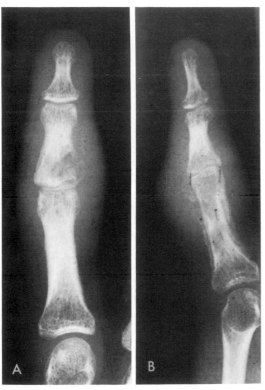

Figure 14–18. Coccidioidomycosis. *A*, A poorly defined destructive focus is seen in the middle phalanx of the index finger. There is considerable soft tissue reaction about it.

B, Periosteal reaction in the proximal phalanx of the fifth finger is associated with some bony destruction. (Courtesy Dr. M. K. Dalinka. Reproduced with permission from *J. Bone Joint Surg.*, 53A:1159, 1971.)

REFERENCES

1. Dalinka, M. K., Dinnenberg, S., Greendyke, W. H., and Hopkins, R.: Roentgenographic Features of Osseous Coccidioidomycosis and Differential Diagnosis. *J. Bone Joint Surg.*, 53A:1157–1164, 1971.
2. Miller, D., and Birsner, J. W.: Coccidioidal Granuloma of Bone. *Am. J. Roentgenol.*, 62:229–236, 1949.
3. Rosen, R. S., and Jacobson, G.: Fungus Disease of Bone. *Sem. Roentgenol.*, 1:370–391, 1966.
4. Sashin, D., Brown, G. N., Laffer, N. C., and McDowell, H. C.: Disseminated Coccidioidomycosis Localized in Bone. *Am. J. Med Sci.*, 212: 565–573, 1946.

Sporotrichosis

This is a relatively rare granulomatous fungus infection caused by *Sporotrichum schenckii.* It is endemic in the Mississippi Valley but has been seen everywhere in the United States and in the remainder of the world. The fungus is a saprophyte on plants, flowers, trees and so forth. The usual mode of infection is through a minor skin wound. Altner and Turner in 1970 reviewed the literature on 24 cases of bone and joint involvement, concluding that in these and in their own cases hand and wrist involvement occurred in 21 per cent of patients. The source of the bone involvement was thought to be dissemination through the blood stream. The infection is chronic.

The radiologic findings of this disorder are variable. The lesions may involve either the bone or the joint. The bone lesions, when present, are multiple, lytic and destructive (Fig. 14–19). The appearance may be similar either to tuberculosis or to pyogenic osteomyelitis. Sporotrichosis is more chronic than pyogenic osteomyelitis. Soft tissue swelling is commonly present. Periosteal reaction may also be seen. The wrist joint may be involved, with carpal bone destruction.

REFERENCES

1. Altner, P. C., and Turner, R. R.: Sporotrichosis of Bones and Joints. Review of the Literature and Report of Six Cases. *Clin. Orthop.*, 68:138–148, 1970.
2. DeHaven, K. E., Wilde, A. H., and O'Duffy, J. D.: Sporotrichosis Arthritis and Tenosynovitis. Report of a Case Cured by Synovectomy and Amphotericin B. *J. Bone Joint Surg.*, 54A:874–877, 1972.
3. Winter, T. Q., and Pearson, K. D.: Systemic Sporotrichosis. *Radiology*, 104:579–583, 1972.

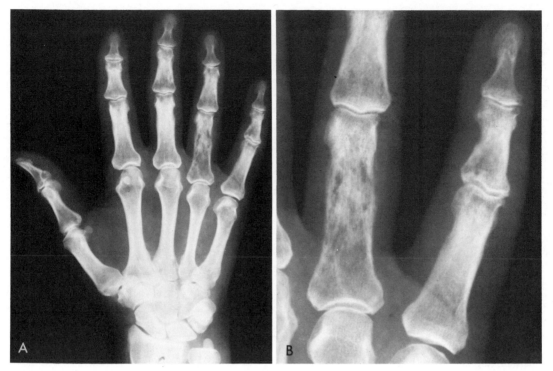

Figure 14–19. Sporotrichosis. A, There is an ill-defined destructive process in the proximal phalanx of the fourth finger, and there is a break in the cortex along the ulnar margin. The middle phalanx of the fifth finger is also involved. This appearance is somewhat atypical of the process.
  B, Close-up view of patient illustrated in A. The destructive lesion in the fourth proximal phalanx is well seen.

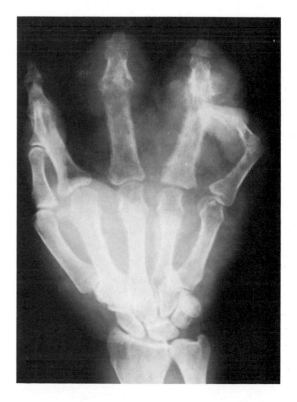

Figure 14–20. Mycetoma of the hand from *Nocardia brasiliensis.* There is gross soft tissue swelling of the hand with irregular destruction of several of the hand bones. There is also flexion deformity of the hand. Some periosteal reaction is seen in the region of the metacarpals. (Film from Ibadan, Nigeria, courtesy Dr. P. Cockshott, Hamilton, Ontario, Canada.)

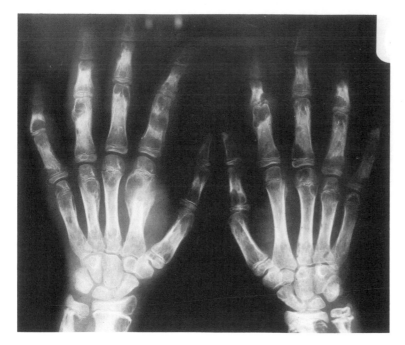

Figure 14-21. Histoplasma duboisii. Both hands are involved by an extensive process of multiple lytic areas which are predominantly metaphyseal. There is some deviation of the digits as the result of the lesions. Considerable periosteal new bone formation is seen in the second metacarpal. (Film from Ibadan, Nigeria, courtesy Dr. P. Cockshott, Hamilton, Ontario, Canada.)

Mycetoma

Mycetoma represents a group of conditions caused by a variety of fungi, including various Actinomycetaceae and Fungi Imperfecti. The lesion most commonly involves the foot but has been seen in the hand.[1] One of the organisms causing this in Ibadan, Nigeria, is *Nocardia brasiliensis.*

Radiographically there is a soft tissue swelling and edema with loss of the fat planes. Eventually there are bone changes with periosteal reaction. Bone involvement can be extensive, with patchy involvement of multiple bones of the hand (Fig. 14-20).

REFERENCES

1. Abbott, P.: Mycetoma in the Sudan. *Trans. R. Soc. Trop. Med. Hyg.,* 50:11–24, 1956.
2. Cockshott, W. P.: Dactylitis and Growth Disorders. *Brit. J. Radiol.,* 36:19–26, 1963.
3. Cockshott, W.P.: Mycetoma. *IN:* Middlemiss, H.: *Tropical Radiology.* Intercontinental Medical Book Corp., Bristol, Great Britain, Chap. IV, pp. 38–48.
4. MacKinnon, J. E., and Artagaveytia-Allende, R. C.: The Main Species of Pathogenic Aerobic Actinomycetes Causing Mycetomas. *Trans. R. Soc. Trop. Med. Hyg.,* 50:31–40, 1956.

Histoplasma duboisii Dactylitis

This is a fungus which occurs in Africa but which differs in its manifestations from the *H. capsulatum.* The hand may be involved as part of a general systemic disease. There may be numerous sites of destruc-

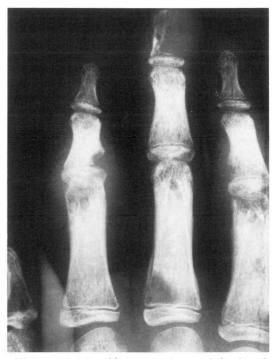

Figure 14-22. Close-up of one of the hands shown in Figure 14-21. The metaphyseal punched-out lesions are more clearly seen, as is the periosteal elevation. The tuft of the distal phalanx of the third finger is destroyed. (Film from Ibadan, Nigeria, courtesy Dr. P. Cockshott, Hamilton, Ontario, Canada.)

tion in the phalanges and metacarpals (Figs. 14–21 and 14–22). The lesions are predominantly metaphyseal and may be well defined.

REFERENCE

1. Cockshott, W. P.: Dactylitis and Growth Disorders. *Brit. J. Radiol.*, 36:19–26, 1963.

OTHER INFECTIONS AND INFESTATIONS

Syphilis

Syphilitic infection may be of the congenital or acquired variety. The hand is not commonly affected except when involvement is most diffuse. In the congenital form the predominant appearance is metaphysitis with destructive foci in the region of the metaphysis (Fig. 14–23). There may be periosteal changes as well. The findings in the hand are similar to those seen in the remainder of the body but usually to a less marked degree.

Acquired syphilis rarely involves the bones of the hand, although chancres on the fingers have been described from human bites; osseous involvement of the hand bones is relatively uncommon.

REFERENCES

1. Boyes, J. H.: *Bunnell's Surgery of the Hand*, 5th ed. J. B. Lippincott Co., Philadelphia, 1970.
2. Caffey, J.: Syphilis of the Skeleton in Early Infancy. The Nonspecificity of Many of the Roentgenographic Changes. *Am. J. Roentgenol.*, 42:637–655, 1939.
3. Cremin, B. J., and Fisher, R. M.: The Lesions of Congenital Syphilis. *Br. J. Radiol.*, 43:333–341, 1970.
4. McLean, S.: Part IV. The Correlation of the Clinical Picture with the Osseous Lesions of Congenital Syphilis as Shown by the X-Rays. *Am. J. Dis. Child.*, 41:1128–1171, 1931.

Yaws

This is a disease occurring in the tropics. It has been seen in Africa and Australia. It

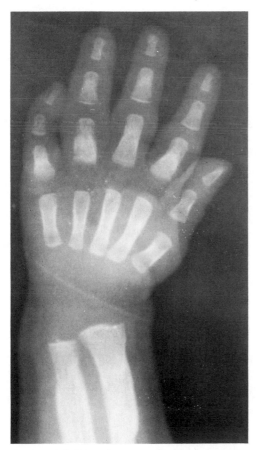

Figure 14–23. Congenital syphilis. Some periosteal cloaking is seen in the radius and ulna. There is also some periostitis and metaphysitis in the proximal phalanx of the fourth finger.

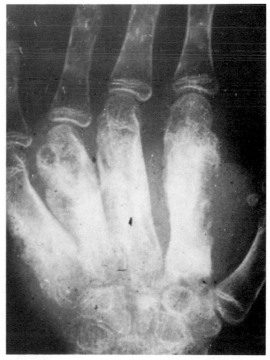

Figure 14–24. Yaws dactylitis involving the metacarpals. There is extensive thickening of the bone and bone sclerosis. (Film from Ibadan, Nigeria, courtesy Dr. P. Cockshott, Hamilton, Ontario, Canada. Reproduced with permission from *Br. J. Radiol.*, 36:19–26, 1963.)

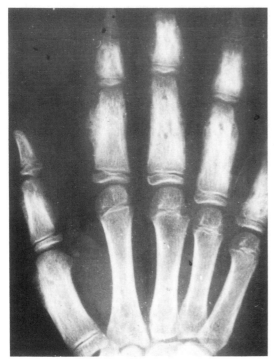

Figure 14-25. Yaws. Extensive protuberant periostitis in some of the phalanges. Radiolucent areas are also seen within the bones. (Film courtesy Dr. P. Cockshott, Hamilton, Ontario, Canada. Reproduced with permission from *Br. J. Radiol.*, 36:19–26, 1963.)

is related to syphilis and is caused by *Treponema pertenue.* The organism is very closely related to the causative organism of syphilis and cannot be reliably distinguished. The disease is acquired by contact, usually extragenital. The lesions occur commonly in children, usually beginning at the end of the first decade.

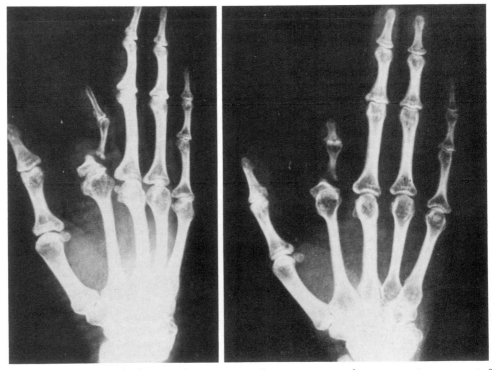

Figure 14-26. Yaws, with doigt en lorgnette configuration secondary to previous yaws infection. (Film courtesy Dr. B. S. Jones. Reproduced with permission from *J. Bone Joint Surg.*, 54B:341–345, 1972.)

The bone lesions are seen in the secondary and tertiary forms of this disorder. The associated dactylitis is seen particularly in the secondary form (Figs. 14–24 and 14–25). The bone lesions are similar to those of syphilis with foci of destruction, periosteal changes and osteitis. Generally, only the tubular bones are involved and the carpals are spared.[1] The distal phalanges are usually not involved.

Most of the osseous lesions resolve rapidly with therapy. However, growth disturbances may occur, resulting in shortening of the digits. An extreme example is called doigt en lorgnette, in which the digits are shortened and the skin is redundant, so that the digits can be pulled out to their full length. Jones[4] reported such a case (Fig. 14–26).

Radiologically, differentiation from syphilis is difficult except that the bone involvement in the hand appears greater than is usually expected in syphilis.

REFERENCES

1. Cockshott, W. P.: Dactylitis and Growth Disorders. Brit. J. Radiol., 36:19–26, 1963.
2. Davies, A. G.: Yaws. IN: Middlemiss, H.: Tropical Radiology. Intercontinental Medical Book Corp., Bristol, Great Britain, 1961, Chap. II, pp. 18–26.
3. Goldmann, C. H., and Smith, S. J.: X-Ray Appearance of Bone in Yaws. Brit. J. Radiol., 16: 234–238, 1943.
4 Jones, B. S.: Doigt en Lorgnette and Concentric Bone Atrophy Associated with Healed Yaws Osteitis. J. Bone Joint Surg., 54B:341–345, 1972.
5. Riseborough, A. W., Joske, R. A., and Vaughan, B. F.: Hand Deformities Due to Yaws in Western Australian Aborigines. Clin. Radiol., 12: 109–113, 1961.

Smallpox (Osteomyelitis Variolosa)

Osteitis and metaphysitis have been seen in association with smallpox, particularly in Africa. The elbow is most often affected, and the hands are the next most frequent site of involvement.[3] The radiographic findings include marked periosteal reaction, transverse destruction of the metacarpals or phalanges and epiphyseal changes. The appearance is rather nonspecific. From histologic studies, Eeckels et al.[3] believed that the basic cause of the lesions was not actually an osteitis, but rather that the lesions were secondary to infarction from a proliferating arteritis that is associated with smallpox. Late films in children with

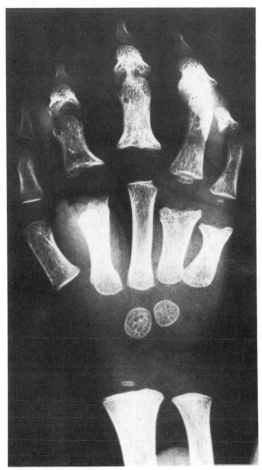

Figure 14–27. Late effects of smallpox dactylitis. There is widening of the bone, bizarre brachydactyly and cone-like epiphyses following smallpox one year previously. (Film from Ibadan, Nigeria, courtesy Dr. P. Cockshott, Hamilton, Ontario, Canada. Reproduced with permission from *Br. J. Radiol.*, 36:19–26, 1963.)

previous smallpox dactylitis show marked deformity of the hand bones with splayed metaphyses and brachydactyly (Fig. 14–27) in a pattern which may also be seen with other causes of vascular phenomena. The cone-like configuration of the ends of the bone also corresponds with the possibility of a vascular lesion.

Harley and Gillespie[4] reported a case of shortening of a digit following congenital vaccinia. It seems possible that this also had a vascular basis.

REFERENCES

1. Cockshott, W. P.: Dactylitis and Growth Disorders. Brit. J. Radiol., 36:19–26, 1963.

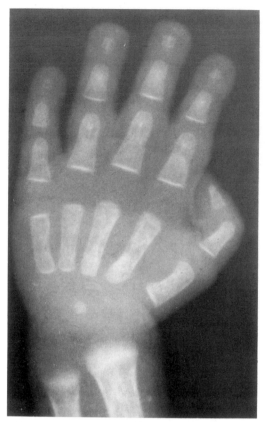

Figure 14–28. Rubella osteitis. There are some ill-defined mottled areas of bone density in the phalanges and metacarpals. They are somewhat linear in configuration. (More definite rubella lesions were seen elsewhere.) These are late changes and were not present at birth. They probably represent the healing phase of the disease.

2. Cockshott, W. P., and MacGregor, M.: The Natural History of Osteomyelitis Variolosa. *J. Faculty Radiol.*, 10:57–63, 1959.
3. Eeckels, R., Vincent, J., and Seynhaeve, V.: Bone Lesions due to Smallpox. *Arch. Dis. Child.* 39:591–597, 1964.
4. Harley, J. D., and Gillespie, A. M.: A Complicated Case of Congenital Vaccinia. *Pediatrics*, 50: 150–153, 1972.

Other Viruses

Viral bone changes are relatively uncommon. Localized osteolytic lesions occurring in parts of the skeleton other than the hands have been reported in cat-scratch disease[1, 2] and in lymphogranuloma venereum.[6] There is some controversy over whether infantile cortical hyperostosis may also have a viral cause, although there is no definite evidence of this. The viruses of rubella cause bony changes, but these rarely involve the hands (Fig. 14–28).[3–5] Similarly, the changes of cytomegalovirus may be seen in the femora but are rarely seen in the hands.

REFERENCES

1. Adams, W. C., and Hindman, S. M.: Cat-Scratch Disease Associated with an Osteolytic Lesion. *J. Pediatr.*, 44:665–669, 1954.
2. Collipp, P. J., and Koch, R.: Cat-Scratch Fever Associated with an Osteolytic Lesion. *New Eng. J. Med.*, 260:278–280, 1959.
3. Poole, C. A., Greenberg, L. A., and Mackey, E. A.: The Late Osseous Manifestations of the Rubella Syndrome: A Case Report and Discussion. *J. Assoc. Canad. Radiol.*, 17:206–210, 1966.
4. Rabinowitz, J. G., Wolf, B. S., Greenberg, E. I., and Rausen, A. R.: Osseous Changes in Rubella Embryopathy. *Radiology*, 85:494–500, 1965.
5. Singleton, E. B., Rudolph, A. J., Rosenberg, H. S., and Singer, D. B.: The Roentgenographic Manifestations of the Rubella Syndrome in Newborn Infants. *Am. J. Roentgenol.*, 97:82–91, 1966.
6. Wright, L. T., and Logan, M.: Osseous Changes Associated with Lymphogranuloma Venereum. *Arch. Surg.*, 39:108–121, 1939.

Seal Finger (Blubber Finger)

Seal finger is an infection which occurs when men slaughter or skin seals. The etiologic agent has not been identified. It enters through a break in the skin. Symptoms include exquisite pain and swelling.

Radiologic findings are minimal. The main finding is a localized demineralization. In 23 cases subjected to radiograms, nine had definite findings. There is evidence of arthritis, which is equally common in the distal and the proximal interphalangeal joints. The metacarpophalangeal joint is almost never involved.

REFERENCES

1. Candolin, Y.: Seal Finger (Spekkfinger) and its Occurrence in the Gulfs of the Baltic Sea. *Acta Chir. Scand.*, Suppl. 177, pp. 7–51, 1953.
2. Skinner, J. S.: Seal Finger. The Report of an Occupational Disease Rare in the United States. *Arch. Dermatol.*, 75:559–561, 1957.

Parasitic Infestations of the Hand

A number of parasites may produce radiographic findings in the hand. Most of these occur in other parts of the world and are not seen in the United States.

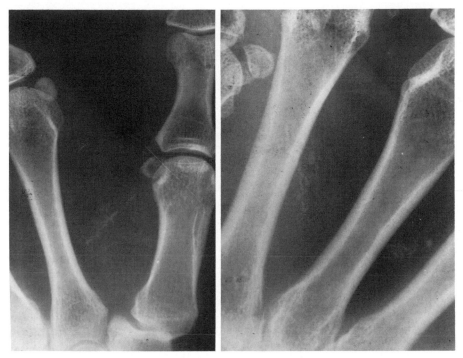

Figure 14–29. *Loa loa.* Calcified parasite is seen in the soft tissues of the hand. (Courtesy Dr. S. Bohrer, Ibadan, Nigeria.)

The filaria *Loa loa* or African eyeworm may cause characteristic radiologic changes. This parasite is endemic to West Africa. Man is infected through the bite of the mango fly, which deposits the infective larvae in the victim's skin. These larvae burrow subcutaneously, where they mature and then produce microfilaria which enter the blood. The migrating adult worms may be seen beneath the skin, and there may be associated soft tissue swelling.

The mature parasites are 3 to 6 cm. in length and less than 0.5 mm. in width. The dead worms commonly calcify (Fig. 14–29) and may be visible on hand radiographs. The characteristic radiologic appearance is a curvilinear small calcification in the soft tissues. Another pattern occasionally seen is a denser calcification, which may represent a capsule around the dead worm.

The guinea worm *(Dracunculus medinensis)* is another parasite which is common in Africa and which may be associated with soft tissue calcification. The mature female worm calcifies after death, producing a longer serpiginous calcification, which is seen much more frequently in the lower than in the upper extremities. It is longer and thicker than *Loa loa.* If death of the worm occurs near a joint, there may be an associated joint effusion or a secondary pyogenic arthritis.

Cysticercosis due to the larval form of the pork tapeworm *Taenia solium* can also cause calcification in the soft tissues. These calcifications are dense, well-defined, rice-grain–shaped opacities and are also less frequently seen in the hands than in other parts of the body.

Filariasis, caused by *Wuchereria bancrofti,* again affects the lower extremities more frequently than the upper extremities. The main radiographic findings are swelling of the soft tissues with marked lymphedema.

REFERENCES

1. Abukhalil, J. M.: Radiography of the Dracunculus Medinensis, the Medina worm. *Radiography,* 37:173–177, 1971.
2. Brailsford, J. F.: Cysticercus Cellulosae – Its Radiographic Detection in the Musculature and the Central Nervous System. *Br. J. Radiol.,* 14: 79–93, 1941.
3. Khajavi, A.: Guinea Worm Calcification: A Report of 83 Cases. *Clin. Radiol.,* 19:433–435, 1968.
4. Reeder, M. M.: Tropical Diseases of the Soft Tissues. *Sem. Roentgenol,* 8:47–71, 1973.
5. Samuel, E.: Roentgenology of Parasitic Calcification. *Am. J. Roentgenol.,* 63:512–522, 1950.
6. Williams, I.: Calcification in Loiasis. *J. Faculty of Radiologists,* 6:142–144, 1954.

Chapter 15

NEOPLASMS AND TUMOR-LIKE CONDITIONS OF THE HAND

Tumors of the hand can arise from any tissue within it. Bone tumors, although of more radiologic interest, are considerably less common than tumors of the soft tissue components. This is borne out by several large series of hand tumors.[1, 2, 4, 7, 10] The benign bone tumors are more common than malignant ones,[1, 6, 8] and they will be discussed first. The most common benign bone tumors occurring in the hand are enchondromas and osteochondromas. However, most of the other benign bone tumors have also been described within the hand. Some tumor-like conditions will be considered, in particular the common epidermoid cyst, but also the rarer hemophilia pseudo-

tumors, the thorn granulomas and the lesions of myositis ossificans.

Soft tissue tumors are also mostly benign and include the most common hand tumors, the ganglia, as well as xanthomas of tendon sheaths, mucous cysts and glomus tumors.[5] Some of these involve bone and present distinct radiologic findings.

Malignant bone tumors are most uncommon in the hand, but malignant soft tissue tumors are more common if one includes skin cancers.

The radiologic diagnosis of bone tumors of the hand is based on criteria similar to those used elsewhere within the skeleton. Our ability to make the diagnosis is based on knowing the relative incidence of certain roentgen signs in each of the tumors. This approach can be computerized, as Lodwick[5] has done. The factors that enter into making the diagnosis include the age and sex of the patient and the location of the lesion, including which bone and which portion of the bone is involved. Diagnosis is also dependent on the degree of mineralization within the tumor and the presence or absence of a small mass outside the bone. The extent and character of the destructive process, including the sharpness and definition of its margins, the type and degree of bone reaction about the tumor and the character of the periosteal reaction, are factors in the evaluation of the rate of growth of the mass. The appearance of the periosteal reaction varies considerably with tumors and may occur in benign disease. A solid periosteal reaction has implications different from those of an interrupted periosteal reaction.[3]

Since the hand is an uncommon site of bone tumors, typical patterns in the hand bones may be poorly defined, and thus differential diagnosis may be more difficult than in other areas of the body. A biopsy of the lesion is usually necessary for confirmation.

Of particular interest where tumors of the hand are concerned are the defects in the distal phalanges. The most common tumor producing such defects is the epidermoid cyst, which accounted for 11 of 35 cases examined by Schajowicz et al.[9] The next most common is the enchondroma. Other lesions which involve the distal phalanx and which can produce a lytic process are the glomus tumors, osteoid osteomas, aneurysmal bone cysts and, occasionally, those due to invasion from a metastatic tumor. Primary malignant processes of the distal phalanges are exceedingly rare; a Ewing's tumor is illustrated in Figure 15–40. Subungual carcinoma and keratoacanthomas can also involve the distal phalanx (Figs. 15–44 and 15–45).

REFERENCES

1. Boyes, J. H.: *Bunnell's Surgery of the Hand*, 5th ed. J. B. Lippincott Co., Philadelphia, 1970.
2. Butler, E. D., Hamill, J. P., Seipel, R. S., and de Lorimier, A. A.: Tumors of the Hand. A Ten-Year Survey and Report of 437 Cases. *Am. J. Surg.*, 100:293–302, 1960.
3. Edeiken, J., Hodes, P. J., and Caplan, L. H.: New Bone Production and Periosteal Reaction. *Am. J. Roentgenol.*, 97:708–718, 1966.
4. Kendall, T. E., Robinson, D. W., and Masters, F. W.: Primary Malignant Tumors of the Hand. *Plast. Reconstr. Surg.*, 44:37–40, 1969.
5. Lodwick, G. S.: *Atlas of Tumor Radiology. The Bones and Joints.* Year Book Medical Publishers, Inc., Chicago, 1971.
6. Mangini, U.: Tumors of the Skeleton of the Hand. *Bull. Hosp. Joint Dis.*, 28:61–103, 1967.
7. Posch, J. L.: Tumors of the Hand. *J. Bone Joint Surg.*, 38A:517–540 and 562, 1956.
8. Salib, P. I.: Tumors of the Bones of the Hand. *Am. J. Orthop. Surg.*, 8:114–121, 1966.
9. Schajowicz, F., Aiello, C. L., and Slullitel, I.: Cystic and Pseudocystic Lesions of the Terminal Phalanx with Special Reference to Epidermoid Cysts. *Clin. Orthop.*, 68:84–92, 1970.
10. Stack, H. G.: Tumours of the Hand. *Br. Med. J.*, I:919–922, 1960.
11. Woods, J. E., Murray, J. E., and Vawter, G. F.: Hand Tumors in Children. *Plast. Reconstr. Surg.*, 46:130–139, 1970.

EPIDERMOID CYST

Epidermoid cysts are lesions probably caused by implantation of epidermal tissue which then grows into a cyst. They are usually located in the distal phalanx of any one of the fingers. Occasionally they have been seen in stumps of other phalanges after amputation. They vary in size from about one to 20 mm. The cysts are probably secondary to previous trauma, which may be either a crush or a penetrating injury. The cysts contain flaky, keratinous debris and are lined with squamous epithelium with a well-defined granulosa layer. They are seen in individuals whose fingers are prone to trauma, such as tailors and machinists.

The symptoms of epidermoid cysts include pain, which may be intermittent or continuous and which has usually been present for several years. The lesions most often appear many years after the initial injury. The finger may be increased in size and there may be some curving of the nail.

Radiologically, the cysts present as a lucent defect in the distal portion of the distal phalanx of the digits (Fig. 15–1). They usually involve the region of the tuft. The margins of the lesion may be sclerotic, or there may be no reactive sclerosis about the lucency. No calcification is seen within the mass. Although many of the cysts are

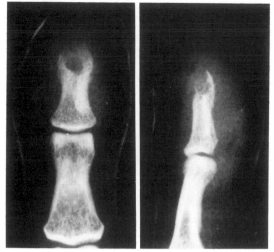

Figure 15–1. Epidermoid cyst. Distal phalanx of a 45 year old woman who drove a needle through it one year previously. There is a lucent defect in the distal phalanx with very little reaction about it. The lesion has broken the cortex along the dorsal and distal aspect. Enostosis along a margin of the shaft of the phalanx is probably unrelated. (Courtesy Dr. E. Krufky, Hartford, Connecticut.)

intraosseous in their appearance, occasionally they seem to erode the finger extrinsically (Fig. 15–2). This is probably due to cysts that arose in the subcutaneous tissues away from the bone.

The differential diagnosis includes enchondromas, which are usually located nearer to the epiphyseal area and may contain some calcification. The lesion may be indistinguishable from a glomus tumor except on clinical grounds. Other destructive lesions in the phalanges, such as metastases, must also be considered.

REFERENCES

1. Byers, P., Mantle, J., and Ralm, R.: Epidermal Cysts of Phalanges. *J. Bone Joint Surg.*, 48B:577–581, 1966.
2. Feulner, R. C., and Marks, J. L.: Epidermoid (Epithelial) Cyst of the Hand. *Am. J. Roentgenol.*, 79:645–647, 1958.
3. Kelly, A. P., Jr., and Clifford, R. H.: Epidermoid Cysts of the Bony Phalanges. *Plast. Reconstr. Surg.*, 17:309–313, 1956.
4. Schajowicz, F., Aiello, C. L., and Slullitel, I.: Cystic and Pseudocystic Lesions of the Terminal Phalanx with Special Reference to Epidermoid Cysts. *Clin. Orthop.*, 68:84–92, 1970.
5. Sieracki, J. C., and Kelly, A. P., Jr.: Traumatic Epidermoid Cysts Involving Digital Bones. *A.M.A. Arch. Surg.*, 78:597–603, 1959.

TUMORS OF VASCULAR ORIGIN

There are a number of tumors of vascular origin which may arise in the hand. These include glomus tumors, hemangiomas of bone, the lesions of skeletal angiomatosis and soft tissue hemangiomas.

GLOMUS TUMOR

These are relatively rare tumors which arise in the neuromyoarterial glomus. The normal glomus is an end-organ apparatus with an arteriovenous anastomosis functioning without an intermediary capillary bed. It plays a role in the control of circulation through the skin and in temperature control.

The glomus tumor is a grossly soft, pink or purple mass, almost always less than one cm. in diameter and usually just a few millimeters in size. It is located most frequently in the subungual region and, next

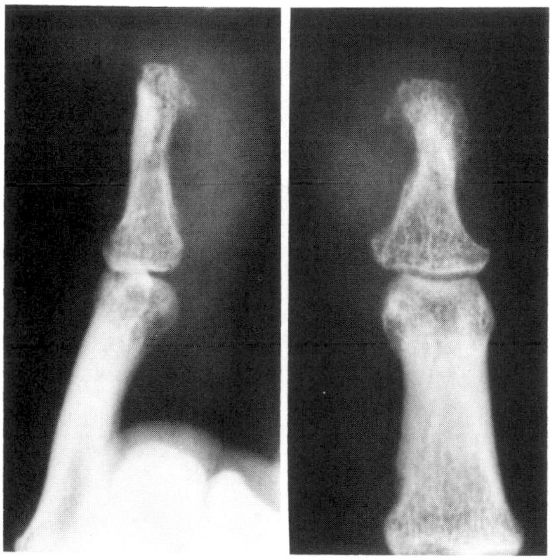

Figure 15–2. Epidermoid cyst. This 50 year old female had a sharp penetrating injury to her finger six months previously and had symptoms of a swollen, painful finger. Radiographically, there is erosion of the lateral aspect of the distal phalanx associated with a soft tissue mass. There is very little reactive bone around the lesion. (Courtesy Dr. E. Krufky, Hartford, Connecticut.)

most commonly, in the palmar lateral aspect of the distal phalanges. Occasionally it can occur in other portions of the hand, such as the palm or the hypothenar area. The subungual tumors in particular are much more common in females than in males.

The symptoms are severe pain, which may either occur for a long time or fluctuate. The area of the tumor is often very tender and is very sensitive to temperature changes, particularly to cold. There may be a visible mass appearing as an area of purple density in the subungual region. Initially the mass may not be visible. It becomes visible or palpable only after a considerable duration of symptoms. The tumors may occur at any age but are seen most often in patients between 30 and 50 years. Occasionally they are seen in children.

Radiologic findings are common. They were seen in 9 of 15 cases of Mathis and Schulz,[3] but in only 4 of 18 cases seen by Carroll and Berman.[1] There may be different types of bone erosion, ranging from a small concave defect (Fig. 15–3) to a sharply defined punched-out lesion seen in the region of the tuft of the phalanx (Fig. 15–4). There is often a thin, sclerotic margin about the defect.

Radiologically the defect can be easily confused with an epidermoid cyst. Usually

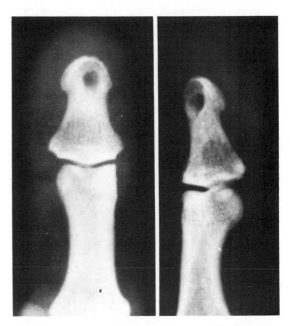

Figure 15–4. Glomus tumor. Under the thumbnail of this 42 year old female was a bluish discoloration that was painful to compression. A well-defined lucent defect is seen along the dorsal aspect of the tuft. (Courtesy Dr. E. Krufky, Hartford, Connecticut.)

its extrinsic origin can be detected and it can, therefore, be distinguished from enchondromas and other osseous lesions.

Mercier et al.[4] reported the use of angiography in the evaluation of these tumors. On angiograms there is evidence of hypervascularity, with rapid venous return and enlargement of the arterial supply to the tumor. There is also evidence of persistence of the contrast medium in the tumor. Angiography could be useful in diagnosing this condition, particularly in cases where tumor is suspected because of the severe pain but is not visible or palpable.

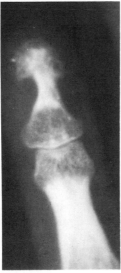

Figure 15–3. Glomus tumor. There is a slight erosion of the lateral aspect of the fourth distal phalanx. (Courtesy Dr. D. Louis, Ann Arbor, Michigan.)

REFERENCES

1. Carroll, R. E., and Berman, A. T.: Glomus Tumors of the Hand. Review of the Literature and Report on Twenty-Eight Cases. *J. Bone Joint Surg.*, 54A:691–703, 1972.
2. Fragiadakis, E. G., and Giannikas, A.: Glomus Tumour in the Fingers. *Hand*, 3:172–174, 1971.
3. Mathis, W. H., Jr., and Schulz, M. D.: Roentgen Diagnosis of Glomus Tumors. *Radiology*, 51: 71–76, 1948.
4. Mercier, R., Bresson, P., Viallet, J. F., and Vanneuville, G.: Intérêt de L Artériographie. Dans les

Tumeurs Glomiques Sous-Unguéales. *J. Radiol. Electrol. Med. Nucl.*, 51:303–304, 1970.
5. Varna, A., and Bojan, L.: Lésions Osseuses Dans les Tumeurs Glomiques Solitaires Chez Les Enfants. *Acta Orthop. Belg.*, 36:362–367, 1970.

HEMANGIOMA OF BONE, HEMANGIOENDOTHELIOMA, ANGIOMATOSIS OF BONE, LYMPHANGIOMATOSIS

Hemangiomas and hemangioendotheliomas of bone are lesions composed of blood vascular channels which may present in various patterns. Skeletal angiomatosis is the multicentric occurrence of vascular tumors of the skeletal system.

The hand is a very uncommon site of bone hemangiomas. Dahlin,[3] in a series of 47 bone hemangiomas, did not have a single case in the hand, nor did Sherman and Wilner[7] in 45 cases, although in the latter series two cases were located in the foot. Gutierrez and Spjut,[4] in a review of 36 cases of skeletal angiomatosis from the literature, found hand involvement in five.

The radiologic appearance of heman-

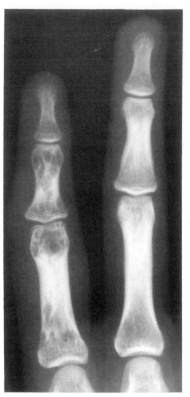

Figure 15–6. Hemangioma of the middle and proximal phalanges. Honeycomb-like structures, with ill-defined areas of radiolucency, are seen in both of these phalanges. The biopsy diagnosis was hemangioma.

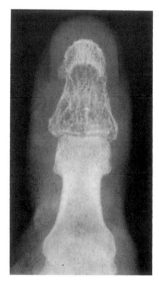

Figure 15–5. Hemangioma of the distal phalanx. The patient had a painful swelling of the distal phalanx of the thumb. A lucency within the distal phalanx involves most of the bone. The honeycomb pattern of the lesion is fairly characteristic of hemangioma. (Courtesy of Dr. W. Reynolds, Henry Ford Hospital, Detroit, Michigan.)

gioma in the hand is similar to its appearance in other tubular bones. There may be increased linear striations parallel to the shaft of the bone, occasionally having a honeycomb appearance (Fig. 15–5). Wide vascular channels in the bone with arteriovenous fistula may sometimes be seen, and were shown angiographically by Trifaud et al.[9] in a metacarpal angioma.

Multiple hemangiomas or multiple hemangioendotheliomas may have an appearance similar to the solitary lesion (Fig. 15–6), or they may be more actively destructive (Fig. 15–7). In cystic angiomatosis the lesions of the bones appear more lytic in nature, producing destructive lesions in many bones. They may mimic histiocytosis X. Cystic lymphangiectasis may also produce a similar appearance.

Rarely, skeletal hemangiomatoses may be associated with hereditary telangiectasia.

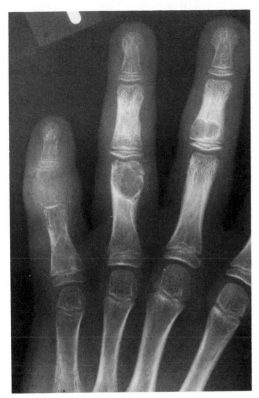

Figure 15-7. Multiple hemangioendotheliomas. There is a destructive lesion in the middle phalanx of the fifth finger which has almost completely destroyed the phalanx. Other lucent defects are seen in several other phalanges. A biopsy was made of the lesion in the middle phalanx, and the consensus of several pathologists was that the defect represented a hemangioendothelioma. (Courtesy Dr. M. Ozonoff, Newington, Connecticut.)

REFERENCES

1. Ackermann, A. J., and Hart, M. S.: Multiple Primary Hemangioma of the Bones of the Extremity. *Am. J. Roentgen.*, 48:47–52, 1942.
2. Boyle, W. J.: Cystic Angiomatosis of Bone. A Report of Three Cases and Review of the Literature. *J. Bone Joint Surg.*, 54B:626–636, 1972.
3. Dahlin, D. C.: *Bone Tumors, General Aspects and Data on 3987 Cases*, 2nd Ed. Charles C Thomas, Springfield, 1967.
4. Gutierrez, R. M., and Spjut, H. J.: Skeletal Angiomatosis. Report of Three Cases and Review of the Literature. *Clin. Orthop.*, 85:82–97, 1972.
5. Hayes, J. T., and Brody, G. L.: Cystic Lymphangiectasis of Bone. A Case Report. *J. Bone Joint Surg.*, 43A:107–117, 1961.
6. Mirra, J. M., and Arnold, W. D.: Skeletal Hemangiomatosis in Association with Hereditary Hemorrhagic Telangiectasia. A Case Report. *J. Bone Joint Surg.*, 55A:850–854, 1973.
7. Sherman, R. S., and Wilner, D.: The Roentgen Diagnosis of Hemangioma of Bone. *Am. J. Roentgenol.*, 86:1146–1159, 1961.
8. Spjut, H. J., and Lindbom, A.: Skeletal Angiomatosis. Report of Two Cases. *Acta Pathol.*, 55:49–58, 1962.
9. Trifaud, A., Bureau, H., and Payan, H.: *Tumeurs Benignes des os et Dystrophies Pseudo-Tumorales.* Masson & Cie, Paris 1959.

HEMANGIOMA OF THE SOFT TISSUES

These are common lesions of the hand, but they are usually of little radiologic importance. Capillary hemangiomas are not visible radiologically. Other forms of hemangioma may be associated with a soft tissue mass, occasionally with phleboliths (Fig. 15–8). There may be bone involvement as well. A number of syndrome-associated conditions may occur with hemangiomas. These include Maffucci's syndrome (page 295), where hemangiomas are associated with enchondromatosis, and the Klippel-Trenaunay-Weber syndrome (page 318), where they are associated with lo-

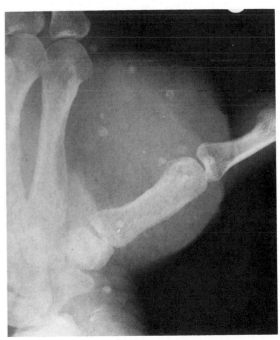

Figure 15–8. Soft tissue hemangioma with bone involvement. There is a large soft tissue mass with multiple calcified phleboliths within it, indicative of hemangioma. There is some erosion of the bony cortex of the second metacarpal. (Courtesy Dr. W. Reynolds, Henry Ford Hospital, Detroit, Michigan.)

calized gigantism. Angiography may be useful in their evaluation (see Chapter 4).

REFERENCES

1. Booher, R. J.: Tumors Arising From Blood Vessels in the Hands and the Feet. *Clin. Orthop.*, 19: 71–96, 1961.
2. Johnson, E. W., Jr., Ghormley, R. K., and Dockerty, M. B.: Hemangiomas of the Extremities. *Surg. Gynec. Obstet.*, 102:531–538, 1956.

BENIGN TUMORS OF CARTILAGINOUS ORIGIN

A number of benign tumors arising from cartilage may be seen in the hand. By far the most common of these are enchondromas, followed by osteochondromas. Others include the periosteal chondroma, the chondromyxoidfibroma and the chondroblastoma.

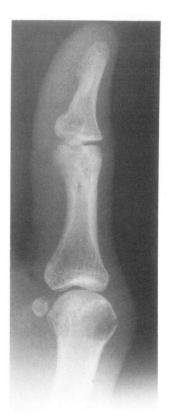

Figure 15–10. Enchondroma in an unusual site. The thumb is a relatively uncommon site for this tumor. There is a pathologic fracture through the lesion in the first metacarpal. There is very little sclerotic bone around its margin.

ENCHONDROMA

These are benign tumors composed of mature hyaline cartilage. When they are located centrally, they have been called enchondromas, but sometimes they appear eccentric or may occur in the periosteum, in which case they have been called periosteal chondromas. They may be isolated or may involve many of the bones. The multiple form of this entity is called Ollier's disease, and when it is associated with hemangiomas of the soft tissues it is called Maffucci's syndrome. The latter two conditions are discussed under the congenital malformation syndromes in Chapter 13.

The enchondroma is the most common bone tumor arising in the hand. The most frequent mode of presentation is that of a painless tumor, although occasionally it may be painful. It may be found incidentally during radiographic examinations for trauma. At times there may be deformity

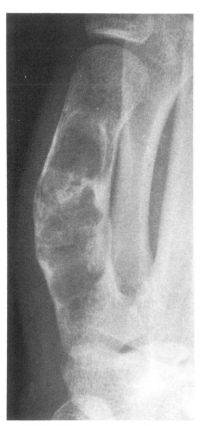

Figure 15–9. Large enchondroma. A typical large enchondroma involves much of the shaft of the metacarpal. (Courtesy Dr. D. Boblitt, Ann Arbor, Michigan.)

or dysfunction, which brings the patient for examination.

The lesions more commonly involve the fingers than the thumb. In 75 monostotic cases studied by Takigawa,[4] only three were in the thumb. The most common site of involvement in the fingers was in the proximal phalanges, with 33 cases, 20 cases were in the metacarpals, 15 were in the middle phalanges, three were in the distal phalanges and one was seen in a carpal. The enchondromas occur more commonly on the ulnar than on the radial side of the hand.

The radiologic appearance is that of a lucent defect which expands and may deform the bone (Fig. 15–9). It has a well-defined margin. The cortex remains intact, although it may be considerably thinned and expanded (Fig. 15–10). Most monostotic cases are central in location (Fig. 15–11). However, a significant percentage are eccentric (Fig. 15–12 A). The appearance in the monostotic cases may be similar to that seen in the multiple form. The loca-

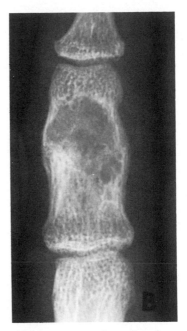

Figure 15–11. Central enchondroma. There is expansion of bone. (Courtesy Dr. D. Boblitt, Ann Arbor, Michgan.)

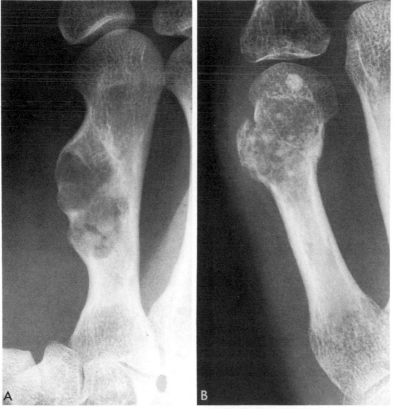

Figure 15–12. A, Eccentric enchondroma. B, Enchondroma. There is some calcification within the tumor. This is a less common manifestation in the hand, but when present is helpful in making the diagnosis of enchondroma. It is more common elsewhere in the body. (Courtesy Dr. D. Boblitt, Ann Arbor, Michigan.)

tion of the lesion is usually in the diaphysis. Occasionally, stippled or mottled calcification may be seen within these lesions (Fig. 15–12 *B*), but this calcification is much less common in lesions of the hand bones than when the lesion occurs in other bones of the body. Pathologic fractures through the enchondroma may be seen (Fig. 15–10), in which case there may be some periosteal new bone formation. In the carpal bones the lesions appear as radiolucencies with sclerotic margins which mimic cystic lesions.

REFERENCES

1. Dahlin, D. C.: *Bone Tumors, General Aspects and Data on 3987 Cases,* 2nd Ed. Charles C Thomas, Springfield, 1967.
2. Jewusiak, E. M., Spence, K. F., and Sell, K. W.: Solitary Benign Enchondroma of the Long Bones of the Hand. Results of Curettage and Packing with Freeze-Dried Cancellous-Bone Allograft. *J. Bone Joint Surg.,* 53A:1587–1590, 1971.
3. Takigawa, K.: Carpal Chondroma. Report of a Case. *J. Bone Joint Surg.,* 53A:1601–1604, 1971.
4. Takigawa, K.: Chondroma of the Bones of the Hand. A Review of 110 Cases. *J. Bone Joint Surg.,* 53A:1591–1600, 1971.

PERIOSTEAL CHONDROMA (JUXTACORTICAL CHONDROMA)

This cartilaginous tumor is related to the chondroma but develops within and beneath the periosteum. The phalanges of the hand are a common site.

The tumors may cause erosion of adjacent bone, or the bone may be uninvolved (Fig. 15–13). There is a soft tissue mass which usually contains calcium.

REFERENCES

1. Nosanchuk, J. S., and Kaufer, H.: Recurrent Periosteal Chondroma. Report of Two Cases and a Review of the Literature. *J. Bone Joint Surg.,* 51A:375–380, 1969.
2. Rockwell, M. A., Saiter, E. T., and Enneking, W. F.: Periosteal Chondroma. *J. Bone Joint Surg.:* 54A:102–108, 1972.

OSTEOCHONDROMA (CARTILAGINOUS EXOSTOSIS)

This is a very common benign bone tumor and has been discussed in Chapter 13 under the title Multiple Cartilaginous Exostoses. Solitary exostoses have an appear-

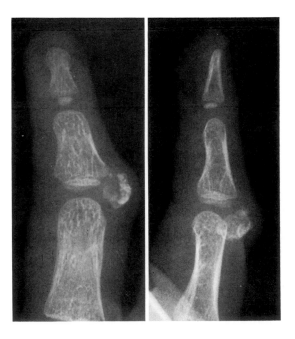

Figure 15–13. Periosteal chondroma. This is a calcified soft tissue mass which does not appear to involve bone. The pathologic diagnosis was periosteal chondroma.

ance similar to the multiple ones. Seven of 414 exostoses seen by Dahlin, and seven of 376 exostoses seen by Mangini were in the hand bones. Almost all are in the phalanges or in the metacarpals. A case of a probable carpal osteochondroma was reported by Heiple. The osteochondromas most peculiar to the hand are the subungual exostoses, which project from the distal portion of the terminal phalanx. Of 37 subungual exostoses seen by Dahlin, four were in the thumb and one was in the index finger, while all the others were in the feet. The subungual exostoses may be more common in females.[1]

Exostoses in the hand are usually asymptomatic unless they project in a region where they may be easily traumatized or unless their location interferes with function. If they are close to the epiphysis, particularly in cases of multiple exostoses,

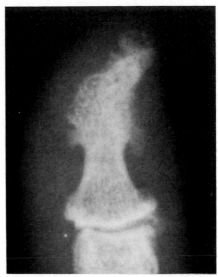

Figure 15–15. Subungual exostosis. Adult female. The subungual exostosis arises from the region of the tuft. (Courtesy Dr. D. Louis, Ann Arbor, Michigan.)

some growth alteration may occur and there may be various curvatures of the fingers.

The radiologic appearance of osteochondromas is that of a broad-based projection arising near the end of a bone (Fig. 15–14). The cortex of the lesion is continuous with the bone in which it is located. The tumor may affect growth at an epiphysis and cause local deformity. They may be confused with enchondromas, particularly when they are broad-based. The subungual exostoses are seen in the region of the tufts (Fig. 15–15).

REFERENCES

1. Dahlin, D. C.: *Bone Tumors, General Aspects and Data on 3987 Cases,* 2nd Ed. Charles C Thomas, Springfield, 1967.
2. Evison, G., and Price, C. H. G.: Subungual Exostosis. *Br. J. Radiol.,* 39:451–455, 1966.
3. Heiple, K. G.: Carpal Osteochondroma. *J. Bone Joint Surg.,* 43A:861–864, 1961.
4. Mangini, U.: Tumors of the Skeleton of the Hand. *Bull. Hosp. Joint Dis.,* 28:61–103, 1967.

CHONDROMYXOID FIBROMA

This is an uncommon tumor derived from cartilage. The hand bones are a relatively

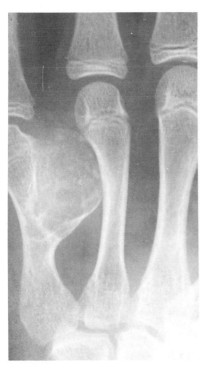

Figure 15–14. Osteochondroma. There is a large bony projection arising from the fifth metacarpal. It partially erodes the fourth metacarpal by pressure. The tumor has a broad base and is attached near the end of the bone. The cortex of the lesion is continuous with that of the fifth metacarpal.

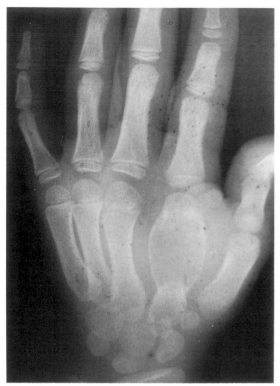

Figure 15–16. Chondromyxoid fibroma. A large lucent defect in the second metacarpal expands the bone. (Courtesy Dr. D. Elzinga and Dr. D. Louis, Ann Arbor, Michigan.)

infrequent site. Phalangeal and metacarpal involvement was seen in eight of 207 cases reviewed by Feldman et al.[1] Mangini reported five such instances, including one occurring in the capitate. The radiographic appearance of the tumor in the small bones is atypical. Although the lesion is a typically circumscribed (Fig. 15–16), eccentrically situated, round or oval metaphyseal defect, some cases, particularly one reported by Feldman, show a rather bizarre appearance. Sometimes the tumor may show evidence of active destruction and may mimic a malignant lesion.

REFERENCES

1. Feldman, F., Hecht, H. L., and Johnston, A. D.: Chondromyxoid Fibroma of Bone. *Radiology,* 94:249–260, 1970.
2. Mangini, U.: Tumors of the Skeleton of the Hand.

Bull. Hosp. Joint Dis., 28:61–103, 1967.
3. Schajowicz, F., and Gallardo, H.: Chondromyxoid Fibroma (Fibromyxoid Chondroma) of Bone. A Clinico-Pathological Study of Thirty-Two Cases. *J. Bone Joint Surg.,* 53B:198–216, 1971.
4. Turcotte, B., Pugh, D. G., and Dahlin, D. C.: The Roentgenologic Aspects of Chondromyxoid Fibroma of Bone. *Am. J. Roentgenol.,* 87:1085–1095, 1962.

CHONDROBLASTOMA

This is a benign tumor with a cartilaginous matrix. It arises in the metaphyseal-epiphyseal area. Neviaser and Wilson[2] reported two cases in the fingers and stated that of 109 cases reported in the literature previously, two appeared in the metacarpal and one in the capitate, with a possible additional one in the proximal phalanx of a finger.

Radiologically there is evidence of an expansive radiolucent process (Fig. 15–17), usually involving the metaphyseal-epiphyseal area. The latter may be intact or broken. The differential diagnosis includes giant cell tumor. Chondroblastomas are, however, very rare in the hand, so there are no well-defined typical manifestations of the lesion in this location.

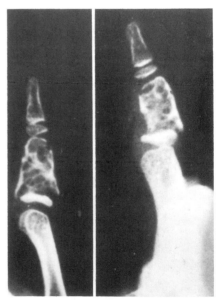

Figure 15–17. Chondroblastoma. Note the bubbly-appearing bone in the middle phalanx. (Courtesy Dr. R. Neviaser, Washington, D.C. Reproduced with permission from *J. Bone Joint Surg.,* 54A:389–392, 1972.)

REFERENCES

1. Mangini, U.: Tumors of the Skeleton of the Hand. *Bull. Hosp. Joint Dis.*, 28:61–103, 1967.
2. Neviaser, R. J., and Wilson, J. N.: Benign Chondroblastoma in the Finger. *J. Bone Joint Surg.*, 54A:389–392, 1972.

OSTEOID OSTEOMA

This is a benign tumor of bone. It is described by Lichtenstein[6] as "a small oval or roundish tumor-like nidus which is composed of osteoid and trabeculae of newly formed bone deposited within a substratum of highly vascularized osteogenetic connective tissue." There is sclerosis about the lesion in many cases.

The symptoms in the hand are pain, which is usually not severe, and possibly swelling. There may be tenderness on compression. Sullivan noted that sweating was increased over the involved fingers, and there may be enlargement of the finger or nail hypertrophy.[8, 10]

Osteoid osteoma does not commonly occur in the hand bones. It was seen in this location in eight of the 102 cases studied by Dahlin.[2] Osteoid osteoma may occur in almost any of the hand bones, including both the phalanges and the carpals.[1, 3, 10] Of the phalanges, the proximal phalanges

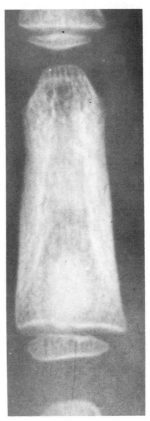

Figure 15-19. Osteoid osteoma of middle phalanx. Thickening and sclerosis of the bone are evident. There is a sclerotic area of increased density in the center of the phalanx. (Courtesy Dr. T. R. Lawrie. Reproduced with permission from *J. Bone Joint Surg.*, 52A:1357–1363, 1970.)

are most commonly involved,[3] although a number of osteoid osteomas are also seen in the middle and distal phalanges.[10] Involvement of almost all of the carpals has also been reported. However, the scaphoid is most commonly affected, followed by the capitate and then the hamate.[9]

Osteoid osteomas are seen mainly in children and young adults. The highest incidence is during the teens and twenties.[3]

The radiologic findings depend somewhat on the location of the lesion. Edeiken et al.[4] described three different types of osteoid osteoma. They include cases with a nidus in the medulla, which has very little sclerosis (Fig. 15-18); with the nidus in the cortex, which has sclerosis (Fig. 15-19); and with the nidus in the periosteal region, which is associated with periosteal reaction. All three forms may occur in the hand bones.

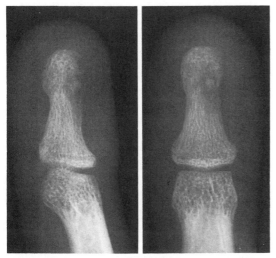

Figure 15-18. Osteoid osteoma in the fingertip. There is a lucency with a central dense nidus. This appearance is characteristic for a medullary location of these lesions. There is no significant sclerosis around the defect.

In the distal phalanges the lesions are often medullary and there is relatively little sclerosis. In the phalanges sclerosis may be quite extensive. The nidus itself is either radiolucent or opaque.

As in other areas of the body, tomography may be useful in localizing the nidus. This is particularly true when there is significant sclerosis or when bone overlap obscures the lesion, as in the carpal bones.[11] Fusion of the adjacent epiphyses may occur as the result of tumor.

Angiograms of osteoid osteomas show increased vascularity in the nidus of the lesion.[7, 10]

Differential diagnosis depends on where the lesions are located. When they are in the distal phalanges, other conditions that may be considered are epidermoid cyst, enchondromas and glomus tumors. Periosteal changes can mimic a wide range of other tumors. Inflammatory processes can sometimes be confused with an osteoid osteoma.

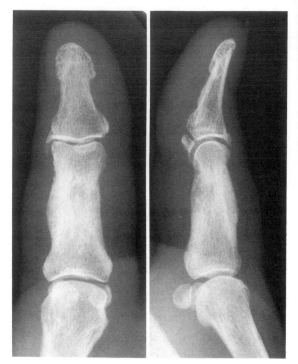

Figure 15–20. Osteoid osteoma or osteoblastoma. There is periosteal thickening of the proximal phalanx; a definite nidus is not identified. Pathologic distinction between the two entities could not be made. (Courtesy Dr. D. Boblitt and Dr. S. Markel, Ann Arbor, Michigan.)

REFERENCES

1. Carroll, R. E.: Osteoid Osteoma in the Hand. *J. Bone Joint Surg.*, 35A:888–893, 1953.
2. Dahlin, D. C.: *Bone Tumors, General Aspects and Data on 3987 Cases*, 2nd Ed. Charles C Thomas, Springfield, 1967.
3. Dunitz, N. L., Lipscomb, P. R., and Ivins, J. C.: Osteoid Osteoma of the Hand and Wrist. *Am. J. Surg.*, 94:65–69, 1957.
4. Edeiken, J., DePalma, A. F., and Hodes, P. J.: Osteoid Osteoma (Roentgenographic Emphasis). *Clin. Orthop.*, 49, 201–206, 1966.
5. Lawric, T. R., Aterman, K., Path, F. C., and Sinclair, A. M.: Painless Osteoid Osteoma. *J. Bone Joint Surg.*, 52A:1357–1363, 1970.
6. Lichtenstein, L.: *Bone Tumors*, 3rd Ed. The C. V. Mosby Co., St. Louis, 1965.
7. Lindbom, A., Lindvall, N., Söderberg, G., and Spjut, H.: Angiography in Osteoid Osteoma. *Acta Radiol.*, 54:327–333, 1960.
8. Rosborough, D.: Osteoid Osteoma. Report of a Lesion in the Terminal Phalanx of a Finger. *J. Bone Joint Surg.*, 48B:485–487, 1966.
9. Spinner, M., Zaleski, A., and Weiner, E.: Osteoid Osteoma of the Hamate. *Bull. Hosp. Joint Dis.*, 33:8–14, 1972.
10. Sullivan, M.: Osteoid Osteoma of the Fingers. *Hand*, 3:175–178, 1971.
11. Verheugen, P.: Ostéome-Ostéoïde du Trapézoïde. *J. Belge Rhumatol. Med. Phys.*, 24:316–321, 1969.

OSTEOBLASTOMA (GIANT OSTEOID OSTEOMA)

This tumor is similar to the osteoid osteoma. However, it does not stay small,

as does an osteoid osteoma, and it frequently lacks a halo of sclerotic bone. Often there may be difficulty in distinguishing it pathologically from an osteoid osteoma (Fig. 15–20). It is a relatively rare lesion. Of 28 patients, Dahlin[1] saw one case in the wrist. Lodwick[2] reported a case in a metacarpal. The typical appearance is that of an expansive process with an intact cortex.

REFERENCES

1. Dahlin, D. C.: *Bone Tumors, General Aspects and Data on 3987 Cases*, 2nd Ed. Charles C Thomas, Springfield, 1967.
2. Lodwick, G. S.: *Atlas of Tumor Radiology. The Bones and Joints.* Yearbook Medical Publishers, Inc., Chicago, 1971.

ANEURYSMAL BONE CYST

An aneurysmal bone cyst is defined as a "benign, usually solitary expansile lesion of bone most often occurring in the metaphysis of long bones and in vertebrae and flat bones. Blood-filled spaces imparting a multicystic appearance, and solid areas with spindled stroma, osteoid, and multinucleated giant cells are characteristically seen."[3]

Some authors think that this does not represent a true bone tumor and that it may be the result of alteration of other preexisting tumors, such as fibro-osseous lesions. Nevertheless, the tumor has a typical radiographic and pathologic appearance. Aneurysmal

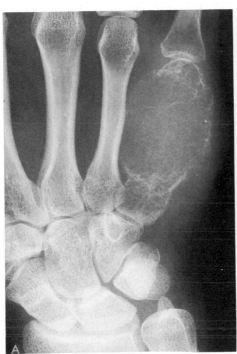
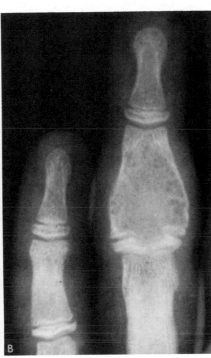
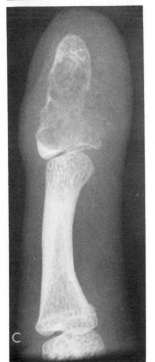

Figure 15–21. Aneurysmal bone cyst.

A, There is an expansile process in the fifth metacarpal of a teenage girl. The bone is markedly expanded, almost paper thin. There is an extremely thin, unbroken cortex about the lesion. There is very little structure within the lesion.

B, This expansile process occurs in the middle phalanx of the fourth finger in a child. The lesion is diaphyseal. There is considerable expansion of the cortex, which is not broken. (Films courtesy Dr. D. Louis, Ann Arbor, Michigan.)

C, Destructive lesion in the distal phalanx. (Film courtesy Mr. W. A. Crabbe. Reprinted with permission from Guys Hosp. Rep., 117:301–308, 1968.)

bone cysts are uncommon in the hand bones. In a study of 95 aneurysmal bone cysts studied by Tillman et al.,[4] only three were located in the hand and wrist bones. Their appearance in this area is similar to that in other bones. Usually they are metaphyseal in location, but occasionally they are diaphyseal. They may even occur in the distal phalanx.[1]

The radiologic appearance is characteristic, consisting of a destructive process in bone with expansion of the cortex (Fig. 15–21). The cortex is usually very thin over the lesion but is usually not broken. The appearance may be similar to that seen in giant cell tumor, bone cyst or occasionally even osteochondroma. The lesion can weaken the bone significantly and fracture may occur.

REFERENCES

1. Murray, R. O., and Jacobson, H. G.: *The Radiology of Skeletal Disorders. Exercises in Diagnosis.* Churchill-Livingstone, Edinburgh, 1971.
2. Slowick, F. A., Jr., Campbell, C. J., and Kettelkamp, D. B.: Aneurysmal Bone Cyst. An Analysis of Thirteen Cases. *J. Bone Joint Surg.,* 50A:1142–1151, 1968.
3. Spjut, H. J., Dorfman, H. D., Fechner, R. E., and Ackerman, L. V.: *Atlas of Tumor Pathology.* 2nd Series. Fascicle 5. Tumors of Bone and Cartilage. Armed Forces Institute of Pathology, Washington, D.C., 1971.
4. Tillman, B. P., Dahlin, D. C., Lipscomb, P. R., and Stewart, J. R.: Aneurysmal Bone Cyst: An Analysis of Ninety-Five Cases. *Mayo Clin. Proc.,* 43:478–495, 1968.

SOLITARY BONE CYST

These lesions are extremely uncommon in the bones of the hand. Mangini[2] reported two cases, from a total of 165, which were located in the hand. Both were in the metacarpals. The appearance of this cyst in the hand is similar to that in other portions of the body. Ewald[1] has reported some questionable cysts in the phalanges.

REFERENCES

1. Ewald, F. C.: Bone Cyst in a Phalanx of a Two-and-a-Half-Year-Old Child. Case Report and Discussion. *J. Bone Joint Surg.,* 54A:399–401, 1972.
2. Mangini, U.: Tumors of the Skeleton of the Hand. *Bull. Hosp. Joint Dis.,* 28:61–103, 1967.

GIANT CELL TUMOR

This neoplasm of uncertain origin probably arises from the mesenchymal cells of the connective tissue framework. The tumor occurs usually after the age of 20 and before the age of 50. The highest incidence is in the third decade. The tumors arise from the epiphysis and may secondarily involve the metaphyseal area. In a review of a number of series, Spjut et al.[4] found that the small bones of the hands were involved in 12 of 419 giant cell tumors. Similarly, of 128 cases, Goldenberg et al.[1] found 11 in the metacarpals and phalanges.

The radiographic appearance is that of an expanding destructive lesion of bone occurring in the region of the epiphysis (Fig. 15–22). Since the tumor is rapidly destructive, there is usually no evidence of sclerosis around its margin and the appearance may be that of a totally lytic defect. Occasionally trabeculation and multiloculation are seen. Periosteal reaction or sclerosis may occasionally occur as a result of healing from associated fracture.

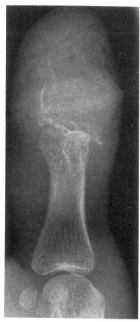

Figure 15–22. Giant cell tumor. ? Histiocytoma. There is marked destruction of the distal phalanx. The tumor contained many giant cells and was thought by the pathologist (Dr. G. Fine) to be a giant cell tumor or histiocytoma of bone. (Courtesy Dr. M. Clark, Henry Ford Hospital, Detroit, Michigan.)

REFERENCES

1. Goldenberg, R. R., Campbell, C. J., and Bonfiglio, M.: Giant-Cell Tumor of Bone. An Analysis of Two Hundred and Eighteen Cases. *J. Bone Joint Surg.*, 52A:619–664, 1970.
2. McGrath, P. J.: Giant-Cell Tumour of Bone. An Analysis of Fifty-Two Cases. *J. Bone Joint Surg.*, 54B:216–229, 1972.
3. Mnaymneh, W. A., Dudley, H. R., and Mnaymneh, L. G.: Giant-Cell Tumor of Bone. An Analysis and Follow-Up Study of the Forty-One Cases Observed at the Massachusetts General Hospital Between 1925 and 1961. *J. Bone Joint Surg.*, 46A:63–75, 1964.
4. Spjut, H. J., Dorfman, H. D., Fechner, R. E., and Ackerman, L. V.: *Atlas of Tumor Pathology.* 2nd Series. Fascicle 5. Tumors of Bone and Cartilage. Armed Forces Institute of Pathology, Washington, D.C., 1971.

GIANT CELL REACTION OF BONE

This is a lesion which somewhat resembles giant cell tumor. It is histologically differentiated from giant cell tumor by

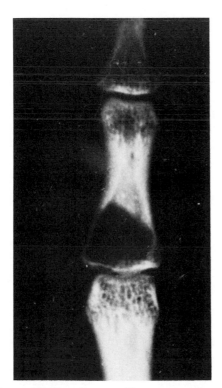

Figure 15-23. Giant cell reaction. The small lucent defect in the middle phalanx is sharply circumscribed (Courtesy Dr. R. D'Alonzo et al. Reproduced with permission from *J. Bone Joint Surg.*, 54A:1267–1271, 1972.)

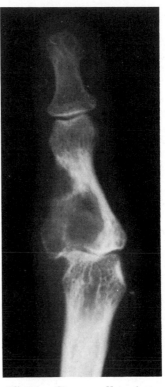

Figure 15-24. Giant cell reaction. This is a more extensive lesion with widening of the bone. (Courtesy Dr. R. D'Alonzo et al. Reproduced with permission from *J. Bone Joint Surg.*, 54A:1267–1271, 1972.)

prominent osteoid production. The lesion produces a phalangeal lucent defect which may be difficult to differentiate from other destructive lesions (Figs. 15–23 and 15–24). It is a benign process which responds to conservative surgical management.

REFERENCES

1. D'Alonzo, R. T., Pitcock, J. A., and Milford, L. W.: Giant-Cell Reaction of Bone. *J. Bone Joint Surg.*, 54A:1267–1271, 1972.
2. Jernstrom, P., and Stark, H. H.: Giant Cell Reaction of a Metacarpal. *Am. J. Clin. Pathol.*, 55:77–81, 1971.

NONOSSIFYING FIBROMA (NONOSTEOGENIC FIBROMA)

These neoplasms are rare in the hand bones. No cases were reported in Dahlin's series.[1] Mangini[2] saw one case in a phalanx of a finger. The lesion caused a small defect in the bone.

REFERENCES

1. Dahlin, D. C.: *Bone Tumors, General Aspects and Data on 3987 Cases*, 2nd Ed. Charles C Thomas, Springfield, 1967.
2. Mangini, U.: Tumors of the Skeleton of the Hand. *Bull. Hosp. Joint Dis.*, 28:61–103, 1967.

NEURILEMOMA (BENIGN SCHWANNOMA)

This is a very rare tumor of nerve sheath origin which occasionally occurs in the hand. It may involve the metacarpals or the phalanges.

The radiographic appearance is that of a lucent defect which is not particularly characteristic (Fig. 15–25). It may be solitary or multiloculated. Erosion of the cortex may occur.

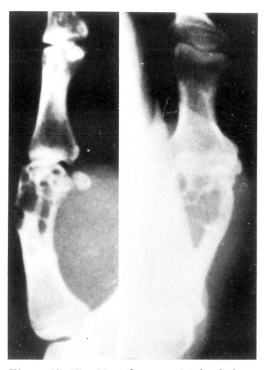

Figure 15–25. Neurilemoma. Multiple lucencies are seen in the distal portion of the first metacarpal. (Courtesy Dr. F. Agha. Reproduced with permission from *Radiology*, 102:325–326, 1972.)

REFERENCES

1. Agha, F. P., and Lilienfeld, R. M.: Roentgen Features of Osseous Neurilemmoma. *Radiology*, 102:325–326, 1972.
2. DasGupta, T. K., Brasfield, R. D., Strong, E. W., and Hajdu, S. I.: Benign Solitary Schwannomas (Neurilemomas). *Cancer*, 24:355–366, 1969.
3. Jacobs, R. L., and Fox, T. A.: Neurilemoma of Bone. A Case Report with a Review of the Literature. *Clin. Orthop.*, 87:248–253, 1972.
4. Lewis, H. H., and Kobrin, H. I.: Neurilemoma of the First Metacarpal. A Case Report. *Clin. Orthop.*, 82:67–69, 1972.

GANGLION OF BONE

Ganglia are one of the most common of the soft tissue tumors of the hand. The soft tissue ganglia are radiographically not significant except on arthrography of the wrist, when they frequently fill with contrast medium (Chapter 5).

Ganglion-like lesions which occur in bone, rather than adjacent to it, have been seen. Most of these lesions lie subchondrally. In the hand and wrist the carpal bones are occasionally involved. Feldman and Johnston[4] reported six cases in the wrist, from a total of 71 cases which included their own cases and a survey of the literature.

The lesions in the wrist are usually well defined with a sclerotic margin. They may be difficult to differentiate from degenerative cysts and from the nonspecific lucent defects which may be occasionally seen in this region (page 130).

REFERENCES

1. Andren, L., and Eiken, O.: Arthrographic Studies of Wrist Ganglions. *J. Bone Joint Surg.*, 53A:299–302, 1971.
2. Crabbe, W. A.: Intra-Osseous Ganglia of Bone. *Br. J. Surg.*, 53:15–17, 1966.
3. Crane, A. R., and Scarano, J. J.: Synovial Cysts (Ganglia) of Bone. Report of Two Cases. *J. Bone Joint Surg.*, 49A:355–361, 1967.
4. Feldman, F., and Johnston, A.: Intraosseous Ganglion. *Am. J. Roentgenol.*, 118:328–343, 1973.
5. Kaplan, E. B.: Intraosseous Ganglion of the Scaphoid Bone of the Wrist. *Bull. Hosp. Joint Dis.*, 32:50–53, 1971.
6. Pellegrino, E. A., Jr., and Olson, J. R.: Bilateral Carpal Lunate Ganglia. *Clin. Orthop.*, 87:225–227, 1972.
7. Sim, F. H., and Dahlin, D. C.: Ganglion Cysts of Bone. *Mayo Clin. Proc.*, 46:484–488, 1971.

NON-NEOPLASTIC BENIGN LESIONS OF BONE

In the differential diagnosis of benign tumors involving the hand bones, certain non-neoplastic conditions must be considered. These include sarcoidosis, tuberous sclerosis, synovial chondromatosis, hemophiliac pseudocyst, myositis ossificans and thorn pseudotumor. Tuberous sclerosis is discussed further in Chapter 13. It can produce punched-out defects throughout the bones of the hand, including the distal phalanges. Lucencies in bone are also seen in sarcoidosis (see Chapter 21). Synovial chondromatosis may be associated with intracortical calcifications and is described further in Chapter 20.

HEMOPHILIAC PSEUDOTUMOR (HEMOPHILIAC CYST OF BONE)

The hand is an uncommon site of these lesions. Several cases have been reported in the literature. The appearance is that of

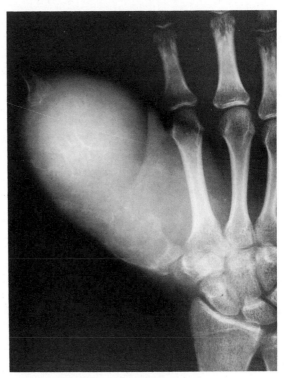

Figure 15–27. Hemophiliac pseudotumor of the thumb. This large destructive lesion has expanded and destroyed the metacarpal and proximal phalanx. (Courtesy Dr. J. Bowerman and Dr. J. Dorst, Baltimore, Maryland. This case was reported by W. Firor and B. Newhall: *Johns Hopkins Med. J.*, 59:237–250, 1936.)

an expanding process of bone with marked destruction (Fig. 15–26). In some cases the bone may be almost totally destroyed (Fig. 15–27). Some sclerosis may occur in older lesions.[2] When the hemorrhage is subperiosteal, elevated periosteum may be noted, forming a ball about the bone. The cyst can occur in any of the tubular bones of the hand. The differential diagnosis will include any aggressively growing benign or malignant process in bone, such as a metastasis, bone cyst, aneurysmal bone cyst and giant cell tumor.

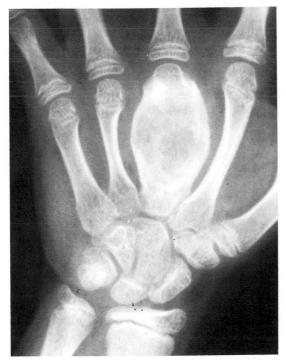

Figure 15–26. Hemophiliac pseudotumor. The expansile lesion in the third metacarpal compresses the adjacent bone. (Courtesy Dr. W. McAllister, St. Louis, Missouri; and Dr. P. Lester, Salt Lake City, Utah.)

REFERENCES

1. Boyes, J. H.: *Bunnell's Surgery of the Hand*, 5th Ed. J. B. Lippincott Co., Philadelphia, 1970, p. 687.
2. Caffey, J.: *Pediatric X-Ray Diagnosis*, 6th ed. Year Book Medical Publishers, Chicago, 1972, Vol. 2, p. 1292.
3. Edeiken, J., and Hodes, P. J.: *Roentgen Diagnosis*

of Diseases of Bone. Williams & Wilkins Co., Baltimore, 1967.

4. Firor, W. M., and Woodhall, B.: Hemophilic Pseudotumor: Diagnosis, Pathology and Surgical Treatment of Hemophilic Lesions in the Smaller Bones and Joints. *Johns Hopkins Med. J.,* 59:237–250, 1936.

5. Steel, W. M., Duthie, R. B., and O'Connor, B. T.: Haemophilic Cysts. Report of Five Cases. *J. Bone Joint Surg.,* 51B:614–626, 1969.

LOCALIZED MYOSITIS OSSIFICANS (EXTRAOSSEOUS LOCALIZED NON-NEOPLASTIC BONE AND CARTILAGE FORMATION)

According to Spjut et al.,[4] this is a "reactive lesion occurring in the soft tissues at times near the bone and periosteum. The lesion is characterized by fibrous osseous and cartilaginous proliferation and metaplasia." It is uncommonly located in the hand. However, Lodwick[2] has reported five cases that include involvement of the metacarpals and phalanges. Histologically there may be a problem in differentiating these lesions from osteosarcomas.

Localized myositis ossificans is usually the result of trauma. Radiologic configuration (Fig. 15–28) depends on the maturation of the lesion. Shortly after trauma, only a soft tissue mass is seen. This mass may be followed by periosteal reaction and rarefaction of bone beneath the tumor. Eventually there is some calcification within the mass. Finally the mass becomes denser and may have a radiolucent center. After several months the mass may shrink somewhat. Norman and Dorfman[3] found that all their cases had a radiolucent zone which separated the lesion from underlying periosteal reaction and cortex. This, however, does not always seem to be true in the hand.

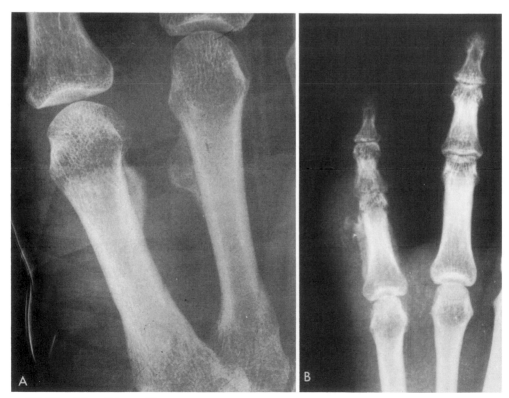

Figure 15–28. Myositis ossificans.

A, A biopsy showed a pseudomalignant soft tissue lesion with ossification. (Courtesy Dr. M. Clark and Dr. G. Fine, Henry Ford Hospital, Detroit, Michigan.)

B, There is localized periosteal reaction and new bone formation in the soft tissues. The pathologic diagnosis was myositis ossificans. (Courtesy Dr. T. Staple and Dr. L. Ackerman, St. Louis, Missouri.)

A related entity is the "turret" exostosis described by Wissinger et al.[5] This is an ossifying subperiosteal hematoma that occurs on the dorsal aspect of the proximal or middle phalanges. The hematoma first appears as a soft tissue mass and then ossifies. It produces a painful lump on the dorsal aspect of the fingers and may interfere with flexion.

REFERENCES

1. Ackerman, L. V.: Extra-Osseous Localized Non-Neoplastic Bone and Cartilage Formation (So-Called Myositis Ossificans). Clinical and Pathological Confusion with Malignant Neoplasms. *J. Bone Joint Surg.*, 40A:279–298, 1958.
2. Lodwick, G. S.: *Atlas of Tumor Radiology. The Bones and Joints.* Year Book Medical Publishers, Inc., Chicago, 1971.
3. Norman, A., and Dorfman, H. D.: Juxtacortical Circumscribed Myositis Ossificans: Evolution and Radiographic Features. *Radiology,* 96: 301–306, 1970.
4. Spjut, H. J., Dorfman, H. D., Fechner, R. E., and Ackerman, L. V.: *Atlas of Tumor Pathology.* 2nd Series. Fascicle 5. Tumors of Bone and Cartilage. Armed Forces Institute of Pathology. Washington, D.C., 1971.
5. Wissinger, H. A., McClain, E. J., and Boyes, J. H.: Turret Exostosis. Ossifying Hematoma of the Phalanges. *J. Bone Joint Surg.,* 48A:105–110, 1966.

THORN PSEUDOTUMOR

In cases of penetrating injury, thorns of palm, yucca, rose and hawthorn may become imbedded in bone. They can cause bone lesions which may be mistaken for bone neoplasm. The foreign body is not radiopaque and is thus not visualized. The symptoms are those of pain and swelling.

Radiologically there is a lucent defect in bone which may have a sharply circumscribed margin, sometimes with a zone of sclerosis. The appearance is often that of a benign bone tumor (Figs. 15–29 and 15–30). In some cases there is mainly a periosteal component and the lesion can be mistaken for Ewing's sarcoma.

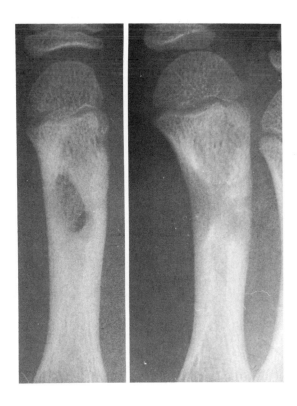

Figure 15–29. Palm thorn granuloma. In the metacarpal there is a lucent defect which appears to extend from the outside of the bone. There is some sclerosis about the bone margin. (Courtesy Dr. J. Gwinn, Los Angeles, California.)

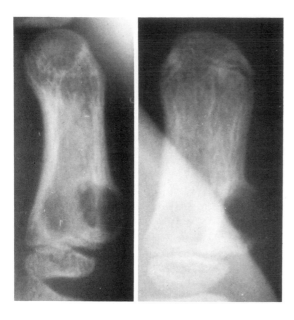

Figure 15–30. Palm thorn granuloma. There is a small, round, localized bone defect in the base of the first metacarpal. The lesion has a well-circumscribed margin and could be misinterpreted as a bone tumor. (Courtesy of Dr. J. Gwinn, Los Angeles, California.)

REFERENCES

1. Borgia, C. A.: An Unusual Bone Reaction to an Organic Foreign Body in the Hand. *Clin. Orthop.*, 30:188–193, 1963.
2. Gerle, R. D.: Thorn-induced Pseudo-tumours of Bone. *Br. J. Radiol.*, 44:642–645, 1971.
3. Maylahn, D. J.: Thorn Induced "Tumors" of Bone. *J. Bone Joint Surg.*, 34A:386–388, 1952.
4. Weston, W. J.: Thorn and Twig-Induced Pseudo-tumours of Bone and Soft Tissues. *Br. J. Radiol.*, 36:323–326, 1963.

LIPOMA

Lipomas of the hand are fatty tumors which are usually well encapsulated. They most often present because of their size, which either interferes with function of the hand or is cosmetically undesirable. Occasionally they may compress nerves with resultant symptoms. According to Paarlberg et al.,[3] less than 5 per cent of benign tumors of the hand are lipomas. They are usually seen in older patients, mostly in the fifth, sixth and seventh decades of life. The tumors are more commonly seen on the volar than on the dorsal aspect of the hand. Some involve the wrist. The localized lipoma is differentiated from a condition of lipomatosis, which may be associated with the Klippel-Trenaunay-Weber syndrome (Chapter 13).

The main radiographic finding is the presence of a relatively radiolucent soft tissue mass (Fig. 15–31). In the Mayo

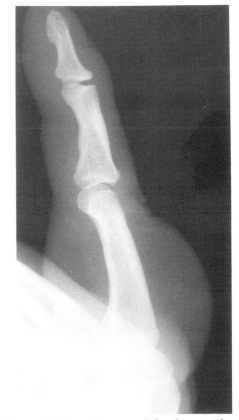

Figure 15–31. Lipoma of the finger. There is a soft tissue swelling about the proximal phalanx. The soft tissue density in the mass is that of fat, which is easily distinguishable from the water density of the skin. Although there was no pathologic proof in this case, the radiologic diagnosis of lipoma could be made.

Clinic series, nine of 28 cases showed radiolucency. There may be some separation of adjacent bones by the tumor. Very rarely is there evidence of bony erosion. The lack of bony erosion is no doubt due to the fact that the tumor is very soft.

Lipofibroma may be seen in the median nerve and may be present as a linear calcification on the volar aspect of the wrist.[2]

REFERENCES

1. Leffert, R. D.: Lipomas of the Upper Extremity. *J. Bone Joint Surg.*, 54A:1262–1266, 1972.
2. Louis, D. S., and Dick, H. M.: Ossifying Lipofibroma of the Median Nerve. *J. Bone Joint Surg.*, 55A:1082–1084, 1973.
3. Paarlberg, D., Linscheid, R. L., and Soule, E. H.: Lipomas of the Hand—Including a Case of Lipoblastomatosis in a Child. *Mayo Clin. Proc.*, 47:121–124, 1972.
4. Phalen, G. S., Kendrick, J. I., and Rodriguez, J. M.: Lipomas of the Upper Extremity. A Series of Fifteen Tumors in the Hand and Wrist and Six Tumors Causing Nerve Compression. *Am. J. Surg.*, 121:298–306, 1971.

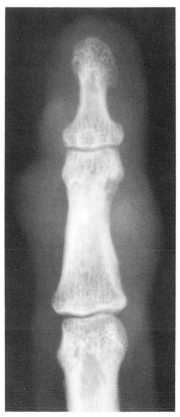

Figure 15–33. Giant cell xanthoma. Several soft tissue swellings are seen in the distal portion of the finger. There are some degenerative changes in the distal interphalangeal joint. Part of the tuft of the phalanx may be eroded.

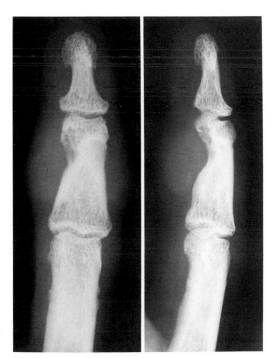

Figure 15–32. Giant cell xanthoma of tendon sheath. There is a soft tissue mass adjacent to the middle phalanx causing some bone erosion. The area of bone erosion has a smooth, well-defined margin. (Courtesy Dr. W. Reynolds, Henry Ford Hospital, Detroit, Michigan.)

GIANT CELL TUMOR OF TENDON SHEATH (FIBROUS XANTHOMA)

This is the second most common hand tumor. It most commonly arises adjacent to the dorsal surface of the distal joint of the index, ring or little fingers, or less commonly from the wrist. It appears as a nontender soft tissue mass. Radiologically there is evidence of a soft tissue mass which may on occasion erode the adjacent bone (four of 13 cases[2]) (Fig. 15–32). Degenerative changes in the adjacent joints are seen, particularly when the distal interphalangeal joint area is involved (18 of 28 cases[1]) (Fig. 15–33). The high frequency of the degenerative changes is greater than that expected from simple chance. Rarely, old xanthomas may calcify (Fig. 15–34).

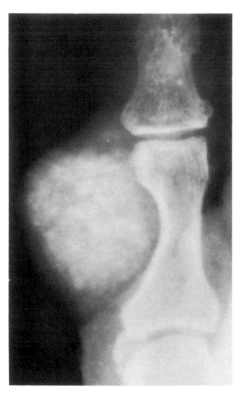

Figure 15–34. Calcified xanthoma. This xanthoma had been present for many years in a 68 year old female. (Courtesy Dr. D. Louis, Ann Arbor, Michigan.)

REFERENCES

1. Jones, F. E., Soule, E. H., and Coventry, M. B.: Fibrous Xanthoma of Synovium (Giant-Cell Tumor of Tendon Sheath, Pigmented Nodular Synovitis). A Study of One Hundred and Eighteen Cases. *J. Bone Joint Surg.,* 51A:76–86, 1969.
2. Phalen, G. S., McCormack, L. J., and Gazale, W. J.: Giant-Cell Tumor of Tendon Sheath (Benign Synovioma) in the Hand. Evaluation of 56 Cases. *Clin. Orthop.,* 15:140–151, 1959.

MUCOUS CYST OF FINGERS

These are thin-walled cysts in the dermis occurring distal to the distal interphalangeal joint. They are located on the dorsal surface of either side of the midline and are seldom greater than 10 mm. in diameter. They are filled with a clear viscid fluid. In the cases of Constant et al.[1] (Fig. 15–35), 26 of 33 patients who had x-rays showed degenerative changes with narrowing and lipping of the joint space.

REFERENCES

1. Constant, E., Royer, J. R., Pollard, R. J., Larsen, R. D., and Posch, J. L.: Mucous Cyst of the Fingers. *Plast. Reconstr. Surg.,* 43:241–246, 1969.
2. Kleinert, H. E., Kutz, J. E., Fishman, J. H., and McCraw, L. H.: Etiology and Treatment of the So-Called Mucous Cyst of the Finger. *J. Bone Joint Surg.,* 54A:1455–1458, 1972.

OTHER SOFT TISSUE BENIGN TUMORS

A variety of other soft tissue benign tumors may be seen, including melanomas, fibromas, epithelial inclusion cysts, extra-abdominal desmoids,[3] papillomas and neuromas. They usually do not affect bone but instead present as soft tissue masses. Occasionally they may be associated with bone growth disturbance (Fig. 15–36).

REFERENCES

1. Boyes, J. H.: *Bunnell's Surgery of the Hand,* 5th Ed. J. B. Lippincott Co., Philadelphia, 1970.

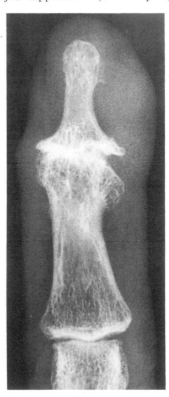

Figure 15–35. Mucous cyst of the finger. The patient had a thin-walled mucous cyst of the finger. The degenerative changes in the distal interphalangeal joint are commonly associated with this condition.

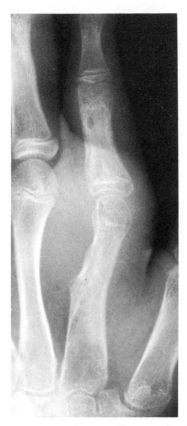

Figure 15–36. Fibroma. ? Juvenile fibroma. This soft tissue mass involves the hypoplastic index finger. There are some defects within the bone. The patient also had a large abdominal mass which was similarly diagnosed. It is not clear whether this should be considered a fibroma or as part of juvenile fibromatosis. (Courtesy Dr. D. Boblitt and Dr. S. Markel, St. Joseph Hospital, Ann Arbor, Michigan.)

2. Butler, E. D., Hamill, J. P., Seipel, R. S., and de Lorimier, A. A.: Tumors of the Hand. A Ten-Year Survey and Report of 437 Cases. *Am. J. Surg.,* 100:293–302, 1960.
3. Cavanagh, R. C.: Tumors of the Soft Tissues of the Extremities. *Seminars Roentgenol.,* 8:73–89, 1973.
4. Ritter, M. A., Marshall, J. L., and Straub, L. R.: Extra-Abdominal Desmoid of the Hand. A Case Report. *J. Bone Joint Surg.,* 51A:1641–1644, 1969.

PRIMARY MALIGNANT BONE TUMORS

Malignant tumors of the hand are usually of cutaneous or soft tissue origin. Primary bone tumors of the hand are exceedingly rare and represent a small proportion of malignant hand tumors. Of 78 malignancies of the hand, Kendall et al.[1] found only two sarcomas of bone. Mangini[2] found five malignant tumors of 152 bone tumors in-

volving the hand. Marcove and Charosky,[3] in a review of the literature in 1972, found 16 cases of chondrosarcoma, 10 cases of osteosarcoma, four cases of fibrosarcoma and three cases of synovial sarcoma in the digits of the hands and feet. Ewing's sarcomas have also been reported.

REFERENCES

1. Kendall, T. E., Robinson, D. W., and Masters, F. W.: Primary Malignant Tumors of the Hand. *Plast. Reconstr. Surg.,* 44:37–40, 1969.
2. Mangini, U.: Tumors of the Skeleton of the Hand. *Bull. Hosp. Joint Dis.,* 28:61–103, 1967.
3. Marcove, R. C., and Charosky, C. B.: Phalangeal Sarcomas Simulating Infections of the Digits. Review of the Literature and Report of Four Cases. *Clin. Orthop.,* 83:224–231, 1972.
4. Netherlands Committee on Bone Tumors: *Radiologic Atlas of Bone Tumors.* Mouton & Co., The Hague, 1966, Vol. 1.

CHONDROSARCOMA

Although they are probably the most common of the malignant bone tumors of the hand, chondrosarcomas at this site are extremely rare. They represent but a minute portion of chondrosarcomas. In Dahlin's series[2] there were three chondrosarcomas of the hand, of a total of 334 seen in various portions of the skeleton. Marcove and Charosky,[9] in a review of phalangeal sarcomas, found 16 cases reported in the digits of the hands and feet. Juxtacortical chondrosarcomas are also rare, and only one case has been reported.[6]

The histologic differentiation between enchondromas of bone and central chondrosarcomas may be ill defined,[5] and this sometimes raises a question regarding the validity of the diagnosis.

As at other sites, chondrosarcomas of the hand bones occur in later life. Of 11 patients reviewed by Jakobson and Spjut,[5] all but one were older than 52 years. The tumors have involved the phalanges and the metacarpals and even a carpal bone. Distant metastases have been described, and metastases from other sites to the soft tissues of the hand have also been seen.[3]

The radiologic appearance of chondrosarcoma is that of an expanding process in bone with a geographic, sometimes irregular, destructive contour (Fig. 15–37). The cortex may be broken and there may be subperiosteal spiculation. Some calcified matrix may be present within the tumor and

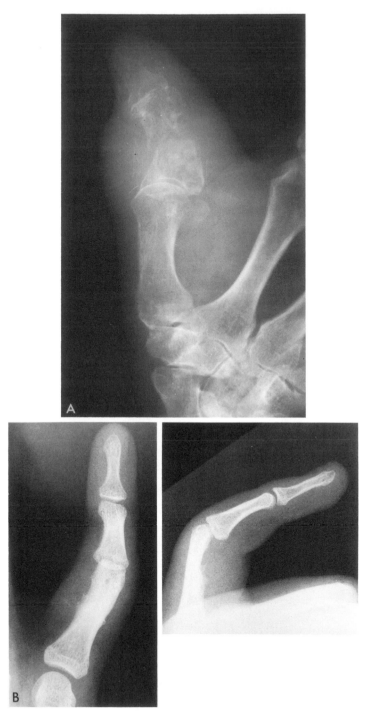

Figure 15–37. A, Chondrosarcoma. There is an active destructive process with considerable soft tissue swelling. There is very little calcification within the tumor, although some localized densities are seen in the base. There is a fracture through the tumor. (Courtesy Dr. T. Staple and Dr. L. Ackerman, St. Louis, Missouri.)

B, Periosteal chondrosarcoma. This 13 year old girl had two biopsies; in both, the lesion was reported as a benign chondroma. The third recurrence biopsy revealed periosteal chondrosarcoma. (Courtesy Dr. C. Campbell, Albany, New York.)

may occur in floccules.[8] Occasionally the tumor can appear radiologically as an enchondroma[10] but later shows active recurrence and destruction.

REFERENCES

1. Cruickshank, A. H.: Chondrosarcoma of a Phalanx with Cutaneous Metastases. *J. Pathol.*, 57: 144–148, 1945.
2. Dahlin, D. C.: *Bone Tumors, General Aspects and Data on 3987 Cases*, 2nd Ed. Charles C Thomas, Springfield, 1967.
3. Froimson, A. I.: Metastatic Chondrosarcoma of the Hand. Report of a Case. *Clin. Orthop.*, 53: 155–160, 1967.
4. Gottschalk, R. G., and Smith, R. T.: Chondrosarcoma of the Hand. Report of a Case with Radioactive Sulphur Studies and Review of Literature. *J. Bone Joint Surg.*, 45A:141–150, 1963.
5. Jakobson, E., and Spjut, H. J.: Chondrosarcoma of the Bones of the Hand. Report of 3 Cases. *Acta Radiol.*, 54:426–432, 1960.
6. Jokl, P., Albright, J. A., and Goodman, A. H.: Juxtacortical Chondrosarcoma of the Hand. *J. Bone Joint Surg.*, 53A:1370–1376, 1971.
7. Lansche, W. E., and Spjut, H. J.: Chondrosarcoma of the Small Bones of the Hand. *J. Bone Joint Surg.*, 40A:1139–1145, 1958.
8. Lodwick, G. S.: *Atlas of Tumor Radiology. The Bones and Joints*. Year Book Medical Publishers, Inc., Chicago, 1971.
9. Marcove, R. C., and Charosky, C. B.: Phalangeal Sarcomas Simulating Infections of the Digits. Review of the Literature and Report of Four Cases. *Clin. Orthop.*, 83:224–231, 1972.
10. Netherlands Committee on Bone Tumors: *Radiologic Atlas of Bone Tumors*. Mouton & Co., The Hague, 1966, Vol. I.

OSTEOSARCOMA

This is another extremely rare primary bone tumor of the hand. In a series of 650 osteogenic sarcomas, Dahlin found three located in the hand. The appearance is that of an actively destructive lesion. Carroll believes that the sarcoma, when present in the hand, carries a better prognosis than when it occurs elsewhere in the body. Drompp[3] reported a bilateral case of osteosarcoma. The appearance of these lesions is not well defined, since so few cases have been reported. The case of Drompp showed a great deal of bone sclerosis associated with the lesion. The radiologic findings are those of an aggressive bone tumor with much destruction and bone formation. Occasionally, when osteosarcoma occurs at multiple sites with bone sclerosis, the hand may be involved.

REFERENCES

1. Carroll, R. E.: Osteogenic Sarcoma in the Hand. *J. Bone Joint Surg.*, 39A:325–331, 1957.
2. Dahlin, D. C.: *Bone Tumors, General Aspects and Data on 3987 Cases*, 2nd Ed. Charles C Thomas, Springfield, 1967.
3. Drompp, B. W.: Bilateral Osteosarcoma in the Phalanges of the Hand. *J. Bone Joint Surg.*, 43A:199–204, 1961.
4. Marcove, R. C., and Charosky, C. B.: Phalangeal Sarcomas Simulating Infections of the Digits. Review of the Literature and Report of Four Cases. *Clin. Orthop.*, 83:224–231, 1972.

PAROSTEAL OSTEOGENIC SARCOMA

This rare form of sarcoma may occasionally be seen in the hands. Stark reviewed the few cases which have been described in the literature and published an example of his own. The tumor encircles the shaft

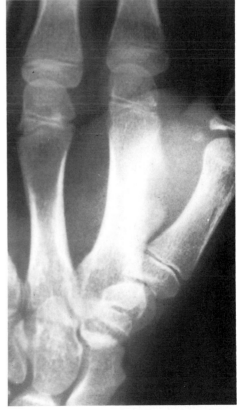

Figure 15–38. Parosteal sarcoma. Eccentric lesion with periosteal reaction. The pathologic diagnosis was parosteal sarcoma. (Courtesy Dr. J. Kuhn and Dr. R. Weiss, Buffalo, New York.)

of the bone without invading it significantly. The appearance of the tumor in the hand is similar to its appearance elsewhere in the body (Fig. 15–38). Sometimes it projects from the bone and resembles myositis ossificans. In some cases the lesion is almost entirely in the soft tissues, with swelling and a region of tumor calcification.

REFERENCES

1. Jacobson, S. W.: Early Juxtacortical Osteosarcoma (Parosteal Osteoma). *J. Bone Joint Surg.*, 40A: 1310–1328, 1958.
2. Mangini, U.: Tumors of the Skeleton of the Hand. *Bull. Hosp. Joint Dis.*, 28:61–103, 1967.
3. Stark, H. H., Jones, F. E., and Jernstrom, P.: Parosteal Osteogenic Sarcoma of a Metacarpal Bone. A Case Report. *J. Bone Joint Surg.*, 53A:147–153, 1971.

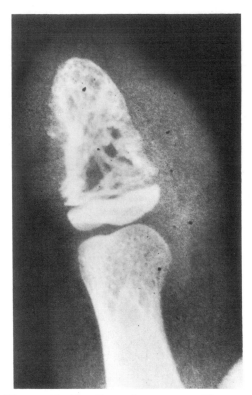

Figure 15–40. Ewing's sarcoma. There is a lacy network with destruction of the distal phalanx. There is some bony destruction of the cortical margins. (Courtesy Dr. H. M. Dick. Reproduced with permission from *J. Bone Joint Surg.*, 53A:345–348, 1971.)

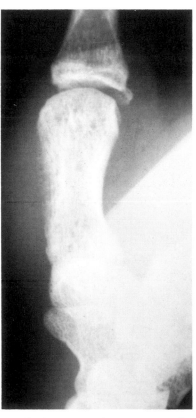

Figure 15–39. Ewing's sarcoma. There is a destructive, permeative process involving the radial aspect of the first metacarpal. The cortex is destroyed by the tumor, and has a lacy network within it.

EWING'S SARCOMA

This is a small, round cell sarcoma of bone. Very few cases have been seen in the hand. Dahlin, in his series of 210 Ewing's tumor, found only one in the hand. In the Netherlands bone tumor series, two of 89 were in the hand. Other cases have also been reported.[2, 4]

Metacarpals and phalanges are involved. The radiologic findings are most often an expansile process in bone with a lacy network within it. There is usually evidence of cortical destruction, and there may be proliferation of the periosteum (Fig. 15–39). Other patterns have also been seen (Fig. 15–40). There may be some associated sclerosis, and there may be bone spicules projecting into the soft tissues.

REFERENCES

1. Dahlin, D. C.: *Bone Tumors, General Aspects and Data on 3987 Cases,* 2nd Ed. Charles C Thomas, Springfield, 1967.
2. Dick, H. M., Francis, K. C., and Johnston, A. D.: Ewing's Sarcoma of the Hand. *J. Bone Joint Surg.,* 53A:345–348, 1971.
3. Netherlands Committee on Bone Tumors. *Radiologic Atlas of Bone Tumors.* Mouton & Co., The Hague, 1966, Vol. 1.
4. Ridings, G. R.: Ewing's Tumor. *Radiol. Clin. North Am.,* 2:315–325, 1964.

OTHER PRIMARY SARCOMAS

Other primary sarcomas in the hand are extremely rare. They include fibrosarcoma[2] and synovial sarcoma.[1, 3] The roentgen appearance of these tumors consists mainly of soft tissue changes, but bone destruction may also be seen.[1]

REFERENCES

1. Anderson, K. J., and Wildermuth, O.: *Clin. Orthop.,* 19:55–69, 1961.
2. Butler, E. D., Hamill, J. P., Seipel, R. S., and de Lorimier, A. A.: Tumors of the Hand. A Ten-Year Survey and Report of 437 Cases. *Am. J. Surg.,* 100:293–302, 1960.
3. Hand, C. R., and McFarland, G. B., Jr.: Synovial Sarcoma of the Hand. *J. La. State Med. Soc.,* 122:1–5, 1970.

MYELOMA AND MULTIPLE MYELOMA

Lytic lesions in myeloma may occur in any portion of the body, but they are not common in the hand. In 80 solitary cases, Griffiths[2] saw only one in the thumb, while in 115 cases with multifocal presentation, there were 13 foci in the forearm and hand. They can involve any bone, including the metacarpals,[1, 3] distal phalanx or carpals.[2] Gompels et al.[1] reported a case with involvement of the distal phalanx of the thumb, and an involved metacarpal was seen in the Netherlands Committee on Bone Tumors series.[3] The appearance, as elsewhere in the body, is that of a lytic destructive process with no significant bone reaction about it (Fig. 15–41). The edges are poorly defined and the cortex may be completely destroyed.

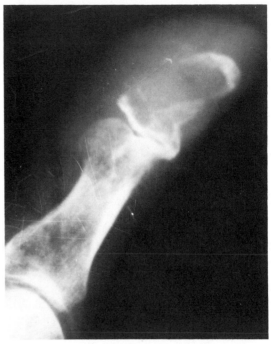

Figure 15–41. Multiple myeloma. There is a destructive process in the terminal phalanx of the thumb, associated with some soft tissue swelling. There is very little bony reaction about the phalanx. There is a break in the cortex. (Courtesy Dr. B. Gompels. Reproduced with permission from *Radiology,* 104:509–514, 1972.)

REFERENCES

1. Gompels, B. M., Votaw, M. L., and Martel, W.: Correlation of Radiological Manifestations of Multiple Myeloma with Immunoglobulin Abnormalities and Prognosis. *Radiology,* 104:509–514, 1972.
2. Griffiths, D. Ll. Orthopaedic Aspects of Myelomatosis. *J. Bone Joint Surg.,* 48B:703–728, 1966.
3. Netherlands Committee on Bone Tumors. *Radiologic Atlas of Bone Tumors.* Mouton & Co., The Hague, 1966, Vol. I.

METASTATIC LESIONS OF THE HAND BONES

Metastatic lesions to the hand bones are not common. They occurred in two of 3000 patients with malignancies studied by Gold and Reefe.[3] Metastatic lesions can occur from many types of tumors, but most commonly they are due to lung cancer. Of 31 cases of metastasis to the hand bones reviewed by Trachtenberg and Roswit,[9] 16 were from bronchogenic cancers, three from breast cancers, two each from parotid and kidney cancers, and one each from cancers of the bladder, uterus, prostate, colon, rectum and skin. There was also a metastasis from a sympathicoblastoma and one from a lymphosarcoma. Esophageal cancer metastatic to the hand bones has also been described.[5]

The metastatic lesions most commonly occur in the tubular bones of the hand, but occasionally carpal metastases have been reported.[1] The metastases may be the first sign of the primary tumor[8] and may present with pain and swelling suggesting infection. Occasionally they present as painless lumps.

The radiologic appearance of the metastasis is most commonly that of an osteolytic lesion of bone with active destruction (Fig. 15–42). The lesions are usually solitary,

particularly in bronchogenic cancer. In other tumors, however, they may be multiple.[6] Occasionally only the soft tissues may be involved. Sclerotic metastases may be seen from carcinoma of the breast or prostate.[3]

REFERENCES

1. Dolich, B. H., Spinner, M., and Kaufman, G.: Isolated Metastasis to the Carpal Bones. Report of a Case. *Bull. Hosp. Joint Dis.*, 31:78–84, 1970.
2. Ferguson, A. D., Chall, H. G., and Shapiro, R. I.: Metastatic Tumors of the Hand. *Grace Hosp. Bull.*, 41:20–22, 1963.
3. Gold, G. L., and Reefe, W. E.: Carcinoma and Metastases to the Bones of the Hand. *J.A.M.A.*, 184:237–239, 1963.
4. Kerin, R.: Metastatic Tumors of the Hand. *J. Bone Joint Surg.*, 40A:263–278, 1958.
5. Murray, R. O., and Jacobson, H. G.: *The Radiology of Skeletal Disorders. Exercises in Diagnosis.* Churchill-Livingstone, Edinburgh, 1971.
6. Panebianco, A. C., and Kaupp, H. A.: Bilateral Thumb Metastasis From Breast Carcinoma. *Arch. Surg.*, 96:216–218, 1968.
7. Smith, R. J.: Involvement of the Carpal Bones with Metastatic Tumor. *Am. J. Roentgenol.*, 89:1253–1255, 1963.
8. Strang, R.: Phalangeal Metastases as a First Clinical Sign of Bronchogenic Carcinoma. *Brit. J. Surg.*, 156:372–373, 1952.
9. Trachtenberg, A. S., and Roswit, B.: Bronchogenic Carcinoma Metastatic to the Hand. *Am. J. Roentgenol.*, 85:886–890, 1961.

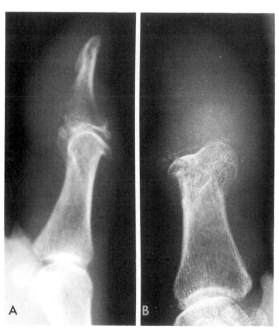

Figure 15–42. Metastases from carcinoma of the lung.

A, The patient presented with soft tissue swelling of the right thumb with pain but without much erythema.

B, Fifty-three days later, the destruction has progressed markedly, with almost complete destruction of the phalanx. There were extensive metastases elsewhere. (Courtesy Dr. M. Clark, Henry Ford Hospital, Detroit, Michigan.)

CARCINOMA OF THE SKIN

Squamous cell cancer is six times more common than basal cell cancer.[1] It accounted for 78 per cent of malignancies seen by Kendall et al.[2] It is five times more common in males than in females.[2] Most patients are over 50 years of age. Of 61 cases seen by Kendall et al., 15 had a history of x-ray exposure and/or evidence of radiodermatitis. A history of exposure to sunlight and chemicals was occasionally seen.[1] Cancers of the skin are more common on the dorsal than on the ventral surface of the hand.

The radiologic findings are significant when there is local bone involvement, which may occur if the tumor is large enough and invasive (Fig. 15–43).

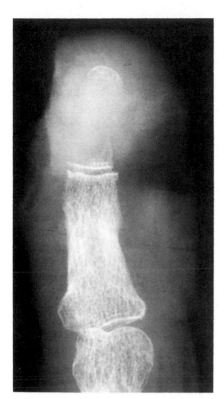

Figure 15–43. Squamous cell carcinoma. A postradiation squamous cell carcinoma of the finger occurred in a physician who received intermittent exposure to his hands over a 20-year period. He had an exophytic tumor of the hand for over three years. The diagnosis was squamous cell carcinoma. There is extensive bony destruction due to the tumor. (Courtesy Dr. M. Clark, Henry Ford Hospital, Detroit, Michigan.)

with localized pain, swelling and inflammation. Subungual squamous cell carcinoma is commonly associated with chronic infection around the nail and previous history of trauma.

Radiologic evidence of pressure erosion of the distal phalanx is seen early in keratoacanthoma, and was present in all cases reviewed by Shapiro and Baraf (Fig. 15–44).[3] Changes are reversible after removal of the tumor. Bony changes are seen in 62 per cent of subungual epidermoid carcinomas and include erosion or destruction (Fig. 15–45). The reason that a greater percentage of change is seen in the subungual keratoacanthoma is most likely the rapidity of growth of this lesion.

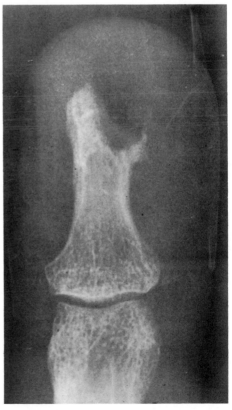

Figure 15–44. Subungual keratoacanthoma. There is a destructive focus in the distal portion of the distal phalanx. (Courtesy Dr. L. Shapiro. Reproduced with permission from *Cancer*, 25: 141–152, 1970.)

REFERENCES

1. Butler, E. D., Hamill, J. P., Seipel, R. S., and de Lorimier, A. A.: Tumors of the Hand. A Ten-Year Survey and Report of 437 Cases. *Am. J. Surg.*, 100:293–302, 1960.
2. Kendall, T. E., Robinson, D. W., and Masters, F. W.: Primary Malignant Tumors of the Hand. *Plast. Reconstr. Surg.*, 44:37–40, 1969.

SUBUNGUAL EPIDERMOID CARCINOMA AND KERATOACANTHOMA

These lesions are masses which grow in the subungual region. They both present

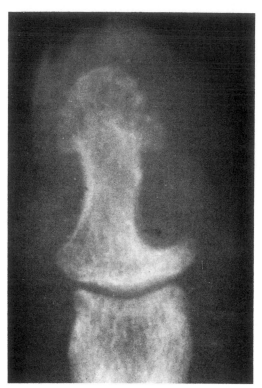

Figure 15–45. Subungual epidermoid carcinoma. Note the smooth erosion and destruction. (Courtesy Dr. L. Shapiro. Reproduced with permission from *Cancer*, 25:141–152, 1970.)

REFERENCES

1. Eibel, P.: Squamous-Cell Carcinoma of the Nail Bed. A Report of Two Cases and a Discussion of the Literature. *Clin. Orthop.*, 74:155–160, 1971.
2. Lamp, J. C., Graham, J. H., Urbach, F., and Burgoon, C. F. Jr.: Keratoacanthoma of the Subungual Region. A Clinicopathological and Therapeutic Study. *J. Bone Joint Surg.*, 46A:1721–1731, 1964.
3. Shapiro, L., and Baraf, C. S.: Subungual Epidermoid Carcinoma and Keratoacanthoma. *Cancer*, 25: 141–152, 1970.

LYMPHOMA

Lymphosarcoma rarely involves bone, but when it does it may produce lytic or blastic lesions. Rarely are the hands involved. Leukemic changes are described in Chapter 19. Lytic changes may be associated with lymphoma cutis.[2] This has the appearance of punched-out lesions or erosion of the shaft of bone in association with soft tissue swelling. This metastatic appearance has also been seen in lymphatic leukemia.[1, 3]

REFERENCES

1. Calvert, R. J., and Smith, E.: Metastatic Acropachy in Lymphatic Leukemia. *Blood*, 10:545–549, 1955.
2. Campbell, J. B., Reeder, M. M., and Sewell, J.: Lymphoma Cutis with Osseous Involvement. *Radiology*, 103:99–100, 1972.
3. Glatt, W., and Weinstein, A.: Acropachy in Lymphatic Leukemia. *Radiology*, 92:125–126, 1969.
4. Schick, A., and Ladd, A. T.: Lymphosarcoma Showing Unusual Bone Manifestations. *Am. J. Roentgenol.*, 79:638–642, 1958.

KAPOSI'S SARCOMA

Idiopathic hemorrhagic sarcoma of Kaposi is a relatively rare disorder with multiple skin nodules that can affect the hand but more commonly involve the feet. The condition, particularly with bone involvement, is much more common in Africa than in the United States. Bone lesions include general rarefaction, cyst-like areas with or without trabeculae, cortical erosions or gross bone destruction.

REFERENCES

1. Davies, A. G. M.: Bone Changes in Kaposi's sarcoma. An Analysis of 15 Cases Occurring in Bantu Africans. *J. Faculty Radiologists*, 8: 32–40, 1956.
2. Davies, A. G.: Sarcoma Idiopathicum Multiplex Pigmentosum. (Kaposi's Sarcoma) In: Middlemiss, H. (Ed.): *Tropical Radiology*. Pages 263–267. Intercontinental Medical Book Corporation, Bristol, Great Britain, 1961.
3. Palmer, P. E. S.: Haemangiosarcoma of Kaposi. *Acta Radiol.*, Supplement 316, pp. 5–30, 1972.

Chapter 16

FRACTURES AND DISLOCATIONS OF THE HAND

by Dean Louis, M.D.

Accurate radiographic diagnosis of injuries to the hand and wrist is an essential part of the complete examination of the traumatized distal upper extremity. Major fractures and dislocations are apparent both radiographically and clinically and do not present a great diagnostic challenge. Lesser degrees of injury, however, may be overlooked both radiographically and clinically and lead to later significant disability out of proportion to the minor trauma that caused them. The finely integrated synchronous functions of the hand depend on skeletal support, ligamentous stabilization and musculotendinous balance. Failure to consider the soft tissue injuries in relation to skeletal trauma may result in delay in diagnosis of ligamentous and musculotendinous injuries. Such a delay may be very costly for the patient, since many soft tissue injuries are better treated early by repair, rather than later by reconstruction. The overriding of fracture fragments, which is acceptable in long bones, would be a disaster in the small bones of the hand.

Likewise, minimal angular and rotational deformities that may be acceptable elsewhere are totally unacceptable in the hand. Modest rotational deformity may compromise the entire hand because of overlapping of digits (Fig. 16–1). Unrecognized closed tendon ruptures may lead to deformities that severely compromise grasp (Fig. 16–2).

Therefore, this chapter places emphasis on the functional radiography of the hand as it relates to trauma. Special emphasis is given to the interpretation of soft tissue injuries that may accompany skeletal trauma. The inclusion in a radiographic report of the suspected tendinous and ligamentous disruption is important because many of these injuries require early operative treatment for an optimal result. The non–life-threatening nature of some of these injuries often results in a cavalier or perfunctory initial treatment by emergency room personnel who are beset with other, more serious problems. The suggestion of significant soft tissue damage in the initial report may prompt appropriate early re-

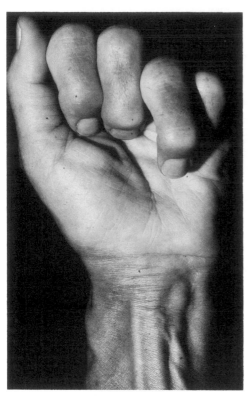

Figure 16-1. Malrotation deformity. This malrotation deformity followed malunion of a proximal phalangeal fracture in the ring finger.

ferral and prevent the necessity for later reconstruction.

In general, posteroanterior, lateral and oblique views of the injured hand or wrist will satisfactorily demonstrate most fractures and dislocations. Special views, as illustrated in Chapter 1 and as described by various authors,[1, 5, 7, 8, 10, 11, 13] may be of occasional value.

REFERENCES

1. Bing, B.: Radiographic Demonstration of the Scaphoid Fracture. *Radiol. Technol.*, 31:380–381, 1960.
2. Böhler, L.: *The Treatment of Fractures*, 4th Ed. William Wood and Co., Baltimore, 1935, pp. 279–299.
3. Boyes, J. H.: Bunnell's Surgery of the Hand, 5th Ed., pp. 581–612, J. B. Lippincott Co., Philadelphia, 1970, pp. 581–612.
4. Brodford, C. H., and Oolphin, J. A.: Fractures of Hand and Wrist. *In* Flynn, S. E. (Ed.): *Hand Surgery.* The Williams & Wilkins Co., Baltimore, 1966, pp. 119–161.
5. Burnam, M.: Anteroposterior Projection of the Carpo-Metacarpal Joint of the Thumb by Radial Shift of the Carpal Tunnel View. *J. Bone Joint Surg.*, 40A:1156–1157, 1958.
6. Eaton, R. G.: *Joint Injuries of the Hand.* Charles C Thomas, Springfield, Illinois, 1971, pp. 1–75.
7. Holly, E. W.: Radiography of the Pisiform Bone. *Radiogr. Clin. Photogr.*, 21:69–70, 1945.
8. Lentino, W., Lubetsky, H., Jacobson, G., and Poppel, M.: The Carpal-Bridge View: A Position for the Roentgenographic Diagnosis of Abnormalities in the Dorsum of the Wrist. *J. Bone Joint Surg.*, 39A:88–90, 1957.
9. Milford, L.: *Campbell's Operative Orthopedics*, 5th Ed. The C. V. Mosley Co., St. Louis, 1971, Vol. I, pp. 190–204.
10. Stetcher, W. R.: Roentgenography of the Carpal Navicular Bone. *Am. J. Roentgenol.*, 37:704–705, 1937.
11. Stripp, W. J.: Radiography of the Ulnar Groove and of the Carpal Tunnel. *Radiography*, 24:277–280, 1958.
12. Vasilas, A., Grieco, V., and Bartone, N.: Roentgen Aspects of Injuries to the Pisiform Bone and Pisotriquetral Joint. *J. Bone Joint Surg.*, 42A:1317–1328, 1960.
13. Wilson, J. N.: Profiles of the Carpal Canal. *J. Bone Joint Surg.*, 36A: 127–132, 1954.

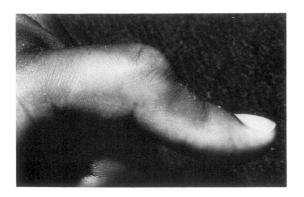

Figure 16-2. Boutonniere deformity. A classic boutonniere deformity followed rupture of the central slip of the extensor tendon.

FRACTURES OF THE DISTAL PHALANX TUFT

Distal tuft fractures typically occur when a heavy object falls on the finger or when the finger is caught in a closing door. Comminution is common, and often these fractures are open. In general, they spare the articular surface, and tendon and ligament disruption is not a problem. Clinical union is expected, since non-union is distinctly rare.

ARTICULAR FRACTURES OF THE DISTAL PHALANX

Baseball finger, mallet finger and drop finger are among the names used to describe this deformity.[3] The extensor apparatus inserts just distal to the dorsal articular margin of the distal phalanx. A sudden flexion force on the actively ex-tended tip may result in one of three deformities: The tendon alone may be avulsed from the distal phalanx, or the tendon and the adjacent dorsal articular margin may be avulsed together with or without dislocation of the distal phalanx (Fig. 16–3). The lateral view is most helpful in determining the extent of the disruption. Flexion of the distal joint and hyperextension of the proximal joint are characteristic. Even when there is no accompanying bony fragment, this posturing of the finger is characteristic. Dorsal soft tissue swelling and joint incongruity may be apparent on the postero-anterior view (Fig. 16–4).

Flexor profundus tendon avulsions are less common injuries.[1, 2] The pathology is obvious when a large volar fragment is present along with the swelling (Fig. 16–5). The swelling alone, however, should lead one to suspect this injury. In eight of 35 cases of flexor profundus avulsion, Carroll and Match[1] noted an avulsed bony

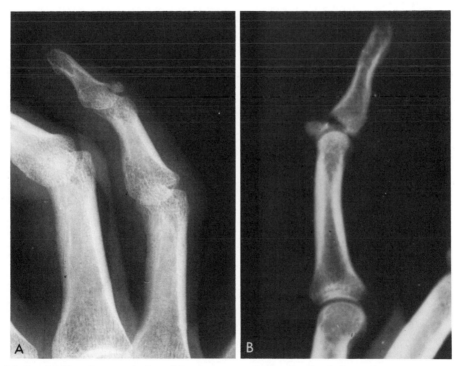

Figure 16–3. Mallet finger. *A,* An oblique view of the distal phalanx demonstrates an avulsed fragment of the distal phalanx associated with loss of active extension.

B, Lateral view of the same patient demonstrates hyperextension deformity of the proximal inter-phalangeal joint, volar displacement of the distal phalanx and a large intra-articular avulsed fragment with its attached extensor tendon.

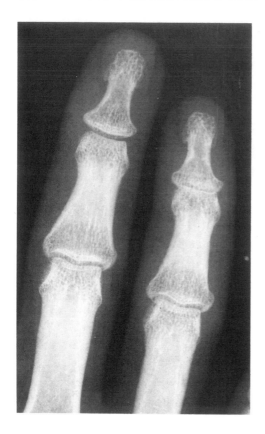

Figure 16–4. Mallet finger. Posteroanterior view of a typical mallet finger demonstrates obliteration of the normal distal interphalangeal joint space due to loss of extension.

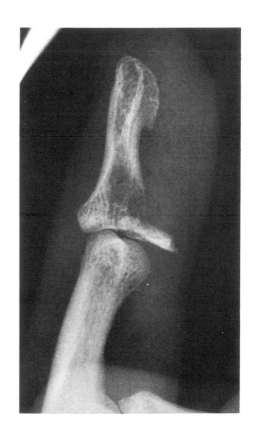

Figure 16–5. Flexor tendon avulsion. The flexor profundus tendon has avulsed a large volar fragment of the distal phalanx.

fragment. Tumors and infections can likewise present as soft tissue swelling at the distal phalangeal level. When a history of trauma is present, however, tendon avulsion should be suspected.

REFERENCES

1. Carroll, R. E., and Match, R. M.: Avulsion of the Flexor Profundus Tendon Insertion. *J. Trauma*, 10:1109–1118, 1970.
2. Folman, R. C., Nelson, C. L., and Phalen, G. S.: Ruptures of the Flexor Tendons in Hands of Non-Rheumatoid Patients. *J. Bone Joint Surg.*, 54A:579–584, 1972.
3. Stark, H. H., Boyes, J. H., and Wilson, J. N.: Mallet Finger. *J. Bone Joint Surg.*, 44A:1061–1068, 1962.

BOUTONNIERE DEFORMITY

The boutonniere or buttonhole deformity is most commonly seen as part of the attritional process that occurs at the proximal interphalangeal joint in rheumatoid arthritis. It may also occur as the result of open or closed trauma at this level. The central slip of the extensor tendon may be cut or may rupture, allowing the lateral bands to slip volar to the flexion axis of the joint.[1] The digit then progressively assumes a typical posture with the proximal joint flexed and the distal joint hyperextended (Fig. 16–2). When a dorsal bony fragment is present, the diagnosis is apparent (Fig. 16–6). However, as with the mallet finger deformity, tendon disruption may occur without bony avulsion. An appreciation of the anatomic possibilities suggested by the characteristic posturing will lead to correct radiographic interpretation.

The early treatment of this deformity is a highly successful surgical endeavor. Treatment of the well-established and fixed boutonniere deformity is far less satisfactory.

REFERENCE

1. Littler, J. W., and Eaton, R. G.: Redistribution of Forces in the Correction of the Boutonniere Deformity. *J. Bone Joint Surg.*, 49A:1267–1274, 1967.

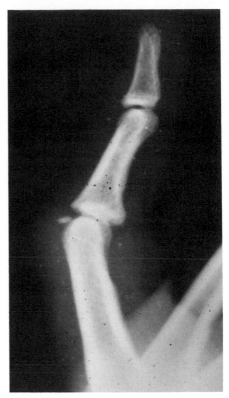

Figure 16–6. Boutonniere deformity. Boutonniere deformity with central slip of the extensor tendon avulsed illustrates distal interphalangeal hyperextension and proximal interphalangeal flexion in the patient shown in Figure 16–2.

METACARPAL NECK FRACTURES

This fracture has been eponymically designated as the boxers' fracture. It may in fact be an uncommon injury in a professional pugilist. It more commonly occurs when the ungloved fist is used. The injury most often involves the small and ring fingers. The fracture line is through the neck of the metacarpal, with volar displacement of the metacarpal head (Fig. 16–7). Less than anatomic reduction is compatible with painless useful function of the hand. This is true even with volar angulation of as much as 40 degrees.[1] Rotation is not acceptable under any circumstances, since overlapping, such as that seen in Figure 16–1, may occur after healing.

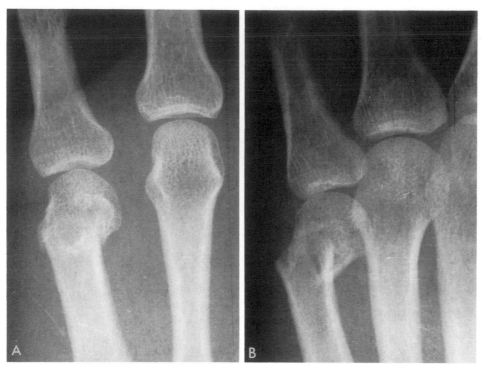

Figure 16–7. Boxers' fracture. *A*, This posteroanterior view of a typical "boxers'" fracture of the distal fifth metacarpal neck demonstrates slight rotation.

B, The oblique projection shows the volar angulation typical of this type of fracture.

REFERENCE

1. Hunter, J. M., and Cowen, N. J.: Fifth Metacarpal Fractures in a Compensation Clinic Population. *J. Bone Joint Surg.*, 52A:1159–1165, 1970.

INTRA-ARTICULAR FRACTURES AT THE BASE OF THE THUMB METACARPAL

In 1882, Bennett[1] first emphasized the significance of this fracture, correlating anatomic specimens with his clinical experience. This fracture dislocation has since received considerable attention.[2, 4–6, 8, 10, 11] The base of the thumb metacarpal has been aptly likened to a rider sitting on the "saddle" of the trapezium. When the oblique fracture occurs through the base of the first metacarpal, the result may be like that in Fig. 16–8. The proximal migration of the major fragment is assisted by the pull of the abductor pollicus longus, which attaches at its base. The ulnar volar ligament retains the minor fragment in position. Since the dislocated metacarpal has no remaining capsular attachments, all of the muscles which arise proximal to the joint and insert distally will encourage dislocation. Varying degrees of displacement may occur, depending on the severity of the trauma. The true extent of the trauma can be demonstrated with techniques described by Billing and Gedda.[2] Lassene et al.[7] have described positioning for evaluation of the thumb carpometacarpal joint.

Because closed reduction of this fracture dislocation is difficult to maintain, open reduction is often undertaken. X-rays through plaster are notoriously difficult to interpret because of the plaster and the superimposed carpus. Tomography may therefore be of value.

The argument has been advanced that degenerative arthritis will ensue if anatomic reduction is not obtained. Considering the myriad times that this joint is used per day,

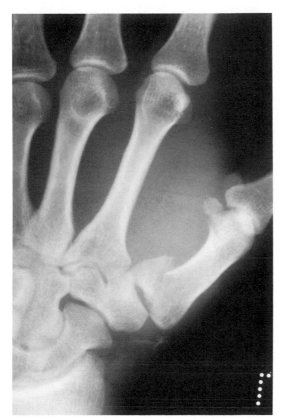

Figure 16–8. Bennett fracture. There is an intra-articular fracture dislocation at the base of the first metacarpal as described by Bennett.

perhaps there is some validity to this view. Orthopedic opinion[3–5, 8, 9, 11] regarding the treatment of this fracture is divided. The papers by Gedda[4] and by Pollen[8] review and represent this polarization.

REFERENCES

1. Bennett, E. H.: Fracture of the Metacarpal Bone of the Thumb. *Dublin J. Med. Sci.*, 73:72–75, 1882.
2. Billing, L., and Gedda, K.: Roentgen Examination of Bennett's Fracture. *Acta Radiol.*, 38:471–476, 1952.
3. Gedda, K. O.: Open Reduction and Osteosynthesis of the So-Called Bennett's Fracture in the Carpo-metacarpal Joint of the Thumb. *Acta Orthop. Scand.*, 22:249, 1953.
4. Gedda, K. O.: Studies on Bennett's Fracture. *Acta Chir. Scand.*, Supplement 193, pp. 1–114, 1954.
5. Griffiths, J. C.: Fractures at the Base of the First Metacarpal Bone. *J. Bone Joint Surg.*, 46B: 712–719, 1964.
6. Johnson, E. C.: Fracture of the Base of the Thumb. A New Method of Fixation. *J.A.M.A.*, 126: 27–28, 1944.
7. Lassene, C., Pausat, D., and Denennes, R.: Osteoarthritis of the Trapeziometacarpal Joint. *J. Bone Joint Surg.*, 31B:534–536, 1949.
8. Pollen, A. G.: The Conservative Treatment of Bennett's Fracture — Subluxation of the Thumb Metacarpal. *J. Bone Joint Surg.*, 50B:91–101, 1968.
9. Spanberg, O., and Thoren, L.: Bennett's Fracture. *J. Bone Joint Surg.*, 45B:732–736, 1963.
10. Wagner, C. J.: Method of Treatment of Bennett's Fracture Dislocation. *Am. J. Surg.*, 80:230–231, 1950.
11. Wagner, C. J.: Transarticular Fixation of Fracture-Dislocations of the First Metacarpal-Carpal Joint. *West. J. Surg. Obstet. Gynec.*, 59:362–365, 1951.

GAMEKEEPERS' THUMB

English gamekeepers subjected the ulnar collateral ligaments of their thumb meta-

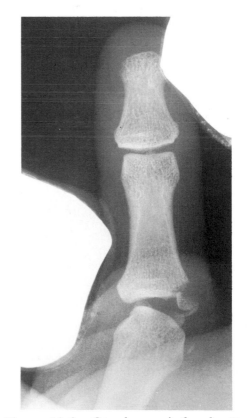

Figure 16–9. Gamekeepers' thumb. Stress view of a "gamekeepers'" thumb demonstrates marked opening of the metacarpophalangeal joint.

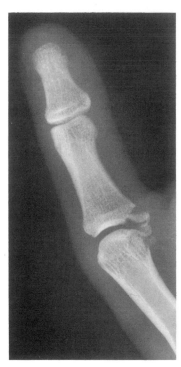

Figure 16–10. Gamekeepers' thumb. Routine posteroanterior view of the metacarpophalangeal joint of the thumb of the patient shown in Figure 16–9.

REFERENCES

1. Campbell, C. S.: Gamekeepers Thumb. *J. Bone Joint Surg.*, 37B:148–149, 1955.
2. Coonrad, R. W., and Goldner, J. L.: A Study of the Pathological Findings and Treatment in Soft-Tissue Injury of the Thumb-Metacarpophalangeal Joint. *J. Bone Joint Surg.*, 50A:439–451, 1968.
3. Frank, W. C., and Dobyns, J.: Surgical Pathology of Collateral Ligamentous Injuries of the Thumb. *Clin. Orthop.*, 83:102–114, 1972.
4. Kaplan, E. B.: *Functional and Surgical Anatomy of the Hand*, 2nd Ed. J. B. Lippincott Co., Philadelphia, 1964, pp. 288.
5. Neviaser, R. J., Wilson, J. N., and Lievano, A.: Rupture of the Ulnar Collateral Ligament of the Thumb (Gamekeepers' Thumb). *J. Bone Joint Surg.*, 53A:1357–1364, 1971.
6. Stener, B.: Displacement of the Ruptured Ulnar Collateral Ligament of the Metacarpophalangeal Joint of the Thumb. *J. Bone Joint Surg.*, 44B:869–879, 1962.

carpophalangeal joints to repetitive stress. This occurred during their particular maneuver of breaking a hare's neck.[1] This same disruption may be seen following acute trauma. A fall upon a hard surface with the thumb outstretched is sufficient to tear the ulnar collateral ligament.[2, 3, 5] This disruption may also involve portions of the joint capsule and extensor hood.[4, 6]

Clinical examination demonstrates the instability, which can also be shown with stress x-rays (Fig. 16–9). Soft tissue swelling is always evident in the acute case. A small chip fracture may be avulsed with the ligament (Fig. 16–10). Failure to recognize this injury early usually leads to surgical arthrodesis for chronic weakness, instability and pain.[3, 5]

INTERPHALANGEAL JOINT DISLOCATION

Dorsal dislocation of the interphalangeal joints is distinctly more common than the volar variety (Fig. 16–11). In order for complete dorsal dislocation to ensue, a disruption of the volar plate must occur. This disruption may be at either attachment of the cartilaginous volar plate or by means of a volar lip articular fracture at the base of the middle phalanx (Fig. 16–12). Instability may be a problem and accurate anatomic reduction is necessary.

Volar dislocations are less common and are often associated with open injuries and extensive soft tissue damage. The central slip of the extensor tendon must be disrupted for volar dislocation to occur. A boutonniere deformity will result if the tendon is not repaired. Collateral ligament avulsion may occur in conjunction with dislocation, as shown in Figure 16–13.

At times the patient, a friend or the initial examining physician will reduce the dis-

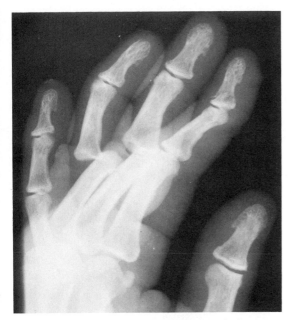

Figure 16–11. Interphalangeal dislocation. Proximal interphalangeal dislocations of the ring and middle fingers with dorsal displacement. Volar dislocation of the metacarpophalangeal joint of the little finger is also present.

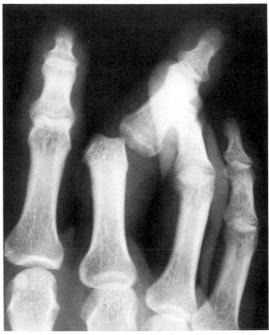

Figure 16–13. Dislocation with collateral ligament disruption. Proximal interphalangeal dislocation is noted, with associated collateral ligament disruption.

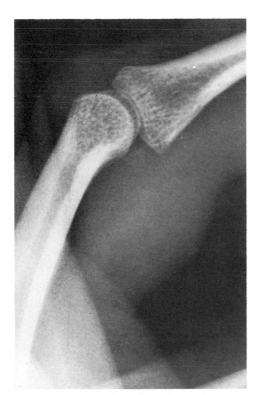

Figure 16–12. Volar plate disruption. There is a volar lip fragment at the base of the middle phalanx with the volar plate attached to the fragment.

location. A visible bony fragment, be it volar (Fig. 16–12) or dorsal (Fig. 16–6), will remain as witness to the prior dislocation. In the absence of bony avulsion, soft tissue swelling alone will persist as the clue.

REFERENCES

1. Curtis, R. M.: Treatment of Injuries of Proximal Interphalangeal Joints of Fingers. *Curr. Pract. Orthop. Surg.*, 2:125–139, 1964.
2. Robertson, R. G., Cawley, J. J., and Fasir, A. M.: Treatment of Fracture-Dislocation of the Interphalangeal Joints of the Hand. *J. Bone Joint Surg.*, 28:68–70, 1946.
3. Selig, S., and Schein, A.: Irreducible Buttonhole Dislocations of the Fingers, *J. Bone Joint Surg.*, 22:436–441, 1940.
4. Wilson, J. N., and Rowland, S. A.: Fracture Dislocation of the Proximal Interphalangeal Joint of the Finger. *J. Bone Joint Surg.*, 48A:493–502, 1966.

METACARPOPHALANGEAL DISLOCATIONS

Dorsal displacement here is likewise more common than the volar variety. Again, rupture of the volar plate is a concomitant

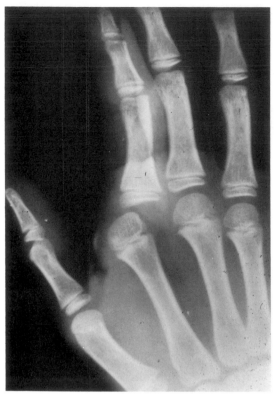

Figure 16–14. Complex metacarpophalangeal dislocation. Oblique view shows a complex dislocation of the metacarpophalangeal joint of the index finger.

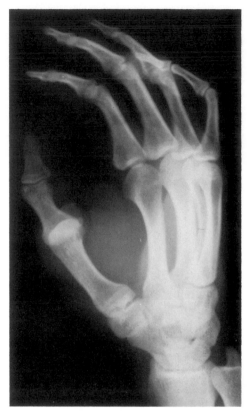

Figure 16–15. Metacarpophalangeal dislocation. Posteroanterior view shows a metacarpophalangeal dislocation of the thumb.

of the trauma. Kaplan[1] has described in detail the pathologic anatomy of the "complex" dorsal dislocation of the metacarpophalangeal joint. In this situation the metacarpal head becomes trapped between four unyielding structures, while the volar plate rests dorsally upon the metacarpal neck. The lumbrical tendon radially, the flexor tendons ulnarly, the natatory ligaments distally and the superficial transverse metacarpal ligaments proximally imprison the metacarpal head. Attempts at closed reduction are uniformly unsuccessful; thus the name "complex" dislocation (Fig. 16–14). Metacarpophalangeal dislocations of the thumb (Fig. 16–15) may become entrapped in the flexor tendons and intrinsic musculature and likewise require open reduction.

REFERENCES

1. Baldwin, L. W., Miller, D. L., Lockhart, L. D., and Evans, E. B.: Metacarpophalangeal-Joint Dislocation of the Fingers. *J. Bone Joint Surg.,* 49A:1587–1596, 1967.
2. Hunt, J. C., Walts, H. B., and Glascow, J. D.: Dorsal Dislocation of the Metacarpophalangeal Joint of the Index Finger with Particular Reference to Open Dislocation. *J. Bone Joint Surg.,* 49A:1572–1578, 1967.
3. Johnson, F. G., and Greene, M. H.: Another Cause of Irreducible Dislocation of the Proximal Interphalangeal Joint of a Finger. *J. Bone Joint Surg.,* 48A:542–544, 1966.
4. Kaplan, E. B.: Dorsal Dislocation of the Metacarpophalangeal Joint of the Index Finger. *J. Bone Joint Surg.,* 39A:1081–1086, 1957.
5. Miller, P. R., Evans, B. W., and Glazer, D. A.: Locked Dislocation of the Metacarpophalangeal Joint of the Index Finger. *J.A.M.A.,* 203: 300–301, 1968.

CARPOMETACARPAL DISLOCATIONS AND FRACTURES

The carpometacarpal joints are shielded from the types of trauma that affect the small joints of the fingers. These injuries are not common. Three views are essential to reveal the extent of disruption, especially when minimal displacement is present (Fig. 16–16). The interosseous ligaments at the carpometacarpal level are very dense and are reinforced by tendon insertions, except for the base of the ring finger metacarpal. The extent of the dorsal dislocation is best determined by a good lateral view (Fig. 16–17). Volar dislocations may be more subtle (Fig. 16–18). Dislocation of the carpometacarpal joint is also occasionally seen (Fig. 16–19).

TRAUMA TO THE WRIST

From childhood to senescence, existence is punctuated by falls on the outstretched upper extremity. The wrist region is commonly involved in such indirect trauma. In childhood, epiphyseal fractures are prevalent. After epiphyseal closure and until the late fifties, scaphoid fractures, intercarpal dislocations and the various patterns of distal radial trauma are the rule. In the later years, with increasing skeletal demineralization, the distal radius is particularly prone to fracture. With the exception of the scaphoid, isolated carpal bone fractures are uncommon at any age.

Scaphoid Fractures

The scaphoid is the carpal bone most often fractured as an isolated injury.[4, 9, 10] Although this injury has been seen prior to skeletal maturity,[3] it is much more common after epiphyseal closure.

The scaphoid is unique for several reasons. First, it has a limited blood supply which enters through its dorsal and distal aspects. The proximal fracture fragment

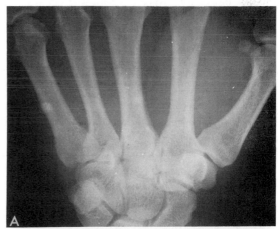
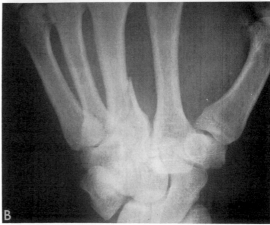

Figure 16–16. Carpometacarpal fracture dislocation. *A*, Posteroanterior view shows fracture dislocations at the base of the index and middle finger metacarpals. The fracture at the base of the third metacarpal is not apparent in this projection; however, the overlapping of the base of the second metacarpal with the trapezoid bone is apparent.

B, This oblique projection more clearly demonstrates the dislocation at the base of the index finger, as well as the fracture through the base of the third metacarpal.

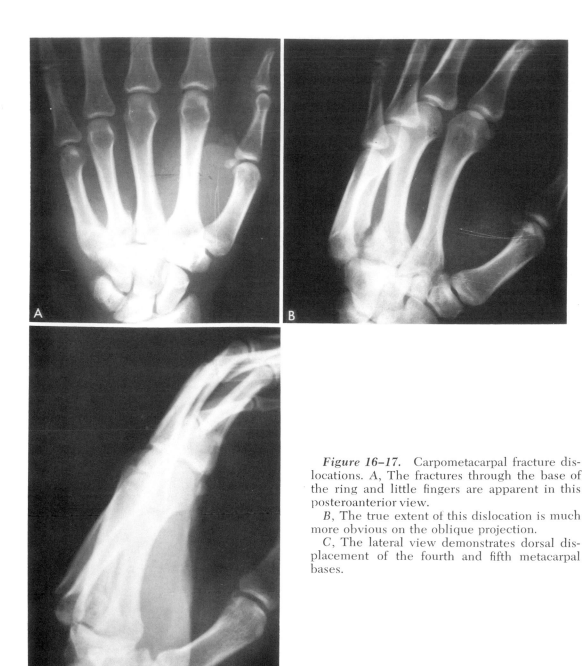

Figure 16–17. Carpometacarpal fracture dislocations. *A,* The fractures through the base of the ring and little fingers are apparent in this posteroanterior view.

B, The true extent of this dislocation is much more obvious on the oblique projection.

C, The lateral view demonstrates dorsal displacement of the fourth and fifth metacarpal bases.

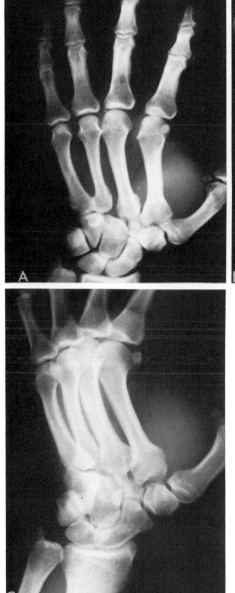

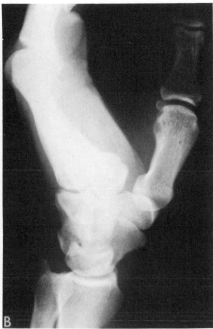

Figure 16–18. Volar metacarpal base dislocations. *A*, Posteroanterior view shows volar dislocations of the bases of the second and third metacarpals. The widened space between the bases of the third and fourth metacarpals is readily apparent.

B, Lateral projection of the hand *A* demonstrates volar displacement of the metacarpal bases.

C, Oblique projection of the same patient again demonstrates volar displacement.

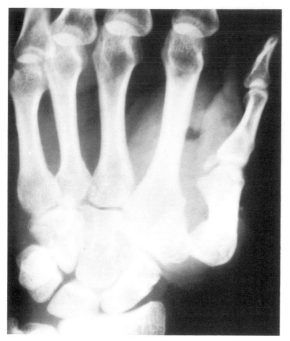

Figure 16–19. Carpometacarpal dislocation of the thumb. All of the interosseous ligaments must be disrupted for this to occur.

must then depend on the blood supply of the distal fragment for healing and re-vascularization. It is precisely for this reason that non-union and avascular necro-

sis are more common with proximal pole fractures, although they represent only 20 per cent of all scaphoid fractures.[2] Further, when the wrist is dorsiflexed, as in an attempt to break a fall, the proximal half of the scaphoid becomes protected under the dorsal overhanging lip of the distal radius. This explains the predominance of fractures through the waist of the scaphoid—70 percent in Bohler's series.[2] Then, because of its relation to the wrist joint and the thumb, the scaphoid is of paramount importance for satisfactory hand function. The voluminous literature relative to trauma involving the scaphoid attests to this. The consequences of late recognition of this fracture have been emphasized repeatedly.[1, 2, 4, 5, 7, 8, 11]

A seemingly innocent fall may be the initial event in an almost predictable sequence of events if treatment is not instituted. Initially, just the persistence of the fracture line may be evident. In the ensuing months and years, cyst formation (Fig. 16–20), eburnation (Fig. 16–21), pseudarthrosis and, later, degenerative arthritis of the radionavicular joint (Fig. 16–22) may be evident.

An adult with a symptomatic wrist after an initial "negative" x-ray has a scaphoid fracture until proved otherwise. Although views in ulnar deviation and in 45 degrees

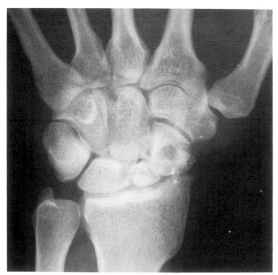

Figure 16–20. Scaphoid fracture. There is an old scaphoid fracture with cyst formation and eburnation of the adjacent fracture surfaces. Hypertrophic changes are also present at adjacent surfaces of the radius and scaphoid.

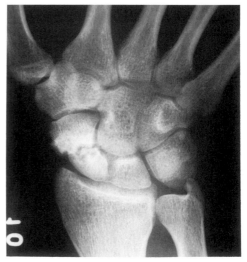

Figure 16–21. Scaphoid non-union. A well-developed non-union of a scaphoid fracture is evident with sclerosis at the bony margins.

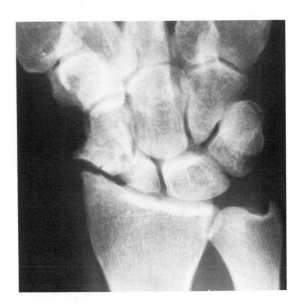

Figure 16–22. Radiocarpal arthritis. There is a pseudarthrosis at the old scaphoid fracture site, with osteophyte formation on the distal pole of the scaphoid, as well as degenerative changes with beaking of the radial styloid.

of pronation and supination may be taken to supplement the three standard initial views, they are not usually necessary. Common orthopedic practice would dictate only the three standard views initially, followed by plaster immobilization of the wrist in the presence of symptoms. Two weeks later, the x-rays are repeated with the plaster removed. At that time, after resorption at the fracture site, the diagnosis will be evident in the majority of cases of occult fracture. Supplemental views at that time will be more likely to aid in diagnosis if they are indeed necessary at all. Fractures through the tuberosity do not present the clinical problems seen with fractures through the waist or proximal pole.

REFERENCES

1. Barnard, L., and Stubbins, S. G.: Styloidectomy of the Radius in the Surgical Treatment of Non-Union of the Carpal Navicular. A Preliminary Report. *J. Bone Joint Surg.*, 30A: 98–102, 1948.
2. Bohler, L.: *The Treatment of Fractures.* Grune & Stratton, Inc., New York, 1956, Vol. I, pp. 827–882.
3. Hill, N. A.: Fractures and Dislocations of the Carpus. *Orthop. Clin. North Am.*, 1:275–284, 1970.
4. Mazet, R., Jr., and Hohl, M.: Fractures of the Carpal Navicular. *J. Bone Joint Surg.*, 45A: 82–112, 1963.
5. Mazet, R., Jr., and Hohl, M.: Radial Styloidectomy and Styloidectomy plus Bone Graft in the Treatment of Old Un-united Carpal Scaphoid Fractures. *Ann. Surg.*, 152:296–302, 1960.
6. McLaughlin, H. L.: Fracture of the Carpal Navicular (Scaphoid) Bone: Some Observations Based on Treatment by Open Reduction and Internal Fixation. *J. Bone Joint Surg.*, 36A: 765–774, 1954.
7. Murray, G.: End Results of Bone-Grafting for Non-Union of the Carpal Navicular. *J. Bone Joint Surg.*, 29:739–756, 1946.
8. Russe, O.: Fractures of the Carpal Navicular. Diagnosis. Non-Operative Treatment and Operative Treatment. *J. Bone Joint Surg.*, 42A:759–768, 1960.
9. Schnek, F. G.: Cited in *Bunnell's Surgery of the Hand.* 5th Ed., J. P. Lippincott Co., Philadelphia, 1970, pp. 590.
10. Snodgrass, L. E.: Cited in *Bunnell's Surgery of the Hand.* 5th Ed., J. P. Lippincott Co., Philadelphia, 1970, pp. 591.
11. Soto-Hall, R., and Haldeman, K. O.: The Conservative and Operative Treatment Fractures of the Carpal Scaphoid (Navicular). *J. Bone Joint Surg.*, 23:841–850, 1945.

Other Carpal Bone Fractures

Compared with the relative frequency of fractures of the scaphoid, isolated fractures of other carpal bones are rare (Figs. 16–23 and 16–24). Fractures of the pisiform and the hook of the hamate may be seen with the carpal tunnel view (Fig. 16–25).[13] The pisiform may also be visualized with an oblique volar projection. Isolated fractures of these bones, as well as of the trapezium, trapezoid, capitate[1] and lunate, are usually

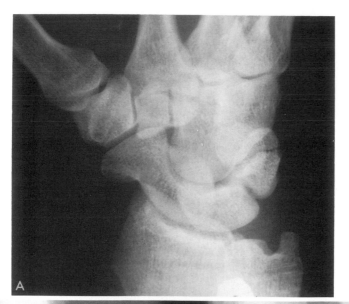

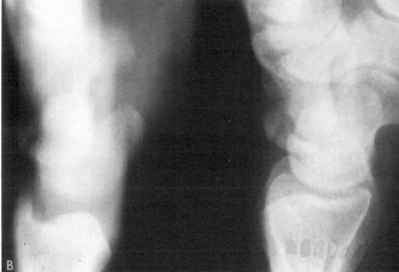

Figure 16–23. Fractured triquetrum. *A,* An oblique projection demonstrates a fracture of the triquetrum.

B, A tomogram and lateral view again show a fracture of the triquetrum.

Figure 16–24. Fractured hamate. An oblique view shows a fracture of the dorsal aspect of the hamate.

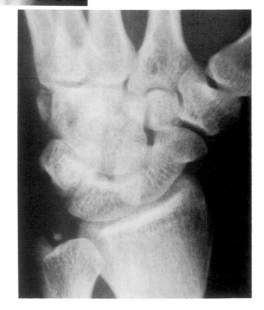

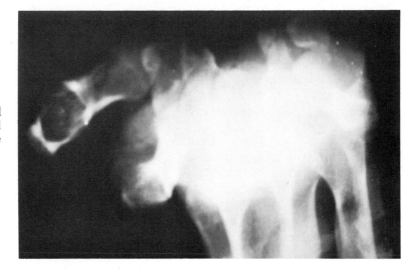

Figure 16–25. Fractured hook of hamate. Carpal tunnel view demonstrates a fracture of the hook of the hamate.

the result of direct trauma in contrast to the indirect trauma that fractures the scaphoid.

REFERENCES

1. Adler, J. B., and Shaftan, G. W.: Fracture of the Capitate. *J. Bone Joint Surg.*, 44A:1537–1547, 1962.
2. Baird, D. B., and Friedenberg, Z. B.: Delayed Ulnar Nerve Palsy Following a Fracture of the Hamate. *J. Bone Joint Surg.*, 50A:570–572, 1968.
3. Bartone, N. F., and Grieco, R. V.: Fractures of the Triquetrum. *J. Bone Joint Surg.*, 38A:353–356, 1956.
4. Bonnin, J. G., and Greening, W. P.: Fractures of the Triquetrum. *Br. J. Surg.*, 31:278–283, 1944.
5. Cordrey, L. J., and Ferrer-Torells, M.: Management of Fractures of the Greater Multangular. *J. Bone Joint Surg.*, 42A:1111–1118, 1960.
6. Howard, F. M.: Ulnar Nerve Palsy in Wrist Fractures. *J. Bone Joint Surg.*, 43A:1197–1201, 1961.
7. Mark, L. K.: Fractures of the Triquetrum. *Am. J. Roentgenol.*, 83:676–679, 1960.
8. McClain, E. J., and Boyes, J. H.: Missed Fractures of the Greater Multangular. *J. Bone Joint Surg.*, 48A:1525–1528, 1966.
9. Persson, M.: Causal Treatment of Lunatomalacia. Further Experiences of Operative Ulnar Lengthening. *Acta Clin. Scand.*, 100:531–544, 1950.
10. Stein, A. H.: Dorsal Dislocation of the Lesser Multangular Bone. *J. Bone Joint Surg.*, 53A:377–379, 1971.
11. Torisu, T.: Fracture of the Hook of the Hamate by a Golfswing. *Clin. Orthop.*, 83:91–94, 1972.
12. Vasilas, A., Grieco, V., and Bartone, N. F.: Roentgen Aspects of Injuries to the Pisiform Bone and Pisotriquetral Joint. *J. Bone Joint Surg.*, 42A:1317–1328, 1960.
13. Wilson, J. N.: Profiles of the Carpal Canal. *J. Bone Joint Surg.*, 36A:127–132, 1954.

Intercarpal Dislocations and Fracture Dislocations

This group of injuries constitutes one of the most interesting complex of articular derangements seen in the upper extremity. Diagnostically, the radiographic changes may be very subtle, especially after manipulation. The fact of the injury usually portends less than normal subsequent function. Less than anatomic reduction is not acceptable here, since it inevitably leads to symptomatic dysfunction. The mechanically deranged carpus will have less than normal motion and is often painful. In time, degenerative arthritis will ensue, which may necessitate arthrodesis of the wrist. Since the majority of these injuries occur in young healthy men, the economic consequences are readily apparent.

The most commonly seen injuries in this group are as follows: trans-scaphoid–perilunate dislocation,[1] lunate dislocation[2] and perilunate dislocation.[6] Dislocation of the scaphoid is seen less frequently, as is the scaphoid-capitate fracture dislocation.[4, 5]

The mechanism of these injuries is probably identical, in that the usual history is one of a fall from a height or a sudden acute hyperextension of the wrist. In all of these injuries the relationship of the lunate to the other carpal bones is the most useful place to look in order to understand the derangements. A good lateral

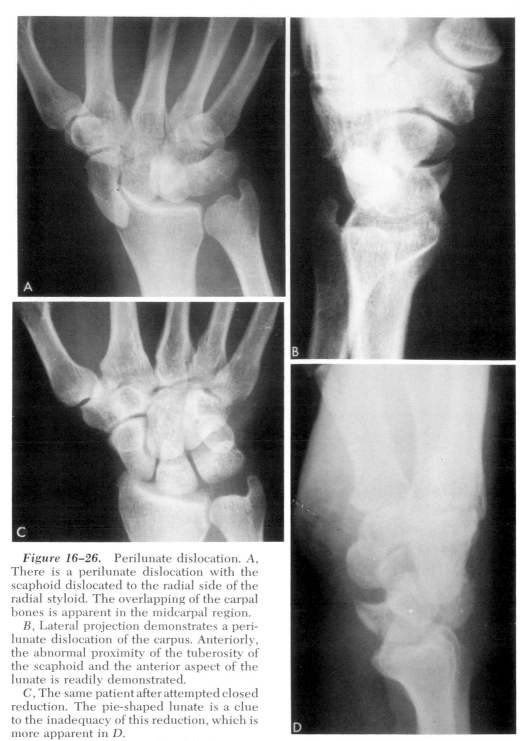

Figure 16–26. Perilunate dislocation. *A*, There is a perilunate dislocation with the scaphoid dislocated to the radial side of the radial styloid. The overlapping of the carpal bones is apparent in the midcarpal region.

B, Lateral projection demonstrates a perilunate dislocation of the carpus. Anteriorly, the abnormal proximity of the tuberosity of the scaphoid and the anterior aspect of the lunate is readily demonstrated.

C, The same patient after attempted closed reduction. The pie-shaped lunate is a clue to the inadequacy of this reduction, which is more apparent in *D*.

D, Note the persistent dorsal dislocation of the carpus, with the lunate maintaining its relationship to the radius.

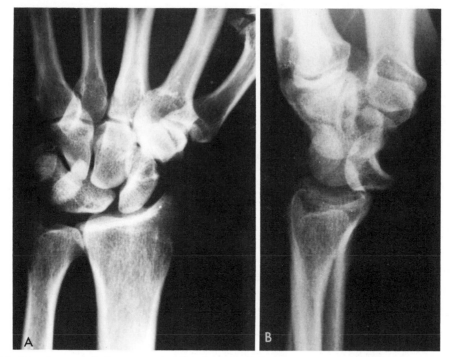

Figure 16–27. Lunate dislocation. A, This lunate dislocation is suggested by the pie-shaped configuration of the lunate seen in this view, as well as by the increased space between the scaphoid and the lunate with ulnar shift of the entire carpus.

B, Lateral view, which demonstrates the lunate resting anterior to the carpus, with the carpus remaining centered over the radius.

view of the wrist is essential (Figs. 16–26 B, 16–26 D, 16–27 B, 16–29 B, 16–30 C and 16–32 B).

Figure 16–26 A shows the posteroanterior projection of a perilunate dislocation. The scaphoid is seen to lie adjacent to the radius and is displaced proximally. The intercarpal relationships are distorted owing to the proximal displacement of all of the carpal bones except the lunate. The capitate is seen to lie between the scaphoid and the lunate on the articular surface of the radius. Figure 16–26 B shows the lateral projection, which confirms the dorsal displacement of the carpus, except for the lunate, which has maintained its relationship with the radius. Figure 16–26 C is a posteroanterior projection after attempted closed reduction. This amply illustrates the subtleties involved with incomplete reduction and the necessity for a good lateral view. In a normal posteroanterior view of the wrist, the lunate is trapezoidal in shape. In this view it appears pie-shaped. Figure 16–26 D, the companion lateral, shows the incomplete reduction of the dislocation. The capitate

is seen to lie posterior to the lunate and the lunate is tilted volarly. It has lost its relationship with the radius, as seen in Figure 16–26 B. Some authorities maintain that this is the true mechanism of lunate dislocation, in which a perilunate dislocation displaces the lunate volarly when reducing spontaneously.

Figure 16–27 A is the posteroanterior view of a lunate dislocation. Again, the pie-shaped configuration of the lunate is seen. In this instance the carpus has shifted ulnarward as well as proximally. Figure 16–27 B confirms the relationships of the volarly displaced lunate, with the capitate lying on the volar surface of the lunate, but centered over the radius.

Trans-scaphoid–perilunate dislocation occurs when the force is sufficient to fracture through the scaphoid. The displacement is usually dorsal, with the lunate and the proximal scaphoid fragment remaining in continuity with the radius. The carpus and distal scaphoid displace dorsally, with additional shifting in either a radial or ulnar direction.

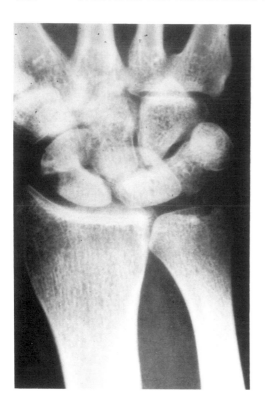

Figure 16–28. Trans-scaphoid–perilunate dislocation. A typical view of a trans-scaphoid–perilunate dislocation. Again, the double density of the lunate and its loss of normal trapezoidal shape indicate the carpal dislocation associated with the fracture.

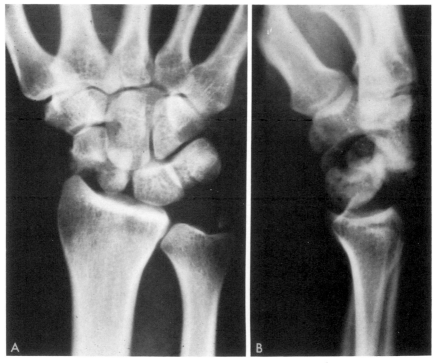

Figure 16–29. Trans-scaphoid–perilunate dislocation. *A,* A trans-scaphoid–perilunate dislocation is evident, with overlapping of the carpal bones in the proximal row and a widely displaced scaphoid fracture.

B, Dorsal displacement of the carpus in relation to the lunate, which is subluxed in relation to the distal radius. The proximal navicular fragment is seen with the lunate.

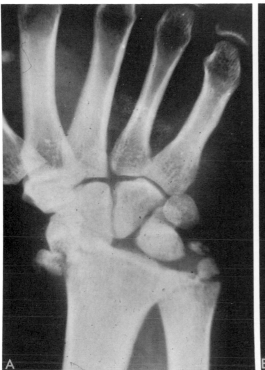

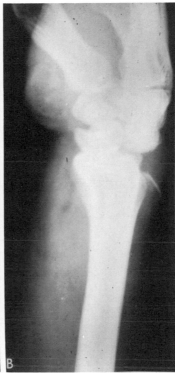

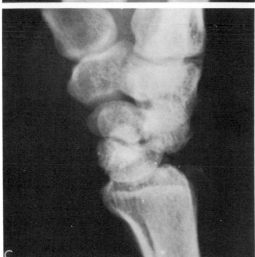

Figure 16–30. Trans-scaphoid–perilunate dislocation. *A,* This is a more severe trans-scaphoid–perilunate dislocation. Here it is associated with fractures of both radial and ulnar styloids.

B, The perilunate displacement of the carpus in relationship to the lunate and the distal radius is further demonstrated.

C, There has been partial improvement by attempted closed reduction. However, the capitate has not been reduced to its normal position with the lunate.

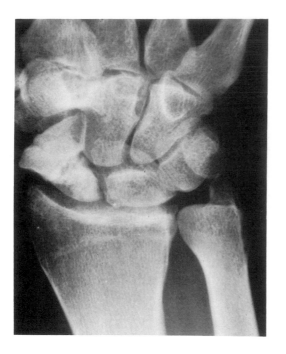

Figure 16–31. Old trans-scaphoid–perilunate dislocation. There persist abnormal relationships of the lunate with the capitate and malrotation of the scaphoid. The tuberosity of the scaphoid is seen in profile as it is rotated on its axis approximately 90 degrees. The capitate is shifted to the radial side of the lunate, and the hamate articulates with the lunate. These abnormal relationships indicate incomplete reduction, and failure to correct scaphoid rotation.

Figure 16–28 clearly shows the scaphoid fracture and overlapping of the capitate, hamate and lunate, as well as ulnar displacement. This is a rather typical posteroanterior view of the disruption, and the carpal overlapping leaves no question regarding the dislocation associated with the scaphoid fracture. The dorsal displacement of the carpus is much more subtle in Figure 16–29 A, although the scaphoid fracture is apparent. Figure 16–29 B reveals the dorsal displacement of the carpus with the capitate sitting well posterior to the lunate. In Figure 16–30 A, all definition of the proximal carpal row is lost with marked radial shifting, so that the third metacarpal is in line with the radial styloid. The lunate is entirely obscured in the posteroanterior view, and its true position is seen only in the companion lateral view (Fig. 16–30 B). Attempted closed reduction in this last case was unsuccessful, as seen in Figure 16–30 C, for although there has been improvement, the capitate has not been satisfactorily reduced to its normal relationship with the lunate. Incomplete reduction with distal scaphoid rotation may be seen late, as in Figure 16–31. The lunate appears wedge-shaped and the distal scaphoid is seen in profile in the posteroanterior view.

This scaphoid rotation is especially important to detect, since it implies displacement with unsatisfactory reduction of the scaphoid.

The unusual scaphoid-capitate fracture dislocation[4, 5] is seen in Figure 16–32. In this instance, an accompanying fracture of the triquetrum is quite apparent also. Figure 16–32 B clearly demonstrates the dorsal displacement of the distal capitate and malrotation of the proximal segment of the capitate in relation to the lunate. Even more bizarre is the complete volar dislocation of the scaphoid and lunate, as seen in Figure 16–33. The diagnosis in this latter instance is readily apparent.

These intercarpal fractures, dislocations and fracture dislocations represent severe trauma to the soft tissues as well as to the osseous structures. Hemorrhage in the area, as well as soft tissue interposition, may block complete reduction. Adequate postreduction views are mandatory and generally require more scrutiny than initial postinjury films. The subtle persistent dislocation or malrotation after attempted closed reduction, as illustrated in the accompanying figures, presents a great challenge, especially when viewed through plaster. Tomography may be most valuable

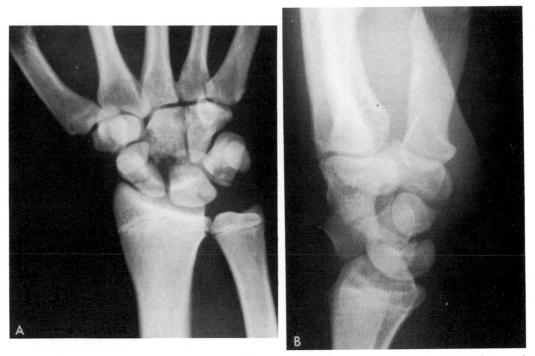

Figure 16–32. Scaphoid-capitate fracture dislocation. *A*, In a posteroanterior view of the scaphoid-capitate fracture dislocation, the proximal capitate is displaced ulnarly.

B, The proximal pole of the capitate, as seen in its relationship with the lunate and the distal part of the capitate, is seen along the dorsal aspect of the lunate.

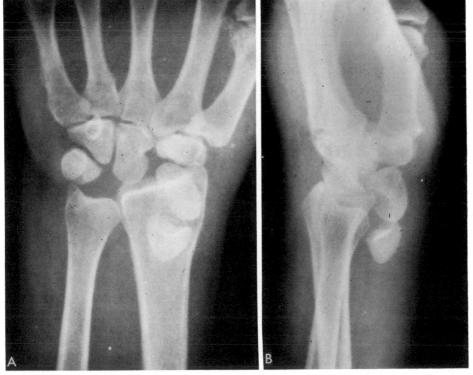

Figure 16–33. Scaphoid-lunate dislocation. *A*, There is a complete dislocation without fracture of the scaphoid and the lunate.

B, This is the lateral view of *A*. Dislocations such as this are distinctly unusual. (Courtesy Dr. R. Carroll, New York, New York.)

in these cases. A recent analysis of the pathomechanics of carpal instability by Linschcid et al.[3] is recommended as an in-depth analysis of these complex problems.

REFERENCES

1. Campbell, R. D., Jr., Thompson, T. C., Lance, E. M., and Adler, J. B.: Indication for Open Reduction of Lunate and Perilunate Dislocations. *J. Bone Joint Surg.*, 47A:915–937, 1965.
2. Hill, N. A.: Fractures and Dislocations of the Carpus. *Orthop. Clin. North Am.*, 1:275–284, 1970.
3. Linscheid, R. L., Dobyns, J. H., Beabout, John W., and Bryan, R. S.: Traumatic Instability of the Wrist: Diagnosis, Classification and Pathomechanics. *J. Bone Joint Surg.*, 54A:1612–1632, 1972.
4. Monahan, P., and Galaski, C.: The Scapho-Capitate Fracture Syndrome. *J. Bone Joint Surg.*, 54B:121–214, 1972.
5. Stein, F., and Siegal, M.: Naviculocapitate Fracture Syndrome. *J. Bone Joint Surg.*, 51A:391–395, 1969.
6. Wagner, C. J.: Perilunar Dislocations. *J. Bone Joint Surg.*, 38A:1198–1207, 1956.

SESAMOID FRACTURES

Fractures of the sesamoids are uncommonly diagnosed injuries and usually are not visualized with routine views. Figure 16–34 shows such a situation in a patient with a painful but stable metacarpophalangeal joint of his right thumb. The fracture was not seen on either the anteroposterior or lateral views. Fractures of the sesamoid may sometimes be confused with bipartite or tripartite ossicles. This is further discussed on page 116.

REFERENCES

1. Reitz, B. G.: Trauma to the Sesamoid Bones of the Thumb. *Am. J. Surg.*, 72:284–285, 1946.
2. Scobie, W. H.: Crush Fracture of Sesamoid Bone of Thumb. *Br. Med. J.*, 2:912, 1941.

EPIPHYSEAL INJURIES

Although epiphyseal injuries involving the long bones have received considerable attention, very little documentation exists pertaining to such injuries in the hand.[1–8] Aiken[1] and Salter and Harris[6] have devised a nomenclature for epiphyseal injuries.

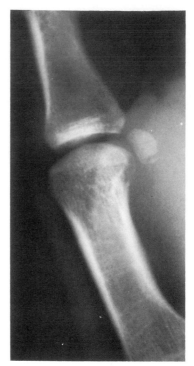

Figure 16–34. Sesamoid fracture. An oblique view of the thumb metacarpophalangeal joint shows a fracture of the ulnar sesamoid.

Based upon clinical and experimental observations, certain facts have been established regarding the nature and fate of these injuries.

The normal epiphyseal plate or physis consists of four distinct zones when viewed in longitudinal section. Proceeding from the epiphysis to the metaphysis, these zones are (1) the zone of resting cells, (2) the zone of proliferation, (3) the zone of hypertrophy and (4) the zone of provisional calcification. The intercellular supporting matrix of collagen fibers lends structural strength to this complex. While this intercellular matrix is abundant in the first two zones, it is relatively deficient in the zone of hypertrophy. The zone of provisional calcification has apparent structural reinforcement due to the calcium deposition.

It is not surprising, then, that the majority of epiphyseal injuries involve separation through the zone of hypertrophy. Experimental as well as clinical experience supports this concept of structural weakness of the hypertrophic zone. The blood supply to the epiphyseal plate is twofold: End capil-

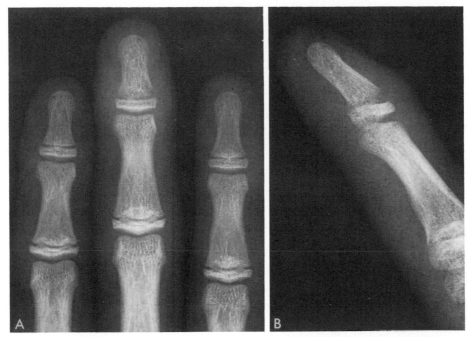

Figure 16–35. Epiphyseal separation. A, There is epiphyseal separation of the distal interphalangeal joint of the middle finger. Soft tissue swelling and obliteration of the distinct cartilaginous zone are evident.

B, An oblique view of A demonstrates the volar angulation of the phalanx in relation to the epiphysis.

lary tufts from the epiphyseal side end in the zone of resting cells. Metaphyseal vessels in a similar fashion end in the zone of provisional calcification. Salter and Harris's[6] work with rabbit epiphyses further amplifies these observations.

If the proliferating resting cells on the epiphyseal side are not injured and the blood supply is not impaired, then longitudinal growth should not be impaired.

Examples of typical epiphyseal injuries in the hand are seen in Figures 16–35 to 16–39. Clinical experience leads to the impression that most epiphyseal injuries in the hand are of the two types illustrated. Either a pure epiphyseal separation occurs through the cartilaginous plate (Figs. 16–36 and 16–38), or a fracture through the adjacent metaphysis accompanies the separation (Figs. 16–37 and 16–39). Growth disturbance does not usually follow these injuries when they are closed. The fact that growth arrest may occur even though separation through the plate did not occur is shown by the case in Figure 16–40. No doubt this represents a crushing injury to the epiphysis itself with resulting avascular necrosis. In the classification of Salter and

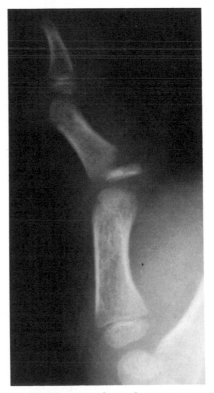

Figure 16–36. Epiphyseal separation. There is a proximal phalangeal epiphyseal separation through the cartilaginous plate.

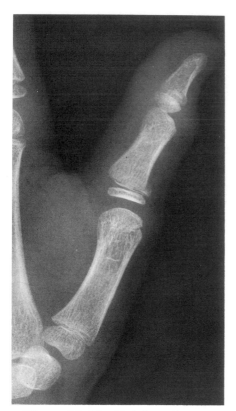

Figure 16–37. Epiphyseal separation. This is an injury similar to that seen in Figure 16–36, except that a portion of metaphyseal bone is attached.

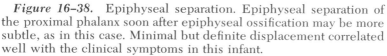

Figure 16–38. Epiphyseal separation. Epiphyseal separation of the proximal phalanx soon after epiphyseal ossification may be more subtle, as in this case. Minimal but definite displacement correlated well with the clinical symptoms in this infant.

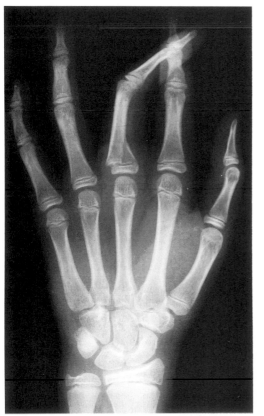

Figure 16–39. Epiphyseal fracture separation. Rotatory epiphyseal fracture separation may present an obvious deformity, as in this case. If correction is not obtained with reduction, late deformity will require osteotomy.

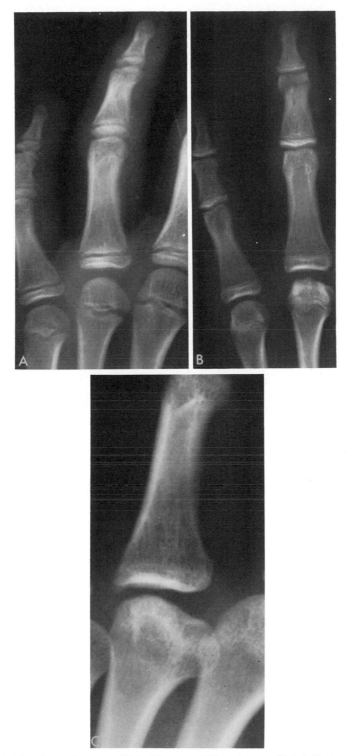

Figure 16–40. A, Epiphyseal injury. This 15 year old boy jammed his left ring finger while playing football. Soft tissue swelling is the only abnormality seen on his initial x-ray.

B, Epiphyseal necrosis. One year later he sustained a fracture of his middle phalanx. The metacarpal head exhibits changes of avascular necrosis.

C, Epiphyseal necrosis. Two years after the injury and with epiphyseal closure, the metacarpal head exhibits persistent deformity.

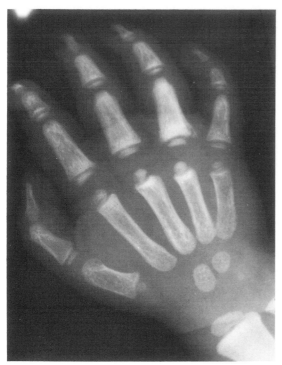

Figure 16–41. Changes from repeated knuckle beating. There is widening of the metaphyses of the fourth proximal phalanx with a small fracture fragment. (Courtesy Dr. W. Berdon, New York, New York.)

Harris,[6] this would represent a type 5 injury, one with a notoriously poor prognosis.

Fractures through the epiphyseal plate may be impossible to diagnose radiologi-cally prior to the onset of ossification of the epiphysis. Only if some metaphyseal avulsion is associated can such fractures be detected. When the epiphysis is small, detection of fractures may also be difficult (Fig. 16–38), since apparent displacement of the epiphyses may be simply due to an eccentric ossification center. Comparison with the opposite side in such cases may be useful.

Epiphyseal fractures may be the result of unrecognized trauma. Punishment of children by repeatedly hitting their knuckles with a stick can cause fractures of the epiphyseal-metaphyseal region (Fig. 16–41).

REFERENCES

1. Aiken, A. P.: Fractures of the Epiphyses. *Clin. Orthop.*, 41:19–31, 1965.
2. Bisgard, J. B., and Mortenson, L.: Fractures of Children. *Surg. Gynec. Obstet.*, 65:464–474, 1937.
3. Blount, W. P.: *Fractures in Children.* The Williams and Wilkins Co., Baltimore, 1955.
4. Dale, G. G., and Harris, W. R.: Prognosis of Epiphyseal Separation. An Experimental Study. *J. Bone Joint Surg.*, 40B:112–116, 1958.
5. Narakas, A.: Interphalangeal Joint Injuries in Children. *The Hand*, 4:163–167, 1972.
6. Salter, R. B., and Harris, W. R.: Injuries Involving the Epiphyseal Palate. *J. Bone Joint Surg.*, 45A:587–622, 1963.
7. Seymour, N.: Juxta-Epiphyseal Fracture of the Terminal Phalanx of the Finger. *J. Bone Joint Surg.*, 48B:347–349, 1966.
8. Stelling, F.: Surgery of the Hand in the Child. *J. Bone Joint Surg.*, 45A:623–641, 1963.

Chapter 17

BURNS, FROSTBITE, FOREIGN BODIES AND OTHER TRAUMATIC LESIONS OF THE HAND

by Dean Louis, M.D.

THERMAL BURNS
ELECTRICAL BURNS
FROSTBITE

FOREIGN BODIES
PENETRATING INJURIES
DRUG ABUSE

Direct trauma may result in the fractures and dislocations discussed in Chapter 16. Other forms of trauma may have indirect effects upon the hand. Among these indirect effects are those seen following thermal burns, electrical burns and cold injury. The radiographic manifestations of these insults are in large part secondary to the injury to adjacent soft tissues and vascular channels. Foreign bodies, crushing injuries and penetrating trauma will also be discussed in this chapter.

Exposure to chemicals and to radiation can cause skin cancer, which is discussed in Chapter 15. Workers in certain chemical industries may develop occupational acro-osteolysis (Chapter 21). Joint disease may result from repeated trauma, particularly in individuals operating vibrating tools. Cystic changes in the carpal bones are an example of the effects of this repetitive trauma, which is discussed in Chapter 20.

Bizarre traumatic lesions in the hand may also be seen in individuals with diminished sensation. Congenital insensitivity to pain, the Lesch-Nyhan syndrome (Chapter 13), and leprosy and syringomyelia, which lead to neuropathic arthropathies, are representative of this group.

THERMAL BURNS

Radiographic changes in patients with burns are well recognized. Thermal as well as electrical burns may result in significant radiographic changes in both skeletal and soft tissues.[1, 5] Schiele and coworkers[8] prospectively analyzed 70 patients with thermal burns of the upper extremities. Joint destruction at the proximal interphalangeal level occurred in 13 per cent of their cases. Loss of soft tissue outlines and osteoporosis are the earliest recognizable changes from direct thermal injury.[3] Later, these may be accompanied by fixed postural deformity, with joint contractures secondary to the extensive soft tissue damage (Fig. 17–1). Acromutilation, as described by Robinson,[7] is a common finding. It occurs when distal soft tissue loss is so extensive that amputation is necessary (Fig. 17–2). The peri-

471

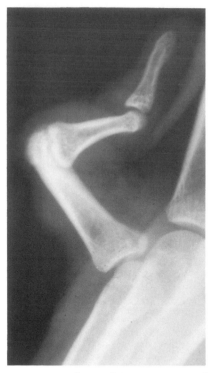

Figure 17-1. Thermal burn. Camptodactyly secondary to soft tissue contracture may follow thermal injuries.

articular ossification that frequently occurs about the elbow in burn patients is not often seen in the hand. Periosteal new bone formation has, however, been observed in the phalanges as a consequence of thermal injury.[3]

The changes visualized early following thermal injury may represent the depth of the acute trauma with loss of soft tissue outlines. Immobilization during early treatment may be responsible for the prominent osteoporosis. Later changes months or years after recovery from the initial thermal insult may reflect static postural deformities as well as disuse osteoporosis. Osteomyelitis is a frequent complication of burns and is discussed further in Chapter 14.

ELECTRICAL BURNS

Electrical burns inflict their tissue destruction in relation to the voltage applied.[6] Currents of less than 1000 volts cause injuries limited to the immediate underlying skin and soft tissue. High voltage here refers to currents in excess of 1000 volts. Such voltages usually cause extensive damage as they travel from the point of entrance to the point of exit. No tissue is immune to the devastating effects of electrical injury; soft tissues, however, exhibit destructive changes earlier than bone. The hand, because of its grasping function, is more commonly involved than any other area of the body. Vascular channels present the path of least electrical resistance; consequently,

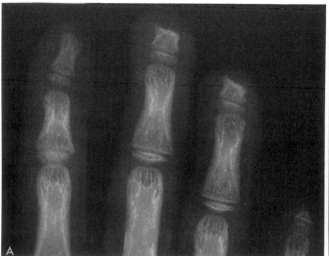

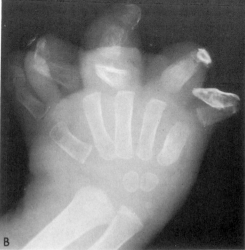

Figure 17-2. Thermal burn. *A,* Acroosteolysis has occurred following thermal burns.
B, This 14 month old child sustained a severe burn. There is demineralization, acroosteolysis and camptodactyly.

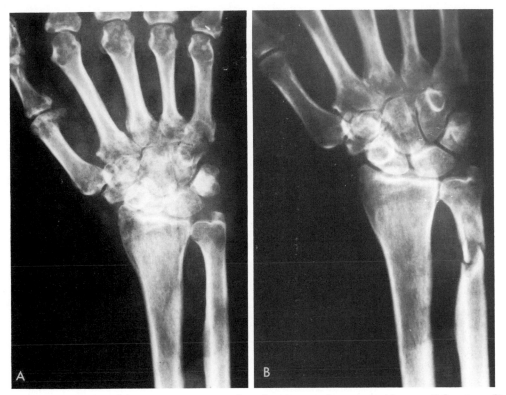

Figure 17–3. Electrical burn. *A,* Four months after injury there is evidence of demineralization with ill-defined areas of radiolucency at the ends of the bone. There is narrowing of the interphalangeal joint of the thumb.

B, Fifteen months after surgery, there is a silent fracture of the ulna. Mineralization has improved. (Courtesy Dr. J. Barber, Cheyenne, Wyoming. Reproduced with permission from *Radiology,* 99: 49–54, 1971.)

superimposed on the direct thermal effects of high voltage injuries are the effects of circulatory damage.

Since skin and bone offer the greatest resistance to current flow, they are the tissues most severely damaged. Bone in the path of an electrical current may be severely damaged although the clinical manifestations may not be apparent for months or years after the initial event.[1] Sequestration, progressive dissolution and segmental bone loss may bear late witness to earlier electrical injury (Fig. 17–3).[2] The combination of direct thermal injury, vascular damage and neurologic interruption leads to late joint and osseous changes. The site of such osseous disruption is usually distant from the entrance and exit locations.

Brinn and Moseley[2] and Jellinek[4] have described changes of mottling rarefaction, medullary widening and fine, discrete zig-zag fracture lines thought to be the result of electrical injury. Of course, disuse osteopenia is also an etiologic factor in the diminished bone density. Barber[1] has emphasized the importance of these late-developing changes.

REFERENCES

1. Barber, J.: Delayed Bone and Joint Changes Following Electrical Injury. *Radiology,* 99:44–54, 1971.
2. Brinn, L. B., and Moseley, J. B.: Bone Changes Following Electrical Injury. Case Report and Review of the Literature. *Am. J. Roentgenol.,* 97:682–686. 1966.
3. Evans, E. B., and Smith, J. R.: Bone and Joint Changes Following Burns: A Roentgenographic Study, A Preliminary Report. *J. Bone Joint Surg.,* 41:785–799, 1959.
4. Jellinek, S.: Changes in Electrically Injured Bones Examined Microscopically and by X-rays. *Br. J. Radiol.,* 31:23–25, 1926.

5. Owens, N.: Osteoporosis Following Burns. *Br. J. Plast. Surg.*, 1:245–256, 1949.
6. Peterson, R. A.: Electrical Burns of the Hand. *J. Bone Joint Surg.*, 48A:407–424, 1966.
7. Robinson, D.: Acromutilation of the Finger, Following Severe Burns. *Radiology*, 77:968–973, 1961.
8. Schiele, H. P., Hubbard, R. B., and Bruck, H. M.: Radiographic Changes in Burns of the Upper Extremity. *Radiology*, 104:13–17, 1972.

FROSTBITE

The effects of prolonged extreme cold exposure to the extremities are well documented.[1-7, 9, 11] Depending on the length of exposure and the prevailing temperature, changes may be seen in soft tissue, bone or both. Initial radiographs taken at the time of injury may fail to show any abnormality. The vascular tree is closed during the time of insult.[2] This anoxic insult is

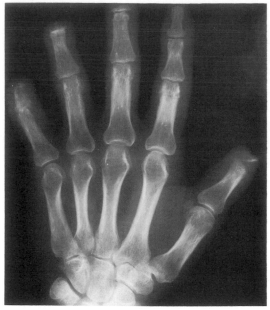

Figure 17–5. Frostbite. Demineralization, cortical bone loss and distal bone loss are seen in this adult's hand. The periarticular bone destruction and cortical punched-out areas in the little finger further typify this injury. (Courtesy Dr. H. Pollack, Minot, North Dakota.)

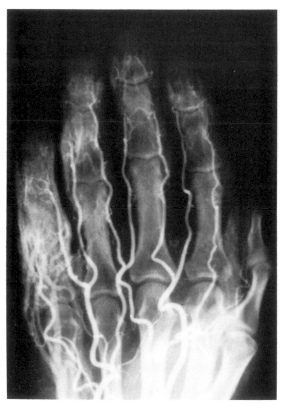

Figure 17–4. Frostbite. An arteriogram following a frostbite shows the diffuse vascular changes typical of prolonged cold exposure. (Courtesy Dr. J. Tishler, Winnipeg, Manitoba. Reproduced with permission from *Radiology*, 102:511–513, 1972.)

responsible for the profound changes seen during recovery. As thawing ensues, vascular channels begin to open, with resulting edema. Direct vascular damage leads to increased permeability, subsequent extravasation and consequent edema. Thrombosis and tissue necrosis may ensue, resulting in eventual amputation.

Hurley[5] has shown that during the recovery phase there is proliferation of abundant collaterals, involving both arterial and venous components (Fig. 17–4).

Blair et al.[3] described four characteristic changes in bone affected by frostbite: (1) variable osteoporosis, (2) acromutilation of tufts due to soft tissue loss (Fig. 17–5), (3) periarticular punched-out areas and (4) punched-out areas with or without marginal sclerosis.

Articular and epiphyseal cartilage may be destroyed or undergo degenerative changes (Figs. 17–5 and 17–6).

Premature epiphyseal closure in childhood (Figs. 17–6 and 17–7) has been de-

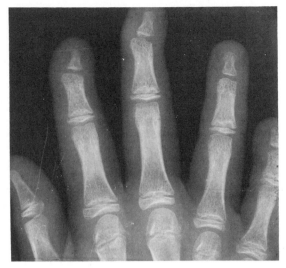

Figure 17-6. Frostbite. In this nine year old girl, the closure of the distal phalangeal epiphyseal growth plate is a characteristic change following frostbite. Deviation of the phalanges is also common.

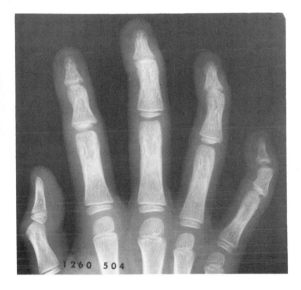

Figure 17-7. Frostbite. This five year old girl had a prolonged cold exposure at the age of two. There is curvature of the fingers and a partial loss of the distal epiphyses.

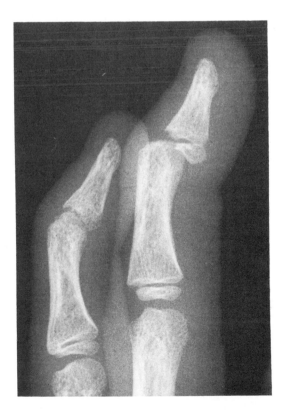

Figure 17-8. Frostbite. Same patient illustrated in Figure 17-7. An oblique view shows that the epiphysis is only partially destroyed. This is most likely the reason for the deviation of the digits.

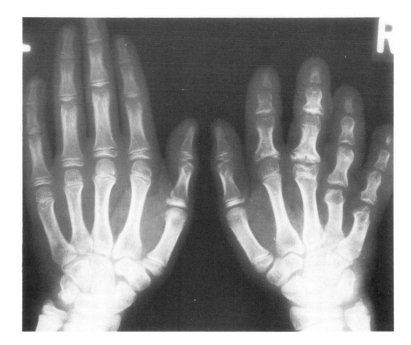

Figure 17–9. Frostbite. This is a severe case of frostbite involving the metacarpals as well as the phalanges. (Courtesy Dr. R. Macpherson, Winnipeg, Manitoba.)

scribed by many authors.[2, 7, 9, 11] The epiphyseal injuries primarily involve the distal phalanges. Occasionally other phalanges are involved, while the metacarpal epiphyses are involved rarely (Fig. 17–9). The thumb is usually spared,[2] since it is clasped within the palm and thereby sheltered from the cold exposure. The surviving hand, which has sustained epiphyseal arrest secondary to cold exposure, is characterized by short distal phalanges. The distal joints may be unevenly involved and thus tend to deviate,[7] sometimes mimicking congenital clinodactyly. The appearance of the hand may also mimic various forms of distal brachydactyly, particularly after the epiphyses have closed (Fig. 17–10). Differentiation from Thiemann's disease is not difficult,[8, 10] since the distribution and type of epiphyseal lesions are different and the condition follows a hereditary pattern (Chapter 13).

Other forms of trauma to the epiphyses, including mechanical means, may produce manifestations in the hand that are similar to those of frostbite, although the distribution is usually different. Occasionally the distribution may be similar, and the true cause of the epiphyseal changes may be difficult to establish (Fig. 17–11).

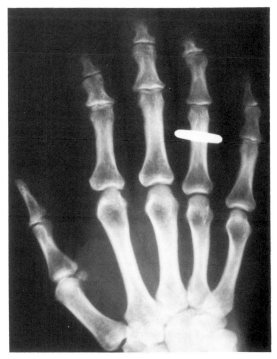

Figure 17–10. Frostbite. The residual broadening, shortening and radial deviation of the distal phalanges are seen in this 20 year old girl who sustained a cold injury at age four. (Courtesy Dr. J. Tishler, Winnipeg, Manitoba.)

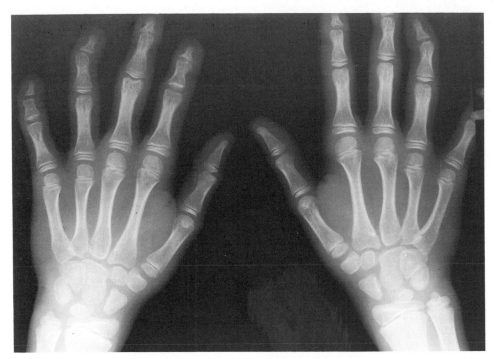

Figure 17-11. Parental abuse with epiphyseal trauma. When he was younger, this child had his hands stomped on by his father. The epiphyseal arrests and phalangeal deviations are probably due to this incident. There was no history of cold exposure. (Courtesy Dr. W. Reynolds, Henry Ford Hospital, Detroit, Michigan.)

REFERENCES

1. Bennet, R. B., and Blount, W. P.: Destruction of Epiphyses by Freezing. *J.A.M.A.*, 105:661–662, 1935.
2. Bigelow, D. R., and Ritchie, G. W.: The Effects of Frostbite in Childhood. *J. Bone Joint Surg.*, 45B:122–131, 1963.
3. Blair, R., Schatzki, R., and Orr, K. D.: Sequelae to Cold Injury in One Hundred Patients. *J.A.M.A.*, 163:1203–1208, 1957.
4. Florkiewica, L., and Kozlowski, K.: Symmetrical Epiphyseal Destruction by Frostbite. *Arch. Dis. Child.*, 37:51–52, 1962.
5. Hurley, L. A.: Angio Architectural Changes Associated with Rapid Rewarming Subsequent to Freezing Injury. *Angiology*, 8:19–22, 1957.
6. Lindholm, A., Nelsson, O., and Svendholm, F.: Epiphyseal Destruction Following Frostbite. *Arch. Environ. Health*, 17:681–684, 1968.
7. Selke, A. C., Jr.: Destruction of Phalangeal Epiphyses by Frostbite. *Radiology*, 93:859–860, 1969.
8. Shaw, E. W.: Avascular Necrosis of the Phalanges of the Hand. (Thiemann's Disease). *J.A.M.A.*, 156:711–713, 1954.
9. Thelander, H. E.: Epiphyseal Destruction by Frostbite. *J. Pediatr.*, 36:105–106, 1950.
10. Thiemann, H.: Idiopathische Erkrankung der Epiphysenknerpel der Fingerphalangen. *Fortschr. Roentgenstr.*, 14:79–87, 1909.
11. Tishler, J.: The Soft-Tissue and Bone Changes in Frostbite Injuries. *Radiology*, 102:511–513, 1972.

FOREIGN BODIES

A seemingly endless list of foreign bodies have found their way into the hand.[22] Solid and semisolid matter are the usual offenders, but liquids and gaseous matter may also be involved. Today, in addition to numerous accidentally introduced foreign bodies, there are a variety of surgical implants that are popular. The majority of these are composed of a silicone rubber and are used for bone or joint replacement (Figs. 17–12 and 17–13). Silicone rubber used for implants usually has a radiopacity similar to that of bone.

Metallic foreign bodies, such as a needle (Fig. 17–14) or a fishhook (Fig. 17–15), are not difficult to identify on a plain film. Mercury globules have been seen in the fingertips following brachial artery sampling using a syringe with a mercury seal.[10]

Paint gun[16, 18] and grease gun injuries[1, 6, 8, 9, 16, 17, 19] are responsible for a num-

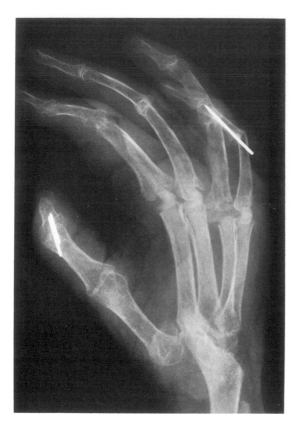

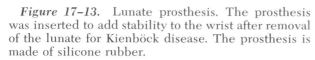

Figure 17-12. Silicone rubber implants in rheumatoid arthritis. Silicone rubber implants have been placed in the metacarpophalangeal joints. Fusion of the interphalangeal and wrist joints has been performed. The implant in the ring finger is malrotated.

Figure 17-13. Lunate prosthesis. The prosthesis was inserted to add stability to the wrist after removal of the lunate for Kienböck disease. The prosthesis is made of silicone rubber.

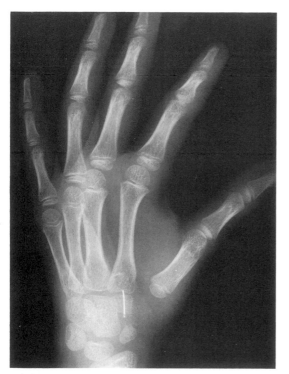

Figure 17-14. Needle in palm. This is a rather typical metallic foreign body found in the hand.

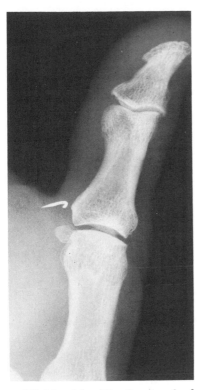

Figure 17–15. Metallic foreign body. This patient's avocation is apparent by the remnant of a fishhook lodged in the soft tissue of his thumb.

Wringers,[13] power mowers,[3] corn pickers[11, 12] and many other machines may cause devastating injuries to the hand.

Glass in the soft tissues can always be demonstrated if the area in question can be projected free from bone. All forms of glass, including those without lead, are more radiopaque than tissue,[4, 7, 14, 20] since the atomic number of glass, which contains silicone, is higher than the atomic number of water. Glass has an opacity similar to that of bone; hence, the importance of multiple views so that all soft tissues may be visualized without overlapping bone. Very small fragments of glass can be visualized (Fig. 17–18).

Most plastics have the same radiopacity as water. With the addition of pigments, however, plastic becomes slightly more opaque. Wood appears somewhat more lucent than the soft tissues but usually can-

ber of digital amputations annually. As pointed out by Stark,[17, 18] early recognition and removal of the foreign matter leads to a higher incidence of finger salvage. If the injected matter has a heavy metal constituent, such as red lead in paint, then its radiopaque trail is easily followed. If such is not the case, the uniform soft tissue swelling may be the telltale sign. When oil is injected, there may be some radiolucency, although edema usually obscures this. The index finger is most commonly involved, since it is the one usually placed over the opening of the nozzle. With accidental discharge, the contents of the gun, under high pressure, dissect a path through tissue planes. This commonly extends along the flexor tendon sheath and may go into the palm. Figure 17–16 illustrates such an injury one hour after the injection of hydraulic fluid into the right index finger. Punch press injuries (Fig. 17–17) may deposit foreign material in the hand, as well as introduce air into the soft tissue.

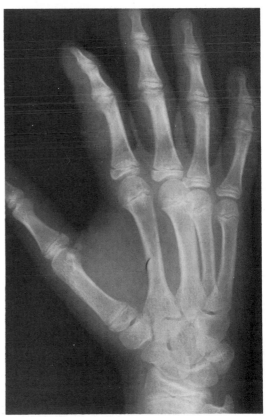

Figure 17–16. Hydraulic fluid injection in soft tissue. No bony abnormality is seen. There is soft tissue swelling of the index finger after this high-pressure injection.

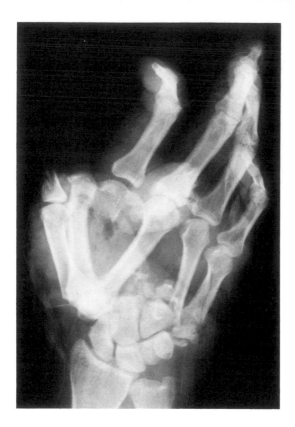

Figure 17-17. Punch press injury. There are multiple fractures and dislocations, and there is air in the soft tissues.

not be identified within bone unless it displaces it (Fig. 17–19).

Xeroradiography[2, 5, 20, 21] is a useful technique for demonstrating foreign bodies that are only slightly opaque or slightly lucent (Fig. 4–4). Wood foreign bodies, for example,[20] are seen much better by means of xeroradiography than with conventional filming (Fig. 17–20). Unusual soft tissue outlines may follow crushing injuries, as seen in Figure 17–21.

PENETRATING INJURIES

Penetrating injuries may require radiography when there is the possibility of a foreign body in the hand. When arterial interruption or penetration has occurred, arteriography may be of great value in delineating the problem. Figure 17–22 depicts a large false aneurysm of the radial artery resulting from a puncture by a fork six months previously. It is quite characteristic for these lesions to present several

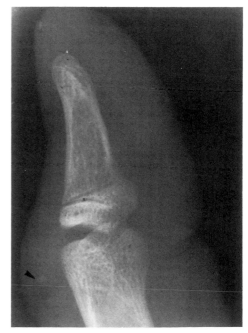

Figure 17-18. Glass foreign body. A minute glass foreign body is seen within the soft tissues dorsal to the interphalangeal joint.

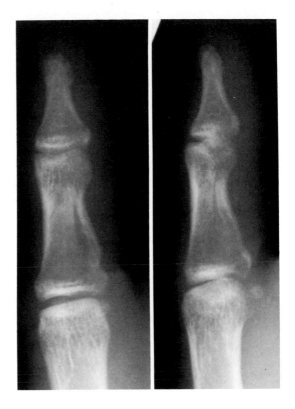

Figure 17-19. Wooden foreign body. A wooden arrow penetrated the middle phalanx and is visible only as an intraosseous lucency. It was surgically removed.

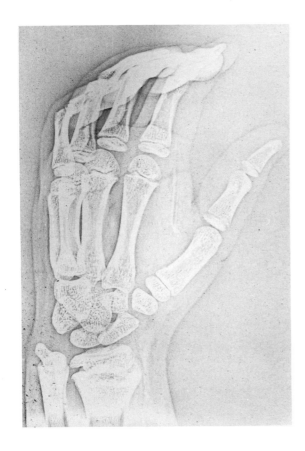

Figure 17-20. Xeroradiogram of wooden foreign body. In the first web space, this xeroradiogram clearly demonstrates a wood splinter that was not visible on conventional films. (Courtesy Dr. M. Ting, Eloise, Michigan.)

Figure 17-21. Avulsed muscle. A punch press crushed this boy's first web space. The abnormal soft tissue density is the avulsed first dorsal interosseous muscle.

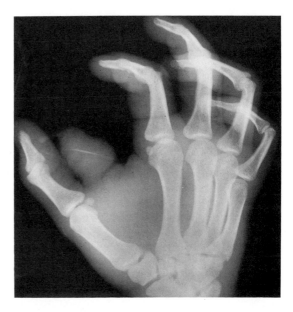

months after such an injury, since soft tissues tamponade the defect early. Arteriography is of great value not only in establishing the diagnosis but also in indicating the therapeutic alternatives. If ligation for such a problem is considered, then the collateral circulation must be assessed preoperatively.

REFERENCES

1. Abernathy, P. J., and Gay, J. G.: An Unusual Injection Injury of the Thumb. *Hand*, 4:173–175, 1972.
2. Campbell, C. J., Roach, J. F., and Jabbur, M.: Xeroroentgenography: Evaluation of its Use in Disease of the Bone and Joints of the Extremities. *J. Bone Joint Surg.*, 41A:271–277, 1959.
3. Danyo, J. J., Lee, K. K., Larsen, R. D., and Posch, J. L.: Power Mower Injuries of the Hand. *Mich. Med.* 67:1061–1062, 1968.
4. Felman, A. N., and Fisher, M. S.: The Radiographic Detection of Glass in Soft Tissue. *Radiology*, 92:1529–1531, 1969.
5. Hills, T. G., Stanford, R. W., and Moore, R. D.: Xeroradiography: Present Medical Application. *Br. J. Radiol.*, 28:545–551, 1955.
6. Jennet, W. B., and Watson, J. A.: The Radiodensity of Glass Foreign Bodies. *Br. J. Surg.*, 46:244–246, 1958.
7. Kaufman, H. D.: The Anatomy of Experimentally Produced High-Pressure Injections of the Hand. *Br. J. Surg.*, 55:340–344, 1968.
8. Kaufman, H. D.: The Clinicopathological Correlation of High Pressure Injection Injuries. *Br. J. Surg.*, 55:214–218, 1968.
9. Kaufman, H. D.: High Pressure Injuries to the Hand. The Problems, Pathogenesis and Management. *Hand*, 2:63–73, 1970.
10. Lathem, W., Lesser, G. T., Messinger, W. J., and Galdston, M.: Peripheral Embolization by Metallic Mercury During Arterial Blood Sampling. *A.M.A. Arch. Int. Med.*, 93:550–555, 1954.
11. Maxim, E. S., Webster, F. S., and Willander, D. A.: The Corn Picker Hand. *J. Bone Joint Surg.*, 36A:21–29, 1954.

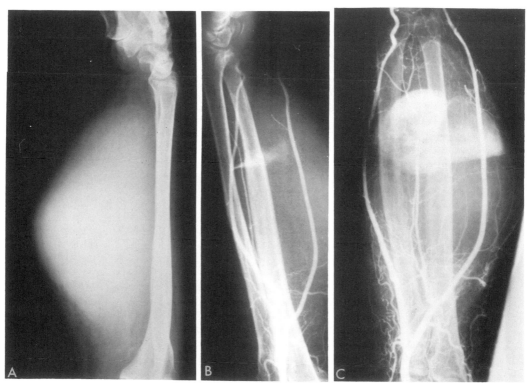

Figure 17–22. Arterial injury after penetrating trauma to the forearm by a fork. *A*, There is marked soft tissue swelling. The mass developed gradually after injury.

B, Early arterial phase shows a leak in the artery.

C, A later film shows the large size of the false aneurysm.

(From Louis, D., and Simon, M.: False Aneurysm of the Radial Artery. *J. Bone Jt. Surg.*, 1974, in press.)

12. Melvin, P.: Cornpicker Injuries of the Hand. *Arch. Surg.*, 104:245–256, 1949.
13. Posch, J. L., Weller, C. N.: Mangle and Severe Wringer Injuries of the Hand in Children. *J. Bone Joint Surg.*, 36A:57–63, 1954.
14. Roberts, W. C.: Radiographic Characteristics of Glass. *Arch. Industrial Health*, 18:470–472, 1958.
15. Shaw, E. W.: Avascular Necrosis of the Phalanges of the Hand. (Thiemann's Disease). *J.A.M.A.*, 156:711–713, 1954.
16. Spak, I.: Finger Injury Caused by Paint Spray Gun. *Acta Chir. Scand.*, 133:331–332, 1967.
17. Stark, H. H., Wilson, J. N., and Boyes, J. H.: Grease Gun Injuries of the Hand. *J. Bone Joint Surg.*, 43A:485–491, 1961.
18. Stark, H. H., Ashworth, C. R., and Boyes, Joseph G.: Paint Gun Injuries of the Hand. *J. Bone Joint Surg.*, 49A:637–647, 1967.
19. Tanzer, R. C.: Grease Gun Injuries of the Hand. *Surg. Clin. North Am.*, 43:1277–1282, 1963.
20. Woesner, M. E., and Sanders, I.: Xeroradiography: A Significant Modality in the Detection of Non-metallic Foreign Bodies in Soft Tissue. *Am. J. Roentgen.*, 115:636–640, 1972.
21. Wolfe, J. N.: Xeroradiography of Bones, Joints, and Soft Tissue. *Radiology*, 93:583–587, 1969.
22. Zatzkin, H. R.: *Roentgen Diagnosis of Trauma.* Year Book Medical Publishers, Inc., Chicago, 1965, pp. 409–438.

COMPLICATIONS OF DRUG ADDICTION

The current widespread abuse of narcotics and other drugs has led to well-recognized sequelae affecting the hands. The intravenous injection of contaminated material or the use of unsterile equipment may lead to local infection, pyarthrosis or osteomyelitis. This is commonly seen in the left hand of a drug addict, but either side may be affected in the chronic, frequent drug user. The puffy hand that is characteristic of chronic drug addiction is seen after venous thromboses and peri-lymphatic fibrosis occur.[3] The accidental or occasionally intentional intra-arterial in-

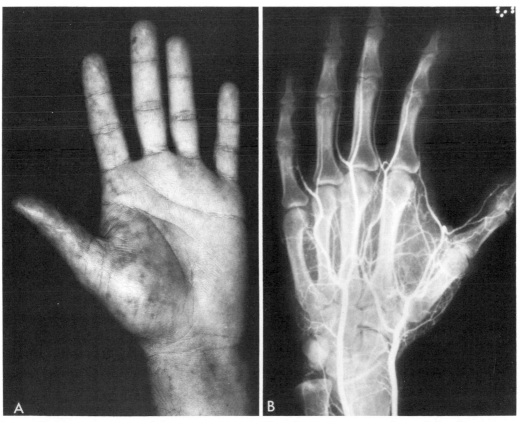

Figure 17–23. Intra-arterial drug injection. *A,* The characteristic mottling of the skin is seen after accidental intra-arterial injection in a drug user. In this case, Methadone mixed with tap water was injected into the radial artery at the wrist 8 hours prior to this picture.

B, This arteriogram shows delayed and diminished filling of the digital artery to the radial side of the index finger in the same patient.

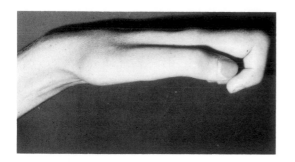

Figure 17-24. Contracture postischemia. This patient lay on his forearm, unconscious, for 24 hours after oral drug abuse. The resulting ischemic contracture seen here is characteristic following prolonged arterial occlusion.

jection of medication may lead to consequences as dire as gangrene of an entire hand.[2] This is particularly likely when medication intended for oral use is injected intra-arterially. Overdosage by either oral or parenteral routes may lead to unconsciousness and to ischemic necrosis of an extremity from prolonged superimposed body weight.[1] Figures 17–23 and 17–24 illustrate the changes consequent to intra-arterial drug injection.

REFERENCES

1. Kaufer, H., Spengler, D. M., Noyes, F. R., and Louis, D. S.: Orthopaedic Implications of the Drug Subculture, in press.
2. Lloyd, W. K., Porter, J. M., Lindell, M. D., Rosch, J., and Dotter, C. T.: Accidental Intraarterial Injection in Drug Abuse. *Am. J. Roentgenol.,* 117:892–895, 1973.
3. Neviaser, R. J., Butterfield, W. C., and Wieche, D. R.: The Puffy Hand of Drug Addiction. *J. Bone Joint Surg.,* 54A:629–633, 1972.

Chapter 18

HEMATOLOGIC DISORDERS AND THE RETICULO-ENDOTHELIOSES

THE ANEMIAS
  Sickle Cell Disease
  Thalassemia (Cooley Anemia, Mediterranean
     Anemia, Erythroblastic Anemia)
  Other Anemias
**MYELOSCLEROSIS (MYELOFIBROSIS, AGNOGENIC
MYELOID METAPLASIA, OSTEOSCLEROTIC
ANEMIA)**
POLYCYTHEMIA

LEUKEMIA
HEMOPHILIA
THE RETICULOENDOTHELIOSES
  Histiocytosis X (Eosinophilic Granuloma,
     Hand-Schüller-Christian Disease
     and Letterer-Siwe Disease)
  Gaucher Disease
  Niemann-Pick Disease

In this chapter we will discuss the anemias, both congenital and acquired, polycythemia, hemophilia, leukemia and the reticuloendothelioses. The congenital malformation syndromes associated with hematologic disturbance, including Fanconi anemia, Blackfan-Diamond anemia and thrombocytopenia–absent radius syndrome, were discussed in Chapter 13. Chronic granulomatous disease of childhood, although it is a disease of the leukocyte, was discussed in Chapter 14 with infections of the hand, which are its primary radiologic manifestations.

THE ANEMIAS

The acquired osseous changes in the anemias are seen both in the congenital anemias, such as sickle cell disease and thalassemia, and in some of the acquired ones, such as iron deficiency anemia. The acquired changes in the hand are of three main types. First, the overactive marrow associated with anemia results in coarsening of the bony trabeculae and failure of tubulation. These phenomena are most marked in thalassemia but may be seen in any of the other forms, and may also occur in other situations where the marrow is

hyperplastic, as in polycythemia or in the storage disorders such as the reticuloendothelioses. The second group of findings is secondary to infarction of bone and occurs mainly in sickle cell disease but can also occur in the others. The third group of findings are nonspecific effects resulting from chronic illness and are manifested by delays in maturation, dwarfism and poor mineralization. There may also be a tendency to infection, particularly in sickle cell anemia.

Sickle Cell Disease

This is a hereditary disorder of hemoglobin transmitted as a mendelian dominant. In its homozygous form (SS hemoglobin) it is associated with a hemolytic anemia. It is seen almost exclusively in blacks. Combinations of sickle cell hemoglobin and other forms may occur, and these mixed hemoglobinopathies may have varying clinical and radiologic manifestations of sickle cell disease. Hemoglobin SC disease[1] is one of the more common of these.

The most characteristic radiologic findings of sickle cell disease are those associated with infarction of bone, the so-called

485

hand-foot syndrome. The clinical manifestations are swelling and tenderness of the hand. The condition occurs almost entirely in infants and young children. It is rarely seen before six months of age, when the children may still have the protection of their fetal hemoglobin.[9] The peak incidence is between six and 24 months, after which it diminishes.[9] The small bones of the hand and feet are most commonly involved in children, although infarction may occur in the long bones as well. The reason for predilection for the hand and foot bones in this age group is not clear, but it may be related to the increase in cellular marrow which may be prone to circulatory stasis.[13] According to Cockshott,[3] the condition is more common in Africa, possibly because babies are carried in a manner that compresses their wrists and ankles.

The true incidence of this infarction is not well documented, and Reynolds[8] states that it may occur in 25 per cent of affected individuals, which is higher than the incidence in the reported series.

At the time of onset of symptoms the radiologic findings are usually nonspecific. There may be coarsening of the trabecular pattern secondary to the anemia, and there is soft tissue swelling. In about two weeks periosteal elevation may become evident. This can vary from a barely perceptible thin line to marked swelling of the shaft. Usually both hands are involved, and several bones in each hand are affected. However, the findings are often asymmetric. In the

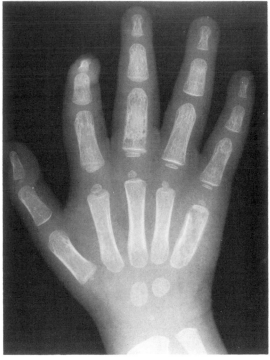

Figure 18–1. Hand-foot syndrome of sickle cell disease. Twenty month old female. Foci of destruction are seen best in the third proximal phalanx and the fifth metacarpal. There is some periosteal elevation in the fifth and second metacarpals. In the opposite hand the destructive changes were in the fifth proximal phalanx and the first metacarpal.

diaphyses there may be areas of bone destruction ranging from minimal to severe (Figs. 18–1 and 18–2). In some patients

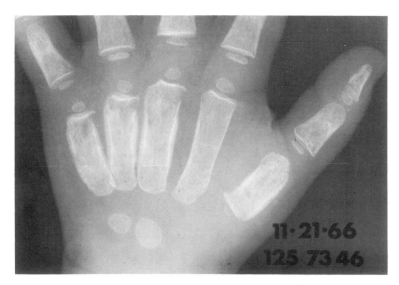

Figure 18–2. Hand-foot syndrome of sickle cell disease. There is extensive periostitis and disphyseal destruction involving a number of bones.

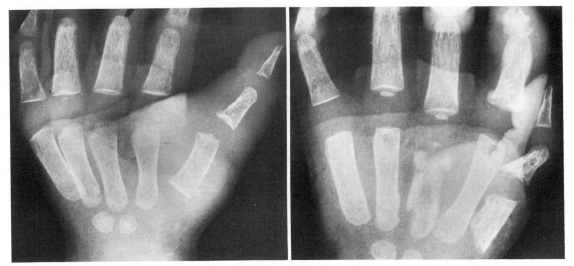

Figure 18–3. Brachydactyly from sickle cell disease. *A*, On the earlier film the first metacarpal is only barely involved.

B, On the subsequent film there is now relative shortening of this metacarpal, as well as a number of new acute lesions. The end of the proximal phalanx of the thumb appears deformed, suggesting that there will be a cone epiphysis at this site. (Courtesy Dr. S. Bohrer, Ibadan, Nigeria.)

there may be relatively few symptoms associated with the infarction. There may be tenderness of one finger, while in other hand bones radiographs show evidence of multiple old infarcts which were previously undetected by the parents or the child.

Differentiation from osteomyelitis is difficult both clinically and radiologically, since the roentgen findings are similar in both conditions. The lack of systemic symptoms and fever may be helpful in diagnosis. Osteomyelitis, particularly due to salmonella but also due to other organisms, such as shigella,[11] occurs more frequently in patients with sickle cell disease than in the general population. Also, infarcted bone may represent a good site for infection. Thus, since infection can never be completely ruled out, the patient should probably be treated as if it were present. Leukemic changes in bone may also have a similar pattern, but the distribution involving the hand and foot only is uncommon in leukemia. Involvement of long bones does, however, occur in some infants and children with sickle cell anemia,[2] so that differentiation is not always possible.

Occasionally the infarcts may result in secondary changes in the epiphyses, resulting in a cone epiphysis (Figs. 18–3 and 18–4). This cone is often associated with

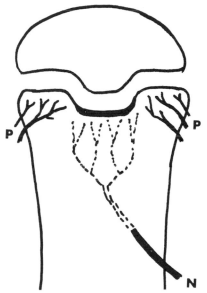

Figure 18–4. Schematic drawing illustrating mechanism of cone formation. The vessels going through the diaphysis supply the central portion of the epiphyseal plate. During infarction of the shaft these vessels are obstructed, with consequent failure of growth of the central portion. The periphery of the epiphyseal plate is supplied by periosteal vessels and remains unaffected. The alteration in growth at the epiphyseal plate causes the cone-shaped epiphysis. (After Reynolds, J., A Re-evaluation of the "Fish Vertebra" Signs in Sickle Cell Hemoglobinopathy. *American Journal of Roentgenology, Radium Therapy and Nuclear Medicine*, 97: 693, 1966. Courtesy of Charles C Thomas, Publisher, Springfield, Illinois.)

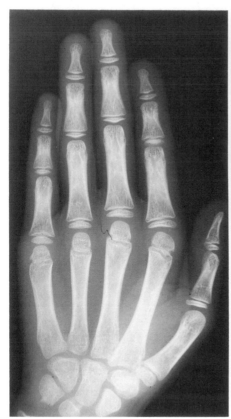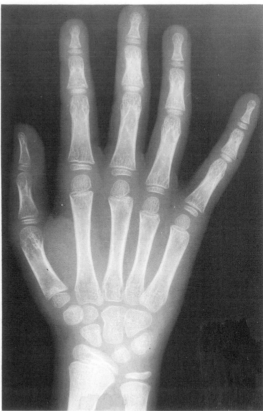

Figure 18–5. Eleven year old girl with sickle cell disease who suffered a stroke at age five with residual paresis of the right side. The right hand is hypoplastic and delayed in maturation when compared to the left. Note also the cone-like indentation on the epiphyseal plate of the first left metacarpal, most likely from an old infarct.

premature fusion that may result in various patterns of brachydactyly (Fig. 18–3),[3, 5, 8] usually with a peculiar distribution which differentiates it from some of the brachydactyly syndromes. If the metacarpals are involved, these changes can mimic those of pseudohyperparathyroidism or related conditions. The mechanism of these changes is that the blood supply to the center of the epiphyseal plate comes through the diaphyseal blood vessels, which may be compressed by the infarction with resultant cessation of growth in this area.[3, 9] The periphery of the epiphyseal plate is supplied by periosteal vessels, which are unaffected. Thus, the central part of the bone does not grow (Fig. 18–4), resulting in a cone epiphysis. The incidence of these secondary findings is not known, since most patients with sickle cell anemia do not have radiographs of the hands when they are older, and the shortening may be difficult to ascertain clinically. It seems likely that this is a rare condition.

The changes of anemia as manifested by coarsening of trabeculation and widening of the shafts are seen mainly in childhood and are most marked between the second and seventh years.[8] There may be an increase in size of the nutrient foramina.[8] These signs are much less marked than in thalassemia. There may also be an overall growth disturbance, with retardation of growth and maturation. Secondary signs in the hand may also be due to stroke, with consequent hypoplasia and demineralization (Fig. 18–5).

Changes in the remainder of the skeleton are well known. They include the stigmata of infarction in the long bones, both in the shaft and in the epiphyseal areas, with necrosis of the femoral heads. The skull may have a granular appearance or there may be widening of the diploic space. Extramedullary hematopoiesis may present as soft tissue masses. Changes in the spine include squarish indentations on the end plates.

REFERENCES

1. Barton, C. J., and Cockshott, W. P.: Bone Changes in Hemoglobin SC Disease. *Am. J. Roentgenol.*, 88:523–532, 1962.
2. Bohrer, S. P.: Acute Long Bone Diaphyseal Infarcts in Sickle Cell Disease. *Br. J. Radiol.*, 43:685–697, 1970.
3. Cockshott, W. P.: Dactylitis and Growth Disorders. *Br. J. Radiol.*, 36:19–26, 1963.
4. Constant, E., Green, R. L., and Wagner, D. K.: Salmonella Osteomyelitis of Both Hands and the Hand-Foot Syndrome. *Arch. Surg.*, 102: 148–151, 1971.
5. Greenfield, G. B.: *Radiology of Bone Diseases.* J. B. Lippincott Co., Philadelphia, 1969.
6. Hewett, B. V., and Nice, C. M., Jr.: Radiographic Manifestations of Sickle Cell Anemia. *Radiol. Clin. N. Am.*, 2:249–259, 1964.
7. Moseley, J. E.: *Bone Changes in Hematologic Disorders (Roentgen Aspects).* Grune & Stratton, Inc., New York, 1963.
8. Reynolds, J.: *The Roentgenologic Features of Sickle Cell Disease and Related Hemoglobinopathies.* Charles C Thomas, Springfield, Illinois, 1965.
9. Reynolds, J.: A Re-evaluation of the "Fish Vertebra" Sign in Sickle Cell Hemoglobinopathy. *Am. J. Roentgenol.*, 97:693–707, 1966.
10. Roberts, A. R., and Hilburg, L. E.: Sickle Cell Disease with Salmonella Osteomyelitis. *J. Pediatr.*, 52:170–175, 1958.
11. Rubin, H. M., Eardley, W., and Nichols, B. L.: *Shigella sonnei* Osteomyelitis and Sickle-Cell Anemia. *Am. J. Dis. Child.*, 116:83–87, 1968.
12. Watson, R. J., Burko, H., Megas, H., and Robinson, M.: The Hand-Foot Syndrome in Sickle-Cell Disease in Young Children. *Pediatrics*, 31: 975–982, 1963.
13. Weinberg, A. G., and Currarino, G.: Sickle Cell Dactylitis: Histopathologic Observations. *Am. J. Clin. Pathol.*, 58:518–523, 1972.

Thalassemia (Cooley Anemia, Mediterranean Anemia, Erythroblastic Anemia)

Thalassemia is a hereditary anemia due to an abnormality in hemoglobin synthesis. It may occur in homozygous form (thalassemia major) or heterozygous form (thalas-

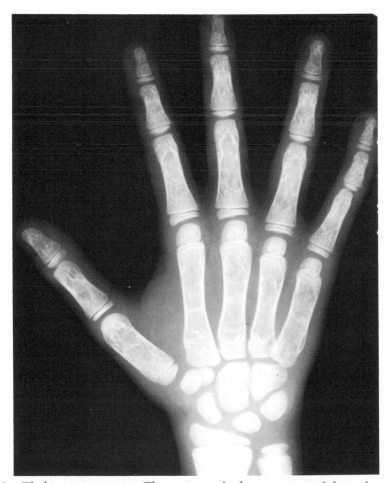

Figure 18–6. Thalassemia major. There is marked coarsening of the trabecular pattern.

semia minor). It is seen mainly in individuals of Mediterranean descent. Thalassemia may also be associated with various hemoglobinopathies. In thalassemia major the anemia is severe and occurs early in childhood. There may be associated splenomegaly and hepatomegaly. Without treatment most patients die in childhood or adolescence.

The radiologic changes in the hand are those of erythroid hyperplasia in the bone marrow, and because of the severity of the anemia in childhood, these changes are usually the most dramatic of those of the anemias (Fig. 18–6). The changes may be seen as early as six months to one year of age,[4] improve with age (Fig. 18–7 *C*), and completely disappear in adolescence.[1] However, the appearance in the hand is nonspecific except on the basis of severity, which if pronounced suggests the possibility of thalassemia rather than of one of the other anemias. The trabecular pattern is coarse and many of the trabeculae are thinned because of resorption due to marrow hyperplasia. There is associated thinning of the cortex and there may be failure of tubulation, particularly in the metacarpals. The nutrient foramina often appear large (Fig. 18–7 *A*).

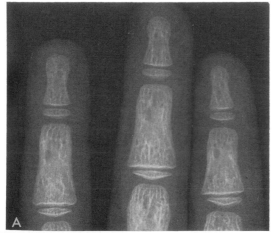

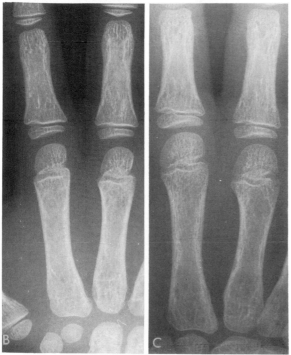

Figure 18–7. Thalassemia major. *A* and *B*, Six year old female. There is coarsening of the trabecular pattern. The nutrient foramina are particularly prominent in the middle phalanges. There is somewhat poor tubulation of the metacarpals.

C, There is an improvement in the trabecular pattern three years later.

There is a generalized failure of growth. Caffey[1] considers this condition to be the most severe example of dwarfism resulting from anemia. Bone maturation may be retarded.[1] Although epiphyseal fusion occurs in the shoulder and other joints, it usually does not occur in the hand.[2] Other skeletal findings include inhibition of pneumatization of the paranasal sinuses, particularly the maxillary. This is fairly characteristic of thalassemia. The maxillary prominence may result in hypertelorism and malocclusion with a rodent-like appearance. The skull findings are similar to those in the other anemias, with widening of the diploic spaces or a hair-on-end appearance. The changes in the long bones may be similar to those in the hand.

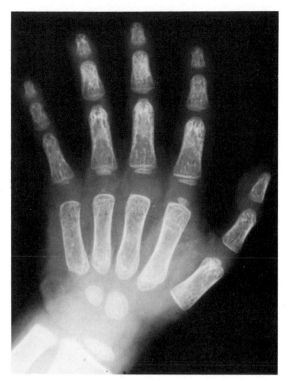

Figure 18–8. Iron deficiency anemia. The coarsened trabecular pattern is nonspecific.

REFERENCES

1. Caffey, J.: Cooley's Anemia: A Review of the Roentgenographic Findings in the Skeleton. Hickey Lecture, 1957. *Am. J. Roentgenol.*, 78:381–391, 1957.
2. Currarino, G., and Erlandson, M. E.: Premature Fusion of Epiphyses in Cooley's Anemia. *Radiology*, 83:656–664, 1964.
3. Logothetis, J., Economidou, J., Constantoulakis, M., Augoustaki, O., Loewenson, R. B., and Bilek, M.: Cephalofacial Deformities in Thalassemia Major (Cooley's Anemia). A Correlative Study Among 138 Cases. *Am. J. Dis. Child.*, 121:300–306, 1971.
4. Moseley, J. E.: *Bone Changes in Hematologic Disorders (Roentgen Aspects).* Grune & Stratton, Inc., New York, 1963.

Other Anemias

Other congenital anemias, including hereditary spherocytosis, hereditary elliptocytosis, pyruvate kinase deficiency and various other hemoglobin abnormalities, may have the nonspecific changes of anemia.[4] Various hemoglobin abnormalities may coexist in the same individual. Severe iron deficiency anemia[1, 3] may produce trabecular changes very similar to those seen in thalassemia or sickle cell disease (Fig. 18–8).

In erythroblastosis fetalis the radiologic findings are nonspecific lucent bands in the metaphysis.[2, 4]

REFERENCES

1. Aksoy, M., Camli, N., and Erdem, S.: Roentgenographic Bone Changes in Chronic Iron Deficiency Anemia. A Study in Twelve Patients. *Blood,* 27:677–686, 1966.
2. Brenner, G., and Allen, R. P.: Skeletal Changes in Erythroblastosis Foetalis. *Radiology,* 80:427–429, 1963.
3. Lanzkowsky, P.: Radiological Features of Iron-Deficiency Anemia. *Am. J. Dis. Child.,* 116:16–29, 1968.
4. Moseley, J. E.: *Bone Changes in Hematologic Disorders (Roentgen Aspects).* Grune & Stratton, Inc., New York, 1963.

MYELOSCLEROSIS (MYELOFIBROSIS, AGNOGENIC MYELOID METAPLASIA, OSTEOSCLEROTIC ANEMIA)

This is a hematologic disorder characterized by fibrous or bony replacement of the bone marrow associated with anemia. It may be preceded by polycythemia, and there may be an associated leukemic blood picture. Most patients are over 50 years of age. The characteristic radiographic picture is of increased bone density, which may be associated with areas of radiolucency. The hands are never[2] or only rarely involved.[3]

REFERENCES

1. Jacobson, H. G., Fateh, H., Shapiro, J. H., Spaet, T. H., and Poppel, M. H.: Agnogenic Myeloid Metaplasia. *Radiology,* 72:716–725, 1959.
2. Leigh, T. F., Corley, C. C., Jr., Huguley, C. M., Jr., and Rogers, J. V., Jr.: Myelofibrosis. The General and Radiologic Findings in 25 Proved Cases. *Am. J. Roentgenol.,* 82:183–193, 1959.
3. Moseley, J. E.: *Bone Changes in Hematologic Disorders (Roentgen Aspects).* Grune & Stratton, Inc., New York, 1963.
4. Pettigrew, J. D., and Ward, H. P.: Correlation of Radiologic, Histologic, and Clinical Findings in Agnogenic Myeloid Metaplasia. *Radiology,* 93:541–548, 1969.

POLYCYTHEMIA

Polycythemia, particularly associated with cyanotic heart disease, can be associated with an increased trabecular pattern similar to that seen in the anemias (Fig. 18–9).

REFERENCE

1. Nice, C. M., Jr., Daves, M. L., and Wood, G. H.: Changes in Bone Associated with Cyanotic Congenital Cardiac Disease. *Am. Heart J.,* 68:25–31, 1964.

LEUKEMIA

Skeletal lesions in leukemia are much more common in children than in adults.[4, 6, 7] The actual incidence varies, depending on how many cases of the late disease are included in the series and also what is defined as an actual bone lesion. Many of the changes in leukemia may be nonspecific.

The radiographic findings in the hand are relatively common, being present in almost 40 per cent of cases that had hand radiographs in Thomas's series.[7] In our own experience, we have seen hand involvement infrequently, even when the distal radius and ulna are markedly involved (Fig. 18–

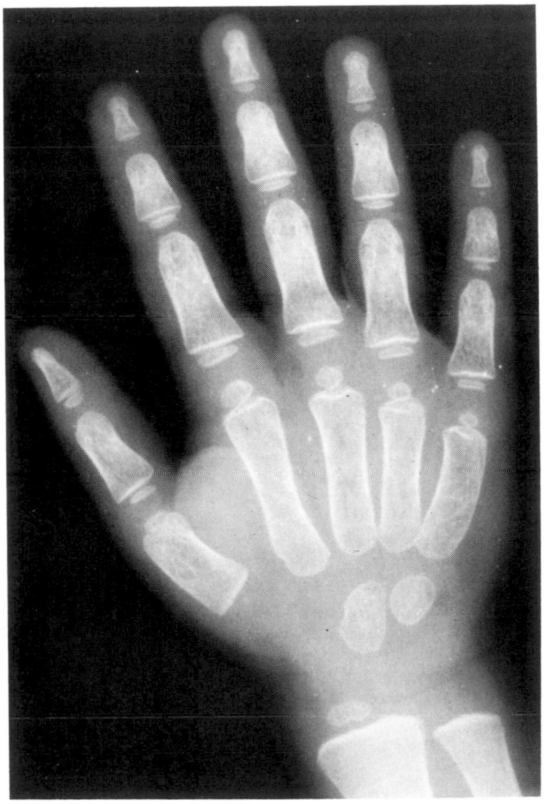

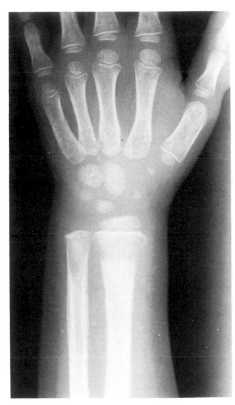

Figure 18–9. Child with polycythemia due to congenital heart disease. Note the thinning of the cortex as well as the increased size of the medullary space, which mimics the anemias.

Figure 18–10. Leukemia. Periosteal reaction is seen in the ulna, and destruction is present in the radius with very little involvement of the hand.

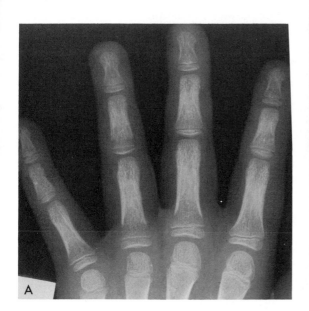
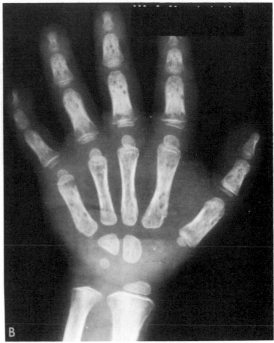

Figure 18–11. A, Acute lymphatic leukemia. Lucencies are seen in several of the metaphyseal regions. (Courtesy Dr. S. Houston, Saskatoon, Saskatchewan.)
B, Monocytic leukemia. Multiple punched-out areas are seen in most of the hand bones.

10). The skeletal findings of leukemia include the following:

1. A line of decreased density in the metaphysis.
2. Osteolytic lesions.
3. Periosteal reaction.
4. Diffuse demineralization.
5. Osteosclerosis.

Although the lucent metaphyseal line is seen commonly in leukemia, it is very nonspecific, particularly if the patient is under two years of age, since many growth disturbances will cause a similar finding.[8] The lines are particularly uncommon in the hand (Fig. 18–11 A). Even in the older age group lucent lines can occasionally be seen in other disorders, such as rheumatoid arthritis.

Osteolytic lesions are common (Fig. 18–11 B). In the early form they are small punctate radiolucencies involving mainly the metaphysis, giving the bone a "motheaten" appearance. These areas may coalesce to form a larger area of destruction. There may even be a well-localized destructive lesion. Periosteal reaction is occasionally seen in the tubular bones of the hand[6] but is much more common in the long bones. Diffuse demineralization is common but is difficult to differentiate from the results of chronic disease. Areas of sclerosis may occasionally be associated with radiolucencies.

An unusual finding in some cases is the presence of acropachy. This has been reported by Glatt and Weinstein[1] and consists of thickening, clubbing and symmetric destruction of the terminal phalanges (Fig. 18–12). In their cases this condition was clinically and radiologically reversible.

Differential diagnosis of the radiologic changes of leukemia in the hand include osteomyelitis and the hand-foot syndrome of sickle cell anemia. Generally speaking, leukemic changes are more diffuse and involve most of the bones more consistently than in osteomyelitis and sickle cell anemia, but sometimes radiologic differentiation may be difficult. Leukemia must also be differentiated from neuroblastoma; the destructive lesions in both of these conditions can be similar, but the metaphyseal line of lucency is rare in neuroblastoma.[3–5, 8]

Changes resulting from various periods

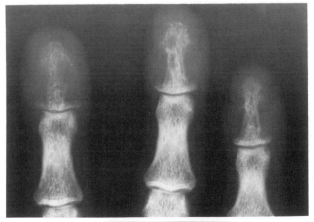

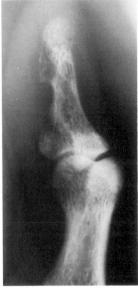

Figure 18-12. Leukemic acropachy. There are erosive changes in the distal phalanges. (Courtesy Dr. W. Glat and Dr. A. Weinstein. Reproduced with permission from *Radiology*, 92:125–126, 1969.)

of disease and remissions may result in a multitude of growth lines in the ends of the bones. The use of systemic chemotherapeutic agents may affect the growth and maturation of bone.

REFERENCES

1. Glatt, W., and Weinstein, A.: Acropachy in Lymphatic Leukemia. *Radiology*, 92:122; 125–126, 1969.
2. Hilbish, T. F., Besse, B. E., Jr., Lusted, L. B., Daves, M. L., Thomas, L. B., and Forkner, C. A.: Acute Leukemia. Skeletal Manifestations in Children and Adults. A.M.A. *Arch. Int. Med.*, 104:741–747, 1959.
3. Lightwood, R., Barrie, H., and Butler, N.: Observations on 100 Cases of Leukaemia in Childhood. *Br. Med. J.*, 1:747–752, 1960.
4. Moseley, J. E.: *Bone Changes in Hematologic Disorders (Roentgen Aspects)*. Grune & Stratton, Inc., New York, 1963.
5. Sherman, R. S., and Leaming, R.: The Roentgen Findings in Neuroblastoma. *Radiology*, 60:837–849, 1953.
6. Simmons, C. R., Harle, T. S., and Singleton, E. B.: The Osseous Manifestations of Leukemia in Children. *Rad. Clin. North Am.*, 6:115–130, 1968.
7. Thomas, L. B., Forkner, C. E., Jr., Frei, E., III, Besse, B. E., Jr., and Stabenau, J. R.: The Skeletal Lesions of Acute Leukemia. *Cancer*, 14:608–621, 1961.
8. Willson, J. K. V.: The Bone Lesions of Childhood Leukemia. A Survey of 140 Cases. *Radiology*, 72:672–681, 1959.

HEMOPHILIA

This disorder of clotting rarely involves bones or joints of the hand. Hemophiliac arthritic changes resulting from repeated hemorrhages may occur in the wrist. Jordan[3] reported wrist involvement in 15 of 56 patients. In the same group, 97 knees and 72 elbows were involved. Intraosseous hemorrhage into the hand or wrist is relatively rare but has occasionally been seen (page 429).[1, 2, 4] It is conceivable that increases in size of the epiphyses may occur in the wrist as they do in other joints, but I have not seen this phenomenon.

REFERENCES

1. Boyes, J. H.: *Bunnell's Surgery of the Hand*, 5th Ed. J. B. Lippincott Co., Philadelphia, 1970, p. 687.
2. Edeiken, J., and Hodes, P. J.: *Roentgen Diagnosis of Diseases of Bone.* The Williams & Wilkins Co., Baltimore, 1967.
3. Jordan, H. H.: *Hemophilic Arthropathies.* Charles C Thomas, Publisher, Springfield, Illinois, 1958.
4. Steel, W. M., Duthie, R. B., and O'Connor, B. T.: Hemophiliac Cysts. *J. Bone Joint Surg.*, 51B: 614–626, 1969.

THE RETICULOENDOTHELIOSES

This topic includes the group of histiocytosis X, as well as the lipid storage disorders: Gaucher disease and Neimann-Pick disease.

Histiocytosis X (Eosinophilic Granuloma, Hand-Schüller-Christian Disease and Letterer-Siwe Disease)

According to Lichtenstein,[5] these three conditions are pathologically related manifestations of the same disorder. There are, however, different clinical pictures, ranging from the isolated eosinophilic granuloma of bone, to the systemic, diffuse acute dis-

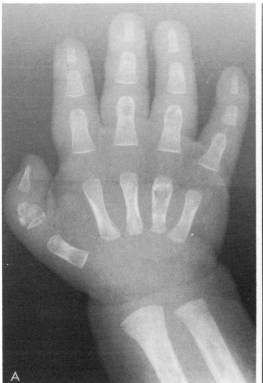 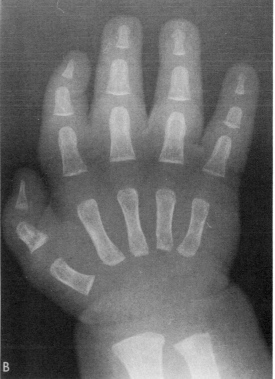

Figure 18–13. Disseminated histiocytosis X. These films were obtained a few months apart.

A, The initial film shows spotty destructive changes in many bones with evidence of bone expansion.

B, On the subsequent film there is rapid response to therapy with marked improvement in modeling and little evidence of previous lesions.

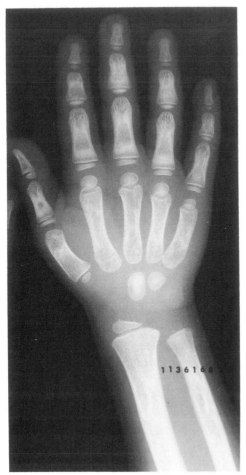

Figure 18–14. Healing stages of histiocytosis X in five year old male. Mottled areas of increased density are the remaining stigmata of previous destructive lesions. There is marked delay of maturation, particularly of the carpals.

often presenting as an external otitis. The classic triad of exophthalmos, diabetes insipidus and holes in the skull is infrequently seen.

These lesions rarely involve the hand bones. Many series do not report occurrence in the hand.[1, 3, 6, 8] Dargeon[2] described cases with hand involvement, and we have seen some, but only in the disseminated form of the disease (Fig. 18–13).

When present in the hand, the manifestations are similar to those in the long bones, ranging from punched-out destructive lesions to areas of sclerosis from healing (Fig. 18–14). Bone modeling may be affected or there may be periosteal reaction. Eosinophilic granuloma can mimic a variety of lesions of bone, including inflammation and neoplasm. Many of these lesions spontaneously resolve, and they are sensitive to both local radiation therapy and systemic chemotherapy.

Another phenomenon which may also be seen in relation to the many phases of

ease of Letterer-Siwe, to the chronic disseminated histiocytosis of Hand-Schüller-Christian disease. Any of the three clinical forms can produce destructive bone lesions that may be radiologically and histologically similar to each other. The incidence of bone lesions is, however, much less common in Letterer-Siwe than in the Hand-Schüller-Christian form.[7]

The lesions are most common in childhood but can occasionally be seen in young adults. The disseminated form is seen usually in younger children and infants. The symptoms are local pain or swelling from the lesion, or they may be due to systemic effects, including hepatosplenomegaly. A common manifestation is a typical rash,

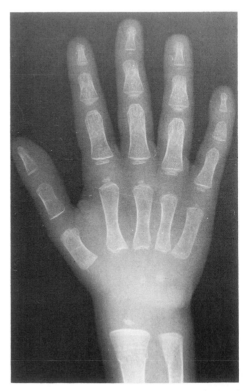

Figure 18–15. Osteoporosis, pathologic fracture and growth lines in a 32 month old male who was treated with 6-mercaptopurine and prednisone for histiocytosis X. These findings are most likely the result of chemotherapy.

recovery and chemotherapy is multiple growth lines in the ends of the bone. These are stigmata of repeated growth arrests and progressions (Fig. 18–15). The steroids and various chemotherapeutic agents can also produce osteoporosis, which may result in pathologic fracture (Fig. 18–15); there is frequently retardation in maturation.

Any bone in the skeleton can be involved in this disease, but the skull is most commonly affected. When the mandible is involved the teeth may be floating.

Gaucher Disease

Gaucher disease is a hereditary disorder of metabolism characterized by storage of abnormal, complex lipids (particularly keratin) in the reticuloendothelial system. Most of the cases reported occur in the Jewish population. There are two clinical forms of the disease: the acute form seen in infancy, and the chronic adult form.

The bone changes in the hand are minimal with some failure of tubulation and coarsening of the trabecular pattern. The appearance is similar to that seen in the anemias.[7] Much more severe changes are seen in other bones: with Erlenmeyer-flask femora, sclerotic changes and bone infarcts, particularly in the femoral heads.

Niemann-Pick Disease

This is another hereditary metabolic disorder. An abnormal lipid lecithin is found in reticuloendothelial systems. It is seen most commonly in the Jewish population. The skeletal changes are due to accumulations of the Niemann-Pick cells in the marrow, with widening of the medullary space and coarsening of the trabeculae. In the hand the osseous changes are similar to those seen in the anemias. There is less of a failure of modeling than in Gaucher disease.[7]

REFERENCES

1. Cheyne, C.: Histiocytosis X. *J. Bone Joint Surg.,* 53B:366–382, 1971.
2. Dargeon, H. W. K.: *Reticuloendothelioses in Childhood. A Clinical Survey.* Charles C Thomas, Publisher, Springfield, Illinois, 1966.
3. Ekert, H., and Campbell, P. E.: Histiocytosis X. A Review of Experience at the Royal Children's Hospital, Melbourne, 1948–1963. *Aust. Paediatr. J.,* 3:139–145, 1966.
4. Fowles, J. V., and Bobechko, W. P.: Solitary Eosinophilic Granuloma in Bone. *J. Bone Joint Surg.,* 52B:238–243, 1970.
5. Lichtenstein, L.: Histiocytosis X (Eosinophilic Granuloma of Bone, Letterer-Siwe Disease, and Schüller-Christian Disease). Further Observations of Pathological and Clinical Importance. *J. Bone Joint Surg.,* 46A:76–90, 1964.
6. McGavran, M. H., and Spady, H. A.: Eosinophilic Granuloma of Bone. A Study of Twenty-Eight Cases. *J. Bone Joint Surg.,* 42A:979–992, 1960.
7. Moseley, J. E.: *Bone Changes in Hematologic Disorders (Roentgen Aspects).* Grune & Stratton, Inc., New York, 1963.
8. Takahashi, M., Martel, W., and Oberman, H. A.: The Variable Roentgenographic Appearance of Idiopathic Histiocytosis. *Clin. Radiol.,* 17: 48–53, 1966.

Chapter 19

ENDOCRINE DISORDERS

HYPOTHYROIDISM
HYPERTHYROIDISM
THYROID ACROPACHY
HYPERPARATHYROIDISM
IDIOPATHIC HYPOPARATHYROIDISM
PSEUDOHYPO- AND
  PSEUDOPSEUDOHYPOPARATHYROIDISM
  (ALBRIGHT HEREDITARY OSTEODYSTROPHY)

GIANTISM AND ACROMEGALY
HYPOPITUITARISM
CUSHING SYNDROME AND STEROID
  THERAPY
SEXUAL PRECOCITY
HYPOGONADISM

A number of endocrine disorders have some influence on the structure of the bones of the hand. Although many of the findings are nonspecific, they can still be useful in making a diagnosis or in excluding it. Skeletal manifestations may be seen in disorders of the thyroid, parathyroid and pituitary glands, in disorders of the adrenal cortex and in abnormalities of the sex hormones. The thyroid and sex hormones predominantly affect the degree of maturation of the hand bones and are thus most noticeable in children.

HYPOTHYROIDISM

A number of forms of hypothyroidism may be seen both in the newborn and in older children.[1, 2] Nongoiterous hypothyroidism beginning in infancy is sometimes called cretinism and is associated with a fairly characteristic facial appearance.

The radiologic manifestations of hypothyroidism are generally independent of the etiology and dependent on the duration of the problem and the time of onset.

The main radiologic finding in hypothyroidism is retardation of skeletal maturation (Fig. 19–1). Thus, it is seen mostly in children and young adults. A number of other signs are related to the relatively slow or uneven ossification and growth. Although many other conditions are associated with retarded maturation (Chapter 3), very rarely

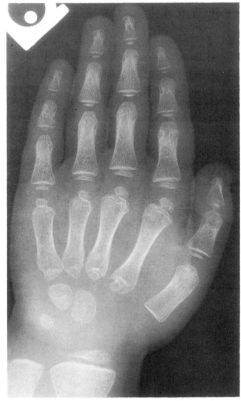

Figure 19–1. Hypothyroidism. This 11 year old female with marked retardation of skeletal maturation was not a cretin at birth. The epiphyses of the middle phalanges are somewhat dense. There are numerous pseudoepiphyses in the metacarpals.

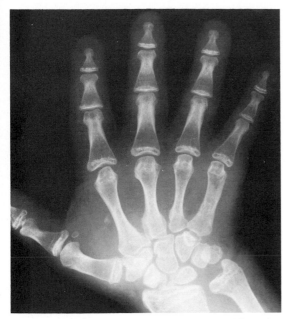

Figure 19–2. Cretinism. 41 year old male. The epiphyseal lines are still evident in the distal phalanges, radius and ulna. There is some fragmentation of ossification of the scaphoid. Note the relative shortening of the metacarpals. (Courtesy Coldwater State Home and Training School, Coldwater, Michigan.)

The epiphyses may show increased radio-pacity (Figs. 19–1 and 19–3), although it is usually not as marked as in the normally occurring "ivory" epiphyses, which are mainly in the distal phalanges (Chapter 6). There may also be increased density in the metaphyses, particularly about the radius and ulna (Fig. 19–4); this may be the result of an inability to handle vitamin D (see Fig. 21–17). Occasionally the end plates may also be irregular (Fig. 19–4), but this disappears after therapy.

One of the helpful diagnostic signs in hypothyroid children is the rapid ossification that results from therapy (Fig. 19–4).

Hypothyroidism causes a severe failure of growth, so that the individual becomes dwarfed. In the hand there is relatively greater shortening of the metacarpals than of the phalanges. This is particularly evi-

is the retardation as severe as it is in long-standing hypothyroidism. The diagnosis of hypothyroidism cannot be entertained in a child with normal maturation! Even when hypothyroidism is associated with precocious puberty, the bone age usually remains retarded.[4, 6] In some cretins that reach adult life, the epiphyseal plates may remain open (Fig. 19–2). In very young infants, radiographs of the knees or feet are usually more useful than those of the hand in the evaluation of hypothyroidism, since the carpal bones are normally not present at birth.

Epiphyseal dysgenesis or fragmented ossification of carpal centers (Figs. 19–2 and 19–3) or phalangeal epiphyses (Fig. 19–3) may occasionally be seen. Epiphyseal dysgenesis is much more common in the hips than in the hand. When the patient is treated, these epiphyses will coalesce. The fragmentation of epiphyses in hypothyroidism must be distinguished from the findings in some of the epiphyseal dysplasias.

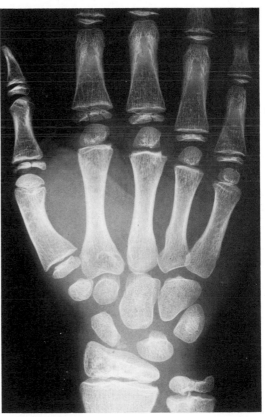

Figure 19–3. Cretinism. There are multiple ossification centers in the phalangeal epiphyses and in the scaphoid. These are a rare manifestation of hypothyroidism. (Courtesy Lapeer State Home and Training School, Lapeer, Michigan.)

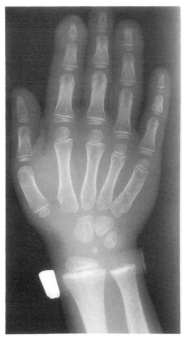 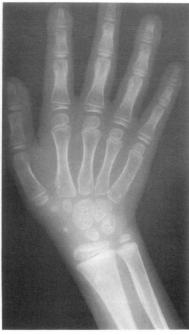

Figure 19–4. Unusual findings in hypothyroidism. There is irregularity of the radial and ulnar metaphysis with some sclerosis. The appearance is somewhat akin to rickets. Calcium and phosphorus levels were normal and the patient responded to thyroid therapy. Soft tissue swelling on the left film was related to monilial infection.

dent in older cretins (Fig. 19–2) and can be demonstrated with pattern profile analysis.

Hypothyroidism may coexist with Down syndrome (trisomy 21), in which case the radiologic findings of both entities may be seen (Fig. 19–5).

REFERENCES

1. Andersen, H. J.: Studies of Hypothyroidism in Children. *Acta Paediatr. Scand.,* 125:7–17, 83–105, 145–150, 1960.
2. Gardner, L. I.: *Endocrine and Genetic Diseases of Childhood.* W. B. Saunders Company, Philadelphia, 1969.
3. Hayles, A. B., Hinrichs, W. L., and Tauxe, W. N.: Thyroid Disease Among Children with Down's Syndrome (Mongolism). *Pediatrics,* 36:608–614, 1965.
4. Pabst, H. F., Pueschel, S., and Hillman, D. A.: Etiologic Interrelationship in Down's Syndrome, Hypothyroidism, and Precocious Sexual Development. *Pediatrics,* 40:590–595, 1967.
5. Rybak, M.: Dysplasie du Squelette et Maturation Osseuse dans L'Insuffisance Thyroïdienne de L'Enfant. Radiology, 13:243–249, 1969.
6. Van Wyk, J. J., and Grumbach, M. M.: Syndrome of Precocious Menstruation and Galactorrhea in Juvenile Hypothyroidism: An Example of Hormonal Overlap in Pituitary Feedback. *J. Pediatr.,* 57:416–435, 1960.
7. Wilkins, L.: Epiphysial Dysgenesis Associated with Hypothyroidism. *Am. J. Dis. Child.,* 61:13–34, 1941.

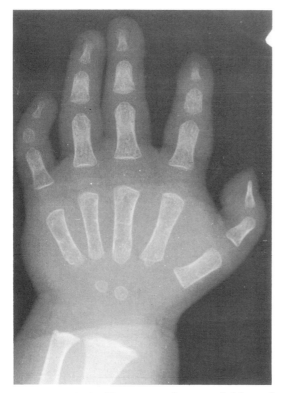

Figure 19–5. Down syndrome child with hypothyroidism. 37 month old female. There is marked retardation of skeletal maturation. There is clinodactyly of the fifth finger with a short middle phalanx. This is a manifestation of trisomy 21.

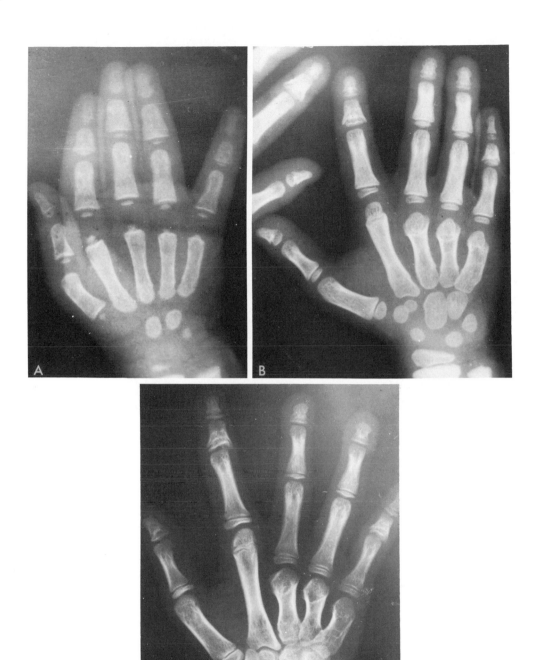

Figure 19–6. Neonatal hyperthyroidism. A, At five weeks there is marked advancement of maturation with ossification of even the phalangeal epiphyses.

B, At age three months the advancement persists. There is some deformation of the epiphyses of the third to fifth metacarpals which has resulted in early closure and consequent brachydactyly. Cone epiphyses of the middle phalanges of the index and fifth fingers are also associated with shortening. There are also cones in the distal phalanges with evidence of shortening.

C, At seven years the brachydactyly has become more prominent and the bone age remains advanced. (Courtesy Dr. W. Riggs, Memphis, Tennessee.)

HYPERTHYROIDISM

As in many endocrine disorders, hyperthyroidism in children is manifested differently from hyperthyroidism in adults. In the infantile form the main radiographic finding is marked advancement of skeletal maturation. In some of the infants the maturational advance is very severe (Fig. 19–6). For example, in one patient of Riggs et al.,[6] the maturation at five weeks of age was about 2½ years, and at 3 months it was 4 years. Similarly, in a case published by Bonakdarpour et al.,[2] three carpal ossification centers were already present at birth, and some phalangeal ossification was also evident. In later childhood the acceleration in skeletal maturation is parallel to acceleration in height, so that hyperthyroidism in childhood may not lead to curtailment of adult height.[8]

In Riggs's patients, cone epiphyses and early fusion led to brachydactyly of some of the metacarpals and middle and distal phalanges.[6]

In the adult patient with hyperthyroidism, the main radiographic findings consist of a severe, permeative type of osteoporosis (Fig. 19–7). According to Bianchi et al.,[1] this is due to marked elevation of the cellular activity and remodeling of bone. With mammographic film and optical magnification, marked striations of the second metacarpal cortex was demonstrated by Meema and Schatz[5] in more than one half of patients with moderately severe thyrotoxicosis. This finding was not present in controls. Striation is not unique for thyrotoxicosis; it is also found in some cases of acromegaly and hyperparathyroidism. The striations in the metacarpals studied by Meema and Schatz[5] correlated well with the mineralization of the distal end of the radius. There was little correlation with metacarpal thickness.

A minor roentgen sign in hyperthyroidism is the visualization of Plummer nails (onycholysis)[3] by demonstrating material collecting under the nail. This is probably of little clinical significance, since it may be visible on casual inspection as well as on the films.

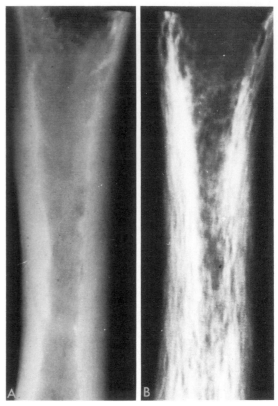

Figure 19–7. Linear striations (*B*) in adult hyperthyroidism, compared to a normal exposure (*A*) made using industrial film. (Courtesy Dr. H. E. Meema, Toronto. Reproduced with permission from *Radiology*, 97:9, 1970.)

REFERENCES

1. Bianchi, G.-S., Meunier, P., Courpron, P., Edouard, C., Bernard, J., and Vignon, G.: Le Retentissement Osseux des Hyperthyroidies. *Rev. Rhum. Mal. Osteoartic.*, 39:19–32, 1972.
2. Bonakdarpour, A., Kirkpatric, J. A., Renzi, A., and Kendall, N.: Skeletal Changes in Neonatal Thyrotoxicosis. *Radiology*, 102:149–150, 1972.
3. Lentino, W., and Poppel, M. H.: The Roentgen Manifestations of Plummer's Nails (Onycholysis) in Hyperthyroidism. *Am. J. Roentgenol.*, 84:941–944, 1960.
4. Meema, H. E., and Meema, S.: Comparison of Microradioscopic and Morphometric Findings in the Hand Bones with Densitometric Findings in the Proximal Radius in Thyrotoxicosis and in Renal Osteodystrophy. *Invest. Radiol.*, 7:88–96, 1972.
5. Meema, H. E., and Schatz, D. L.: Simple Radiologic Demonstration of Cortical Bone Loss in Thyrotoxicosis. *Radiology*, 97:9–15, 1970.
6. Riggs, W., Jr., Wilroy, R. S., Jr., and Etteldorf, J. N.: Neonatal Hyperthyroidism with Accelerated Skeletal Maturation, Craniosynostosis, and Brachydactyly. *Radiology*, 105:621–625, 1972.
7. Samuel, S., Pildes, R. S., Lewison, M., and Rosenthal, I. M.: Neonatal Hyperthyroidism in an Infant Born of an Euthyroid Mother. *Am. J. Dis. Child.*, 121:440–443, 1971.

8. Schlesinger, S., MacGillivray, M. H., and Munschauer, R. W.: Acceleration of growth and bone maturation in childhood thyrotoxicosis. *J. Pediatr.*, 83:233–236, 1973.

THYROID ACROPACHY

This unusual manifestation of thyroid disease is seen in about one percent of patients with thyrotoxicosis. The disorder may occur following treatment of hyperthyroidism or may occur during hyperthyroidism. It has also been seen in euthyroid and hypothyroid patients.[4] The word acropachy, derived from two Greek words, means thickening of the extremities. The clinical signs are digital clubbing, soft tissue swelling of the hands and feet and periosteal new bone formation. Occasion-

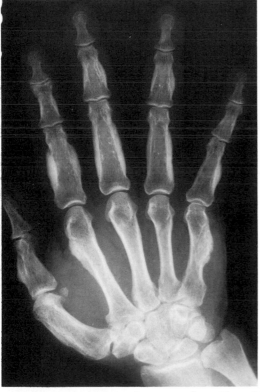

Figure 19–8. Thyroid acropachy. This 64 year old female had known hypothyroidism for 20 years and had been receiving 3 grains of thyroid daily. There is periosteal new bone in the metacarpals and phalanges. It appears somewhat more solid than is sometimes seen in patients with thyroid acropachy following hyperthyroidism.

ally the fingertips are spared. Most of the swelling is over the middle and proximal phalanges.[6]

Males and females are equally affected, which is significant since hyperthyroidism is much more common in females than in males. Almost all cases have had exophthalmos, which was often progressive. Many also had pretibial myxedema.

The radiographic changes are active periosteal involvement of the metacarpals and of the proximal and middle phalanges. The periosteal reaction may be dense and solid, or it may be feathery. It involves only the diaphysis (Fig. 19–8).

The differential diagnosis includes pulmonary osteoarthropathy, in which the periosteal reaction is lamellar and oriented parallel to the long axis of the shaft rather than perpendicular to it as in thyroid acropachy. When the periosteal reaction is solid, differentiation of the two entities may be difficult. Pachydermoperiostosis also may be similar to pulmonary osteoarthropathy. Periosteal changes of vascular disease and Van Buchem disease show some differences from thyroid acropachy.

REFERENCES

1. Gimlette, T. M. D.: Thyroid Acropachy. *Lancet*, 1:22–24, 1960.
2. King, L. R., Braunstein, H., Chambers, D., and Goldsmith, R.: A Case Study of Peculiar Soft-Tissue and Bony Changes in Association with Thyroid Disease. *J. Clin. Endocrinol.*, 19:1323–1330, 1959.
3. Moule, B., Grant, M. C., Boyle, I. T., and May, H.: Thyroid Acropachy. *Clin. Radiol.*, 21:329–333, 1970.
4. Nixon, D. W., and Samols, E.: Acral Changes Associated with Thyroid Diseases. *J.A.M.A.*, 212:1175–1181, 1970.
5. Scanlon, G. T., and Clemett, A. R.: Thyroid Acropachy. *Radiology*, 83:1039–1042, 1964.
6. Torres-Reyes, E., and Staple, T. W.: Roentgenographic Appearance of Thyroid Acropachy. *Clin. Radiol.*, 21:95–100, 1970.

HYPERPARATHYROIDISM

Increased activity of the parathyroid gland may have various causes. Primary hyperparathyroidism may be due to adenomas, general hyperplasia or, occasionally, carcinoma. Hyperparathyroidism may be secondary to rickets, severe renal insufficiency, osteomalacia of sprue or other problems in absorption. Primary hyperparathyroidism is most common in the third to fifth decade and is three times more common in women than in men. It has, however, been seen in infancy.[3]

The hand is probably the most useful portion of the body for radiologic evaluation of this disorder. The hand is almost always involved whenever there is any bone involvement. The radiologic findings include periosteal resorption, tuft erosion, cystic lesions, joint calcification, demineralization and sclerosis (Fig. 19–9). Although the incidence of these various findings is somewhat different in primary and secondary hyperparathyroidism, all of them can occur in either of the forms. Generally speaking, the cystic lesions are relatively uncommon in secondary hyperparathyroidism, while the increased bone density and metastatic calcification are more common in secondary hyperparathyroidism. One

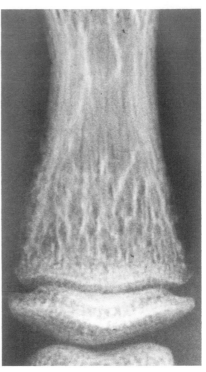

Figure 19–10. Subperiosteal resorption in a patient with secondary hyperparathyroidism from renal disease. A lacy appearance of the periosteum is seen.

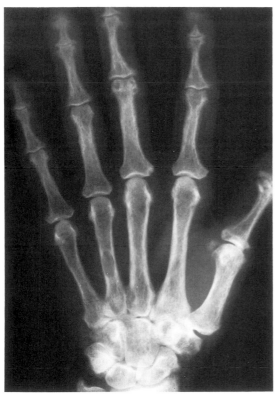

Figure 19–9. Primary hyperparathyroidism. Severe. There are extensive subperiosteal erosions, particularly in the middle phalanges. Lucent defects are seen, such as the one in the fourth metacarpal and in some carpals.

abnormality that occurs mainly in secondary hyperparathyroidism and renal osteodystrophy is separation at the epiphysis,[5] which occasionally may occur in the bones of the hands.

Subperiosteal bone resorption is the most significant radiologic finding in both primary and secondary hyperparathyroidism (Figs. 19–9 and 19–10). It was originally described by Pugh.[8] There is a lace-like appearance of bone beneath the periosteum, with loss of a well-defined cortical margin. The bone resorption may be seen in almost any of the bones but is most commonly noted on the radial side of the middle phalanges. It is not always symmetrical. Occasionally, some phalanges are involved while others are not. The subperiosteal resorption can be best detected by using a fine-grain film, such as mammography film (Fig. 19–11).[7] Without periosteal resorption, it is very difficult to make a radiologic diagnosis of hyperparathyroidism.

Tuft resorption is also seen in primary and secondary forms of hyperparathyroid-

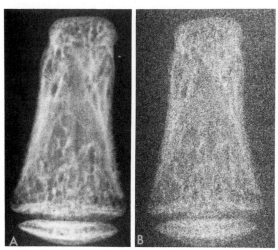

Figure 19–11. In *A*, there is minimal subperiosteal erosion, taken on mammography film (RPM Kodak), in a patient with secondary hypoparathyroidism. The detail is clearly visible. In *B*, which was taken on fast film (nonscreen exposure—RPR Kodak), the grain pattern interferes with visualization.

ism (Fig. 19–12). It must be differentiated from the normal irregularity of the tufts.

Cyst-like lesions are seen more commonly in primary than in secondary hyper-

parathyroidism (Figs. 19–9 and 19–13). These localized areas of destruction may involve multiple bones of the hand. They have also been called brown tumors or osteoclastomas.

Joint calcification is a relatively uncommon finding in this disorder. In Dodds and Steinbach's series[1] it was seen in 12 of 91 patients with hyperparathyroidism. Usually the calcification is in the region of the triangular ligament adjacent to the ulna. The calcification tends to occur in older individuals. It is, however, not simply a manifestation of old age, since it was present in only 2.5 per cent of normal individuals who had a mean age of 69.

Generalized "demineralization" is common. There is evidence of a fine trabecular pattern in the cortex of the metacarpals and linear striations throughout it. These anatomic findings are more significant than actual measurement of the amount of cortex.[6] Sclerosis of bone is occasionally seen in primary hyperparathyroidism, but it is much more common in the form associated with uremia, as is metastatic calcification in the soft tissues (Fig. 19–14). This soft tissue calcification usually occurs about the joints and, as previously mentioned, in the joint cartilages surrounding the wrist.

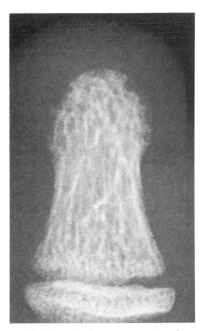

Figure 19–12. Tuft erosion in the patient described in Figure 19–10. There are small defects in the tuft.

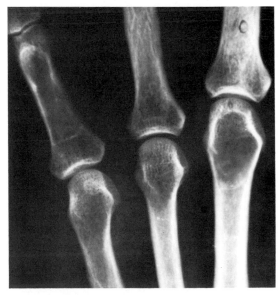

Figure 19–13. Brown tumor in hyperparathyroidism due to adenoma. There is a lucent defect in the third metacarpal and another in the fifth proximal phalanx.

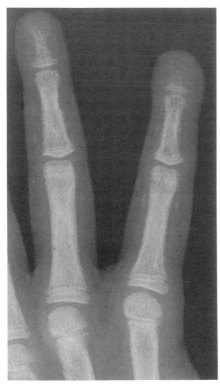

Figure 19–14. Calcification in secondary hyperparathyroidism. There is also extensive tuft erosion and subperiosteal resorption.

REFERENCES

1. Dodds, W. J., and Steinbach, H. L.: Primary Hyperparathyroidism and Articular Cartilage Calcification. *Am. J. Roentgenol.*, 104:884–892, 1968.
2. Doyle, F. H.: Some Quantitative Radiological Observations in Primary and Secondary Hyperparathyroidism. *Br. J. Radiol.*, 39:161–167, 1966.
3. Du Bois, R., Farriaux, J. P., Maillard, E., and Maillard, J. P.: Hyperparathyroidisme Primitif Chez un Nouveau-né. *Ann. Radiol.*, 12:407–412, 1969.
4. Gleason, D. C., and Potchen, E. J.: The Diagnosis of Hyperparathyroidism. *Radiol. Clin. North Am.*, 5:277–287, 1967.
5. Kirkwood, J. R., Ozonoff, M. B., and Steinbach, H. L.: Epiphyseal Displacement after Metaphyseal Fracture in Renal Osteodystrophy. *Am. J. Roentgenol.*, 115:547–554, 1972.
6. Meema, H. E., and Meema, S.: Comparison of Microradioscopic and Morphometric Findings in the Hand Bones with Sensitometric Findings in the Proximal Radius in Thyrotoxicosis and in Renal Osteodystrophy. *Invest. Radiol.*, 7:88–96, 1972.
7. Meema, H. E., Rabinovich, S., Meema, S., Lloyd, G. J., and Oreopoulos, D. G.: Improved Radiological Diagnosis of Azotemic Osteodystrophy. *Radiology*, 102:1–10, 1972.
8. Pugh, D. G.: Subperiosteal Resorption of Bone. A Roentgenologic Manifestation of Primary Hyperparathyroidism and Renal Osteodystrophy. *Am. J. Roentgenol.*, 66:577–586, 1951.
9. Steinbach, H. L., Gordan, G. S., Eisenberg, E., Crane, J. T., Silverman, S., and Goldman, L.: Primary Hyperparathyroidism: A Correlation of Roentgen, Clinical, and Pathologic Features. *Am. J. Roentgenol.*, 86:329–343, 1961.
10. Vix, V. A.: Articular and Fibrocartilage Calcification in Hyperparathyroidism: Associated Hyperuricemia. *Radiology*, 83:468–471, 475, 1964.
11. Zimmerman, H. B.: Osteosclerosis in Chronic Renal Disease. Report of 4 Cases Associated with Secondary Hyperparathyroidism. *Am. J. Roentgenol.*, 88:1152–1169, 1962.

IDIOPATHIC HYPOPARATHYROIDISM

Primary hypoparathyroidism is a rare entity that has few significant radiologic findings in the hand. There may be some bone demineralization, and there may be some soft tissue calcification. Occasionally there may be signs of hyperparathyroidism as well.

REFERENCES

1. Costello, J. M., and Dent, C. E.: Hypo-Hyperparathyroidism. *Arch. Dis. Child.*, 38:397–407, 1963.
2. Taybi, H., and Keele, D.: Hypoparathyroidism: A Review of the Literature and Report of Two Cases in Sisters, One with Steatorrhea and Intestinal Pseudo-Obstruction. *Am. J. Roentgenol.*, 88:432–442, 1962.

PSEUDOHYPO- AND PSEUDO-PSEUDOHYPOPARATHYROIDISM (ALBRIGHT HEREDITARY OSTEODYSTROPHY)

Pseudohypoparathyroidism is defined as a congenital abnormality which is characterized by hypocalcemia and hyperphosphatemia similar to that seen in hypoparathyroidism, but which does not respond to parathyroid hormone. The patients are usually short, obese and mentally retarded, and may have brachydactyly. Pseudopseudohypoparathyroidism is similar to pseudohypoparathyroidism in clinical and radiologic findings, but it is associated with normal blood chemistry. There is evidence that both of these conditions are probably different manifestations of the same disorder. Both pseudohypoparathyroidism and pseudopseudohypoparathyroidism have been seen in the same family. Also, the blood chemistry in the same individual may change from abnormal to normal and vice versa. This disease is probably X-linked or possibly autosomal dominant.[8]

Radiologic findings in the hand include calcification or ossification of the skin or subcutaneous tissues, shortening of the bones, and, occasionally, changes of secondary hyperparathyroidism. There may be a reduction in the carpal angle in this condition.[2] Cone epiphyses are also commonly seen.

The soft tissue calcification in this condition (Fig. 19–15) occurs in approximately 55 per cent of patients with pseudohypoparathyroidism, and 40 per cent of patients with pseudopseudohypoparathyroid-

ism.[7] The calcifications may be present at birth, are superficial in location, may often be palpable and are usually periarticular in their distribution. They are particularly common in the hands and feet but may be asymmetric. On examination they may appear small and punctate or they may coalesce into plaques. The soft tissue calcification can accumulate without abnormalities of calcium and phosphorus in the blood.

All of the metacarpals and phalanges may appear relatively short, although no measurements in a large series of cases exist at this time. There may be disproportionate shortening of the metacarpals. The fourth and fifth metacarpals in particular are commonly short in about 80 to 90 per cent of cases.[7] The other metacarpals may also be short. The pattern of metacarpal shortening is not necessarily symmetrical. Although the metacarpal sign (Chapter 3) may be used for evaluation, it is unreliable since

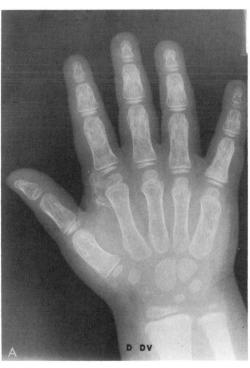
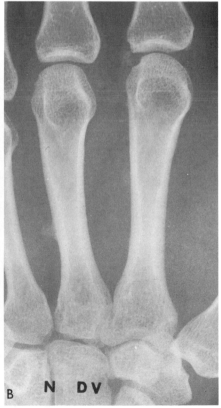

Figure 19–15. Familial pseudohypoparathyroidism. *A,* In this four year old female there is soft tissue calcification, some thinning of the bony cortex and a generally small hand.

B, This is the mother of the patient in *A.* There is a bony spur in the metacarpal, which is nearer midshaft than is the usual exostosis. Periarticular soft tissue calcification is also evident.

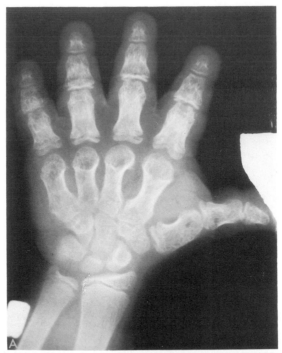

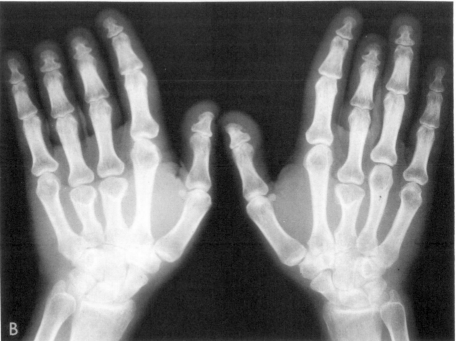

Figure 19–16. Pseudohypoparathyroidism (PHP) and pseudopseudohypoparathyroidism (PPHP) in mother and daughter. *A,* The daughter has a chemical abnormality (PHP). The hand bones are uniformly short with cone epiphyses. The appearance is somewhat suggestive of acrodysostosis.

B, The mother has a normal chemistry (PPHP). There is asymmetric shortening of the metacarpals and phalanges.

This family illustrates the spectrum of abnormality in this condition. (Courtesy Dr. W. McAlister, St. Louis, Missouri.)

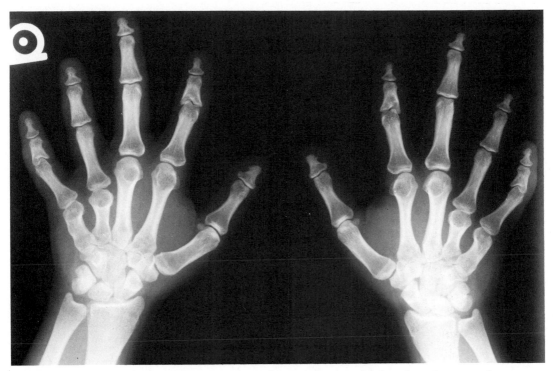

Figure 19-17. Pseudopseudohypoparathyroidism. 16 year old female. There is shortening of the fourth and fifth metacarpals bilaterally, and there is evidence of an old cone epiphysis in the second and fifth middle phalanges.

the third metacarpal as well as the fourth is often short. Premature fusion of the metacarpals and phalangeal epiphyses is seen in many cases. Short phalanges were also common, according to Steinbach et al.,[6] and these most often occurred in the distal phalanges, although many cases also showed middle phalangeal shortening, particularly in the second digit. There may be deformity at the base of the phalanx due to a previous cone epiphysis (Fig. 19-17). Exostoses are also sometimes seen in this condition. They differ from those in multiple exostoses in that they are more central and project at right angles to the shaft of the bone (Fig. 19-15 *B*).[7]

Hyperparathyroidism as a secondary manifestation of hypoparathyroidism can occur both in the pseudo and in the primary hypoparathyroidism.[7]

The radiologic findings may sometimes be difficult to distinguish from acrodysostosis (Fig. 19-16 A).

REFERENCES

1. Christiaens, L., Fontaine, G., Farriaux, J. P., and Biserte, G.: Le Pseudohypoparathyroidisme Chronique. A Propos de Trois Cas Familiaux. *Acta Paediatr. Belg.*, 21:5–70, 1967.
2. Goeminne, L.: Albright's Hereditary Poly-Osteochondrodystrophy. (Pseudo-Pseudo-Hypoparathyroidism with Diabetes Hypertension, Arteritis and Polyarthrosis). *Acta Genet. Med.*, 14:226–281, 1965.
3. Gwinn, J. L., Lee, F. A., Frech, R. S., and McAlister, W. H.: Radiological Case of the Month. *Am. J. Dis. Child.*, 119:447–448, 1970.
4. Kolb, F. O., and Steinbach, H. L.: Pseudohypoparathyroidism with Secondary Hyperparathyroidism and Osteitis Fibrosa. *J. Clin. Endocrinol.*, 22:59–69, 1962.
5. Lee, J. B., Tashjian, H., Jr., Streeto, J. M., and Frantz, A. G.: Familial Pseudohypoparathyroidism. Role of Parathyroid Hormone and Thyrocalcitonin. *New Eng. J. Med.*, 279:1179–1184, 1968.
6. Steinbach, H. L., Rudhe, U., Jonsson, M., and Young, D. A.: Evolution of Skeletal Lesions in Pseudohypoparathyroidism. *Radiology*, 85:670–676, 1965.

7. Steinbach, H. L., and Young, D. A.: The Roentgen Appearance of Pseudohypoparathyroidism (PH) and Pseudo-Pseudohypoparathyroidism (PPH). Differentiation From Other Syndromes Associated with Short Metacarpals, Metatarsals, and Phalanges. *Am. J. Roentgenol.*, 97:49–66, 1966.
8. Spranger, J. W.: Skeletal Dysplasias and the Eye: Albright's Hereditary Osteodystrophy. *Birth Defects, Original Article Series*, 5:122–128, 1969.

GIANTISM AND ACROMEGALY

Excessive growth hormone production, such as that caused by an eosinophilic adenoma of the pituitary, will have different manifestations depending on the age of the patient. When it occurs in childhood it results in giantism; in adolescence it produces a tall acromegalic individual; and in adulthood it produces simply the syndrome of acromegaly.

The radiologic findings in acromegaly are much better defined than those in giantism. Giantism is much rarer than acromegaly, and most of the roentgen findings are not as well developed, except perhaps for the increase in the length of the hand bones and the alteration in maturation during adolescence.

Human growth hormone appears to have little effect on skeletal maturation (Fig. 3–1). Most cases of giantism resulting from pituitary eosinophilic adenoma have normal skeletal maturation in childhood. During adolescence and into young adult life, their epiphyses remain open, which allows them to grow to extreme heights. Determination of skeletal maturation is useful in the evaluation of giants in that when maturation is advanced, it implies a cause other than pituitary overactivity. Conditions with increased size and advanced maturation include cerebral giantism (Chapter 13), lipodystrophy syndrome (Chapter 13), some cases of hyperthyroidism and occasionally constitutional giantism. Of course, occasionally pituitary adenomas can co-exist with another endocrine tumor. Poznanski and Stephenson[7] described a boy who had pituitary giantism, but his bone age was advanced due to an associated functioning testicular tumor.

The other radiologic manifestations in growth hormone overactivity seen in the hand include prominent tufts of the fingers, accentuation of tendon attachment, thick bones, large sesamoids, degenerative changes about the joints, exostoses and a coarse trabecular pattern. A number of soft tissue findings may also be seen, including increased width of the fingers and increased thickness of the joints. These findings are seen predominantly in adult acromegalics; the child with giantism usually does not have them,[10] although the extent of these changes in childhood is not well documented, probably because of the rarity of the condition.

Widening of the tufts of the distal phalanges (Fig. 19–18) is a well-recognized sign of acromegaly. However, this sign must be considered in terms of sex and occupation, since tufts are more prominent in males than in females, and more prominent in individuals who do heavy manual labor than those of more sedentary habits. Sharp spikes at the edges of the tufts are seen in older individuals and are not very useful in differentiation from normal. Anton[1] found the width of the tuft in normal individuals to be 8.5 mm. in males and 7.4 mm. in females (with standard deviations of 1.0 mm. and 0.9 mm., respectively). In acromegalics, most tufts measured more than 3 S.D. above the mean for sex.

Cortical thickening in the proximal phalanges may be a manifestation of increased appositional growth.[6] Exostoses may be present, particularly around the area of the

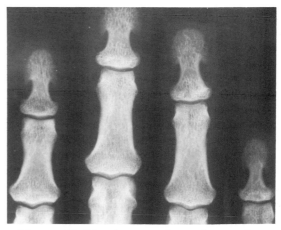

Figure 19–18. Acromegaly with prominent tufts. 39 year old male. There are prominent spikes at the sides of the tufts. Bony spurs are seen at the bases of the second and fifth distal phalanges. The soft tissues are thick.

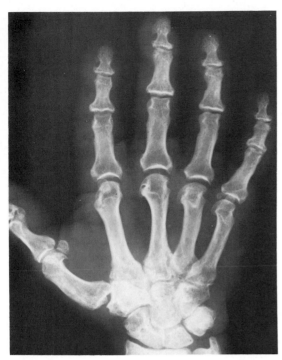

Figure 19-19. Acromegaly. Note the increased width of the metacarpophalangeal joints associated with degenerative changes. The tufts appear wide. The sesamoids appear larger than usual. The soft tissues are thick.

metacarpal and proximal phalangeal heads. This finding was seen by Lin and Lee[6] in approximately 60 per cent of acromegalic patients, particularly in those who showed a metacarpophalangeal joint widening greater than 2 mm. The spurring about the joints may give rise to locking of the finger joints and produce arthritic symptoms. One of the ways in which acromegalic joint changes can be differentiated from degenerative arthritis is that in acromegaly the joint thickness usually is increased, while in osteoarthritis it is narrowed (Fig. 19-19).

The sesamoid bones, particularly around the first metacarpophalangeal joint, appear enlarged (Fig. 19-19). There is normally a rather large sex difference in the size of the sesamoids. Figures for their measurement are given by several authors.[1, 5, 6] This is probably not as useful a sign as it was once thought to be because of the considerable overlap in the distribution between the acromegalic and the control group.[6]

There appears little evidence that there is indeed bone loss in acromegaly. Although there is evidence of a coarsened trabecular structure, studies by Doyle[2] show that mineralization in the ulna is within normal limits. There is evidence of a high turnover of cortical bone. Periosteal apposition may occur, which may thicken the bone. In 10 acromegalic patients, we found the total diameter, T, of the second metacarpal to be 1.73 S.D. above normal for age and sex, the medullary diameter, M, to be 1.83 S.D. above normal, and the cortical thickness, C, to be essentially normal (0.09 S.D. below mean).

The soft tissue changes in acromegaly are interesting in that they are probably the most discriminatory finding between the normal and abnormal patients,[6] and are the second most useful criterion after heel pad thickness.[6, 11] The greatest soft tissue thickening appears to be in the region of the proximal midphalanges[6.] The width in acromegalic males was 27.3 mm. (range 24 to 30 mm.), and in females it was 25.9 mm. (range 23 to 29 mm.).[6] In the normal control group, on the other hand, the mean was 23.1 mm. in males (range 18 to 28) and 20.4 mm. in females (range 18 to 26). Change in the soft tissue thickness of the hand is also a useful parameter of the effectiveness of therapy, since it responds faster than the bone.

Another useful measurement in the hand of acromegalics is the thickness of the cartilage (Fig. 19-19). The thickening is due either to thickening of the articular cartilage or to thickening of the synovial membrane, and is particularly prominent in the metacarpophalangeal joints. It is particularly useful in that there is no difference between the sexes. In acromegaly, the width of the metacarpophalangeal joint of the index finger ranged from 2 to 3 mm. (mean 2.4 mm., S.D. ± 0.4 mm.)[6] In the control group, the width ranged from 1 to 2.5 mm. (mean 1.6 mm., S.D. ± 0.3 mm.).[6]

As in many radiologic findings, it is often the combination of roentgen signs that is useful in the diagnosis. For example, increased soft tissue width can be due to lymphedema, myxedema, obesity and so forth. However, in these patients there is rarely evidence of increased width of the joint space. Similarly, exostoses and degenerative changes can be seen in osteoarthritis, but when the joint is also widened, this is further evidence that these findings may be due to acromegaly.

REFERENCES

1. Anton, II. C.: Hand Measurements in Acromegaly. *Clin. Radiol.*, 23:445–450, 1972.
2. Doyle, F. H.: Radiologic Assessment of Endocrine Effects on Bone. *Radiol. Clin. North Am.*, 5: 289–302, 1967.
3. Hurxthal, L. M.: Pituitary Gigantism in a Child Five Years of Age: Effect of X-Radiation, Estrogen Therapy and Self-Imposed Starvation Diet During an Eleven-Year Period. *J. Clin. Endocrinol.*, 21:343–353, 1961.
4. Kellgren, J. H., Ball, J., and Tutton, G. K.: The Articular and Other Limb Changes in Acromegaly. A Clinical and Pathological Study of 25 Cases. *Quart. J. Med.*, 45:405–424, 1952.
5. Kleinberg, D. L., Young, I. S., and Kupperman, H. S.: The Sesamoid Index. An Aid in the Diagnosis of Acromegaly. *Ann. Int. Med.*, 64: 1075–1078, 1966.
6. Lin, S. -R., and Lee, K. F.: Relative Value of Some Radiographic Measurements of the Hand in the Diagnosis of Acromegaly. *Invest. Radiol.*, 6:426–431, 1971.
7. Poznanski, A. K., and Stephenson, J. M.: Radiographic Findings in Hypothalamic Acceleration of Growth Associated with Cerebral Atrophy and Mental Retardation (Cerebral Gigantism). *Radiology*, 88:446–456, 1967.
8. Saxena, K. M., and Crawford, J. D.: Acromegalic Gigantism in an Adolescent Girl. *J. Pediatr.*, 62:660–665, 1963.
9. Sotos, J. F.: *In* Gardner, L. I.: *Endocrine and Genetic Diseases of Childhood.* W. B. Saunders Company, Philadelphia, 1969, p. 142.
10. Spence, H. J., Trias, E. P., and Raiti, S.: Acromegaly in a 9½-Year-Old Boy. Pituitary Function Studies Before and After Surgery. *Am. J. Dis. Child.*, 123:504–506, 1972.
11. Steinbach, H. L., Feldman, R., and Goldberg, M. B.: Acromegaly. *Radiology*, 72:535–549, 1959.

HYPOPITUITARISM

The radiographic findings of hypopituitarism are not particularly characteristic. The main finding is a decrease in length of the hand bones, which parallels the general dwarfism associated with this condition. There is usually moderately severe retardation of skeletal maturation. However, the bone age is usually greater than the height age unless there is a pronounced secondary hypothyroidism.[5] According to Kaplan et al.,[2] height-age–bone-age ratio was 0.69 in isolated hyposomatotropism, and 1.28 in multiple tropin deficiencies. A bone-age–chronological-age ratio of 2:3 in patients suggests pituitary dwarfism.

Another condition that has a similar radiographic and clinical appearance is pseudohypopituitary dwarfism with normal or elevated plasma growth hormones.[3, 4] In these children, too, the bone age is retarded. The bones have been described as small and delicate.

REFERENCES

1. Clayton, B. E., Tanner, J. M., Newns, G. H., White-house, R. H., and Renwick, A. G. L.: Differential Diagnosis of Children with Short Stature not Associated with Metabolic, Chromosomal, or Gross Nervous System Defects. *Arch. Dis. Child.*, 42:245, 1967.
2. Kaplan, S. L., Goodman, H. G., and Grumbach, M. M.: Isolated Growth Hormone Deficiency in Childhood. *In International Symposium on Growth Hormone*, Milan, 1967. Excerpta Medical Foundation, Int. Congr. Series No. 142, p. 42.
3. Laron, Z., Pertzelan, A., and Mannheimer, S.: Genetic Pituitary Dwarfism with High Serum Concentration of Growth Hormone. A New Inborn Error of Metabolism? *Isr. J. Med. Sci.*, 2:152–155, 1966.
4. New, M. I., Schwartz, E., Parks, G. A., Landey, S., and Wiedemann, E.: Pseudohypopituitary Dwarfism with Normal Plasma Growth Hormone and Low Serum Sulfation Factor. *J. Pediatr.*, 80:620–626, 1972.
5. Trygstad, O.: Human Growth Hormone and Hypopituitary Growth Retardation. *Acta Paediatr. Scand.*, 58:407–419, 1969.

CUSHING SYNDROME AND STEROID THERAPY

The main radiologic manifestation of increased cortical glucosteroids, either iatrogenic or on the basis of Cushing syndrome, is evidence of osteoporosis. In the child, Cushing syndrome usually depresses skeletal maturation as well as growth, and produces some demineralization.

REFERENCES

1. Murray, R. O.: Radiological Bone Changes in Cushing's Syndrome and Steroid Therapy. A Paper Read Before the British Institute of Radiology on November 19, 1959. *Br. J. Radiol.*, 33:1–19, 1960.
2. Strickland, A. L., Underwood, L. E., Voina, S. J., French, F. S., and Van Wyk, J. J.: Growth Retardation in Cushing's Syndrome. *Am. J. Dis. Child.*, 123:207–213, 1972.

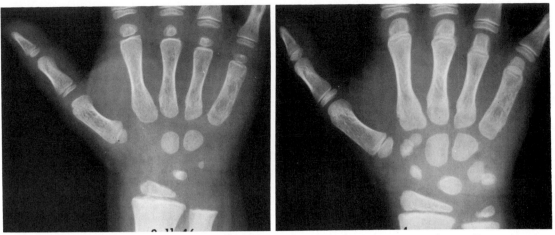

Figure 19–20. Functioning adrenal cortical carcinoma with precocious puberty. Patient at ages 3 and 4 years. Note the rapid advance in maturation in the 14 month interval between the films.

SEXUAL PRECOCITY

There are many causes of sexual precocity; these are well illustrated in various texts.[3] The radiologic findings in most of the abnormalities are identical. Usually what is seen is an advancement of skeletal maturation that is greater than the advancement in the size of the hand. Depending on the duration of the precocious puberty, the bone age may be markedly advanced (many years) or just slightly advanced. Slightly advanced bone age particularly occurs when tumors cause sexual precocity, since the precocity is of relatively recent onset; the bone age does not change as much as in the isosexual type of precocity, although with time the rate of increase in maturation can be dramatic (Fig. 19–20). Other radiologic manifestations may be seen in the hand. For example, in the sexual precocity of polyostotic fibrous dysplasia, the changes of fibrous dysplasia may also be noted (page 300). Occasionally, sexual precocity can be seen with maturational retardation. This has occurred in some cases of Silver syndrome, where the bone age is normally markedly retarded, while in children with this syndrome who have some sexual precocity it may be slightly below normal or normal. Hypothyroid children with sexual precocity or children with Down syndrome with sexual precocity may have retarded maturation.

REFERENCES

1. Kaplan, S. A., Ling, S. M., and Irani, N. G.; Idiopathic Isosexual Precocity. *Am. J. Dis. Child.,* 116:591–598, 1968.
2. Sigurjonsdottir, T. J., and Hayles, A. B.: Precocious Puberty. A Report of 96 Cases. *Am. J. Dis. Child.,* 115:309–321, 1968.
3. Van Der Werff Ten Bosch, J. T.: *In* Gardner, L. I.: *Endocrine and Genetic Diseases of Childhood.* W. B. Saunders Company, Philadelphia, 1969, p. 544.

HYPOGONADISM

Skeletal maturation is usually decreased in conditions with hypogonadism. The appearance is usually nonspecific. In some of the chromosomal abnormalities associated with hypogonadism, osseous abnormalities may be seen. (See Turner syndrome, page 224, and the XXXXY syndrome, page 228.)

Chapter 20

JOINT DISORDERS

by Tom W. Staple, M.D.

DEGENERATIVE JOINT DISEASE

The terms osteoarthritis, arthritis deformans and hypertrophic arthritis are misnomers, since no inflammatory reaction is apparent microscopically or clinically. It is rather a process of breakdown of cartilage with secondary changes in synovium and bone. Degenerative changes in the hands may be a manifestation of generalized systemic disease such as primary osteoarthritis or occur in a patchy fashion in separate joints of the hand as a part of aging. It may appear in single joints following trauma with or without associated fracture of an adjoining bone.

Whatever the etiology, the manifestations are similar. Articular cartilage fibrillates and gradually fragments. Subchondral cysts containing synovial fluid, gelatinous material or necrotic tissue form in the subjacent bone. The overlying cartilage gradually wears away and subchondral tissue responds by adding new bone, causing increased density called eburnation. Osteophytes form at the joint periphery and widen the articular surfaces. The clinical manifestation of osteophyte formation is called Heberden nodes (Fig. 20–1) in the distal interphalangeal joints and Bouchard nodes (Fig. 20–2) in the proximal interphalangeal joints.[1]

The distal and proximal interphalangeal joints are most commonly involved. The first carpometacarpal joint may develop a painful degenerative change severe enough to produce muscle atrophy of the thenar eminence and inability to oppose the thumb (Fig. 20–3). Surgical fusion to relieve pain has been in my experience the most common cause of fusion of the first carpometacarpal joint in the adult.

The initial roentgen manifestation of degenerative joint disease is slight narrowing of the joint space as cartilage is lost. The joint may swell. The bone soon produces subchondral sclerosis and volar and dorsal growth of osteophytic spurs (Fig. 20–1 C). Calcification in degenerated cartilage and the joint capsule is occasionally present (Fig. 20–4). Demineralization is absent since joint motion is only mildly limited. Generalized demineralization is usually due to age or postmenopausal osteoporosis. Subluxation occurs, but is more common when rheumatoid arthritis or trauma has altered or destroyed the adjacent capsule, ligaments or tendons. Joint fusion may occasionally occur, but is much more likely to be due to juvenile rheumatoid arthritis,

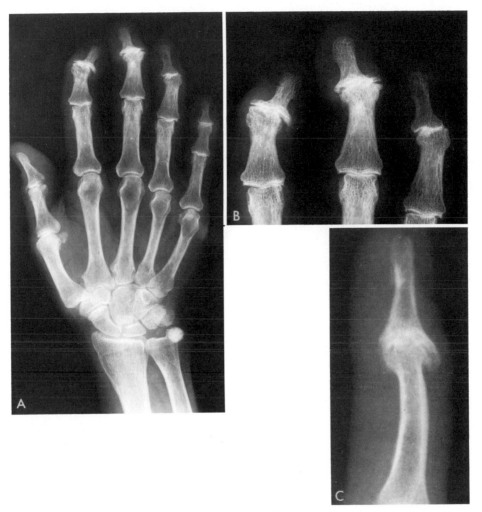

Figure 20–1. Degenerative joint disease. *A*, Principally distal interphalangeal joint disease caused subluxation and deviation of the fingers.

B, Detail of distal and proximal interphalangeal joint space narrowing. Widening of the bases of the distal phalanges and of the heads of the middle phalanges create palpable Heberden nodes. The subchondral bone is dense.

C, Spurs form a cap over dorsum of articulation producing Heberden nodes.

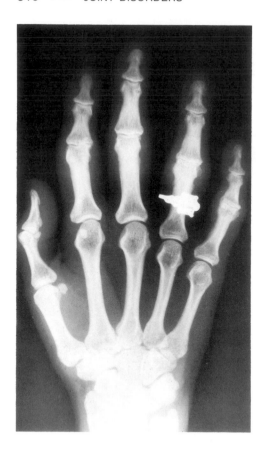

Figure 20–2. Degenerative joint disease. Bouchard nodes. Soft tissue thickening about the proximal interphalangeal joints causes clinically apparent nodules. The interphalangeal joints are slightly narrowed.

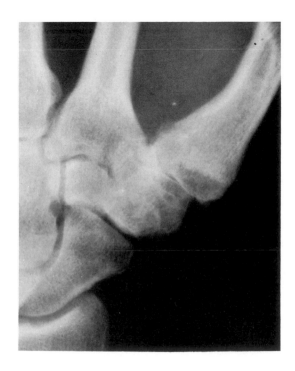

Figure 20–3. Degenerative joint disease. The first carpometacarpal joint space is narrowed. There is a small osteophyte at the base of the first metacarpal.

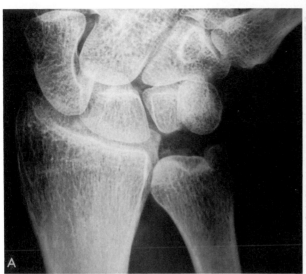
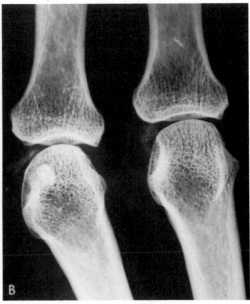

Figure 20–4. Degenerative joint disease. There is cartilage calcification in the (A) radiocarpal, ulnocarpal and (B) metacarpophalangeal articulations. This was a 70 year old woman with minimal complaints and no acute exacerbations.

psoriatic arthritis, infection or surgery.[2] Infection, trauma, aseptic necrosis, arthritides, tumors, and congenital epiphyseal dysplasias all cause joint surface incongruity. Before dismissing any deformative changes in the hand as primary degenerative joint disease, these processes should be considered as factors producing a secondary rather than a primary disease response.

REFERENCES

1. Jaffe, H. L.: *Metabolic, Degenerative, and Inflammatory Diseases of Bone and Joints.* Lea and Febiger, Philadelphia, 1972.
2. Smuckler, N., Edeiken, J., and Giuliani, V. J.: Ankylosis in Osteoarthritis of the Finger Joints. *Radiology,* 100:525–530, 1971.

EROSIVE OSTEOARTHRITIS

Erosive osteoarthritis is a disease of middle-aged postmenopausal women. Its onset and course are more rapid than primary degenerative arthritis, although it affects the same areas, namely, the distal interphalangeal joints and, to a lesser degree, any of the proximal interphalangeal or the first carpometacarpal joints.[1, 2]

The roentgen appearance is one of progressive destruction and subluxation occurring over a number of years (Fig. 20–5). Erosions are not surrounded by sclerosis. The base of the distal phalanx may broaden, but osteophytes are not common. The lesions are asymmetrically distributed. Only one joint may be affected at first, to be followed by others several years later. The disease is self-limited, usually healing partially with some residue resembling degenerative joint disease but without bony ankylosis. In spite of severe erosions, neither the bones nor the muscles are atrophied.

Biopsy of the joints shows osteoarthritic changes and only rarely alterations suggesting rheumatoid disease.

Erosive osteoarthritis involves only the hands while primary degenerative joint disease affects the weight-bearing joints, namely, the hips, knees and lumbar spine in addition to the hands. The disease differs from rheumatoid arthritis because the rheumatoid factor and sedimentation rate are normal, the process does not involve the intercarpal and metacarpophalangeal joints and the patient has no systemic symptoms. It may be mistaken for psoriatic arthritis because of distal interphalangeal in-

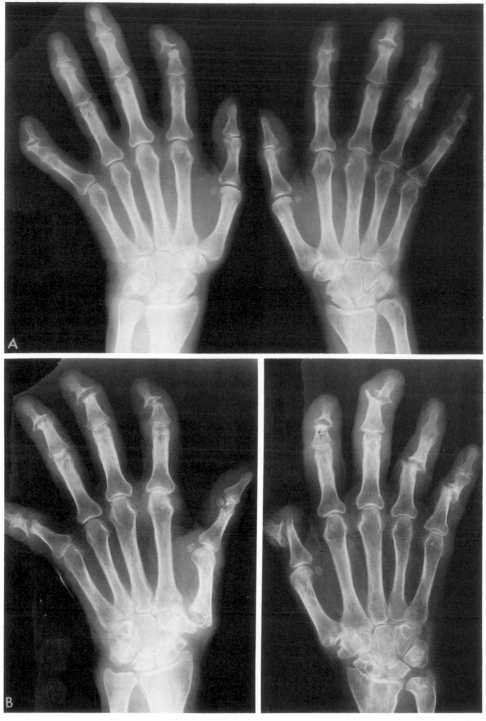

Figure 20–5. Erosive osteoarthritis. This 67 year old woman had pain, redness and swelling about the distal interphalangeal joints of both hands for two years. There is recent-onset deformity of the fingers of the left hand.

A, Note the asymmetric erosive changes in the distal interphalangeal joints. The distal phalanx of the left index finger is subluxed ulnarward. The proximal interphalangeal joints of the right ring finger and of the right and left little fingers are narrowed. Bone mineralization has been maintained.

B, Two years later, destruction involves all the distal and most of the proximal interphalangeal, radiocarpal and first carpometacarpal joints bilaterally. The left first metacarpal, multiple phalanges and the distal phalanx of the right thumb are subluxed. The distal interphalangeal joint of the right ring finger is fused.

(*Figure continued on opposite page.*)

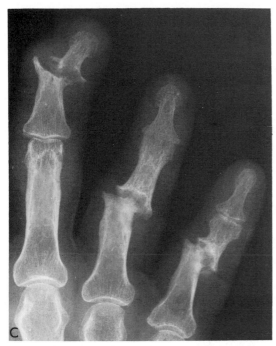

Figure 20–5. Continued. C, Detail view of the distal interphalangeal joints of the right hand. The patient had a negative rheumatoid factor, no subcutaneous nodules and no psoriatic lesions.

volvement, but the other roentgen and clinical features should support the latter diagnosis.

REFERENCES

1. Kidd, K. K., and Peter, J. B.: Erosive Osteoarthritis. *Radiology*, 86:640–647, 1966.
2. Peter, J. B., Pearson, C. M., and Maramor, L.: Erosive Osteoarthritis of the Hands. *Arthritis Rheum.*, 9:365–388, 1966.

RHEUMATOID ARTHRITIS

The primary process in rheumatoid arthritis is synovial proliferation with secondary erosion of joint cartilage and bone.[1, 3] The metacarpophalangeal, proximal interphalangeal, radiocarpal and intercarpal joints are most often involved. The index and middle finger metacarpophalangeal joints are affected earlier and more frequently. The intercarpal joints, except for the pisitriquetral, become involved as a group because they share a common synovial cavity. The distal radioulnar and ulnotriquetral joints are often involved as well.

Periarticular bone demineralization and synovial thickening are early roentgen signs of rheumatoid arthritis (Fig. 20–6 *A*). Synovial thickening can be demonstrated by low kilovoltage soft tissue roentgenography or mammographic techniques. Such thickening is symmetric and diffuse (Figs. 20–6 *B* and 20–7). If the proliferation is profuse, the joint capsule distends and capsular extensions may appear as subcutaneous masses. Such an extension from under the transverse carpal ligament is not uncommon in severe or moderately severe rheumatoid arthritis (Figs. 20–9 and 20–10).

The synovium proliferates around the joint, beginning at the juncture of the capsule and the articular cartilage. It is at the joint periphery where the articular cartilage is thinnest that early bone erosion is commonly demonstrated (Fig. 20–6 *C*). Erosions at the metacarpophalangeal joints begin on the volar aspect of the metacarpal heads and are best demonstrated with the hand supinated with 45° of internal rotation. Nonscreen type M industrial film gives the best detail to demonstrate early very small breaks or "skip areas" in the subchondral cortex. As synovial proliferation continues, the corners of the articular surfaces are eroded. The proliferation also extends over the joint surface and may break through the articular plate. As the synovium breaks through the subchondral cortex, it spreads out, producing cysts in cancellous bone (Fig. 20–9 *B*).

Subluxation, dislocation and deformities supervene as a result of joint disruption and associated tendon and capsular weakness. Flexion is often the characteristic deformity at the distal interphalangeal joints, and hyperextension is characteristic at the proximal interphalangeal joints (Fig. 20–9 *A*). The reverse may also occur. The carpus may rotate so that the scaphoid lies within the hollow of the radius (Fig. 20–9 *C*). The distal radioulnar joint separates, and the ulna may dislocate dorsally (Fig. 20–9 *C*). The intercarpal joints may fuse (Fig. 20–9 *B*). The fingers tend to drift into ulnar deviation because of unbalanced muscle pull, combined with laxity of the joint capsules and retaining structures of the tendons (Fig. 20–9 *A* and *C*).

Attachments of ligaments and tendons may develop similar erosions. These are particularly evident at the base of the distal phalanx attachment of the flexor pollicis

(*Text continued on page 524.*)

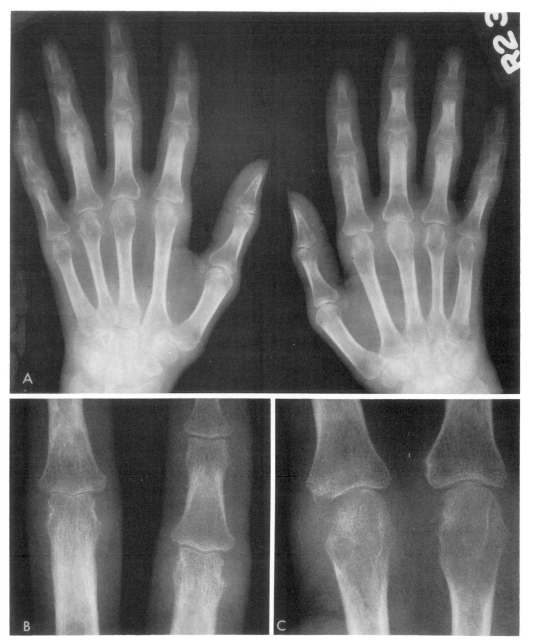

Figure 20–6. Rheumatoid arthritis. *A,* General demineralization is more apparent about the joints. *B,* The proximal interphalangeal joint space is narrowed and the synovium is thickened. The corners of the proximal phalangeal heads are eroded.

C, The metacarpophalangeal joint spaces are narrowed. There are erosions of the radial aspect of the metacarpal heads and the base of the second proximal phalanx. The synovium is thickened.

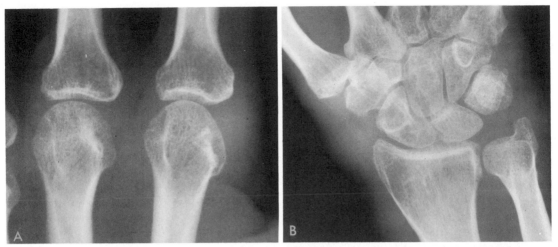

Figure 20–7. Rheumatoid arthritis. *A,* The synovium is thickened about the metacarpophalangeal joints. The left metacarpal head contains small subchondral cysts. *B,* The synovium about the carpus is markedly thickened. The bone is mildly demineralized.

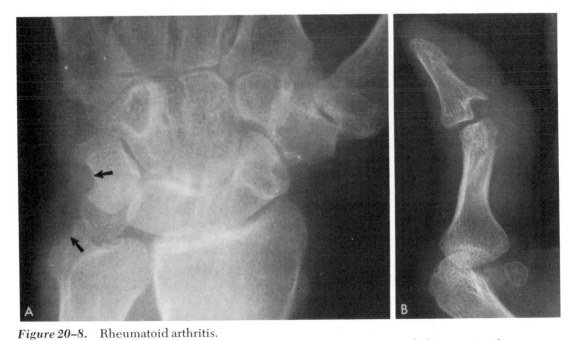

Figure 20–8. Rheumatoid arthritis.
A, The ulnar styloid and the ulnar aspect of the triquetrum are eroded (*arrows*). The synovium thickened.
B, There is erosion of the base of the distal phalanx of the thumb at the insertion of the flexor pollicis longus. The synovium produces a soft tissue mass at the distal interphalangeal joint.

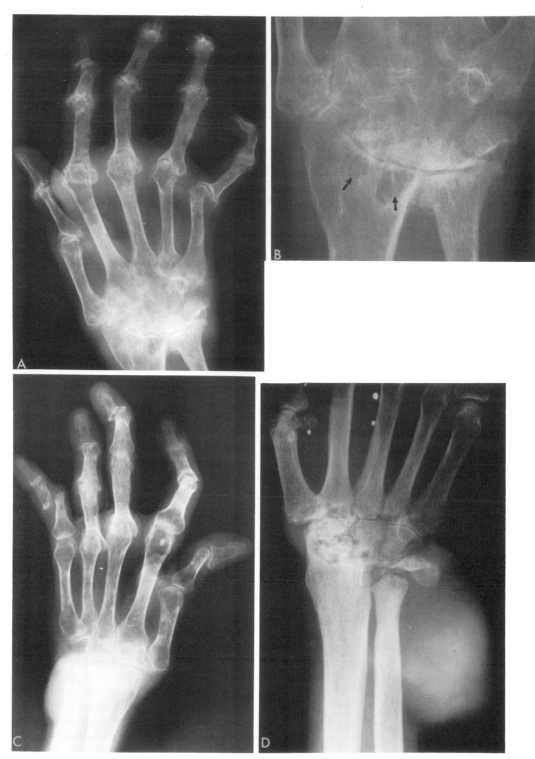

Figure 20-9. Advanced rheumatoid arthritis. *A,* Note the ulnar deviation of the fingers and the flexion deformities at the distal interphalangeal joints. The bases of many of the phalanges are cupped. The thenar and hypothenar eminences are atrophic.

B, The intercarpal and carpometacarpal joints are fused, and the radiocarpal and radioulnar joints are narrowed. There are two subchondral cysts in the radius (*arrows*).

C, The phalanges of many of the fingers are subluxed, the thumb is hyperextended, the proximal carpal row is partially eroded and subluxed, and the tip of ulna is completely destroyed. Extension of synovium forms a mass about the ulna.

D, Rheumatoid arthritis. A large synovial cyst extends from a severely destroyed carpus. The bases of the metacarpals are eroded. Despite extensive destruction, there is little new bone formation.

522

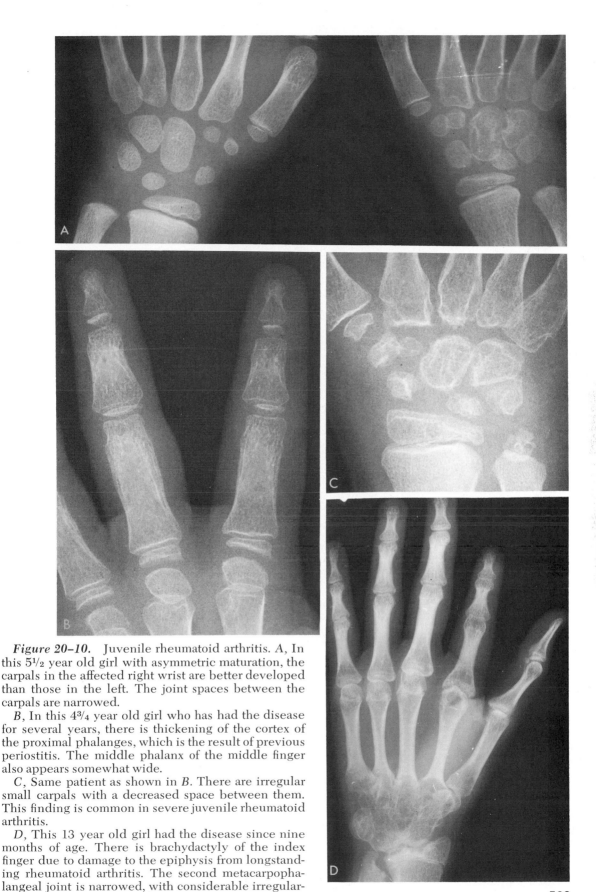

Figure 20–10. Juvenile rheumatoid arthritis. *A,* In this 5½ year old girl with asymmetric maturation, the carpals in the affected right wrist are better developed than those in the left. The joint spaces between the carpals are narrowed.

B, In this 4¾ year old girl who has had the disease for several years, there is thickening of the cortex of the proximal phalanges, which is the result of previous periostitis. The middle phalanx of the middle finger also appears somewhat wide.

C, Same patient as shown in *B*. There are irregular small carpals with a decreased space between them. This finding is common in severe juvenile rheumatoid arthritis.

D, This 13 year old girl had the disease since nine months of age. There is brachydactyly of the index finger due to damage to the epiphysis from longstanding rheumatoid arthritis. The second metacarpophalangeal joint is narrowed, with considerable irregularity of the second metacarpal and poorly developed phalanges. Extensive carpal fusion is evident.

523

longus to the thumb (Fig. 20–8 B) and at the styloid attachment of the ulnar collateral ligament (Fig. 20–8 A). A similar erosive change can narrow the waist of the carpal scaphoid and the triquetrum (Fig. 20–8 A). Following severe destructive changes, muscular stress may also precipitate further erosion of the weakened articular surface, causing a cupping deformity between adjacent bones (Fig. 20–9 A). Periosteal new bone formation is occasionally found along the attachment of the capsule into the periosteum or at the attachment of ligaments or tendons. It is usually a very fine, minimal reaction and later may result in thickening of the bones of the hand (Fig. 20–10 B). It is more common and profuse in juvenile rheumatoid arthritis than in the adult and may also occur in juvenile psoriatic arthritis (Fig. 20–16 G). Juvenile rheumatoid arthritis will locally alter the epiphyseal growth pattern about joints. Hyperemia causes early appearance and closure

of epiphyses (Fig. 20–10 A), so that the growth centers are more mature than the unaffected epiphyses about other joints. Early epiphyseal closure or joint fusion may cause shortening of a ray or digit (Fig. 20–10 D).

Surgical alterations may simulate destructive processes in rheumatoid arthritis. Arthroplasty at the metacarpophalangeal joints results in a flattened and shortened metacarpal head and phalangeal base (Fig. 20–11 A). Prostheses of radiolucent silicone require similar surgical remodeling at the metacarpophalangeal joint and can be seen if the radiographic technique demonstrates the adjacent soft tissue (Fig. 20–11 B).[2]

REFERENCES

1. Berens, D. L., Lin, R., and Lockie, L. M.: *Roentgen Diagnosis of Rheumatoid Arthritis*. Charles C Thomas, Publisher, Springfield, Illinois, 1969.
2. Calenoff, L., and Stromberg, W. B.: Silicone Rubber Arthroplasties of the Hand. *Radiology*, 107: 29–34, 1973.
3. Martel, W.: The Pattern of Rheumatoid Arthritis in the Hand and Wrist. *Radiol. Clin. North Am.*, 2:221–234, 1964.
4. Martel, W., Holt, J. F., and Cassidy, J. T.: Roentgenologic Manifestation of Juvenile Rheumatoid Arthritis. *Am. J. Roentgenol.*, 88:400–423, 1962.

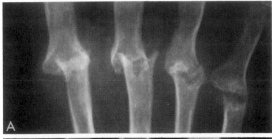
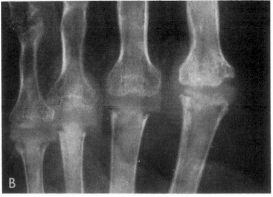

Figure 20–11. Rheumatoid arthritis. Surgical alterations. *A,* Arthroplasty of each metacarpophalangeal joint produces a squared-off appearance of the metacarpal heads and phalangeal bases.

B, Swanson prostheses. The metacarpal heads and phalangeal bases have been replaced by silicone joint spacers.

GOUT

The hand is affected less frequently than the lower extremities. In fact, hand without foot involvement is rare. Radiographs may show only joint effusion. The periarticular bones are normally mineralized since immobilizing pain and hyperemia is episodic, in contrast to the chronic progressive arthritides such as rheumatoid joint disease.[2] Periarticular demineralization develops if extensive destruction causes persistent hyperemia and painful immobilization.

The destructive changes in the joints are produced in two ways. First, intra-articular urate crystals stimulate synovial proliferation into and onto articular cartilage, particularly at the periphery of the joint. The thin cartilage in this area is quickly destroyed with subsequent bone erosion.

Secondly, urate crystals are deposited as

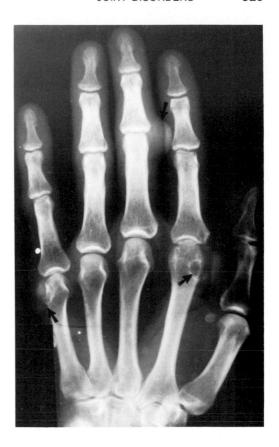

Figure 20–12. Gout. The proximal interphalangeal joint of the middle finger is asymmetrically and eccentrically enlarged by a tophus (*arrow*). A calcified tophus erodes the radial aspect of the second metacarpal head (*arrow*). Another calcified tophus is adjacent to the ulnar aspect of the fifth metacarpal head (*arrow*).

tophi in subchondral bone. They begin as oval lucencies with a slightly sclerotic border. As these tophi enlarge, they break through the bony cortex into the joint or adjacent to it. These expanded tophi are often surrounded by a feathery-like thin sclerotic rim and often contain calcifications (Fig. 20–12). On occasion, the enlargement of these tophi may cause metaphyseal widening, simulating an aneurysmal bone cyst or enchondroma (Fig. 20–13). Since gout involves both sides of the joint, differentiation of such bony enlargement by a tophus from tumor is readily apparent. Tumors tend to be singular and affect only one side of the joint.

Tophi within synovium may form a mass which will create asymmetric enlargement (Fig. 20–12). In fact, such asymmetry in periarticular soft tissues indicates a mass, since joint fluid is distributed evenly, creating a fusiform enlargement. If the asymmetrically swollen joint also contains calcifications in the swollen area, the diagnosis of a gouty tophus can be made with virtual certainty. A small intra-articular tophus will not cause asymmetry if it is hidden by a larger joint effusion. Severe deformity of the hand may simulate rheumatoid arthritis. However, the necrobiotic nodules of rheumatoid arthritis never contain calcifications, and calcified nodules indicate that the joint deformities are due to gout rather than to rheumatoid disease (Fig. 20–13 *B*).

Gout may incite the carpal tunnel syndrome when a tophus deposited on the flexor tendons compresses the median nerve against the transverse carpal ligament. It usually occurs in patients with tophaceous gout of severe degree and long duration. Erosions in the wrist bones will give a clue as to the gouty cause of the carpal tunnel syndrome. The carpal tunnel view may, on

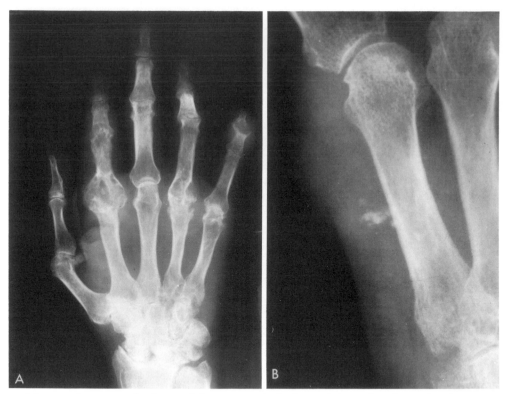

Figure 20–13. Gout. *A*, The base of the proximal phalanx of the index finger has been expanded by a large tophus which has destroyed the joint. There are similar changes in the metacarpophalangeal joint of the ring finger, and in the distal interphalangeal joint of the fifth finger. There are also multiple erosions in the carpus and in the radiocarpal joints.

B, Opposite hand of patient in *A*. A calcified tophus extends along the ulnar aspect of the fifth metacarpal.

a rare occasion, be helpful if calcified tophi can be demonstrated about the flexor tendon group under the transverse carpal ligament. In general, however, no calcification is discernible and gout can only be suspected on clinical grounds.[1]

REFERENCES

1. O'Hara, L. J., and Levin, M.: Carpal Tunnel Syndrome and Gout. Arch. *Intern. Med.,* 120: 180–184, 1967.
2. Talbott, J. H.: *Gout.* Grune and Stratton, Inc., New York, 1967.

PSEUDOGOUT

Pseudogout is characterized by recurrent acute attacks of pain and joint effusion precipitated by calcium pyrophosphate dihydrate crystals in the synovium and joint fluid. The crystals are also deposited in fibrocartilage and hyaline cartilage along the articular surface. The wrist is affected in half the patients. It is usually bilateral and involves the triangular cartilage at the ulnocarpal articulation of the cartilage of the radiocarpal joint (Fig. 20–14). The symphysis pubis, hips, shoulders, and elbows are affected in about half the patients.[1] Pubic involvement is characterized by a linear calcification running down the center of the symphysis. Similar calcifications are also present in patients with hyperparathyroidism, ochronosis, gout and degenerative joint disease.

The diagnosis is made when calcium pyrophosphate dihydrate crystals are demonstrated in the joint fluid by polarizing microscopy.

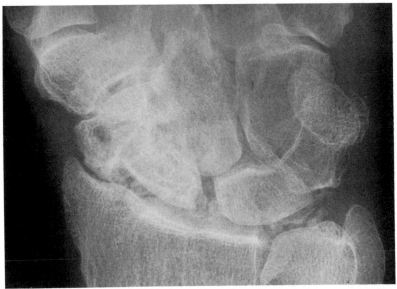

Figure 20–14. Pseudogout. Calcifications are distributed in the triangular cartilage and in the radiocarpal joint. The patient had bouts of severe joint pain. Calcium pyrophosphate dihydrate crystals were obtained from other joints.

REFERENCE

1. McCarty, D. J., and Haskin, M. E.: The Roentgenographic Aspects of Pseudogout. *Am. J. Roentgenol.*, 90:1248–1257, 1963.

REITER SYNDROME

The combination of conjunctivitis, urethritis and arthritis is referred to as Reiter syndrome. While the etiology is unclear, the symptoms usually appear shortly after an episode of dysentery or sexual intercourse.

The knees, ankles and feet are involved more often than the hands, a differential point from rheumatoid arthritis. Diaphyseal periosteal new bone of either linear or a fluffy woolly type appears in 30 per cent of cases (Fig. 20–15). The former appears in acute cases of a few weeks' to a few months' duration, while the latter is common after a prolonged disease. Similar periosteal new bone develops much less frequently in psoriatic arthritis. The periarticular bone is demineralized in 75 per cent of acute cases and in over 50 per cent of all joints involved. The periarticular tissues enlarge in over 80 per cent of cases with acute symptoms and in 69 per cent of all cases (Fig. 20–15).[2]

Joint narrowing or destruction is characteristic of the hand and wrist, frequently in acute cases of less than a year's duration and in 43 per cent of chronic cases. More than 50 per cent of joints with narrowing will have some permanent change.

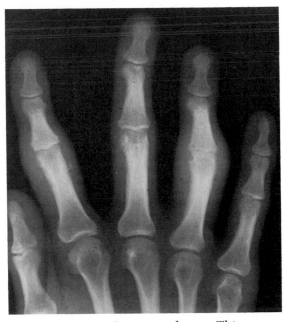

Figure 20–15. Reiter syndrome. This young man had repeated urethritis, arthritis, and mucosal lesions of Reiter disease in the hard palate. The soft tissues about the index and ring fingers are swollen. Each affected bone shows periosteal reaction of moderate degree.

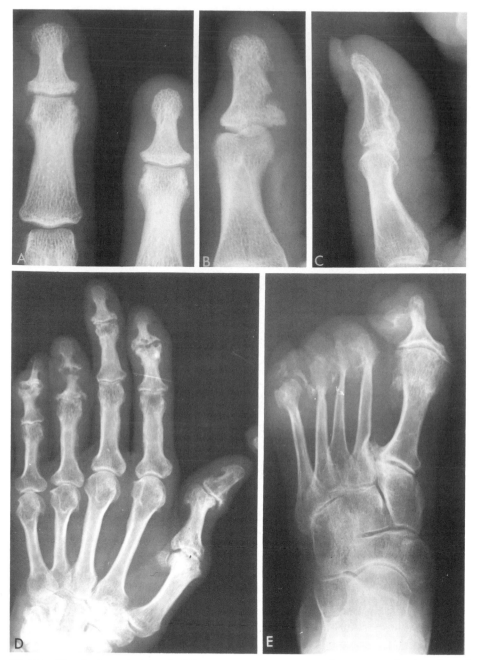

Figure 20–16. Psoriatic arthritis. *A,* There are early erosive changes on both sides of the two distal interphalangeal joints. The soft tissue about the joint is thickened.

B, In the thumb of same patient, there are erosive changes of the metaphysis of the base of the distal phalanx, and convexity of the proximal phalangeal head. The periarticular soft tissue is thickened.

C, This is another patient with a thickened thumbnail.

D, There is advanced disease, with marked erosion of all distal and the proximal ring finger interphalangeal joints.

E, Left foot of patient shown in *D.* The distal phalanx of the great toe is almost entirely destroyed. The proximal phalangeal head is pointed, and its base is broadened. Similar changes occur in the hand in some patients with psoriatic arthritis.

(*Legend and figure continued on opposite page.*)

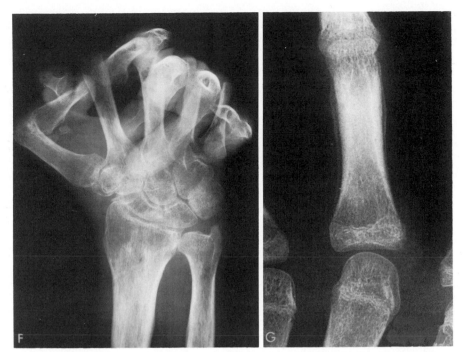

Figure 20–16. *Continued. F,* Arthritis mutilans in a man who had psoriasis for many years. *G,* Note periosteal elevation in the proximal phalanx of a patient with juvenile psoriatic arthritis. This degree of periosteal reaction is unusual.

Tendon calcification can develop about the knee, shoulder and foot but has not been reported in the hand and wrist.

REFERENCES

1. Moskowitz, R. W., and Kath, D.: Chondrocalcinosis and Chondrocalsynovitis (Pseudogout Syndrome). *Am. J. Med.,* 43:322–334, 1967.
2. Peterson, C. C., Jr., and Silbiger, M. L.: Reiter's Syndrome and Psoriatic Arthritis. *Am. J. Roentgenol.,* 101:860–871, 1967.

PSORIATIC ARTHRITIS

Psoriatic arthritis is a polyarticular process in which the skin disease usually precedes and only rarely follows arthritis. The articular disease is usually asymmetric and most commonly involves the distal interphalangeal joints of the hands and feet. The arthritic symptoms wax and wane with the course of the skin disease. The remissions are more frequent and complete than those of rheumatoid arthritis. The rheumatoid factor is normal and patients have neither systemic symptoms nor subcutaneous nodules.

A distinctive pattern of roentgenographic changes occurs in approximately 25 per cent of patients. These are as follows: (1) destructive arthritis primarily affecting the distal interphalangeal joints of the fingers and toes, creating abnormally wide spaces with destroyed, well-demarcated adjacent bony surfaces (Fig. 20–16 *D*); (2) bony ankylosis of the affected interphalangeal joints; (3) interphalangeal joint destruction of the great toe accompanied by bony proliferation at the base of the distal phalanx; and (4) resorption of the tufts of the distal phalanges of the hands and feet (Fig. 20–16 E).[1] Asymmetric distal interphalangeal joint involvement differentiates psoriatic from typical rheumatoid arthritis. Ankylosis in psoriatic arthritis does not affect the carpus. Severe destruction results in marked deformity of the hands or "arthritis mutilans" (Fig. 20–16 F). Microscopic examination demonstrates complete destruction of the bone end, which is enclosed in a fibrous tissue collar, maintaining a space between the affected parts.

Early pathologic changes demonstrate marginal overgrowth at tendon insertions and pale, edematous granulation tissue extending out from the joint and along the metaphysis, destroying bone. There are no rheumatoid granulomas in the synovium.

Twenty-five per cent of patients have roentgenographic changes simulating those of rheumatoid arthritis. It is of note that some patients with rheumatoid arthritis also have distal interphalangeal joint destruction, and some observers feel that these are variant lesions of rheumatoid arthritis. This postulate is supported by the fact that the symptoms of psoriatic arthritis recede during pregnancy, and that the leukocytes of some patients contain rheumatoid factor, as occurs in rheumatoid arthritis.[3]

Psoriatic arthritis may simulate juvenile rheumatoid arthritis. The average onset of psoriatic arthritis in children is 12.5 years, compared with 6.8 years in juvenile rheumatoid arthritis. Children with psoriatic arthritis have prominent distal interphalangeal joint involvement and no systemic symptoms (Fig. 20–16 A and B). Periosteal elevation similar to that in rheumatoid arthritis may be seen (Fig. 20–16 G). The nails show changes varying from minimal thickening and ridging to "pepper-pot" pitting, discoloration and onycholysis (Fig. 20–16 C). The rheumatoid factor, antinuclear antibody titers and serum uric acid levels are normal.[2]

Occasionally the pustular lesions of psoriasis cannot be distinguished from the skin lesion keratodermia blennorrhagica of Reiter syndrome. Both diseases may have similar nail changes and peripheral and spinal joint involvement. However, there is a predilection for the feet, ankles and knees in Reiter syndrome. Roentgen changes in joints rarely appear in adults before psoriatic skin changes. If they do, skin lesions will appear within one to two years.[3]

REFERENCES

1. Avila, R., Pugh, D. G., Slocumb, C. H., and Winkleman, R. K.: Psoriatic Arthritis: A Roentgenologic Study. *Radiology,* 75:691–702, 1960.
2. Peterson, C. C., and Silbiger, M. L.: Reiter's Syndrome and Psoriatic Arthritis—Their Roentgen Spectra and Some Interesting Similarities. *Am. J. Roentgenol.,* 101:860–871, 1967.
3. Sigler, J. W.: Psoriatic Arthritis. *In:* Hollander, H. L. (Ed.): *Arthritis and Allied Conditions.* Lea & Febiger, Philadelphia, 1972, pp. 724–735.

TABLE 20–1.   Comparative Incidence of Roentgen Changes*

	SCLERODERMA		OTHER COLLAGEN DISEASES		PRIMARY RAYNAUD DISEASE
	% without Raynaud	% with Raynaud	% without Raynaud	% with Raynaud	%
	(23)†	(29)†	(39)†	(4)†	(22)
Bone Erosion	39	41	3	0	14
Calcification	22	14	0	0	0
Atrophy	17	55	0	25	36
Any of the above roentgen changes	52	72	3	25	41
Combined	63		5		

*Data after Yune, H. Y., et al.: Early Fingertip Changes in Scleroderma. *J.A.M.A.,* 215:1113–1116, 1971.
†Number of cases with roentgenograms.

SCLERODERMA

Scleroderma in the hand is characterized by soft tissue resorption and fibrosis, joint contractions, thin skin and subcutaneous calcifications. Yune et al.[1] compared the hand roentgenograms of 52 patients with scleroderma, 53 patients with other collagen disease exluding rheumatoid arthritis, and 22 patients with primary Raynaud disease. The details are tabulated in Table 20–1. The roentgenograms were those available from a group of 508 patients, of which 132 had scleroderma, 296 other forms of collagen disease and 80 primary Raynaud disease.

Roentgen changes of bone erosion, soft tissue atrophy, or subcutaneous calcifications could be detected in 63 per cent of patients with scleroderma, in only 3 per cent of those with other collagen diseases and in 41 per cent of patients with primary Raynaud disease (Fig. 20–17). Soft tissue resorption or atrophy of a fingertip is pres-

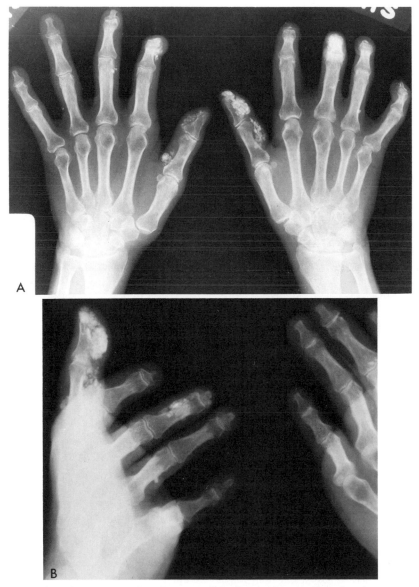

Figure 20–17. Scleroderma. *A,* The fingers of both hands are flexed. There are multiple subcutaneous calcifications, particularly about the fingertips.

B, Resorption of fingertips and distal phalanges is demonstrated by detailed positioning.

ent radiographically when the vertical distance between the tip of a normal distal phalanx and the skin surface is less than 20 per cent of the transverse diameter of the base of the same distal phalanx on an anteroposterior film of the digit. Amorphous calcifications form small subcutaneous nodules and plaques. This calcification may involve either the subcutaneous tissues or the periarticular capsule.

Bone erosion occurs in 40 per cent of patients with scleroderma. The tufts of the distal phalanges resorb to a pencil-like deformity. Erosions develop at the margins of the distal interphalangeal joints. Subsequently, the joint surfaces become irregular and deformed and ankylosis may develop. As a result of the chronic disease and immobilization, the bones of the hand may demineralize in the later stages of scleroderma.

Raynaud phenomenon occurs in 42 percent of patients with scleroderma and in 3 per cent of patients with other collagen diseases. Bone erosion and soft tissue calcification in scleroderma occur with equal frequency, regardless of vascular involvement, but Raynaud phenomenon appreciably increases the incidence of soft tissue atrophy; in primary Raynaud disease, it is the most common finding. Of some note is the absence of soft tissue calcification in patients with either other collagen diseases or with primary Raynaud disease. Therefore, patients with digital soft tissue calcifications and suspected collagen disease very likely have scleroderma.

Yune[1] discovered with some surprise that bone erosions or soft tissue calcifications developed in the fingers of 35 per cent of patients within six months of the onset of scleroderma. Soft tissue calcification and osseous resorption occur simultaneously only in scleroderma. Similar resorption of bone and soft tissue without calcification occurs in leprosy, Buerger disease, lupus erythematosus, Raynaud disease, diabetes mellitus, frostbite and ainhum.

REFERENCE

1. Yune, H. Y., Vix, V. A., and Klatte, E. C.: Early Fingertip Changes in Scleroderma. *J.A.M.A.*, 215:1113–1116, 1971.

STEROID ARTHROPATHY

Subchondral bone destruction following systemic administration of steroids occurs most often in weight-bearing joints, particularly the knees and hips.[1, 4] Of the non-weight-bearing joints, the shoulder is primarily affected. The wrist and hand rarely develop steroid arthropathy.

The roentgenographic findings are similar to aseptic necrosis from a variety of causes. The process is initially a bone disease involving one joint component. Joint destruction is a secondary phenomenon. The most common roentgen findings are subcortical mottling due to loss of definition of trabeculae or localized subchondral rarefaction surrounded by a thin rim of sclerosis. Sometimes areas of increased and decreased density adjoin each other. A "rim sign" is produced as a lucent line adjacent and parallel to the subchondral cortex by a sliver of fragmented bone. With progression, the articular cortex is depressed so that a normally convex bone becomes flat or concave (Fig. 20–18).[3] As the process advances, large portions of the bone may resorb, resulting in a "bite sign." Periosteal new bone apposition often develops as a fine ossification at the metaphysis of the involved bone.

The cause of aseptic necrosis following steroid therapy is unknown. We do know that steroids increase blood coagulability and viscosity and that fat emboli can be found in necrotic bone lesions after steroid administration. In most instances, long-term, large doses of exogenous steroid produce these changes. Very rarely do patients with Cushing's disease develop osteonecrosis, suggesting a different response of bone to exogenous and endogenous steroids. It has been postulated that fluctuation in exogenous steroids may be a contributing factor.[3]

Avascular necrosis of bone may be common in patients receiving high doses of steroid following renal transplantation.[1] Harrington et al.[2] reported an incidence of over 30 per cent in patients receiving massive doses.[2] During a 3¼ year period, 50 patients received 120 to 200 mg. of prednisone daily for three weeks following transplantation, and were then tapered to a daily average dosage of 30 mg. The three-week average total dose was 2960 mg. Six-

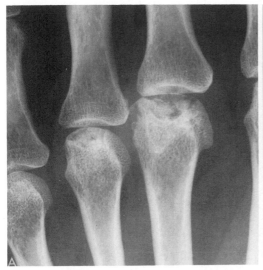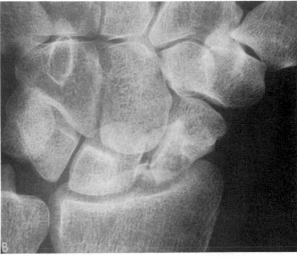

Figure 20–18. A, Steroid arthropathy. This 45 year old woman with systemic lupus erythematosus was treated with corticosteroids for six years. The heads of the third and fourth metacarpals partially collapsed following necrosis of subchondral bone. The appearance is similar to aseptic necrosis of the femoral head. Both femoral heads and both humeral heads were also affected in this patient.

B, Same patient as shown in A. There is aseptic necrosis in the navicular bone.

teen of the 50 patients developed aseptic necrosis in one or more bones. Thereafter, 101 patients received 120 to 200 mg. of prednisone daily for two to four days, after which the dose was reduced rapidly to 30 mg. a day. The average four-day dosage was 1180 grams. In this group, only two patients developed osteonecrosis. Both groups of patients were treated identically in other respects. The authors felt that the high initial dosage of the first group contributed to aseptic necrosis.

Of the patients in Harrington's series, six had osteonecrosis in one bone, seven in two bones, and five in more than two bones. Forty-seven bones were involved, and only 12 non-weight-bearing bones were affected. The phalanges and carpal bones were involved four times.

REFERENCES

1. Fisher, D. E., and Bickel, W. H.: Corticosteroid–Induced Avascular Necrosis: A Clinical Study of Seventy-Seven Patients. *J. Bone Joint Surg.*, 53A:859–873, 1971.
2. Harrington, K. D., Murray, W. R., Kountz, S. L., and Belzer, F. O.: Avascular Necrosis of Bone after Renal Transplantation. *J. Bone Joint Surg.*, 53A:203–215, 1971.
3. Martel, W., and Sitterley, B. H.: Roentgenologic Manifestations of Osteonecrosis. *Am. J. Roentgenol.*, 106:509–522, 1969.
4. Miller, W. T., and Restifo, R. A.: Steroid Arthropathy. *Radiology*, 86:652–657, 1966.

LUPUS ERYTHEMATOSUS

At some time 90 per cent of patients with lupus erythematosus have polyarthralgia with little or no inflammation. Often the muscles about the joint atrophy.

Radiographic joint changes are rare, although synovial biopsy demonstrates diffuse periarticular inflammation and microvascular obliteration by large endothelial cells, intraluminal inflammatory cells or platelet fibrin thrombi.[5] Patients may develop a Jaccoud-like postrheumatic fever deformity of the hands. Kramer et al.[4] reported 14 patients with ulnar deviation of the fingers which could be voluntarily and passively reduced and in which no erosive changes could be demonstrated radiographically (Fig. 20–19).[4] Other joints were symptomatic and the disease had been present an average of 14½ years. Twelve had a positive Schirmer test, suggesting that patients with deformities of the hands and

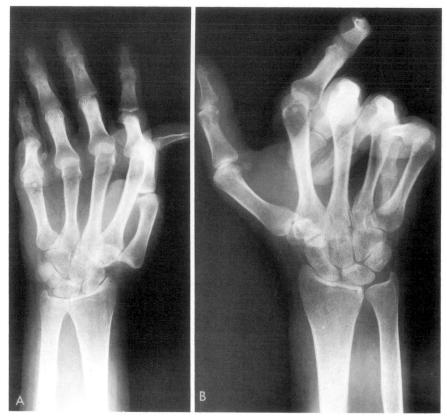

Figure 20–19. Lupus erythematosus in a 32 year old woman. *A*, Left hand. The fingers are sub-luxed volarward and deviated ulnarward. The distal phalanx of the thumb is hyperextended. *B*, Right hand. There are flexion contractures of the last three fingers, and ulnar deviation and volar sub-luxation of the index finger.

The first metacarpals of both hands are subluxed dorsally. Despite the severe deformities, there are no erosive bony changes.

lupus erythematosus may also have Sjö-gren syndrome. The authors predict that more patients will develop such hand de-formities as the length and incidence of survival increases.

Steroid arthropathy or avascular necrosis due to the collagen disease is more common in the weight-bearing joints than in the hands.[1] Confusion with rheumatoid arth-ritis is unlikely. It is of some interest that the rheumatoid factor in patients with lupus erythematosus is positive in about half the patients when measured using whole serum, but it is present in only 3 per cent when the same test is made with a cold precipitable fraction.[6] Kellgren and Ball[3] reported positive sheep cell tests in some patients with prominent articular or periph-eral vascular lesions in lupus.[3] Between 0 and 27 per cent of patients with rheumatoid arthritis will have a positive LE prepara-tion. However, there is a marked variation in response of these individuals, and it is generally not thought to be due to lupus erythematosus. Subcutaneous and synovial rheumatoid necrobiotic nodules occur in 5 to 7 per cent of patients with systemic lupus erythematosus. Three patients in the series of Dubois et al.[2] also had post-rheumatic fever or Jaccoud type arthritis. Eight of the nine patients had positive LE preparations and the other had typical clini-cal findings of LE. The rheumatoid factor was positive in four patients and negative in five.

REFERENCES

1. Dubois, L., and Cozen, L.: Avascular (Aseptic) Necrosis Bone Process Associated With Sys-temic Lupus Erythematosus. *J.A.M.A.*, 174: 966–971, 1960.

2. Dubois, E. L., Friou, G. J., and Chandor, S.: Rheumatoid Nodules and Rheumatoid Granulomas in Systemic Lupus Erythematosus. *J.A.M.A.*, 200:515–518, 1972.
3. Kellgren, J. H., and Ball, J.: Clinical Importance of the Rheumatoid Serum Factor. *Br. Med. J.*, 1:523–530, 1959.
4. Kramer, L. S., Ruderman, J. E., Dubois, E. L., and Friou, G. J.: Deforming, Nonerosive Arthritis of the Hands in Chronic Systemic Lupus Erythematosus (SLE). *Arthritis Rheum.*, 13: 239–330, 1970.
5. Labowitz, R., and Schumacher, H. R.: The Articular Manifestations of Systemic Lupus Erythematosus (SLE): A Clinico-Pathologic Study. *Arthritis Rheum.*, 13:330, 1970.
6. Svartz, N., and Schlossman, K.: Agglutination of Sensitized Sheep Erythrocytes in Disseminated Lupus Erythematosus. *Ann. Rheum. Dis.*, 16: 73–75, 1957.

NEUROPATHIC ARTHROPATHY

Neuropathic joint disease is a chronic, progressive degenerative arthropathy developing as a complication of a variety of neurological disorders. The knees, hips, ankles and spine are most often affected secondary to tabes dorsalis or diabetes. Syringomyelia and tabes dorsalis produce upper extremity joint changes. The shoulder and elbow are usually affected, while the hand and wrist are infrequently involved. Isolated wrist involvement in syringomyelia is rare. At least one other joint in the same extremity is also affected. Swelling and mild pain are the clinical hallmarks of the disease. Pain is especially mild, considering the severity of joint destruction.

The principle roentgenographic features are effusion, subluxation and bone destruction with normal or increased periarticular mineralization. Early roentgen findings are joint swelling and subluxation. Later, joint cartilage fragments and, thereafter, the subchondral bone fractures, scattering pieces of bone throughout the joint. Portions of the synovium ossify. Identification of such ossification microscopically is characteristic of the neuropathic joint. Spurs may form at the periphery of the wrist joint but are not as apparent as in the spine and larger weight-bearing articulations.

Bone resorption begins as erosions at the periphery of the epiphysis, undermining the subchondral cortex. Later the articular surface and the entire head or base are destroyed, leaving a pencil-like diaphy-

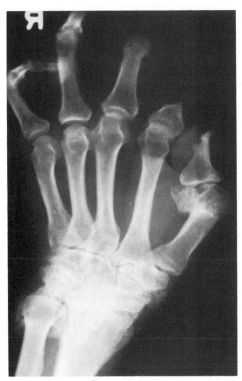

Figure 20–20. Syringomyelia. Neuropathic joint. The bones of many resorbed fingers have a "penciling" deformity. The wrist joint is normally mineralized. Multiple small fragments of bone are imbedded about the synovium of the carpus and the radiocarpal and radioulnar joints. (Courtesy Dr. R. Rapp, Veterans Administration Hospital, Ann Arbor, Michigan.)

sis (Fig. 20–20). Again, mineralization is normal despite severe destruction.[1, 3]

The soft tissues of the fingers are resorbed and may ulcerate following trauma incited by the neurologic deficit. The tufts of the distal phalanges undergo resorption simultaneously. If an ulceration overlies the destroyed bone, osteomyelitis may be an additional cause of bone destruction.

Joint destruction is a gradual process that accelerates once fragmentation occurs. However, sometimes extensive changes from a normal roentgenographic appearance to marked disorganization can take place in as little as nine days to three weeks.[2]

REFERENCES

1. Eichenholz, S. J.: *Charcot Joints.* Springfield, Charles C Thomas, Publisher, Springfield, Illinois, 1966.

2. Norman, A., Robbins, H., and Milgram, J. E.: The Acute Neuropathic Arthropathy—A Rapid, Severely Disorganizing Form of Arthritis. *Radiology*, 90:1159–1164, 1968.

3. Staple, T. W.: Radiology of the Diabetic Foot. *In: The Diabetic Foot.* The C. V. Mosby Co., St. Louis, 1973.

JACCOUD ARTHROPATHY

This asymptomatic deforming arthropathy of the hands and feet is associated with previous attacks of rheumatic fever. Its appearance is similar to that of rheumatoid arthritis, but bone adjacent to the joint is changed very little.

The major clinical and roentgenographic manifestations are ulnar deviation and volar subluxation of the fingers at the metacarpophalangeal joints. The hand may be deviated medially at the wrist. Subluxation of the proximal phalanges may cause slight degenerative changes and a hook-like deformity on the volar aspect of the metacarpal heads. Of particular significance is the severe hand deformity which produces little roentgenographic change in the bones of the involved joints. The alteration can be corrected actively or passively (Fig. 20–21).[2]

The disease is recognized late because of its asymptomatic character. Usually, repeated attacks and occasionally only one bout of rheumatic fever precedes the joint disease. The articular process is probably active simultaneous with heart disease, but because of its very insignificant progression, it is usually not discovered until much later. In fact, some patients are unaware of deforming changes in the hand until they are pointed out by their physician. At that time, cardiac examination will demonstrate a murmur of mitral or aortic valve disease.

Biopsy of the joint capsule demonstrates fibrosis of the periarticular tissues with a normal synovium. It has been postulated that the deformities are due to laxity about the joint or to scarred and fibrosed cords pulling the joints into their deformed state.

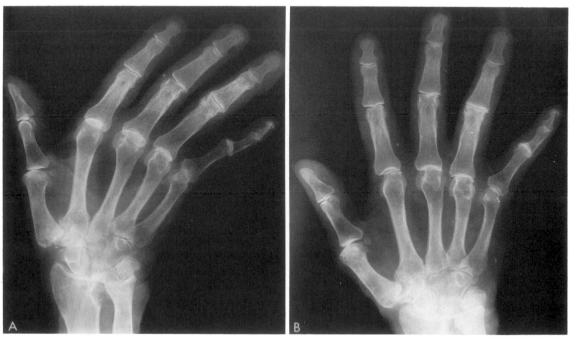

Figure 20–21. Jaccoud arthropathy. *A*, There is marked subluxation of the fingers at the metacarpophalangeal joints with minimal erosive changes. The fingers are deviated ulnarward.

B, The deformity has been reduced passively. (Reproduced with permission from *Am. J. Roentgenol.*, 118:300–307, 1973.)

Such deformities may also be due to fibrosis about the joints, which does not allow normal repositioning of the involved parts.

The erythrocyte sedimentation rate is normal and the rheumatoid factor is negative. The diagnosis is made on the basis of previous attacks of rheumatic fever associated with minimal residual joint symptoms and insidious and painless onset of joint deformity. Similar deformities develop with long-standing lupus erythematosus, but the clinical findings of LE have been present for at least five years.[1]

REFERENCES

1. Kramer, L. S., Ruderman, J. E., Dubois, E. L., and Friou, G. J.: Deforming Nonerosive Arthritis of the Hands in Chronic Systemic Lupus Erythematosus (SLE). *Arthritis Rheum.*, 13: 329–330, 1970.
2. Murphy, W., and Staple, T. W.: Jaccoud's Arthropathy Reviewed. *Am. J. Roentgenol.*, 118:300–307, 1973.

PIGMENTED VILLONODULAR SYNOVITIS AND GANGLION

In 1941, Jaffe et al.[2] described a lesion of joints, bursae and tendons containing pigmented villous and nodular proliferation of the synovium which seemed to be inflammatory in origin.[2] The lesion most commonly affects the knee, hip, ankle, tarsus, carpus, elbow and shoulder, in decreasing order of frequency. It rarely affects more than one joint.

The clinical manifestations are a diffuse, mildly painful swelling which may be associated with palpable nodular masses or synovial thickening. Joint effusion is common and the fluid is xanthochromic or serosanguineous. All the standard laboratory tests for arthritis are normal. The joint fluid is usually high in cholesterol content, but the blood cholesterol levels are normal.

In most instances the only roentgen manifestations are joint effusion or an accompanying noncalcified soft tissue mass.[4] A few of the lesions erode bone.[1] The erosion is extrinsic, creating a defect in the cortex and the underlying medullary bone. The ero-

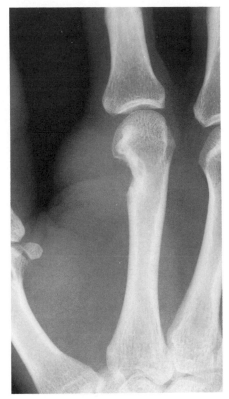

Figure 20–22. Villonodular synovitis. Tendon sheath. A soft tissue mass erodes the ulnar aspect of the proximal phalanx. The rim of new bone indicates a benign process of erosion from the tendon sheath.

sion is surrounded by a thin border of sclerotic bone, indicating slow progression as would be found in a benign lesion (Fig. 20–22). In isolated instances, the masses may attain considerable size, destroying a large portion of bone adjacent to the joint. The periarticular structures are usually normally mineralized since the lesion is relatively painless and motion is only mildly limited.

A ganglion results when the collagenous tissue of a joint capsule or tendon sheath undergoes myxoid degeneration and cystic softening.[3] Such ganglia are most common in the dorsum of the wrist and can also extend from the carpal joint under the transverse carpal ligament. It forms a multi-loculated cyst of varying size. Its connection with the wrist joint can be demonstrated by arthrography (Fig. 20–23).

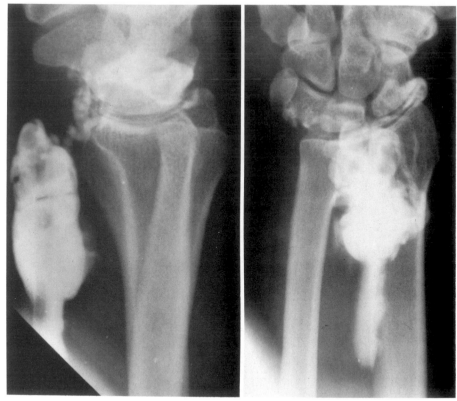

Figure 20–23. Ganglion. Wrist arthrogram shows extension of synovium along the flexor tendons.

REFERENCES

1. Breimer, C. S., and Freiberger, R.: Bone Lesions Associated With Villonodular Synovitis. *Am. J. Roentgenol.*, 79:618–629, 1958.
2. Jaffe, H. L., Lichtenstein, L., and Sutro, C. G.: Pigmented Villonodular Synovitis, Bursitis, and Tenosynovitis. *Arch. Path.*, 31:731–765, 1941.
3. Lichtenstein, L.: *Disease of Bone and Joints.* The C. V. Mosby Co., St. Louis, 1970.
4. Smith, J. H., and Pugh, D. G.: Roentgenographic Aspects of Pigmented Villonodular Synovitis. *Am. J. Roentgenol.*, 87:1146–1156, 1962.

SYNOVIAL CHONDROMATOSIS

Osseous metaplasia of synovium is a common occurrence in the knee, shoulder and elbow. In fact, any synovial joint, even the temporomandibular, may develop osteochondromatosis. Wrist and hand involvement is rare.[1]

The process begins as focal metaplastic growths of normal-appearing cartilage in the synovium. Portions of these bodies may be attached to stalks, and others may be completely detached and become loose bodies. When these bodies calcify and ossify, the condition is called synovial osteochondromatosis.[3]

Pain, joint swelling or clicking sensations are clinical manifestations. If calcified or ossified, the cartilaginous masses can be seen roentgenographically (Fig. 20–24). Recurrent effusion may cause extension of the synovium under the transverse carpal ligament, producing a cystic mass of the volar aspect of the wrist. Purely cartilaginous masses may be detected by injection of the bursa to demonstrate the lobulation in the synovium (Fig. 20–25). Without calcifications, such lobulation cannot be differentiated from villonodular synovitis or synovial hypertrophy. In the latter conditions, the roentgenographic appearance of the wrist may help define the cause of the synovial enlargement. Chondromatosis is a benign lesion and only rarely undergoes malignant change.[2]

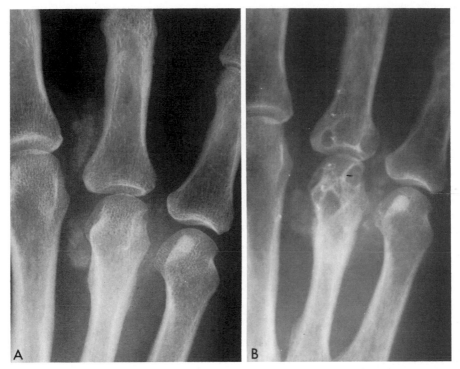

Figure 20–24. Osteochondromatosis. *A*, Osseous and noncalcified cartilage masses were found in this expanded joint at surgery.

B, Eight years later, synovial proliferation causes secondary bone erosion. New bone fragments have formed.

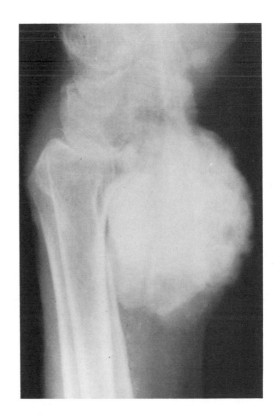

Figure 20–25. Synovial chondromatosis. In this 50 year old woman with a painless, nontender wrist mass, a contrast material injection of the mass demonstrates multiple, histologically proved cartilaginous nodules.

REFERENCES

1. Feist, J. H., and Gibbons, T. G.: Osteochondromatosis of the Temporomandibular Joint. *Radiology*, 74:291–293, 1960.
2. King, J. W., Spjut, H. J., Fechner, R. E., and Vanderpol, D. W.: Synovial Chondrosarcoma of the Knee Joint. *J. Bone Joint Surg.*, 49A:1389–1396, 1967.
3. Lichtenstein, L.: *Diseases of Bone and Joints*. The C. V. Mosby Co., St. Louis, 1970.

DE QUERVAIN DISEASE AND OTHER FORMS OF TENDINITIS

Inflammatory and degenerative processes may occur in any tendon, tendon sheath or accompanying bursa. De Quervain disease, or stenosing tendinitis of the abductor pollicis longus, is the only one of these processes with a specific name. The disease causes pain, swelling, tenderness and roentgenographic changes about the radial styloid process. Soft tissue roentgenography will demonstrate a lateral bulge of the skin near the radial styloid. Accumulation of synovial fluid within the tendon sheath enlarges the sheath complex and deviates the subcutaneous fatty layer. When edema occurs, the usually well-defined subcutaneous tissue planes are obliterated. No changes in the underlying bone are apparent.[3]

Patients with calcific tendinitis about the wrist present an easily recognizable clinical history. A nontraumatic, moderately severe pain begins fairly suddenly and increases rapidly. The wrist is tender, swollen

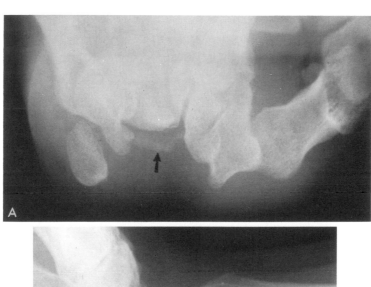

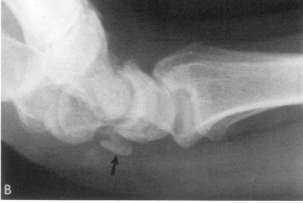

Figure 20–26. Calcific tendinitis. *A*, Carpal tunnel view. *B*, Lateral view. In this 25 year old woman, who had sudden wrist pain, swelling and tenderness, there is calcification in the flexor tendon sheath (*arrow*).

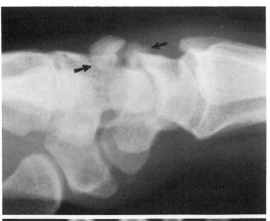

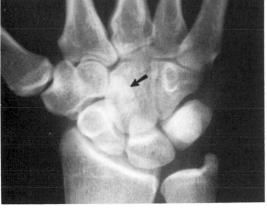

Figure 20–27. Calcific tendinitis. Calcification (*arrows*) in the extensor tendons has occurred. There were periodic episodes of tenderness and swelling in the dorsum of the wrist. (Courtesy Dr. W. Walker, St. Louis, Missouri.)

and red. The pain increases to such an extent that a fracture is suspected clinically (Figs. 20–26 and 20–27). The roentgenographic examination will demonstrate calcification within one of the tendons about the wrist, suggesting an avulsion fracture. However, a source of the fragment cannot be located and the patient will invariably deny any trauma to the wrist despite a rather dramatic sudden onset of pain. The history is quite similar to that of a patient with calcific tendinitis of the shoulder, except that in this instance the physical findings may be more dramatic because the involved tendons are not covered by as great a thickness of subcutaneous tissue.

The calcific tendinitis may simulate gout. Thompson et al.[2] reported eight patients with acute monarticular arthritis, four of

whom had calcific tendinitis of the fingers or wrists.[2] The serum uric acid levels were normal in each instance, but colchicine or phenylbutazone therapy relieved the symptoms dramatically. Biopsy of one of the calcified masses showed material composed of hydroxyapatite. No uric acid or urates could be found. Their excellent experience compels them to recommend colchicine therapy for calcific tendinitis once joint aspiration to exclude pyarthrosis has been performed.

Gondos[1] reported eight patients with calcified wrist tendons. In four patients the calcification was near the pisiform in the flexor carpi ulnaris tendon, while in the remaining four the flexor carpi radialis, common flexor and extensor carpi ulnaris tendons were affected. Two tendons can be involved simultaneously. Pain is not always sudden and severe, while tenderness over the involved tendon is common.

REFERENCES

1. Gondos, B.: Calcification About the Wrist Associated with Acute Pain (Periarthritis Calcarea). *Radiology,* 60:244–251, 1953.
2. Thompson, G. R., Ming Ting, Y., Riggs, G., Fenn, M. E., and Denning, R. J.: Calcific Tendinitis and Soft Tissue Calcification Resembling Gout. *J.A.M.A.,* 203:464–472, 1968.
3. Weston, W. J.: De Quervains Disease: Stenosing Fibrosis Tendovaginitis at the Radial Styloid Process. *Br. J. Radiol.,* 40:446–448, 1967.

HYPERTROPHIC PULMONARY OSTEOARTHROPATHY

Hypertrophic pulmonary osteoarthropathy is a syndrome consisting of clubbing of the fingers and toes, periosteal bone formation about the shaft and metaphyses of cylindrical bones of the extremities, and a form of osteoarthritis. The disease is most often associated with pulmonary tumors, either carcinoma of the lung or pleural mesothelioma (Fig. 20–28). It also occurs with long-standing suppurative disease of the lung (i.e., bronchiectasis, abscess, empyema or tuberculosis), cyanotic congenital heart disease, chronic diarrheal gastrointestinal disease, or jaundice due to atresia of the bile ducts. Osteosarcoma

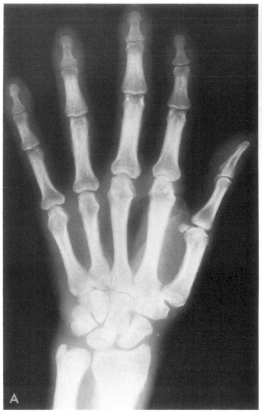

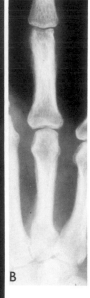

Figure 20–28. Hypertrophic pulmonary osteoarthropathy secondary to bronchogenic carcinoma. *A,* Periosteal new bone extends in a fine lace-like pattern around the diaphyses of the proximal phalanges, the metacarpals and the distal radius and ulna.

B, Detail of *A.*

metastatic to the lung can also incite the periosteal response (Fig. 20–29).

Clinically, the hand, wrist, foot and ankle joints are mildly stiff and painful. Indeed, the patient with a pulmonary neoplasm may initially complain of "arthritis" about the wrists or ankles. The condition uncommonly affects only one joint. Careful questioning will usually indicate that the patient has more joints involved than those of which he initially complained. On a rare occasion, the polyarthritis may be severe and accompanied by fever.[2]

A roentgenogram of the hand will show periosteal new bone about the metaphyses and diaphyses of the phalanges, metacarpals and distal radius and ulna. In fact, the entire radius and ulna and even the humerus may be involved. The feet, tibias and femurs may be similarly affected. The process begins as a thin, smooth layer of periosteum added to the diaphyseal and metaphyseal cortices. As the layer becomes thicker, it is often slightly rough and irregular, but with further progression the added new bone assumes a smooth, slightly lobulated configuration. A fine, lucent line is often discernible between the original and the added new bone. This line contains fibrous tissue from which the new bone is formed. Occasionally, actual marrow spicules may be present in this area. Soft tissue thickening about the tufts of the fingers may be visualized radiographically.

Microscopy of the bulbous enlargement of the tuft or tip of the finger shows only some hyperemia and edema, and a mild infiltration of lymphocytes and plasma cells. The bone of the distal phalanx is atrophic but the periosteum is normal.

The periosteum of the shafts of the involved bones lays on spicules perpendicular to the cortical surface and imbedded in a loose fibrous matrix. These spicules become incorporated in a parallel lamellae, and marrow tissue appears. Outside the

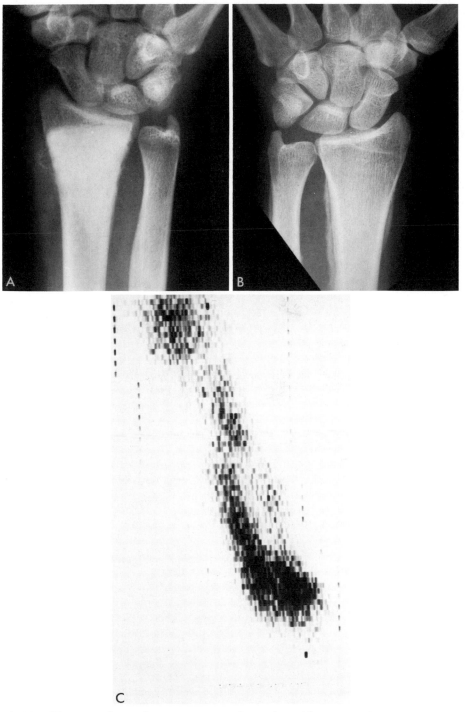

Figure 20-29. Hypertrophic pulmonary osteoarthropathy with metastatic osteosarcoma. *A,* There is a sclerotic primary osteosarcoma within and extending from the distal radius.

B, The patient had pain in the opposite wrist 1½ years after amputation of tumor-containing forearm. There is fine periosteal new bone around the diaphyses of the radius and ulna.

C, Fluorine-18 scan of radius shows activity in area of pulmonary osteoarthropathy. The patient also had hypertrophic osteoarthropathy in other bones and ossified pulmonary metastases.

medullary portion of the periosteal new bone, the cortex becomes progressively thickened.

The changes in the synovial membrane show vascular sclerosis and fibrosis very much like those of a mild villonodular synovitis. Fibrosis thickens the capsule, while the articular cartilage becomes degenerated, causing some narrowing. Far-advanced cases may develop changes similar to those of rheumatoid arthritis with eventual destruction of the cartilage and ankylosis.[1]

Removal of the inciting pulmonary tumor will reverse the symptoms within several days, while the bony manifestations resolve after several months.

REFERENCES

1. Aegerter, E., and Kirkpatrick, J. A.: *Orthopedic Diseases*. W. B. Saunders Company, Philadelphia, 1968.
2. Brunner, W.: Subacute Polyarthritis with Bronchogenic Carcinoma—A Paraneoplastic Syndrome. *Schweiz. Med. Wochenschr.*, 97:611–612, 1967.

Chapter 21

METABOLIC BONE DISEASE AND OTHER ABNORMALITIES OF THE HAND

OSTEOPOROSIS AND OSTEOPENIA

The terminology of the various conditions associated with loss or poor formation of bone is confusing. Precise definition of the terms is difficult. The term osteoporosis literally means porous bone and usually refers to a condition in which there is a less than normal amount of bone, and the bone that is present is qualitatively normal. Usually the term refers to postmenopausal osteoporosis. The term osteopenia means poor bone and is even less well defined. These two conditions differ from osteomalacia, in which osteoid is normally laid down but cannot be adequately calcified. The term bone loss has also been used for all these conditions. However, this is not an ideal term since the problem may not necessarily be a loss of bone but instead a lack of formation of adequate bone.

The number of causes of osteoporosis is great (Figs. 21–1 to 21–6). Perhaps the most common is the so-called postmenopausal or senile osteoporosis. A number of acquired conditions may be similar to osteoporosis. These include protein malnutrition, vitamin C deficiency (Fig. 21–3), endocrine disorders (Chapter 19),[3] disuse (Fig. 21–4), reflex neurovascular problems, and copper deficiency. A number of congenital conditions may be similar to osteoporosis. These include osteogenesis imperfecta (Chapter 13), many of the congenital malformation syndromes and in particular the chromosomal disorders. Various drugs can also cause osteoporosis.

RADIOLOGIC FINDINGS. The radiologic manifestations of bone loss or osteoporosis include changes in the cortex and in cancellous bone.

The cancellous changes include coarsening of some of the trabeculae, a decreased number of bony trabeculae and thinning of many of the trabeculae. The bone appears more lucent, and the cortex, although thin, stands out against the lucent cortex (Fig. 21–5). These changes are subjective and difficult to quantitate (Chapter 2). They may also be indistinguishable from changes due to normal aging.

The bony cortex is a much more useful part of the hand for evaluation of bone loss. As discussed in Chapter 2, the measurement of the second metacarpal at its midpoint is clinically useful, since much normative data are available for all ages and for various populations. By measuring the width of the bone at this location (T) and the width of the medullary space (M), it is possible to calculate the cortical thickness (C = T − M), the cortical area and the percentage of cortical area. With these measurements it is possible to determine whether bone has been lost or gained and whether this has occurred on the inside or the outside of the bone. This information may be of value in differentiating different types of bone loss, since various conditions lose bone in different ways (Table 21–1).

In senile osteoporosis, most of the bone loss occurs at the inner surface of the bone, while the overall thickness (T) may slightly increase in size with age. The medullary cavity enlargement results in a decrease in cortical thickness and in the percentage of cortical area. Different patterns of bone loss may occur in other conditions. For example, an overall bone loss may be due both to the decrease in bone formation (as manifested by a small outside diameter) and to the increase in bone resorption (as manifested by an increased medullary width). This situation exists in the XXXXY syndrome, in Turner syndrome and in juvenile trisomy 21 patients. Decreased bone formation is manifested by a decrease in the outside diameter and a decrease in bone loss as manifested by a decrease in medullary cavity size. This is seen in osteogenesis imperfecta, in adult trisomy 21 and in medullary stenosis of normal individuals. Increased bone formation together with increased bone loss is shown by a large outside diameter and a decrease in the medullary cavity. This is present in the XYY syndrome and in cerebral giantism and really is not a bone loss.

Although the various measurements of the cortex of the second metacarpal are useful parameters of bone mineralization and usually correlate well with results using

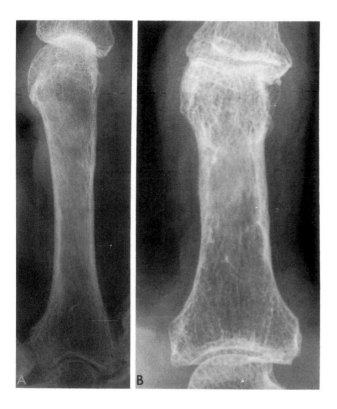

Figure 21–1. Osteoporosis in a 91 year old woman with hip fracture. *A,* In the second metacarpal, the cortex is extremely thin and the trabecular pattern is coarse.

B, In the fifth proximal phalanx the trabecular pattern is coarse.

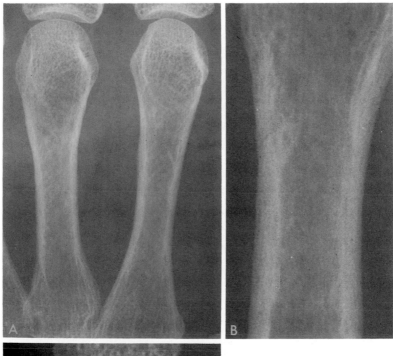

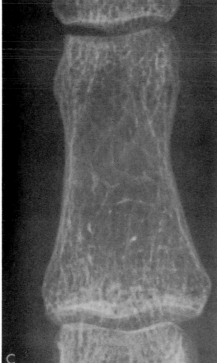

Figure 21-2. Postgastrectomy sprue in adult female. A, There is coarsening of the trabecular pattern. The bony cortex is thin, particularly on its inner aspect.

B, Close-up view of the metacarpal from A shows the permeative type of bone resorption to better advantage.

C, The coarse trabecular pattern is best seen in this film. This manifestation is probably a combination of both osteoporosis and osteomalacia.

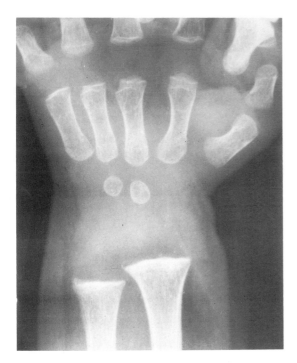

Figure 21–3. Scurvy. There is osteoporosis with a very thin bony cortex. The carpals have a rim of dense sclerosis, which is often present in this disorder. The osteoporosis is otherwise not different from that due to other causes.

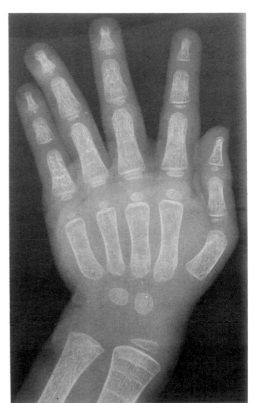

Figure 21–4. Osteoporosis of disuse. This $4^{3}/_{12}$ year old was quadriplegic. There is marked retardation of maturation and the cortex appears very thin.

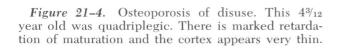

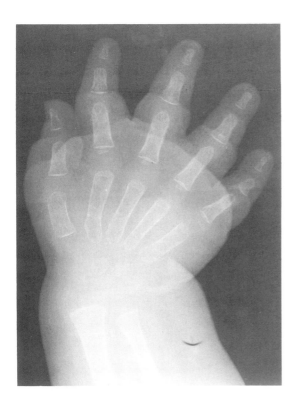

Figure 21–5. Atrophy of disuse. This is another example of a very thin bony cortex due to lack of motion.

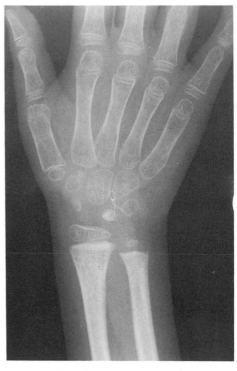

Figure 21–6. Bone demineralization associated with Volkmann contracture. This child had a supercondylar fracture with associated contracture. There is marked demineralization of the bones of the hand, while the radius and ulna are relatively well mineralized.

methods such as isotope absorptiometry, they do not necessarily reflect the state of bone loss within the rest of the skeleton, since some forms of bone loss affect mostly the spongy bone rather than the cortical bone. Also, in some conditions, i.e., thyrotoxicosis and immobilization, the bone loss is more permeative in type with lucent streaks seen within the cortex. In this type of bone loss, the cortical measurements are difficult to obtain since the limits of the cortex are poorly defined. Even when obtained, they will show relatively little change, although other methods suggest that the bone loss is great.

In spite of these limitations, the evaluation of the second metacarpal remains probably the most practical approach to the

TABLE 21–1. Comparison of Subperiosteal and Endosteal Surface Remodeling in Various Bone Conditions*

| ENDOSTEAL SURFACE | SUBPERIOSTEAL SURFACE APPOSITION | | |
	Reduced T	*Normal T*	*Increased T*
Below normal resorption or increased apposition (decreased M)	Normal medullary stenosis; juvenile osteogenesis imperfecta	—	Paget disease; osteopetrosis
Normal resorption	Adult trisomy G; some cases of adult osteogenesis imperfecta	Normal bone	—
Increased endosteal surface resorption (increased M)	XO; Noonan syndrome; XXXXY; juvenile 47 trisomy G; immobilization states; juvenile hypophosphatasia	Adult bone loss; post-castration loss; adult malabsorption states; vitamin D–resistant rickets; adult dialysis patients; acute protein-calorie malnutrition	XYY; juvenile cerebral giants; acromegaly; intestinal bypass

*From Garn, S. M., Poznanski, A. K., and Nagy, J. M.: Bone Measurement in the Differential Diagnosis of Osteopenia and Osteoporosis. *Radiology,* 100:509–518, 1971.

evaluation of bone mineralization. It does not require any specialized equipment or skill. A technician can be easily trained to perform these measurements. The measurements are easily reproduced and easily stored and transmitted, and they give relatively little radiation to the patient.

REFERENCES

1. Al-Rashid, R. A., and Spangler, J.: Neonatal Copper Deficiency. *N. Engl. J. Med.*, 285:841–843, 1971.
2. Dequeker, J.: *Bone Loss in Normal and Pathological Conditions.* Leuven University Press, Belgium, 1972.
3. Doyle, F. H.: Radiologic Assessment of Endocrine Effects on Bone. *Radiol. Clin. North Am.*, 5:289–302, 1967.
4. Frost, H. M.: Postmenopausal Osteoporosis: The Evolution of our Concepts of its Cause. *Henry Ford Hosp. Med. J.*, 20:83–90, 1972.
5. Garn, S. M.: The Earlier Gain and the Later Loss of Cortical Bone. In Nutritional Perspective. Charles C Thomas, Publisher, Springfield, Illinois, 1970.
6. Garn, S. M.: The Course of Bone Gain and the Phases of Bone Loss. *Orthop. Clin. North Am.*, 3:503–520, 1972.
7. Garn, S. M., and Poznanski, A. K.: Transient and Irreversible Bone Losses. *In:* Barzel, U. S. (Ed.): *Osteoporosis.* Grune & Stratton, Inc., New York, 1970.
8. Garn, S. M., Poznanski, A. K., and Nagy, J. M.: Bone Measurement in the Differential Diagnosis of Osteopenia and Osteoporosis. *Radiology*, 100:509–518, 1971.
9. Karpel, J. T., and Peden, V. H.: Copper Deficiency in Long-Term Parenteral Nutrition. *J. Pediatr.*, 80:32–36, 1972.
10. Smith, D. A., Anderson, J. B., Shimmins, J., Speirs, C. F., and Barnett, E.: Changes in Metacarpal Mineral Content and Density in Normal Male and Female Subjects with Age. *Clin. Radiol.*, 20:23–32, 1969.
11. Smith, R. W., Jr., Eyler, W. R., and Mellinger, R. C.: On the Incidence of Senile Osteoporosis. *Ann. Intern. Med.*, 52:773–781, 1960.
12. Steinbach, H. L.: The Roentgen Appearance of Osteoporosis. *Radiol. Clin. North Am.*, 2: 191–207, 1964.

RICKETS AND OSTEOMALACIA

These two conditions are simply the child and adult forms of the same disorder. The adult form is called osteomalacia and in the hand is radiographically indistinguishable from osteoporosis. In the child, however, when new bone is still being laid down, the appearance is that of rickets, which can be easily distinguished radiologically from osteoporosis.

The causes of rickets are many. It may be dietary, due to lack of vitamin D or poor absorption of vitamin D and calcium. Dietary lack of vitamin D is rare in the United States because of the widespread vitamin supplementation of milk. Dietary rickets may, however, occur in the premature infant receiving a vitamin D–enriched formula, since the infant does not consume enough of the formula to get an adequate amount of vitamin D, and his requirement for the vitamin is the same as that of a term infant.[5]

There are a number of renal causes of rickets. The term "renal rickets" is unsatisfactory; it does not differentiate among the various types and probably should be dropped. Renal failure with an elevated B.U.N. level can result in renal osteodystrophy, a significant component of which is rickets. Renal tubular acidosis can also be associated with rickets. Tubular defects in the kidneys may result in vitamin D–resistant rickets (phosphate diabetes, hypophosphatemic rickets). Vitamin D–dependent rickets is another condition resulting from relative insensitivity of the body to vitamin D.[1, 8] Children with this type of rickets may be treated by a moderate increase in vitamin D lower than that required in vitamin D–resistant rickets. Rickets may also be secondary to anticonvulsant therapy, particularly to the use of Dilantin.

RADIOLOGIC FINDINGS. The radiologic appearance in all of the various forms of rickets is basically the same. The findings are due to a lack of calcification of osteoid, which is still being laid down. The result is an increased width of the epiphyseal space with irregularity and cupping of the end of the metaphysis (Fig. 21–7). In the shaft a similar process occurs, with uncalcified bone along the outer shaft. This results in a poorly defined radiolucent cortex which often has streaks of permeative type demineralization. In severe cases the shadow cast by the bone is barely detectable on the film (Fig. 21–8). Demineralization of a shaft causes it to become weaker and more prone to fracture, although fractures are less common in the hand than in the long bones.

During the phases of healing, the region

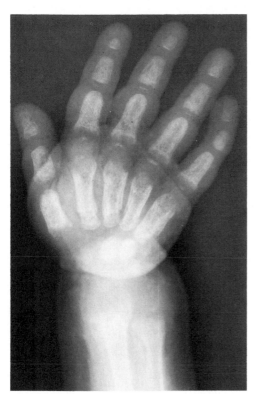

Figure 21-7. Refractory rickets. Severe. This is a classic appearance of rickets, with widening of the epiphyseal plates, cupping of the metaphyses and permeative radiolucency throughout the bones. There is some widening of the metacarpal shaft. This is due to calcification of periosteum and is a manifestation of healing. The epiphyses are markedly irregular.

between the proliferating cartilage and the ossified metaphysis becomes rapidly calcified. The calcification often starts at the edge of the epiphyseal plate and may produce a dense line with a lucency between it and the remainder of the metaphysis (Fig. 21-10). A similar phenomenon in the shaft of the bone can give an appearance of periosteal elevation in the shaft (Fig. 21-9).

All of the manifestations of rickets are less prominent in the hand than in the distal radius and the femora.

Another radiologic feature of rickets is an apparent retardation of skeletal maturation. This is due to failure of the epiphyses to ossify. During therapy a remarkably rapid recovery may be seen. A rare phenomenon in rickets is asymmetry of the findings; the cause is not known (Fig. 21-14).

The cause of rickets cannot be determined by radiologic appearance alone, since the basic pathologic process is the same in all cases. The age of the patient, however, is a useful factor in differentiating among the various types. Rickets occurring in premature infants (Fig. 21-12) is usually due to inadequate intake of vitamin D. In older infants the various forms are indistinguishable, but they can be distinguished by their response to treatment with vitamin D. Patients with vitamin D deficiency respond rapidly to doses of vitamin D only slightly higher than the daily requirement. Vitamin D–resistant rickets, on the other hand, will require much higher doses of vitamin D (above 50,000 units) and may respond poorly even to this dose. Vitamin D–dependent rickets responds completely to dosages intermediate between those of vitamin D–deficiency rickets and vitamin D–resistant rickets.

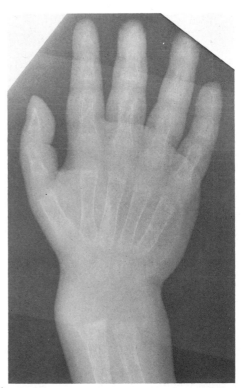

Figure 21-8. Extremely severe rickets. Type unknown. Although this boy has been on anticoagulants, his rickets required a large dose of vitamin D before it responded. This most likely represents a vitamin D–dependent rickets. The bone is barely visualized on the radiograph and has a frayed, irregular appearance.

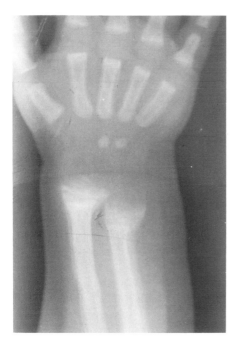

Figure 21-9. Vitamin D—dependent rickets with some healing. Severe rachitic changes are more noticeable in the radius and ulna than in the metacarpals. There is some periosteal cloaking both of the metacarpals and of the radius and ulna, which is evidence of healing. There is evidence of a fracture of the forearm.

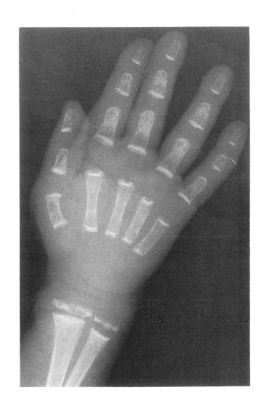

Figure 21-10. Healing rickets of prematurity. This infant did not receive supplemental vitamin D for about six weeks after birth. He showed extremely rapid healing on small doses of vitamin D, resulting in band-like densities at the end of each bone.

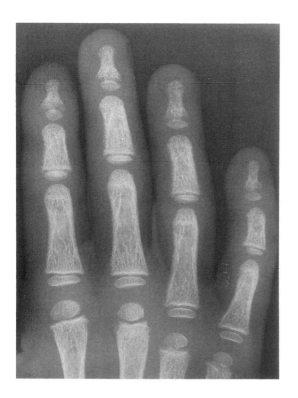

Figure 21-11. Renal osteodystrophy with rachitic changes. There is widening of the epiphyseal plates of the distal phalanges. Subperiosteal resorption, a manifestation of hyperparathyroidism, is noted.

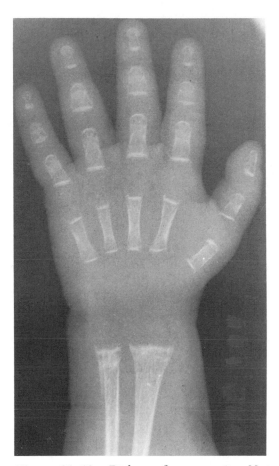

Figure 21–12. Rickets of prematurity. Note the cupped metaphyses. The infant had low vitamin D intake. In these conditions, one is never certain whether the patient actually has rickets or is developing the so-called premature bone disease of infancy.

In the older child, chronic renal disease is probably the most common cause of rickets seen in children's hospitals today (Fig. 21–11). This type of rickets, however, is not a diagnostic problem, since the renal failure is usually obvious. In older children without uremia, the main cause of rickets is the vitamin D–resistant form (hypophosphatemic rickets).

The rickets seen in renal osteodystrophy due to chronic renal disease is often associated with secondary hyperparathyroidism. This is discussed in Chapter 19. The severity of the rickets in renal osteodystrophy ranges from minimal to severe and seems unrelated to the severity of the secondary hyperparathyroidism. The radiologic appearance of the rickets is similar to that from other causes, except that there is a greater tendency for fracture across the epiphysis. Although this phenomenon is more commonly seen in the region of the femoral epiphysis, it can occur in some of the epiphyses in the hand. Other radiologic findings in renal osteodystrophy include bone sclerosis, dense epiphyses and soft tissue calcification.

Small stature is commonly associated with rickets, particularly in the familial hypophosphatemic or vitamin D–resistant type. This decrease in stature is most often limited to the lower extremities; the diminution in size of the hands is usually not striking.

The differential diagnosis of rickets is limited to two conditions. The first is hypophosphatasia, a familial disorder of alkaline

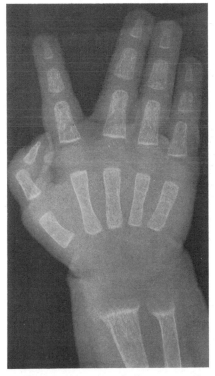

Figure 21–13. Copper deficiency with ricket-like changes. This infant had a massive bowel resection and developed copper deficiency because of long-term intravenous alimentation without copper supplementation. The ricket-like changes are seen mainly in the distal radius and ulna and, to a lesser degree, in the other bones. The picture of copper deficiency has some of the characteristics of both rickets and osteoporosis.

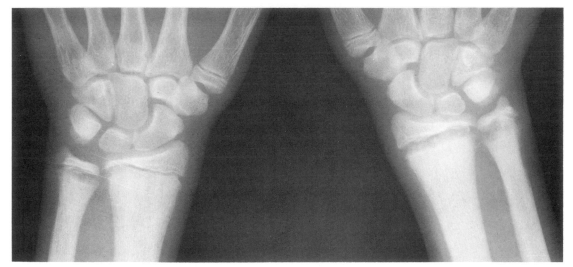

Figure 21–14. Asymmetric rickets in renal osteodystrophy. There is marked asymmetry of the rachitic changes in the radius and ulna. The reason for this asymmetry is unknown.

phosphatase which in some ways is a type of rickets (Chapter 13). The other condition that can have similar radiologic findings is metaphyseal dysostosis. This may be difficult to differentiate from some of the forms of the vitamin D–resistant rickets, particularly when the metaphyseal dysostosis is mild, as in the Schmidt type (Chapter 13). Differences in the blood chemistry may be useful to separate these two conditions; however, this is not an entirely valid method since a biochemical disturbance may exist in some patients with the Jansen type of metaphyseal dysostosis.

REFERENCES

1. Arnaud, C., Kaijer, R., Reade, T., Scriver, C. R., and Whelan, D. T.: Vitamin D Dependency: An Inherited Postnatal Syndrome with Secondary Hyperparathyroidism. *Pediatrics,* 46: 871–880, 1970.
2. Arnstein, A. R., and Frame, B.: Primary Hypophosphatemic Rickets and Osteomalacia: A Review. *Clin. Orthop.,* 49:109–118, 1966.
3. Borgstedt, A. D., Bryson, M. F., Young, L. W., and Forbes, G. B.: Long-Term Administration of Antiepileptic Drugs and the Development of Rickets. *J. Pediatr.,* 81:9–15, 1972.
4. Caffey, J.: *Pediatric X-Ray Diagnosis,* 6th Ed. Year Book Medical Publishers, Chicago, 1972, Vol. 2.
5. Lewin, P. K., Reid, M., Reilly, B. J., Swyer, P. R., and Fraser, D.: Iatrogenic Rickets in Low-Birth-Weight Infants. *J. Pediatr.,* 78:207–210, 1971.
6. Lussier-Lazaroff, J., and Fletcher, B. D.: Rickets and Anticonvulsant Therapy in Children: A Roentgenologic Investigation. *J. Can. Assoc. Radiol.,* 22:144–147, 1971.
7. McNair, S. L., and Stickler, G. B.: Growth in Familial Hypophosphatemic Vitamin-D-Resistant Rickets. *N. Engl. J. Med.,* 281:511–516, 1969.
8. Scriver, C. R.: Vitamin D Dependency. *Pediatrics,* 45:361–363, 1970.
9. Steinbach, H. L., and Noetzli, M.: Roentgen Appearance of the Skeleton in Osteomalacia and Rickets. *Am. J. Roentgenol.,* 91:955–972, 1964.
10. Weller, M., Edeiken, J., and Hodes, P. J.: Renal Osteodystrophy. *Am. J. Roentgenol.,* 104: 354–363, 1968.

FIBROGENESIS IMPERFECTA

This is an extremely rare condition which is due to an abnormality in collagen of bone. Histologically there is a marked reduction in the birefringence normally seen in collagen fibers of bone when examined with the polarizing microscope. There is a marked increase in the number of osteoid seams and a reduced bone appositional rate characteristic of osteomalacia.[1] The disease is associated with skeletal pain, tenderness and occasionally fractures.

RADIOLOGIC FINDINGS. The radiologic findings are characteristic and include widening of the bones in their outer diameter with a relatively thin cortex; and a markedly coarsened trabecular pattern, giving the appearance of increased bone density (Fig. 21–15) in spite of the fact that histologically there is osteomalacia. All the hand bones are usually involved, and similar findings may be seen in the remainder of the skeleton. The main entities in the differential diagnosis are Paget disease and hyperphosphatasia.

REFERENCES

1. Baker, S. L., Dent, C. E., Friedman, M., and Watson, L.: Fibrogenesis Imperfecta Ossium. *J. Bone Joint Surg.*, 48B:804–825, 1966.
2. Frame, B., Frost, H. M., Pak, C. Y., Reynolds W., and Argen, R. J.: Fibrogenesis Imperfecta Ossium. *N. Engl. J. Med.*, 285:769–772, 1971.
3. Thomas, W. C., and Moore, T. H.: Fibrogenesis Imperfecta Ossium. *Trans. Am. Clin. Climatol. Assoc.*, 80:54–62, 1968.

ACCIDENTAL EXPOSURE TO VARIOUS SUBSTANCES

Excess amounts of certain chemical substances can cause radiologic changes in the hand. These include the vitamins A and D and a number of substances which are normally not present in the diet, such as lead, phosphorous, bismuth and fluorine. Exposure to certain chemicals can also cause a chemical acroosteolysis.

HYPERVITAMINOSIS A

Excess vitamin A can produce acute or chronic symptoms. The acute symptoms are due to a single large ingestion and produce no radiologic changes. Chronic ingestion produces tender, firmly fixed swellings over

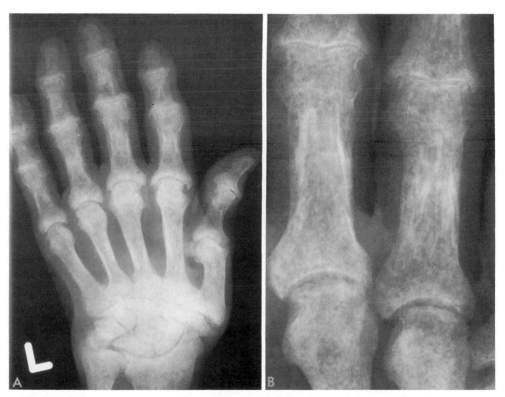

Figure 21–15. Fibrogenesis imperfecta osseum. Left hand in a 51 year old male.

A, There is widening of the phalanges with a bizarre, coarse trabecular pattern. Extensive degenerative changes are seen about the fingers, and there is a flattening and deformity of the carpal bones.

B, Close-up view of the proximal phalanges shows the coarsening of the trabecular pattern and the area of increased sclerosis.

(Courtesy Dr. W. Reynolds and Dr. B. Frame, Henry Ford Hospital, Detroit, Michigan. Reproduced with permission from *N. Engl. J. Med.*, 285:769–772, 1971.)

the bone associated with irritability of the child.

The main radiologic finding of chronic vitamin A poisoning is evidence of cortical hyperostosis, which most commonly occurs in the ulna and metatarsals and rarely involves the hand; Caffey's classic paper on this subject described seven patients in whom the metacarpals were only rarely involved. Most cases of vitamin A poisoning are seen in children, although Frame et al.[2] have seen a teen-aged boy with extensive bizarre periosteal changes involving the metacarpals, as well as some adults without roentgen manifestations. Periosteal elevation in their patient was quite marked, with the periosteum appearing as rounded protuberances from the bone. In animals, Wolbach[4] found damage to the epiphyseal plate with focal areas of premature closure. Pease[3] described similar findings in children's lower extremities with resultant shortening of the limbs. It is conceivable that brachydactyly could be caused in this way.

REFERENCES

1. Caffey, J.: Chronic Poisoning Due to Excess of Vitamin A. *Am. J. Roentgenol.*, 65:12–26, 1951.
2. Frame, B., Jackson, C. E., Reynolds, W., and Umphney, J. E.: Hypercalcemia and Skeletal Effects in Chronic Hypervitaminosis A. *Ann. Int. Med.*, January, 1974, in press.
3. Pease, C. N.: Focal Retardation and Arrestment of Growth of Bones due to Vitamin A Intoxication. *J.A.M.A.*, 182:980–985, 1962.
4. Wolbach, S. B.: Vitamin-A Deficiency and Excess in Relation to Skeletal Growth. *J. Bone Joint Surg.*, 29:171–192, 1947.

HYPERVITAMINOSIS D

Excess intake of vitamin D may be associated with both clinical and radiologic signs and symptoms. In childhood, doses of 50,000 units per day can be toxic. The toxic dose in adults may be higher. There may be some relationship between hypervitaminosis D in a mother and the hypercalcemia of infancy;[3] the manifestations of hypercalcemia of infancy are similar to those of vitamin D poisoning (Chapter 13).

It is often difficult to be certain that the toxic symptoms are due entirely to vitamin D and not due to associated vitamin A or possibly fluorine.

RADIOLOGIC FINDINGS. In the child there are increased bands of density with thickening of the cortex (Figs. 21–16 A and 21–17).[2] Rarefaction of bone has also been

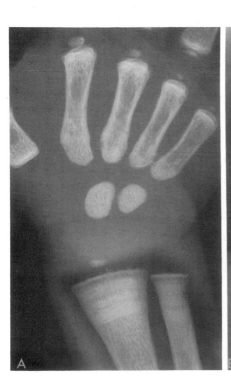
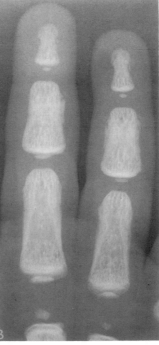

Figure 21–16. Hypervitaminosis D. This two year old male was treated with 50,000 units of vitamin D per day for 1½ years for physiologic bowing of the legs.

A, There are zones of sclerosis in the radius and ulna and in the metacarpals. The cortex of the metacarpals appears thick.

B, The cause of periosteal changes about the phalanges is not clear. They do not have the appearance of renal osteodystrophy, and the boy did not receive toxic levels of either fluorine or vitamin A.

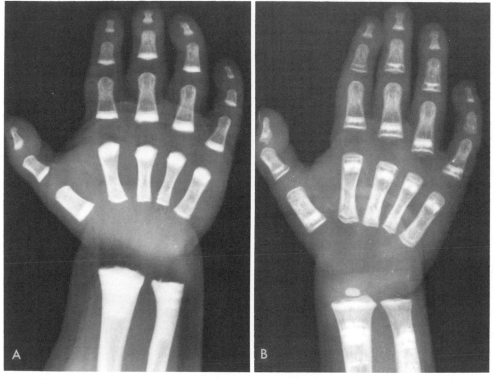

Figure 21–17. Hypervitaminosis D in a 4 year old cretin. *A,* Dense lines are seen at the ends of the bones.

B, Seven months after institution of thyroid therapy, the dense lines have moved significantly down the shafts of the bones. No radiologic abnormality was seen 23 years later.

reported, as has periosteal thickening (Fig. 21–16 *B*).[4] In the adult there may be areas of metastatic calcification in blood vessels in both the extremities and the viscera. Periarticular calcification has been seen also, but this occurs mainly in patients who have been treated for rheumatoid arthritis and may be related to this disease. A generalized osteoporosis has also been described. Another radiologic finding of vitamin D poisoning is calcification of the falx cerebri.

REFERENCES

1. Christensen, W. R., Liebman, C., and Sosman, M. C.: Skeletal and Periarticular Manifestations of Hypervitaminosis D. *Am. J. Roentgenol.,* 65:27–41, 1951.
2. DeWind, L. T.: Hypervitaminosis D with Osteosclerosis. *Arch. Dis. Child.,* 36:373–380, 1961.
3. Lowe, C. U., Coursin, D. B., Heald, F. P., Holliday, M. A., O'Brien, D., Owen, G. M., Pearson, H. A., Scriver, C. R., Filer, L. J., Jr., and Kline, O. L.: The Relation Between Infantile Hypercalcemia and Vitamin D – Public Health Implications in North America. *Pediatrics,* 40:1050–1061, 1967.
4. Ross, S. G.: Vitamin D Intoxication in Infancy. A Report of Four Cases. *J. Pediatr.,* 41:815–822, 1952.

FLUOROSIS

This condition has different manifestations, depending on the source of the fluoride. Endemic skeletal fluorosis has been seen in certain parts of India as well as other countries where there is a high fluoride level in the drinking water. This condition affects both adults and children.[2] The radiologic findings in the hand include a combination of osteosclerosis and osteoporosis, with a thick cortical margin and coarse trabeculae within bone (Fig. 21–18).

Soriano and Manchón[1] described a somewhat different manifestation of fluorosis due to habitual drinking of wine containing fluorine in Spain. They felt that the

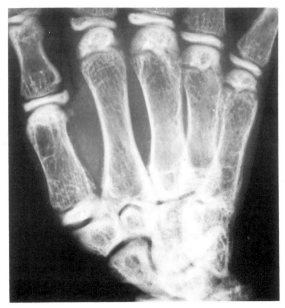

Figure 21-18. Endemic fluorosis. This individual lived in an area in which the water had a high content of fluoride. The bones are dense with marked cortical thickening, particularly in the carpals. There is some coarsening of the trabeculae. (Courtesy Dr. M. Teotia, Lucknow, India.)

radiologic findings in this type of fluorosis were pathognomonic: a bizarre phalangeal periostitis, which was very localized to certain phalanges and which spared other phalanges. The periosteum was irregular and in some places was as wide as the bony shaft. Other changes described were condensing osteitis with porotic and malacic aspects.

REFERENCES

1. Soriano, M., and Manchón, F.: Radiological Aspects of a New Type of Bone Fluorosis, Periostitis Deformans. *Radiology*, 87:1089–1094, 1966.
2. Teotia, M., Teotia, S. P. S., and Kunwar, K. B.: Endemic Skeletal Fluorosis. *Arch. Dis. Child.*, 46:686–691, 1971.

LEAD INTOXICATION

Chronic lead intoxication may result in radiologic findings. These include zones of increased bone density at the ends of the bones, mainly affecting the knees. The hands are much less frequently involved. The increased bone density is probably due to the laying down of calcium rather than lead. The amount of lead measured within bone is so small that it would most likely not cast a shadow. Radiology plays a very small role in the evaluation of lead poisoning, since in most cases the lead lines are indistinguishable from the normally dense ends of the metaphyses. Sometimes several episodes of lead poisoning have occurred, resulting in multiple lead lines separated by lucent areas. Another manifestation of lead poisoning may be some failure of modeling of the bones, which is particularly noticeable in the femora.

REFERENCES

1. Leone, A. J., Jr.: On Lead Lines. *Am. J. Roentgenol.*, 103:165–167, 1968.
2. Pease, C. N., and Newton, G. G.: Metaphyseal Dysplasia Due to Lead Poisoning in Children. *Radiology*, 79:233–240, 1962.

POISONING FROM INGESTION OF OTHER SUBSTANCES

Phosphorus poisoning can cause dense metaphyseal lines but is rarely seen today. Bismuth poisoning can also cause dense bone lines, as can other heavy metals.

REFERENCE

1. Edeiken, J., and Hodes, P. J.: *Roentgen Diagnosis of Diseases of Bone.* The Williams & Wilkins Co., Baltimore, 1967.

OCCUPATIONAL ACROOSTEOLYSIS

This disorder is seen in workers involved in the polyvinylchloride polymerization process. It occurs in the hand cleaning of the polymerizers. The clinical findings are those of Raynaud phenomenon, which antecedes the osteolytic lesions. Radiologic findings include erosion of the tips of the tufts (Fig. 21–19 A). There is often a lucent band between the tip of the tuft and the remainder of the phalanx (Fig. 21–19 B). With removal from exposure to the causative chemicals, there is ultimate healing which may result in shortening and widening of the distal phalanges (Fig. 21–19 C). The differential diagnosis of the tuft findings includes both congenital and ac-

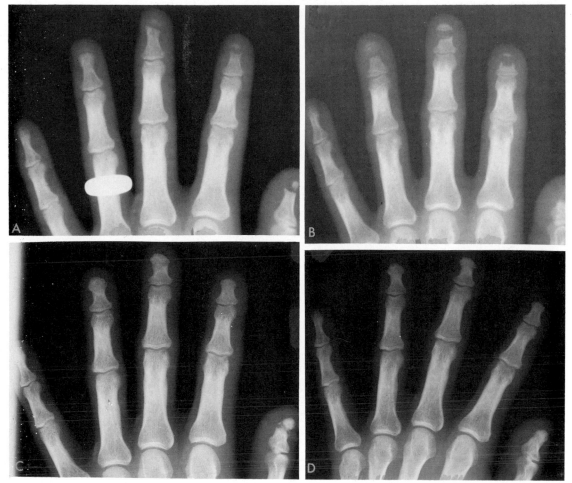

Figure 21–19. Occupational acroosteolysis. This is an adult male who was employed in a polyvinylchloride polymerization process.
A through *D*, Films over a four year interval. The earliest film shows tuft erosions. Subsequently there is some regeneration of the tuft with resultant shortening of the distal phalanges.

quired conditions. Among the congenital conditions are familial acroosteolysis (Cheney syndrome), progeria and pycnodysostosis. These are further discussed in Chapter 13. Acquired conditions include Raynaud disease, scleroderma and various neurotropic conditions such as leprosy and syringomyelia.

REFERENCES

1. Cook, W. A., Giever, P. M., Dinman, B. D., and Magnuson, H. J.: Occupational Acroosteolysis. II. An Industrial Hygiene Study. *Arch. Environ. Health*, 22:74–82, 1971.
2. Dinman, B. D., Cook, W. A., Whitehouse, W. M., Magnuson, H. J., and Ditcheck, T.: Occupa-
tional Acroosteolysis. I. An Epidemiological Study. *Arch. Environ. Health*, 22:61–73, 1971.
3. Dodson, V. N., Dinman, B. D., Whitehouse, W. M., Nasr, A. N., and Magnuson, H. J.: Occupational Acroosteolysis. III. A Clinical Study. *Arch. Environ. Health*, 22:83–91, 1971.
4. Markowitz, S. S., McDonald, C. J., Fethiere, W., and Kerzner, M. S.: Occupational Acroosteolysis. *Arch. Derm.*, 106:219–223, 1972.
5. Wilson, R. H., McCormick, W. E., Tatum, C. F., and Creech, J. L.: Occupational Acroosteolysis. *J.A.M.A.*, 201:577–581, 1967.

SOFT TISSUE CALCIFICATION

Calcification may occur in any of the soft tissues of the hand and may be due to many different etiologic agents. The terminology

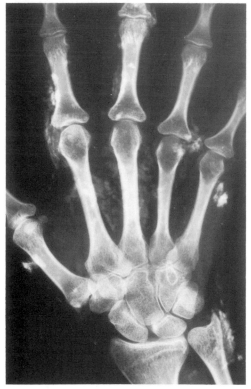

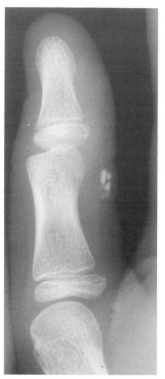

Figure 21–20. There is extensive soft tissue calcification in a patient with dermatomyositis.

Figure 21–21. Minimal calcification in the finger of a patient with burned-out dermatomyositis. The other calcifications in the body were also decreasing at this time.

used for soft tissue calcification is often confusing. Terms like "calcinosis universalis," "calcinosis cutis" and "osteoma cutis" are descriptive terms rather than specific pathologic entities. Often the cause of calcification is not clear from the radiograph (Fig. 21–22). Calcification may simply be an end stage of a previous disease, particularly dermatomyositis (Figs. 21–20 and 21–21). Scleroderma (Fig. 21–23), which is further described in Chapter 20, can produce diffuse calcification or may involve simply the region of the fingertips. Other conditions that may be associated with definite soft tissue calcification include idiopathic hypercalcemia (Fig. 21–24), hypervitaminosis D, hyperparathyroidism and hypoparathyroidism (Chapter 19). Extravasation of calcium gluconate infusion will cause the deposition of calcium in the soft tissues within a few days of the injection (Fig. 21–25).

Extensive large foci of calcification may be the result of chronic renal disease, particularly in patients undergoing hemo-

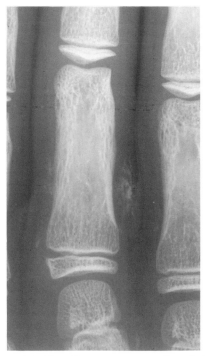

Figure 21–22. Osteoma cutis. This child had multiple areas of calcification. The cause was unknown.

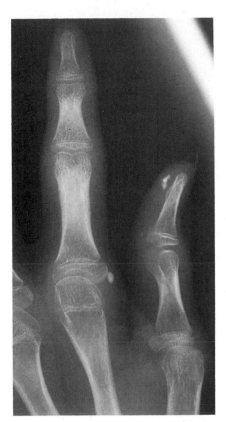

Figure 21-23. Scleroderma. Some soft tissue calcification is seen in the tips of the fingers.

seen in any patient with arteriosclerosis and is particularly common in diabetes mellitus (Fig. 21–27). It may be seen in other conditions, particularly vitamin D toxicity and hyperparathyroidism. Arterial calcification is also sometimes seen after extravasation of calcium gluconate injection (Fig. 21–25).[2]

Calcified phleboliths may be seen in the hand associated with hemangiomas (Chapter 15). Tumor calcification may also be seen in a variety of soft tissue tumors, particularly periarticular chondromas and synoviomas.

Parasites are a rare cause of soft tissue calcification in the United States but can be seen in other parts of the world (Chapter 14).

A number of skin disorders may also be associated with skin calcification. Bizarre calcium collections can be seen in benign proliferative skin lesions.[5] The calcified

dialysis.[7] The entity of tumoral calcinosis may have associated changes in the hand; its etiology is not clear.

Calcification within and around joints is further described in Chapter 20. These calcifications may be within joint cartilage, as in the pseudogout syndrome and degenerative arthritis; it may be within the joint space itself, as in osteochondromatosis and lipocalcinogranulomatosis; or it may be periarticular, as in tuberculosis (Chapter 14). Joint calcification may also be present in many of the generalized causes of calcification previously described.

Calcification in the ligaments in the region of the wrist may be posttraumatic in origin, and when it occurs in an area of little space, as in the region of the carpal tunnel, it can interfere with the structures running through it. Trauma to other structures may also result in calcification (Fig. 21–26).

Arterial calcification in the hand may be

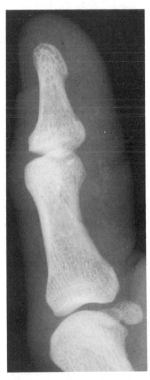

Figure 21-24. Idiopathic hypercalcemia. This patient had hypercalcemia of infancy and was originally reported in the *Am. J. Med.*, 26:9–36, 1959.

On follow-up radiographs as an adult, there is some soft tissue calcification remaining in the fingers. (Courtesy Dr. R. Hall, Detroit, Michigan.)

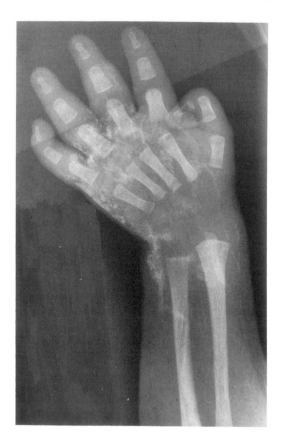

Figure 21–25. Calcification in soft tissue resulting from extravasation of calcium gluconate. The calcification was located on the dorsum of the hand. There was associated soft tissue necrosis. Arterial calcification in the forearm is also present.

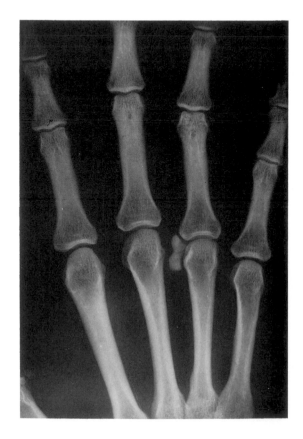

Figure 21–26. Traumatic calcification. This young man sustained trauma to his hand eight weeks previously while playing football. At biopsy there was only calcification in the collateral ligament. (Courtesy Dr. D. Louis, Ann Arbor, Michigan.)

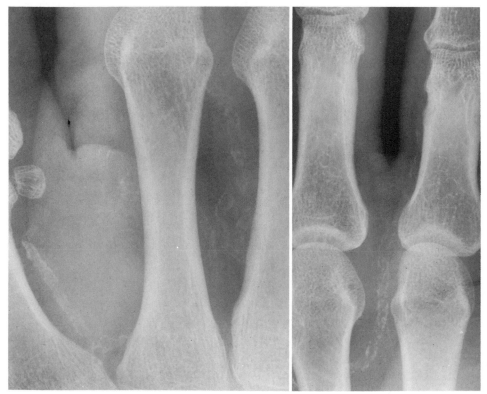

Figure 21-27. Diabetic with extensive arterial calcification. The patient had longstanding diabetes mellitus.

mass in some of these patients is several times larger than the bones of the hand. A clinical presentation in these patients is that of hyperkeratosis and verrucae of the so-called mutilating type.

REFERENCES

1. Baldursson, H., Evans, E. B., Dodge, W. F., and Jackson, W. T.: Tumoral Calcinosis with Hyperphosphatemia. A Report of a Family with Incidence in Four Siblings. *J. Bone Joint Surg.*, 51A:913–925, 1969.
2. Berger, P. E., Heidelberger, K. P., and Poznanski, A. K.: Extravasation of Calcium Gluconate as a Cause of Soft Tissue Calcification in Infancy, in press.
3. Collard, M.: Une Forme Familiale de Lipocalci-granulomatose Avec Calcinose Arterielle. *J. Radiol. Electrol. Med. Nucl.*, 47:31–40, 1966.
4. Dodds, W. J., and Steinbach, H. L.: Triangular Cartilage Calcification in the Wrists: Its Incidence in Elderly Persons. *Am. J. Roentgenol.*, 105:850–852, 1969.
5. Greenfield, G. B., Rosado, W., and Rothbart, F.: Benign Proliferative Skin Lesions Causing Destructive and Resorptive Bone Changes. *Am. J. Roentgenol.*, 97:733–735, 1966.
6. Harkess, J. W., and Peters, H. J.: Tumoral Calci-

nosis. A Report of Six Cases. *J. Bone Joint Surg.*, 49A:721–731, 1967.
7. Johnson, C., Graham, C. B., and Curtis, F. K.: Roentgenographic Manifestations of Chronic Renal Disease Treated by Periodic Hemodialysis. *Am. J. Roentgenol.*, 101:915–926, 1967.
8. Maclean, G. D., Main, R. A., Anderson, T. E., and Best, P. V.: Connective Tissue Ossification Presenting in the Skin. *Arch. Derm.*, 94:168–174, 1966.
9. Palmer, P. E. S.: Tumoural Calcinosis. *Br. J. Radiol.*, 39:518–525, 1966.
10. Sutro, C. J.: Carpal Tunnel Syndrome Caused by Calcification in the Deep or Volar Radio-Carpal Ligament. *New York Hospital for Joint Diseases*, 30:23–27, 1969.
11. Whiting, D. A., Simson, I. W., and Dannheimer, I. P. L.: Unusual Cutaneous Lesions in Tumoral Calcinosis. *Arch. Derm.*, 102:465–473, 1970.

PAGET DISEASE (OSTEITIS DEFORMANS)

This is a well-known condition in other bones, but it is very seldom seen in the hand. Its origin is unknown. Most series of Paget disease do not describe hand in-

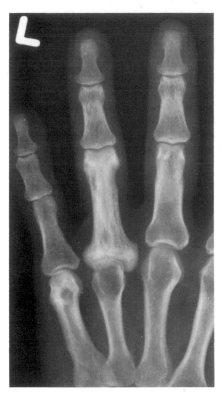

Figure 21-28. Paget disease. There are typical pagetoid changes in the fourth proximal phalanx and, to a lesser degree, in the fifth metacarpal. Note widening of the affected bones with coarsening of the trabeculae. (Courtesy Dr. D. Wilner and Dr. R. S. Sherman. From *Medical Radiography and Photography*, published by Radiography Markets Division, Eastman Kodak Company.)

volvement;[2] however, individual cases have been seen by various authors.[1, 3]

The radiologic findings in the reported cases of Paget disease have been mainly those of the sclerotic form with cortical thickening and widening of the bone (Fig. 21-28). However, so few cases of the lytic type have been reported that it is uncertain how often this form occurs. In some cases with lucent changes (Fig. 21-29), the diagnosis is uncertain unless extensive pagetoid changes are seen in the remainder of the skeleton.

REFERENCES

1. Haverbush, T. J., Wilde, A. H., and Phalen, G. S.: The Hand in Paget's Disease of Bone. Report of Two Cases. *J. Bone Joint Surg.*, 54A:173–175, 1972.
2. Steinbach, H. L.: Some Roentgen Features of Paget's Disease. *Am. J. Roentgenol.*, 86:950–964, 1961.
3. Wilner, D., and Sherman, R. S.: Roentgen Diagnosis of Paget's Disease (Osteitis Deformans). The Usual – The Unusual – The Complications. *Med. Radiogr. Photogr.*, 42:35–78, 1966.

SARCOIDOSIS

Skeletal manifestations of sarcoidosis are not common. The incidence of bony change is different in various series. In the cases of Holt and Owens,[2] 16.9 per cent had bone involvement. The bone changes are predominantly in the hand and involve the middle and distal phalanges. Other bones of the hand, the foot and other portions of the skeleton can also be involved.

Several types of osseous lesions may be seen in sarcoidosis. The most common type is the diffuse change in which there is widening of the medullary portion of bone with a honeycomb or lattice-work configuration (Fig. 21-30). The periosteum is usually

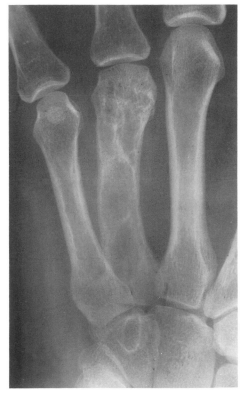

Figure 21-29. Paget disease. Lucent phase. There are areas of radiolucencies in the fourth metacarpal. There is widening of the shaft of the bone. This patient had extensive pagetoid changes in the remainder of the skeleton. (Courtesy Dr. M. Clark, Henry Ford Hospital, Detroit, Michigan.)

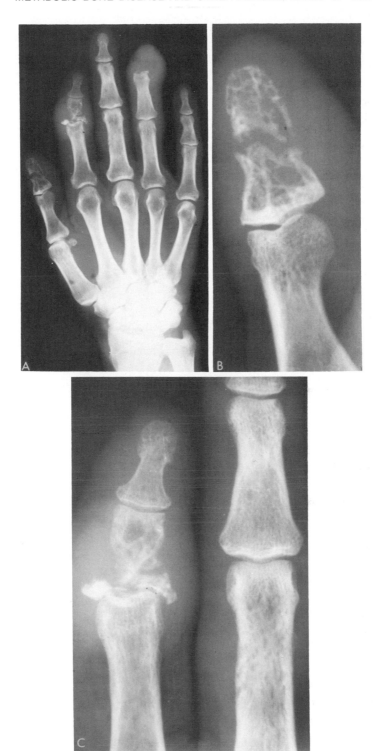

Figure 21–30. Sarcoidosis in an adult male. Extensive destructive changes. *A,* The distal phalanx of the fourth finger is completely destroyed. The lack of periosteal elevation is typical of sarcoidosis.

B, Close-up view of the distal phalanx of the thumb shows a honeycomb-like structure of the trabeculae with a fracture through it.

C, Destruction and secondary sclerosis is seen in the middle phalanx of the index finger.

(Courtesy Dr. J. F. Holt. Reproduced with permission from *Radiology,* 53:11–30, 1949.)

not affected, although periosteal elevation may occasionally be seen. The lack of periosteal involvement is a helpful sign in the diagnosis of sarcoidosis. Another type of lesion occurs when several of the lucent areas coalesce and form more localized, cyst-like vacuoles (Fig. 21–31). These well-defined radiolucencies are less common, and when associated with healing they may have a sclerotic margin. A third type of lesion occurs with marked mutilation and destruction of the ends of the bone (Fig. 21–30). In some patients the bone may completely disappear; in others there may be significant collapse of the bone with retention of the normal cutaneous structure, producing a main en lorgnette appearance (Fig. 21–32). This is a relatively rare phenomenon, as are the sclerotic changes in the distal phalanges.[1]

When the lesions are not pronounced, complete healing may occur. When the destruction is great, residual changes will remain after healing.

The differential diagnosis of sarcoidosis

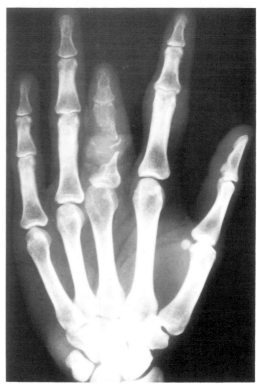

Figure 21–32. Sarcoidosis. Doigt en lorgnette. There is marked destruction of the bones in the third finger with relative uninvolvement of the skin, which gives a clinical appearance of main en lorgnette.

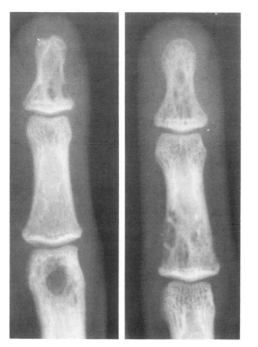

Figure 21–31. Sarcoidosis. 17 year old male. There is a well-defined lucent defect in the proximal phalanx, and less well-defined lucencies are seen in other bones. There is some loss of the distal tuft in the film on the left. (Courtesy Dr. J. F. Holt. Reproduced with permission from *Radiology*, 53:11–30, 1949.)

may be difficult, since tuberculosis and other inflammatory processes, as well as tumors, can mimic its appearance, particularly when destructive changes are present. Differentiation can be made in many inflammatory conditions because subperiosteal changes are more common in inflammatory disease than in sarcoidosis. The involvement of multiple bones and the presence of the honeycomb appearance is useful in separating sarcoidosis from other disorders. Sarcoidosis may also be very difficult to diagnose when there is evidence of joint involvement,[5] in which case it can mimic some of the arthritides.

REFERENCES

1. Bonakdarpour, A., Levy, W., and Aegerter, E. E.: Osteosclerotic Changes in Sarcoidosis. *Am. J. Roentgenol.*, 113:646–649, 1971.
2. Holt, J. F., and Owens, W. I.: The Osseous Lesions of Sarcoidosis. *Radiology*, 53:11–30, 1949.
3. FitzGerald, P., and Meenan, F. O. C.: Sarcoidosis

of Hands. *J. Bone Joint Surg.*, 40B:256–261, 1958.

4. Knutsson, F.: Skeletal Changes in Sarcoidosis. *Acta Radiol.*, 51:429–432, 1959.

5. Sokoloff, L., and Bunim, J. J.: Clinical and Pathological Studies of Joint Involvement in Sarcoidosis. *N. Engl. J. Med.*, 260:841–846, 1959.

6. Stein, G. N., Israel, H. L., and Sones, M.: A Roentgenographic Study of Skeletal Lesions in Sarcoidosis. *Arch. Intern. Med.*, 97:532–536, 1956.

URTICARIA PIGMENTOSA (MASTOCYTOSIS)

Urticaria pigmentosa is a chronic skin disorder which usually begins in the first year of life but may start in adolescence or even in adult life. The appearance is that of oval, pigmented, yellowish to red-brown macular, papular and occasionally nodular lesions which occur particularly on the back. The lesions may also be seen on the face, scalp, palms and soles. Histologically, the upper one-third to two-thirds of the dermis is replaced by a zone of mast cells which obscures the normal dermal landmarks. There is involvement of most organs that contain the reticuloendothelial systems. The bone lesions are produced by tissue mast cell proliferation in the bone marrow and are of two different types: there may be thickening of the trabecular structure, giving the appearance of osteoporosis; or, more rarely, there may be calcified deposits in decalcified areas. Most of the bone lesions are in the central skeleton; the hand changes are usually minor, since there is only a small amount of bone marrow in the adult hand. Hand changes can occur in children, however, since there is still residual bone marrow present.[2]

REFERENCES

1. Bendel, W. L., Jr., and Race, G. J.: Urticaria Pigmentosa with Bone Involvement. *J. Bone Joint Surg.*, 45A:1043–1055, 1963.

2. Cole, A. R. C.: Mastocytosis. Report of a Case in a 15½-Week-Old Infant with Cutaneous and Generalized Skeletal Changes. *Arch. Dis. Child.*, 40:677–683, 1965.

3. Jensen, W. N., and Lasser, E. C.: Urticaria Pigmentosa Associated with Widespread Sclerosis of the Spongiosa of Bone. *Radiology*, 71:826–832, 1958.

4. Schorr, S., Loewenthal, M., Berlin, C., Rabinowitz, M., and Efrati, P.: Mastocytosis: Urticaria Pigmentosa, Myelofibrosclerosis and Occlusive Panarteritis. *Clin. Radiol.*, 15:84–89, 1964.

AMYLOIDOSIS

Radiographic changes in the hand in this condition are extremely rare. Amyloid lesions of bone can present in two different forms. First, a joint form, which is associated with deposits of amyloid in the synovium and joint capsule. This form may cause a carpal tunnel syndrome or may cause subluxation. Some of these synovial deposits may invade para-articular bone, producing small radiolucencies without sclerotic margins. This type of involvement has been seen in the wrist.[2] The other form of amyloidosis is that of bone marrow infiltration with amyloid deposits. Since there is relatively little bone marrow in the hand, this finding is usually not seen in the hand bones. Since amyloidosis is frequently associated with multiple myeloma, it may be difficult to be certain whether the lucent defect in the bone is that of myeloma or of amyloid deposit. An

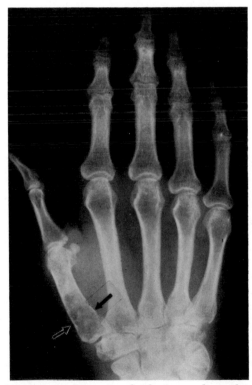

Figure 21–33. Amyloidosis and multiple myeloma. It is difficult to be certain whether the lucent defect (*arrows*) in the bone is due to the multiple myeloma or to amyloid disease. (Pear, B., The Radiographic Manifestations of Amyloidosis. *American Journal of Roentgenology, Radium Therapy and Nuclear Medicine*, 111: 821, 1971. Courtesy of Charles C Thomas, Publisher, Springfield, Illinois.)

example of this is illustrated by Pear (Fig. 21–33).[3]

REFERENCES

1. Axelsson, U., Hallén, A., and Rausing, A.: Amyloidosis of Bone. Report of Two Cases. *J. Bone Joint Surg.*, 52B:717–723, 1970.
2. Grossman, R. E., and Hensley, G. T.: Bone Lesions in Primary Amyloidosis. *Am. J. Roentgenol.*, 101:872–875, 1967.
3. Pear, B. L.: The Radiographic Manifestations of Amyloidosis. *Am. J. Roentgenol.*, 111:821–832, 1971.
4. Strauss, R. G., Schubert, W. K., and McAdams, A. J.: Amyloidosis in Childhood. *J. Pediatr.*, 74:272–282, 1969.
5. Weinfeld, A., Stern, M. H., and Marx, L. H.: Amyloid Lesions of Bone. *Am. J. Roentgenol.*, 108:799–805, 1970.

BONE LESIONS IN PANCREATITIS

Fat necrosis in bone, probably resulting from elevated lipase due to pancreatitis of various etiologies, may result in roentgenographically demonstrable bone lesions. The most dramatic lesions visible during the acute phase of this process are lytic areas (Fig. 21–34). There may be associated periosteal reaction (Fig. 21–35), particularly in children. Soft tissue swelling may be present. Occasionally, osteosclerosis can occur. Arthritis may be another manifestation.[3] The lesions may heal completely without disturbance, or there may be a small residual epiphyseal abnormality (Fig. 21–35 C). In children the lesions must be distinguished from those caused by infections and from sickle cell dactylitis.

REFERENCES

1. Boswell, S. H., and Baylin, G. J.: Metastatic Fat Necrosis and Lytic Bone Lesions in a Patient with Painless Acute Pancreatitis. *Radiology*, 106:85–86, 1973.
2. Keating, J. P., Shackelford, G. D., Shackelford, P. G., and Ternberg, J. L.: Pancreatitis and Osteolytic Lesions. *J. Pediatr.*, 81:350–353, 1972.
3. Mullin, G. T., Caperton, E. M., Jr., Crespin, S. R., and Williams, R. C., Jr.: Arthritis and Skin Lesions Resembling Erythema Nodosum in Pancreatic Disease. *Ann. Intern. Med.*, 68:75–87, 1968.

WEBER-CHRISTIAN DISEASE

Bone changes have been associated with Weber-Christian disease (relapsing febrile nodular nonsuppurative panniculitis). These have included enlargement of the medullary space associated with intra-

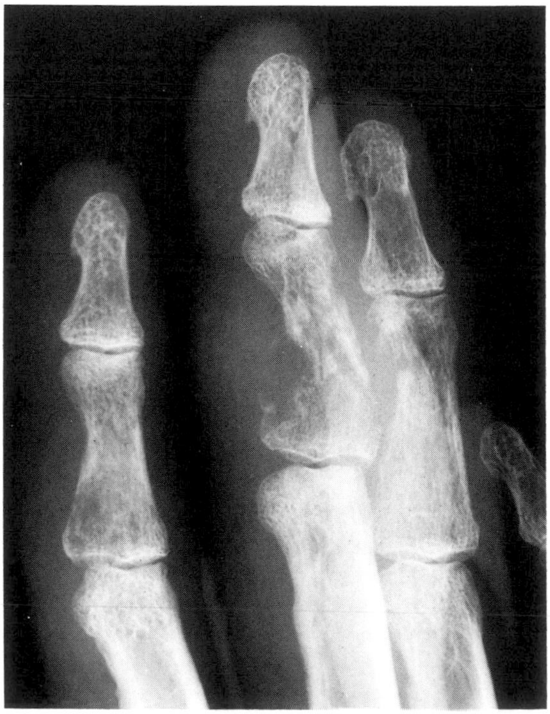

Figure 21–34. Pancreatitis with metastatic fat necrosis. There is extensive destruction of bone in a 44 year old alcoholic with pancreatitis. (Courtesy Dr. S. Boswell and Dr. G. Baylin. Reproduced with permission from *Radiology*, 106:85–86, 1973.)

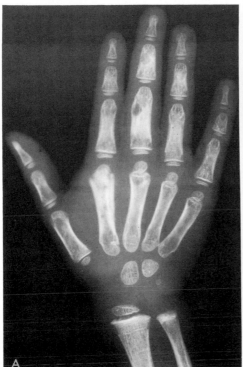
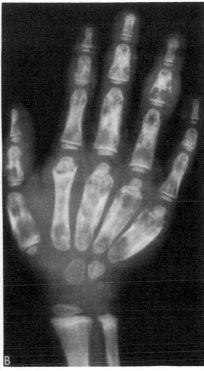
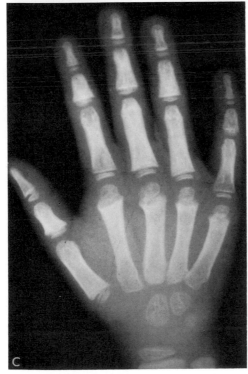

Figure 21–35. Pancreatitis and metastatic fat necrosis. This 3½ year old Negro female had post-traumatic pancreatitis. Her hemoglobin was AA phenotype.

A, Six weeks after admission, there are multiple osteolytic lesions.

B, At eleven weeks there is a marked increase in periosteal reaction and an increase in the number of destructive lesions.

C, One year after admission, there is marked resolution of the destructive lesions with only small epiphyseal abnormalities of the metacarpals remaining.

(Courtesy Dr. G. Shackelford, Washington University School of Medicine. Reproduced with permission from Keating, J. P., et al.: *J. Pediatr.,* 81:350–353, 1972.)

medullary fat necrosis[2] and lytic lesions in the phalanges.[1] The appearance may be similar to that seen in fat necrosis associated with pancreatic disease.

REFERENCES

1. Bismuth, V., Duperrat, B., Gaquiere, A., Bard, M., and Bourdon, R.: Maladie de Weber-Christian. A Détermination Mésentérique et Osseuse. *Ann. Radiol.*, 7:197–210, 1964.
2. DeLor, C. J., and Martz, R. W.: Weber-Christian Disease with Bone Involvement. *Ann. Intern. Med.*, 43:591–598, 1955.

ASEPTIC NECROSIS OF THE BONES OF THE HAND

This is a somewhat heterogeneous group of conditions, the etiology of which is not clear. In fact, many different etiologic agents may be present. Thiemann's disease is probably a congenital entity and was discussed in Chapter 13. Kienböck disease (of the lunate) may be a traumatic lesion. The scaphoid is uncommonly affected. Aseptic necrosis of the metacarpal heads is less common and is probably an acquired rather than a congenital process. It may be associated with repeated trauma and has been seen in lupus erythematosus[1] and in association with steroid therapy. These two situations are further discussed in Chapter 20.

REFERENCES

1. Carstam, N., and Danielsson, L. G.: Aseptic Necrosis of the Head of the Fifth Metacarpal. *Acta Orthop. Scand.*, 37:297–300, 1966.
2. Lightfoot, R. W., Jr., and Lotke, P. A.: Osteonecrosis of Metacarpal Heads in Systemic Lupus Erythematosus. Value of Radiostrontium Scintimetry in Differential Diagnosis. *Arthritis Rheum.*, 15:486–492, 1972.

Kienböck Disease (Aseptic Necrosis of the Lunate)

The etiology of this entity is far from clear. There is strong evidence that it may be simply a traumatic lesion, since many cases are preceded by trauma and the condition is seen frequently in individuals using pneumatic tools.[2] Also, occasionally the necrosis may occur following dislocation of the lunate. A significant portion of cases, however, are not associated with known trauma. Hulten[3] found that in 74 per cent of his cases the ulna was somewhat shorter than the radius, the so-called ulna-minus variant. Therkelsen and Andersen[7] also found a greater incidence of ulna-minus variant in their patients with Kienböck disease. Sobel and Sobel[6] reported a bilateral case without associated trauma, and Ringted[7] has reported a bilateral case in brothers.

The radiologic findings include increased density of the lunate, which may house a focal area of radiolucency within it (Fig. 21–36). Fragmentation of the lunate is common (Fig. 21–37). According to Gentaz et al.,[2] fragmentation is seen more commonly when lateral tomograms are obtained; there is usually a posterior fragment which can be easily missed in the frontal projection. The lunate is often flattened and decreased in size. The commonly associated presence of the relatively short ulna (Fig. 21–36) may also be seen radiologically. Degenerative changes in the wrist are seen in a significant percentage of cases (23 of 61).[7]

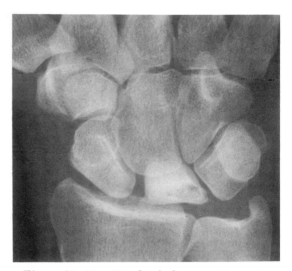

Figure 21–36. Kienböck disease. The patient had trauma to the wrist prior to this film. There is sclerosis of the lunate with an area of radiolucency within it. At surgery the lunate appeared flat, discolored and soft. It broke into several pieces on removal.

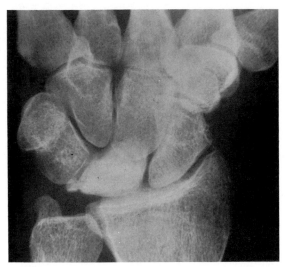

Figure 21–37. Kienböck disease. Note the sclerotic lunate in a 24 year old male with painful wrist. The ulna is shorter than the radius, which is common in this condition. There is a small fragment of the lunate present.

REFERENCES

1. Cave, E. F.: Kienböck's Disease of the Lunate. *J. Bone Joint Surg.*, 21:858–866, 1939.
2. Gentaz, R., Lespargot, J., Levame, J.-H., and Poli, J.-P.: La maladie de Kienböck. Approche tomographique. Analyse de 5 cas. *La Nouvelle Presse Médicale*, 1:1207–1210, 1972.
3. Hulten, O.: Über die Entstehung und Behandlung der Lunatummalazie (Morbus Kienböck). *Acta Chir. Scand.*, 76:121–135, 1935.
4. Jaffe, H. L.: *Metabolic Degenerative and Inflammatory Diseases of Bones and Joints.* Lea and Febiger, Philadelphia, 1972.
5. Kienböck, R.: Über traumatische Malazie des Mondbeins und ihre Folgezustände: Entartungsformen und Kompressionsfrakturen. *Fortschr. Geb. Roentgenstr. Nuklearmed.*, 16: 77–103, 1910.
6. Sobel, A., and Sobel, P.: Un Cas de Maladie de Kienboeck Bilatérale. *J. Radiol. Electrol.*, 31: 13–14, 1950.
7. Therkelsen, F., and Andersen, K.: Lunatomalacia. *Acta Chir. Scand.*, 97:503–526, 1949.

INDEX